AIDS in Asia

AIDS in Asia

Edited by

Yichen Lu, PhD

Principal Research Scientist,
Harvard AIDS Institute
Harvard School of Public Health
Boston, Massachusetts, USA

Special Professor,
Nankai University
Tianjin, China

Max Essex, DVM, PhD

Chairman, Harvard AIDS Institute
Chairman, Department of Immunology and Infectious Diseases
Mary Woodard Lasker Professor of Health Sciences,
Harvard School of Public Health
Boston, Massachusetts, USA

Managing Editor

Ellen Stiefvater, MPP

Harvard AIDS Institute
Harvard School of Public Health
Boston, Massachusetts, USA

Springer-Science+Business Media, LLC

Library of Congress Cataloging-in-Publication Data

AIDS in Asia / [edited by] Yichen Lu and Max Essex.
p. ; cm.
Includes bibliographical references and index.

1. AIDS (Disease)—Asia. I. Lu, Yichen. II. Essex, Myron.
[DNLM: 1. Acquired Immunodeficiency Syndrome—epidemiology—Asia. 2. Developing Countries—Asia. 3. HIV Infections—prevention & control—Asia. 4. Population Surveillance—Asia. WC 503.4 JA1 A2882 2004]
RA643.86.A78A537 2004
362.196'9792'0095—dc22 2004046116

ISBN 978-1-4419-3452-9 ISBN 978-0-306-48536-7 (eBook)
DOI 10.1007/978-0-306-48536-7

Originally published by Springer Science+Business Media, Inc. in 2004
Softcover reprint of the hardcover 1st edition 2004

springeronline.com

10 9 8 7 6 5 4 3 2

A C.I.P. record for this book is available from the Library of Congress

This book is dedicated to the memory of Dr. Natth Bhamarapravati of Thailand, who contributed immensely to the fight against HIV/AIDS in his country and the world. Although he did not live to see the publication of this book, he shared his hope with us about making available to other Asian countries the successes and lessons of Thailand in the battle against HIV/AIDS.

Contributors

Iyanthi Abeyewickreme, MBBS, MSc, MD, Dip Ven, Consultant Venereologist, Director, National STD/AIDS Control Programme, Ministry of Health, Colombo, Sri Lanka

Marcus Altfeld, MD, PhD, Assistant Professor, Harvard Medical School; Partners AIDS Research Center, Massachusetts General Hospital, Boston, Massachusetts, USA

Anthony Amoroso, MD, Assistant Professor of Medicine, Institute of Human Virology, University of Maryland, Baltimore, Maryland, USA

Bai Li-shi, MS, Professor, Heilongjiang Provincial Center for Disease Control and Prevention, Harbin, China

Kruavon Balachandra, PhD, Principal Investigator, Department of Medical Sciences, Ministry of Public Health, Nonthaburi, Thailand

Tony Barnett, MA, PhD, Economic and Social Research Council Professorial Research Fellow, Development Studies Institute, London School of Economics and Political Science, London, UK

Chris Beyrer, MD, MPH, Associate Research Professor, Departments of Epidemiology and International Health, Johns Hopkins Bloomberg School of Public Health, Baltimore, Maryland, USA

Natth Bhamarapravati, MD, DSc, Professor of Pathology, Center for Vaccine Development, Mahidol University Salaya, Nakhonpathom, Thailand

Deborah L. Birx, MD, Director, US Military HIV Research Program, Rockville, Maryland, USA

Robert C. Bollinger, MD, MPH, Assistant Professor of Medicine, Division of Infectious Diseases, Department of International Health, Johns Hopkins Bloomberg School of Public Health, Baltimore, Maryland, USA

Jotika Boonlong, PhD, Chief of Division of International Affairs, Department of Medical Sciences, Ministry of Public Health, Nonthaburi, Thailand

Prudence Borthwick, Regional Project Officer, HIV/AIDS, UNICEF East Asia Pacific Regional Office, Bangkok, Thailand

Arthur E. Brown, MD, MPH, Chief, Department of Retrovirology, Armed Forces Research Institute of Medical Sciences, Bangkok, Thailand

Raywadee Butraporn, PhD, Head, Division of Experimental Animals Research, Department of Medical Sciences, Ministry of Public Health, Nonthaburi, Thailand

Huyen Cao, MD, Director, California Department of Health Services, Richmond, California, USA

Suk-yan Chan, MBA, Deputy Chief Executive, Programs, Hong Kong AIDS Foundation, Shaukeiwan, Hong Kong

Donna K. F. Chandler, PhD, Deputy Director, Division of Vaccines and Related Products Applications, Office of Vaccines Research and Review, Center for Biologics Evaluation and Research, Food and Drug Administration, Rockville, Maryland, USA

Jie Chen, MD, Deputy Director, Guangxi Centers for Disease Control and Prevention, Nanning, Guangxi Province, China

Yi-Ming Arthur Chen, MD, ScD, Professor and Director, AIDS Prevention and Research Center, Chairman, Institute of Public Health, National Yang-Ming University, Taipei City, Taiwan

Intira Collins, MSc, Institut de Recherche pour le Developpement 054 Perinatal HIV Prevention Trial Group, Chiang Mai, Thailand

Therese Cvetkovich, MD, Senior Medical Reviewer, Division of Vaccines and Related Products Applications, Office of Vaccines Research and Review, Center for Biologics Evaluation and Research, Food and Drug Administration, Rockville, Maryland, USA

Nicholas Daniels, MD, MPH, Associate Clinical Professor, General Internal Medicine, University of California, San Francisco, California, USA

Charles E. Davis, MD, Assistant Professor of Medicine, Institute of Human Virology, University of Maryland, Baltimore, Maryland, USA

Mark S. de Souza, PhD, MPH, Principal Scientist, Armed Forces Research Institute of Medical Sciences, Bangkok, Thailand

Ding Jian-ping, MD, STD/AIDS Prevention Section, Jiangsu Province Center for Disease Control and Prevention, Nanjing, Jiangsu Province, China

Arwind R. Diwan, PhD, Department of Tropical Medicine & Medical Microbiology, John A. Burns School of Medicine, University of Hawaii at Manoa, Honolulu, Hawaii, USA

Scott Dowell, MD, MPH, Director, International Emerging Infections Program, Thailand Ministry of Public Health-U.S. Centers for Disease Control and Prevention Collaboration, Nonthaburi, Thailand; U.S. Centers for Disease Control and Prevention, Atlanta, Georgia, USA

Du Yaping, MD, Vice Director, Jingjiang Epidemic Prevention and Health Station, Jingjiang, Jiangsu Province, China

Rebecca J. Garten, PhD Candidate, Department of Molecular Microbiology and Immunology, Johns Hopkins Bloomberg School of Public Health, Baltimore, Maryland, USA

Antonia Geber, MD, Supervisory Medical Officer, Division of Vaccines and Related Products Applications, Office of Vaccines Research and Review, Center for Biologics Evaluation and Research, Food and Drug Administration, Rockville, Maryland, USA

Bruce L. Gilliam, MD, Assistant Professor of Medicine, Institute of Human Virology, University of Maryland, Baltimore, Maryland, USA

Karen L. Goldenthal, MD, Director, Division of Vaccines and Related Products Applications, Office of Vaccines Research and Review, Center for Biologics Evaluation and Research, Food and Drug Administration, Rockville, Maryland, USA

Ganesh Gurung, MA, Sociologist and Executive Chair, Nepal Institute of Development Studies, Kathmandu, Nepal

Han Mengjie, MPH, MSc, Assistant Director, Office of State Council AIDS Committee, Chinese Ministry of Public Health, Beijing, China

Takaichi Hamano, PhD, Researcher, AIDS Research Center, National Institute of Infectious Diseases, Tokyo, Japan

Takashi Hara, Researcher, AIDS Research Center, National Institute of Infectious Disease, Tokyo, Japan

H.M.S.S.D. Herath, MBBS, FRCP, MRCP, DTPH, DIH, MFOM, Consultant, National HIV/AIDS Prevention Project, Ministry of Health, Colombo, Sri Lanka

Mitsuo Honda, MD, PhD, Head, Vaccine Research and Development Group, AIDS Research Center, National Institute of Infectious Diseases, Tokyo, Japan

Hamamal Jayawardena, MBBS, MSc, MD, LLM, Consultant HIV/AIDS, World Health Organization, Dhaka, Bangladesh

Yasuyuki Izumi, Researcher, AIDS Research Center, National Institute of Infectious Diseases, Tokyo, Japan

Gonzague Jourdain, MD, MS, Harvard School of Public Health, Boston, Massachusetts, USA; Institut de Recherche pour le Developpement 054 Perinatal HIV Prevention Trial, Chiang Mai, Thailand

William H.F. Kam, DMS, MSocSc, Deputy Chief Executive, Corporate Affairs, Hong Kong AIDS Foundation, Shaukeiwan, Hong Kong

Phyllis J. Kanki, DVM, SD, Professor of Immunology and Infectious Disease, Harvard School of Public Health, Harvard AIDS Institute, Boston, Massachusetts, USA

Stephen G. Karel, MPH, DPH, Former WHO staff member, Western Pacific Regional Office; Former Executive Director, Pacific Island Health Officers Association, Honolulu, Hawaii, USA

June-Myung Kim, MD, PhD, Professor, Division of Infectious Diseases, Department of Internal Medicine, Yonsei University College of Medicine, Seoul, Korea

Chaiyos Kunanusont, MD, MPH, MS, PhD, HIV/AIDS/STI Advisor, UNFPA/CST for East and South-East Asia, Bangkok, Thailand

Shenghan Lai, MD, MPH, Associate Research Professor, Department of Epidemiology, Johns Hopkins Bloomberg School of Public Health, Baltimore, Maryland, USA

Marc Lallemant, MD, MS, Harvard School of Public Health, Boston, Massachusetts, USA; Institut de Recherche pour le Developpement 054 Perinatal HIV Prevention Trial, Chiang Mai, Thailand

Sophie Le Coeur, MD, PhD, Institut National d'Etudes Demographiques, Institut de Recherche pour le Developpement 054 Perinatal HIV Prevention Trial Group, Paris, France

Jongkoo Lee, MD, PhD, Department of Infectious Disease Control, Korea Center for Disease Control and Prevention, Seoul, Korea

Joo-Shil Lee, PhD, Head, Center for AIDS Research, Department of Virology, National Institute of Health, Seoul, Korea

William C. Levine, MD, MSc, Associate Director, Global AIDS Program-Thailand, Thailand Ministry of Public Health-U.S. Centers for Disease Control and Prevention Collaboration, Nonthaburi, Thailand; U.S. Centers for Disease Control and Prevention, Atlanta, Georgia, USA

Khanchit Limpakarnjanarat, MD, MPH, Adjunct Director, International Emerging Infections Program, Thailand Ministry of Public Health-U.S. Centers for Disease Control and Prevention Collaboration, Nonthaburi, Thailand

Mario Consorcia Lim-Quizon, MD, Project Leader, Infectious Disease Surveillance and Control Project, National Epidemiology Center, Manila, Philippines

Oi-chu Lin, MA, Chief Executive, Hong Kong AIDS Foundation, Shaukeiwan, Hong Kong

Xiaojun Lin, MD, MBA, Senior Biomedical Engineer, Eastern Home Pharmaceuticals, Chengdu, China

Liu Kangmai, Professor, National Center for STD/AIDS Prevention and Control, Chinese Center for Disease Control, Beijing, China

Wei Liu, MD, Director, Guangxi Centers for Disease Control and Prevention, Nanning, Guangxi Province, China

Liu Yan-Cheng, MD, Professor, Heilongjiang Provincial Center for Disease Control and Prevention, Harbin, China

Yichen Lu, PhD, Principal Research Scientist, Harvard AIDS Institute, Harvard School of Public Health, Boston, Massachusetts, USA; Special Professor, Nankai University Vaccine Laboratory, Tianjin, China

Fan Lv, PhD, Associate Professor, National Center for AIDS and STD Prevention and Control, Chinese Center for Disease Control and Prevention, Beijing, China

Marina Mahathir, President, Malaysian AIDS Council, Kuala Lumpur, Malaysia

Timothy D. Mastro, MD, Deputy Director, Global AIDS Program, U.S. Centers for Disease Control and Prevention, Atlanta, Georgia, USA

Kazuhiro Matsuo, PhD, Researcher, AIDS Research Center, National Institute of Infectious Diseases, Tokyo, Japan

Francine McCutchan, PhD, Chief, Global Molecular Epidemiology Program, US Military HIV Research Program, Rockville, Maryland, USA

Kenneth McIntosh, MD, Professor of Pediatrics, Harvard Medical School; Professor of Immunology and Infectious Diseases, Harvard School of Public Health; Chief Emeritus, Division of Infectious Diseases, Children's Hospital Boston, Boston, Massachusetts, USA

John G. McNeil, MD, MPH, HIV Vaccine Advanced Development Project, US Military HIV Research Program, Rockville, Maryland, USA; Vaccine Research Center, National Institute of Allergy and Infectious Diseases, National Institutes of Health, Bethesda, Maryland, USA

Shruti H. Mehta, MPH, PhD, Assistant Research Professor, Department of Epidemiology, Johns Hopkins Bloomberg School of Public Health, Baltimore, Maryland, USA

Syed Abdul Mujeeb, MBBS, M Phil, Assistant Professor, Blood Bank; In charge, HIV/AIDS Surveillance Centre; Jinnah Postgraduate Medical Centre, Karachi, Pakistan

Tadashi Nakasone, MD, PhD, Principal Investigator, AIDS Research Center, National Institute of Infectious Diseases, Tokyo, Japan

Nicole Ngo-Giang-Huong, PharmD, PhD, Harvard School of Public Health, Boston, Massachusetts, USA; Institut de Recherche pour le Developpement 054 Perinatal HIV Prevention Trial, Chiang Mai, Thailand

Tung Nguyen, MD, Associate Clinical Professor, General Internal Medicine, University of California, San Francisco, California, USA

Wiput Phoolcharoen, MD, MPH, Health Systems Research Institute, Ministry of Public Health, Nonthaburi, Thailand

Pilaipan Puthavathana, PhD, Professor, Siriraj Hospital, Mahidol University, Bangkok, Thailand

Punnee Pitisuttithum, MBBS, DTM&H, FRCPT, Associate Professor, Chief, Clinical Infectious Disease Research Unit, Department of Clinical Tropical Medicine, Mahidol University, Bangkok, Thailand

Duanthanorm Promkhatkaew, PhD, Principal Investigator, Department of Medical Sciences, Ministry of Public Health, Nonthaburi, Thailand

Robert R. Redfield, MD, Director of Clinical Care and Research, Institute of Human Virology, University of Maryland, Baltimore, Maryland, USA

Philip O. Renzullo, PhD, MPH, Epidemiologist, US Military HIV Research Program, Rockville, Maryland, USA

Bryan Roberts, D Phil, President, Parallel Solutions, Inc., Cambridge, Massachusetts, USA

Kiat Ruxrungtham, MD, PhD, Associate Professor, Chulalongkorn University, Bangkok, Thailand

Yiming Shao, MD, PhD, Professor, National Center for AIDS and STD Prevention and Control, Chinese Center for Disease Control and Prevention, Beijing, China

Sharaf Ali Shah, MBBS, MSPH, Provincial Program Manager, Sindh AIDS Control Program, Karachi, Pakistan

Rebecca L. Sheets, PhD, Vaccine Scientific and Regulatory Specialist, Vaccine Research Center (VRC) and Division of AIDS (DAIDS), National Institutes of Health (NIH), Bethesda, Maryland, USA

Shen Jie, Director, National Center for STD/AIDS Prevention and Control; Vice Director, Chinese Center for Disease Control, Beijing, China

Taweesap Siraprapasiri, MD, MPH, Adjunct Director, Thailand Ministry of Public Health-U.S. Centers for Disease Control and Prevention Collaboration, Ministry of Public Health, Nonthaburi, Thailand

Nopporn Sittisombut, MD, PhD, Associate Professor, Chiang Mai University, Chiang Mai, Thailand

Busarawan Sriwanthana, PhD, Principal Investigator, Department of Medical Sciences, Ministry of Public Health, Nonthaburi, Thailand

Henry Stephens, PhD, Head of Tissue Typing, Institute of Urology and Nephrology, University College London, The Middlesex Hospital, London, UK

Ruengpung Sutthent, MD, PhD, Professor, Siriraj Hospital, Mahidol University, Bangkok, Thailand

B. K. Suvedi, MBBS, MPH, Senior Medical Officer, Ministry of Health, Kathmandu, Nepal

Viroj Tangcharoensathien, MD, PhD, Director, International Health Policy Program, Health Systems Research Institute, Ministry of Public Health, Nonthaburi, Thailand

Jordan W. Tappero, MD, MPH, Director, Thailand Ministry of Public Health-U.S. Centers for Disease Control and Prevention Collaboration, Nonthaburi, Thailand; U.S. Centers for Disease Control and Prevention, Atlanta, Georgia, USA

Vallop Thaineua, MD, Permanent Secretary, Ministry of Public Health, Bangkok, Thailand

Visanu Thamlikitkul, MD, Professor of Medicine, Faculty of Medicine Siriraj Hospital, Mahidol University, Bangkok, Thailand

Sombat Thanprasertsuk, MD, MPH, Director, Bureau of AIDS, Tuberculosis and Sexually Transmitted Infections, Department of Disease Control, Ministry of Public Health, Nonthaburi, Thailand

Sodsai Tovanabutra, PhD, Scientist, US Military HIV Research Program, Rockville, Maryland, USA

Srikanth P. Tripathy, MBBS, MD, Deputy Director, National AIDS Research Institute, Pune, India

Sriram P. Tripathy, MBBS, MD, FAMS, Director General (retired), Indian Council of Medical Research (ICMR), Chairman, ICMR HIV-TB Special Task Force, Pune, India

Julienne M. Vaillancourt, R Ph, MPH, Senior Project Manager, Division of Vaccines and Related Products Applications, Office of Vaccines Research and Review, Center for Biologics Evaluation and Research, Food and Drug Administration, Rockville, Maryland, USA

Bruce D. Walker, MD, Director, Division of AIDS, Harvard Medical School; Professor of Medicine, Harvard Medical School; Partners AIDS Research Center, Massachusetts General Hospital, Boston, Massachusetts, USA

Paijit Warachit, MD, PhD, Inspector General, Ministry of Public Health, Nonthaburi, Thailand

Alan Whiteside, D Econ, Director, Health Economics and HIV/AIDS Research Division, University of KwaZulu-Natal, Durban, South Africa; Visiting Professor, School of Tropical Medicine, University of Liverpool, UK; Visiting Fellow, School of Development Studies, University of East Anglia, UK

Jane S. Wilson, Dip Ed, PhD, UNAIDS Country Programme Advisor, Joint United Nations Program on HIV/AIDS, Jakarta, Indonesia

Wu Yu-Hua, MD, Professor, Heilongjiang Provincial Center for Disease Control and Prevention, Harbin, China

Xu Hua, MD, Secretary General, Chinese Foundation for Prevention of STD and AIDS, Beijing, China

Naoki Yamamoto, MD, PhD, Director, AIDS Research Center, National Institute of Infectious Diseases, Tokyo, Japan

Shudo Yamazaki, MD, PhD, Emeritus Director, National Institute of Infectious Diseases, Tokyo, Japan

Yang Haitao, MD, Chief, STD/AIDS Prevention Section, Jiangsu Province Center for Disease Control and Prevention, Nanjing, Jiangsu Province, China

Naoto Yoshino, PhD, Researcher, AIDS Research Center, National Institute of Infectious Diseases, Tokyo, Japan

Xiao-Fang Yu, MD, D Sc, Associate Professor, Department of Molecular Microbiology and Immunology, Johns Hopkins Bloomberg School of Public Health, Baltimore, Maryland, USA

Xu G. Yu, MD, MSc, Research Fellow, Partners AIDS Research Center, Massachusetts General Hospital, Boston, Massachusetts, USA

Zeng Yi, MD, Chief Scientist, National Center for Prevention and Control of STD and AIDS; President, Chinese Foundation for Prevention of STD and AIDS; President, China Preventive Medicine Association, Beijing, China

Zhang Fujie, Director, Division of Treatment and Care, National Center for STD/AIDS Prevention and Control, Chinese Center for Disease Control, Beijing, China

Zhang Jiaxi, MD, Vice Secretary General, China Preventive Medicine Association, Beijing, China

Zhao Zhong-hou, MD, Professor, Heilongjiang Provincial Center for Disease Control and Prevention, Harbin, China

Foreword

Asian nations face urgent choices on HIV/AIDS. In recent years, many of these nations have been flourishing and appear to be on track for further robust growth. But individual and family well-being, health systems, and social development are in danger of being undermined by HIV/AIDS. The Asian HIV/AIDS epidemic seems unlikely to reach the proportions seen in sub-Saharan Africa, where the disease threatens entire countries with economic and institutional collapse. Yet, local and national epidemics that fall well short of that level can inflict enormous suffering and losses on countries. In much of Asia, a window of opportunity exists to launch highly effective control strategies before the virus gains a firm hold in the broad population. The opportunity will not last long. The following chapters analyze the specific epidemiology of HIV in this region now, assess what is at stake, and make the case for rapid, concerted action.

About 7 million people in Asia are infected with HIV, and the virus is spreading quickly in many countries. Asia being home to 60% of the world's population, current trends could have devastating global implications. The impact of the epidemic on individuals, families, and health systems is growing. More than half a million Asians die of AIDS each year. In Asian countries with high HIV prevalence, annual AIDS mortality is expected to increase the total number of annual deaths in the population aged 15–49 by up to 40%. Effective interventions exist, but they need to be used systematically and on a large scale. Otherwise, some models suggest that as many as 40 million people in Asia might be infected with HIV by 2010.

In Asia, as elsewhere, HIV risk is not distributed evenly across whole populations. Certain social groups bear a disproportionate burden. Epidemics have taken their greatest toll in groups such as commercial sex workers, intravenous drug users, and men who have sex with men. Special measures must be taken to provide members of these vulnerable groups with the knowledge and the means to protect themselves, and with the treatment that can extend and improve their lives if they have become infected.

Some take the current concentration of HIV risk in socially marginalized groups as a sign that Asian epidemics will probably remain limited in their spread. But those at heightened risk represent between 7 and 25% of the adult population in Asian countries, meaning that even if the risk is limited to them, the threat of severe, generalized epidemics throughout the region is real. Epidemics that begin by affecting specific subgroups cross over increasingly into the wider population.

Some countries, such as Thailand and Cambodia, have used targeted outreach to sex workers and their clients as a key component of national programmes and have registered important successes in slowing the spread of

HIV. Yet, even in these countries, outreach to intravenous drug users and men who have sex with men has been much less effective, and rates of condom use among young people remain low. Much must still be done to shut down these other pathways of transmission.

This substantial volume will strengthen understanding of the specific dynamics of HIV/AIDS in Asian contexts and lead to focused action guided by evidence. It analyzes and links a range of key issues for HIV/AIDS work in the region. It brings together the surveillance data and projections needed to convince decision-makers of the need for action and to help design well-targeted programmes. It takes up the issues of testing and diagnosis that can lead to stronger prevention and open doors to proper care. It shows how, by implementing effective prevention programs, Asian countries can contain their HIV epidemics, as Thailand and Cambodia have demonstrated. Other chapters emphasize the crucial lesson that effective prevention, care, treatment, and support to people living with HIV/AIDS form an integrated whole. Prevention and treatment strengthen each other, and Asian countries can begin to apply this lesson immediately. Care and treatment should be scaled up rapidly, ultimately to reach all those who need them, regardless of social position or economic circumstances. The contributions show how basic science builds the future of both prevention and care, and they make a strong case for increased investment in research.

Both in their content and in the way they have been put together, these studies reflect another essential component of HIV/AIDS work: international collaboration. Where we are making headway against HIV/AIDS, this is happening through an intensive dialogue and exchange of knowledge between continents, countries, institutions, communities, and individuals. As Asian countries move to scale up their response to HIV/AIDS, they draw on accumulated knowledge from other parts of the world affected earlier by the epidemic. At the same time, Thailand, for example, has shared its expertise in fields such as HIV prevention and ARV drug production with several African countries. Such cross-fertilization and learning must be intensified.

The successful battle to contain SARS in early 2003 demonstrated the importance of international cooperation in epidemiological surveillance and response. It showed that coordinated effort among national and local health authorities and international organizations can overcome health emergencies. The time has come to apply these lessons and mobilize a similar commitment to controlling HIV/AIDS.

In September 2003, WHO and its partners in the UN system declared lack of access to antiretroviral (ARV) therapy for HIV/AIDS a global health emergency. We launched the "3 by 5" Initiative, which aims to give three million people in developing countries access to ARVs by the end of 2005. Evidence shows that expanding ARV therapy reduces the stigma and discrimination attached to HIV disease and markedly increases the uptake of voluntary counselling and testing, thereby reinforcing HIV prevention. The necessity of such an integrated approach is increasingly recognized by health officials and political leaders. Countries in the Asia-Pacific region are committing themselves to providing HIV/AIDS care, including antiretroviral treatment. China, India, Thailand, and others have recently pledged to expand rapidly the availability of ARV therapy. WHO is working with them to drive this process forward. *AIDS in Asia* will be an extremely valuable resource as leaders and stakeholders move to set up integrated HIV/AIDS control programmes. It will help them to enlist the latest evidence in support of fair treatment for the vulnerable, which is the foundation of all adequate public health policy.

When I was working on polio eradication in the Western Pacific Region, I saw Asian political leaders, health professionals, and communities mobilize to carry out highly effective mass immunization activities. During the SARS crisis I visited political leaders and health staff in Beijing, and witnessed similar skill and dedication. HIV/AIDS is a threat to Asia's peoples and to the region's future, but it can be beaten. The pages that follow provide detailed and extensive evidence that the knowledge and tools to do so exist. Many countries in the region have formidable resources at their disposal, including strong political leadership, large numbers of skilled health professionals, sophisticated production capacities for pharmaceuticals and other medical technologies, and a robust civil society. Where one or more of these advantages are lacking, regional and international partners must be ready to assist. With swift and coherent action now, millions of infections can be prevented. This will extend the lives and protect the families of innumerable people, and avert vast damage in the world's most populous region. The success of Asia's battle with HIV/AIDS will be felt far beyond the region itself. A wealth of information on how to achieve it is made available by the following studies.

Lee Jong-Wook
Director-General,
World Health Organization

Preface

Just three decades ago, many international health experts predicted that epidemics of infectious diseases were soon to be relics of the past. Efficacious vaccines for polio and the common childhood infections were available and widely used. Smallpox was in the process of being eradicated. Potent drugs to treat malaria, TB, and bacterial infections were widely available. Research and teaching on infectious diseases was no longer deemed to be important to medicine and public health.

Soon after, health experts had to rethink and retrench as the era of newly emerging and re-emerging infections began. Many of the wonder drugs seemed less wonderful as drug resistant variants of TB and malaria rapidly spread around the globe. New diseases appeared. Some, such as the hemorrhagic fevers, were frightening in infected individuals, but limited as epidemics. HIV/AIDS was frightening to both individuals and public health officials. It would soon progress to become the most serious new epidemic since the bubonic plague. It would also become the leading cause of death in Africa, a region already known for high rates of death from other infectious diseases.

HIV/AIDS has already killed tens of millions, and infected 40 million more. In Africa it has severely damaged economies, posed threats to national security, and disrupted the structure of family life. In some countries, childhood mortality rates have increased 3–5 fold, and life expectancy has fallen by decades. For southern Africa, it has reversed a half-century of progress in public health.

HIV/AIDS has not yet wreaked the same degree of havoc in Asia. On a per capita basis, it seems unlikely that it will. However, the population of Asia is much larger than that of Africa. For China to reach the same rate of infection as, for example, the Republic of South Africa, would translate into 145 million cases of HIV/AIDS. Even if Asia as a whole only reaches rates of infection comparable to those in sub-Saharan Africa's lower-prevalence countries, there would be over 100 million HIV infections in the region.

In the pathway of the global epidemic of HIV/AIDS, Asia is now at a pivotal juncture, with "only" about 7 million infections. Aggressive action now can cause the epidemic to plateau and eventually decrease. A lack of action could result in disaster. Some clear lessons are provided from the African experience. Two model countries stand out as clear examples. Senegal, where aggressive education began soon after the epidemic was detected, now has rates that are only a small fraction of those seen in the rest of Africa. Uganda, which had some of the highest rates in Africa 15 years ago, now has a prevalence that is considerably lower than the mean for sub-Saharan Africa. The success stories of Senegal and Uganda were most notable for their examples of strong government leadership. While some other governments in Africa were in denial—denial of the presence and potential of the epidemic; even denial of HIV as the cause of AIDS—Senegal and Uganda were openly seeking cooperation and support from international partners. Countries that were forthcoming in this way experienced a surge of support from both private and public donor agencies.

Thailand was the first country to be hard hit by HIV/AIDS in Asia, but it also became one of the few examples of successful control. This was again exemplified by strong governmental commitment and a proportionately strong response by the international community. What began as a double digit prevalence in young adults in the north of Thailand soon plateaued and diminished as Thailand became a strong leader in education and research. Many other countries in the region are now experiencing the beginning of an epidemic of HIV/AIDS. Countries such as Cambodia and Myanmar now have higher rates of infection than Thailand. The very large countries of India and China are now experiencing major expansions in restricted subpopulations. The need for action is acute. Comprehensive strategic surveillance is particularly important. The epidemic in China, for example, is characterized by the presence of new recombinant viruses, whose potential for expansion is unknown. It is also characterized by a combination of transmission routes—rapid spread by injection drug users combined with sexual transmission. Widespread surveillance should be combined with focused measures for prevention.

This book represents a key resource that documents the current status of HIV/AIDS in Asia. We are fortunate to have contributions from most of the leaders in the war against HIV/AIDS in Asia. The countries and regions of Asia are represented by the words of local and regional experts with direct experience. The book contains two significant contributions from Natth Bhamarapravati, some of the last words he wrote on the topic before his untimely death. Natth was a giant in AIDS research. He was an eloquent spokesman for AIDS in Asia, a supreme leader in a country that led by example, the embodiment of a multinational collaborator who sought cooperation from all while never forgetting his roots in Thailand.

This book explores the geographical and epidemiological aspects of AIDS, and attempts to interpret the impact of the epidemic in the context of other infectious diseases of importance in Asia. Research on HIV vaccines is addressed in detail, as are the options for the use of antiretroviral drugs for both chemoprevention and therapy. Very recently, we have observed rapid progress in reducing the cost of antiretroviral drugs, and utilizing AIDS treatment as another means for control of HIV in developing countries is now much closer to becoming reality.

The available measures to prevent and control HIV/AIDS represent expanding and exciting opportunities. The need for action in Asia is imminent. It is our hope that this book can provide information and encouragement to those physicians, nurses, researchers, public health officials, governmental leaders, and all others who use their expertise to prevent and control the HIV/AIDS epidemic in Asia.

Max Essex
Harvard AIDS Institute

Acknowledgments

The editors thank Elizabeth Perry and Molly Holme for enormous help with the editing process. Thanks are also due to Julie Stiefvater, Nancie Koenigsberg, Ann Frenning, Monique Wyatt, Kim Alexander, Jennifer Dochterman and Kimberley Morrisseau for editorial assistance; Elizabeth Liao and Helia Morris for departmental support; Chong Jing, Kou Yang, Luo Ling, Leng Jin, and Li Shu of Nankai University for translation; Bill Tucker and his team at Kluwer for their encouragement and guidance; and Desmond Avery and his colleagues at WHO for their assistance.

In preparing this volume, as in its other work, the Harvard AIDS Institute's China Project has relied on the support and encouragement of Mrs. William McCormick Blair, Jr. and the financial support of the Marx family and Saks Jandel, Jane Hitchcock and Jim Hoagland, and Buffy and Bill Cafritz.

Contents

I: SNAPSHOTS OF HIV/AIDS IN ASIA

III: DIAGNOSIS, SURVEILLANCE, AND PROJECTED SCENARIOS

IV: PREVENTION EFFORTS AND TREATMENT OPTIONS

V: THE DECISIVE BATTLEGROUND

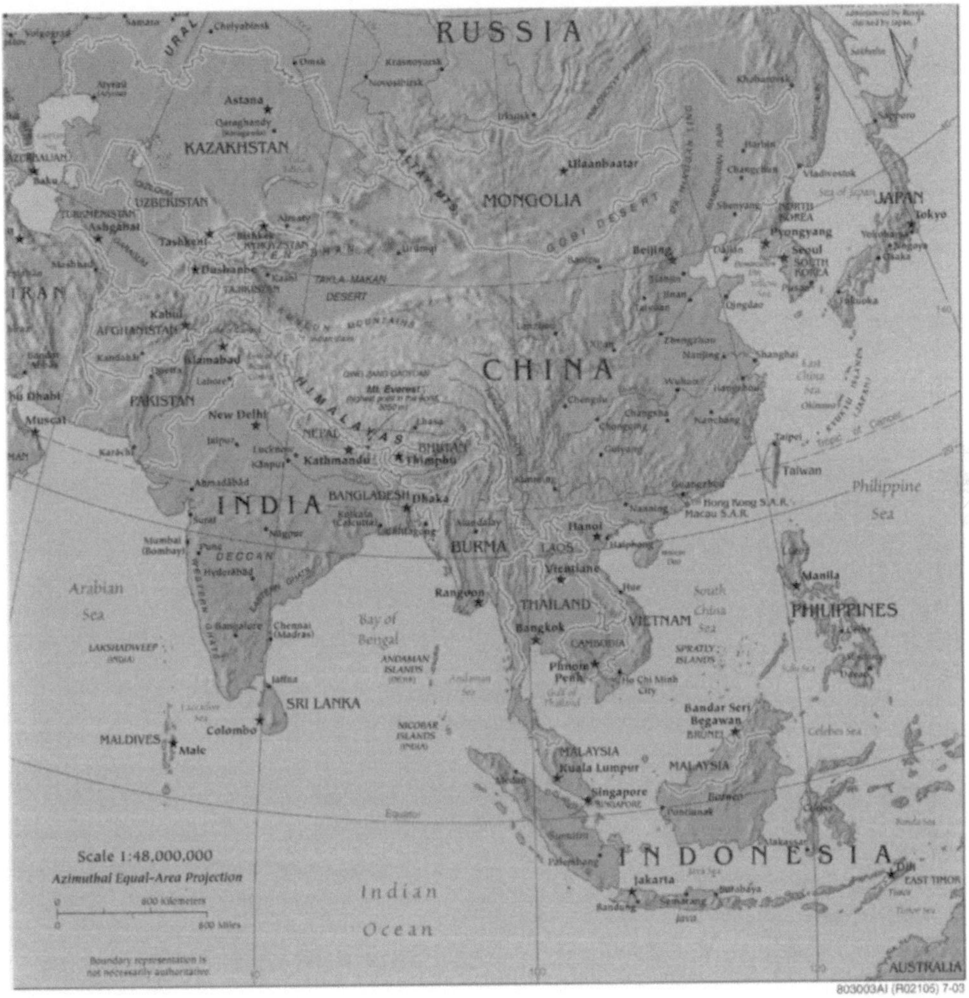

803003AI (R02105) 7-03

I

Snapshots of HIV/AIDS in Asia

1

HIV/AIDS in Thailand

Wiput Phoolcharoen[1], Chaiyos Kunanusont[2], Punnee Pitisuttithum[1], and Natth Bhamarapravati[1]

[1]*Mahidol University, Bangkok, Thailand*
[2]*UNFPA/CST for East and South East Asia, Bangkok, Thailand*

EVOLUTION OF THE HIV/AIDS PROGRAM IN THAILAND

Introduction

The rapid growth of the HIV/AIDS epidemic in Thailand began in the late 1980s, as in many other countries in Asia, but with a subsequently more rapid upsurge in HIV prevalence than in the other countries. Some factors provided fertile ground for HIV transmission in Thailand, including an extensive sex industry that drew its male clientele from across the socioeconomic spectrum. This coincided with high levels of several other sexually transmissible infections (STI), and the widespread practice of injecting illicit drugs. These risk factors have been exacerbated by a certain societal reticence to publicly acknowledge the ubiquity of sexual and drug use practices that represent potential pathways for HIV transmission.

The first visible evidence of HIV in Thailand was the diagnosis of AIDS in a man returning from overseas and receiving treatment in Bangkok in 1984. Within the first few years of the epidemic, a handful of other cases were reported, predominantly among men having sex with men (MSM) who had contracted the virus locally. Concerned that HIV might spread throughout the country, a few small-scale HIV sero-surveillance studies were conducted in populations with high-risk behaviors between 1984 and 1987. These studies only sporadically detected HIV, most commonly in male sex workers, at low levels of between 1% and 2%, or in injecting drug users (IDU) at less than 1%, as well as only one case in a female sex worker (FSW). This was followed by the detection, in 1989, of a high HIV prevalence in FSW in the northern provinces (Phoolcharoen, 1991). The subsequent waves of the Thai epidemic, as it moved through the clients of sex workers to their wives and children, have been well documented (Phoolcharoen, 1991).

As information on the behavior, epidemiology, and underlying determinants of the epidemic became increasingly clear in the early 1990s, the social and behavioral roots of the epidemic became more apparent. While Thailand initially responded to HIV as a health problem confined to a few, the virus was recognized as a serious national development issue in the early 1990s. As a result, Thailand's response to the HIV epidemic evolved in interaction with the concerns raised by various sectors of society, such as the government, nongovernmental organizations (NGOs), private businesses, communities, community-based organizations, and universities. Thailand's response was also influenced by the interaction of these various sectors with international agencies responding to the HIV epidemic.

Policy Evolution

Thailand's HIV/AIDS prevention and care strategy has evolved through a number of stages since the beginning of the epidemic. Initial steps were characterized by programs that focused on individual risk and responsibility through the provision of information, awareness-raising campaigns, and sometimes delivery of fear-invoking messages. As the epidemic progressed, it became clear that effective messages needed to focus on sustaining safe behaviors. Better understanding of the cultural and social dimensions of behavior were crucial to developing more sophisticated responses, aimed at facilitating community support for changed behavior.

The evolution of Thailand's HIV/AIDS policy may be categorized into three main phases: confrontation of the new epidemic, creation of unified alliances, and alleviation of the consequences.

Confrontation of the New Epidemic (1984–1990)

Although the development of AIDS policy was in its infancy and there was little evidence of the AIDS epidemic in Thailand in 1985, the Ministry of Public Health took initial steps to deal with the AIDS issue. By Ministerial Announcement, under the umbrella of the Infectious Diseases Act, AIDS was classified as a notifiable disease. This was followed by the establishment of an AIDS voluntary reporting system under the responsibility of the Epidemiology Division, in order to track the epidemic. These and other health-related activities focused on epidemiological risk groups, such as IDU, MSM, and FSW.

In 1987, the Department of Communicable Disease Control (CDC) of the Ministry of Public Health (MOPH) expanded AIDS-related health activities through the coordination of other sectors, as well as NGOs, under the National Advisory Committee on AIDS. The World Health Organization (WHO) initiated technical and financial support in the form of a short-term HIV/AIDS program in 1988. Implementation of the national sentinel surveillance system to monitor HIV infection in key population groups in 1989, and the public dissemination of results, made it difficult to maintain an official position of denial and helped initiate the changes in social norms necessary to change behavior.

The first evidence that HIV could spread rapidly in the Thai population did not appear until 1988, when HIV testing was introduced into government methadone treatment centers for heroin addicts. This coincided with the development of a short-term AIDS plan. It was followed by Cabinet approval of the Medium Term Program for the Prevention and Control of AIDS 1989–1991, which followed the WHO/Global Programme on AIDS (GPA) guidelines. The plan intended to provide a working framework for government, NGOs, and private initiatives, and included measures for program management, health education, counseling, training, surveillance, monitoring, medical and social care, and laboratory and blood safety control. However, the majority of the funds to support the AIDS activities in this period were from external sources, including international organizations and bilateral aid. The internal resources mobilized were very limited, since the focus of HIV/AIDS policy was still controversial.

The explosive spread of HIV in IDU (Thanyarak Hospital reported that about 30% of IDU patients had HIV in 1987) prompted both the Royal Thai Army and the Epidemiology Division of the MOPH to launch HIV surveillance of specific groups of the population in 1989. In mid-June 1989, testing was launched in 14 provinces in samples of 100–200 people from each of several sentinel groups of the population—IDU, brothel-based FSW, male sex workers, male patients at STI clinics, blood donors, pregnant women, new prisoners and ex-prisoners. This testing was then expanded to all 73 provinces in 1990. Simultaneously, the Royal Thai Army launched biannual testing of the 60,000 21-year-old army conscripts chosen annually by national lottery, finding an HIV prevalence rate of 0.5% during the first round (Myers, 1991). Since then, the prevalence of HIV and reported risky sexual behavior among Thai conscripts have been used to estimate infection rates in young male adults.

As a result of the very limited information available on the extent of the HIV risk behaviors of the general population, the first national survey of behavioral risks for HIV infection (Partner Relations Survey) was launched in 1990, sponsored by the WHO and conducted by the Thai Red Cross and Chulalongkorn University (Sittitrai, 1992). The finding that HIV infection already had a foothold in the Thai population (Thai Trial Working Group on HIV/AIDS Projection, 2001) again emphasized that the virus posed a threat to the whole population.

The public availability of epidemiological surveillance results helped NGOs to accelerate their prevention, treatment, and human rights activities in at-risk populations and created an important constituency and lobbying group so that effective AIDS policy could be formulated. An NGO consortium on AIDS was formed in 1989 to empower civil society and the community for active moves against the AIDS epidemic. Nevertheless, there were still segments of the media that wanted to downplay the danger because of concerns about the possible impact on tourism, and because government financial support for the AIDS program was meager. In addition, several repressive measures had already been implemented or were under debate. For example, an immigration law required HIV testing upon entry into the country, and there was an initiative to enact a law to prevent people living with HIV/AIDS (PLWHA) from leaving the country.

Despite the growing evidence of the epidemic's spread, the government continued to downplay its significance in the general population. They encouraged, or at least did nothing to correct, the public perception that AIDS was likely to affect only marginal groups like MSM, male sex workers, and IDU. The prevention activities that were undertaken focused only on smaller, marginalized groups, and not on the general population.

Creation of Unified Alliances (1991–1997)

In 1991, under the short transitional government of Prime Minister Anand Panyarachun (1991–1992), AIDS prevention and control became a national priority at the highest level, emphasizing progressive policies to encourage safer behavior, and galvanizing the efforts of many sectors, including NGOs. Four important developments during the Anand administration had profound and lasting effects on AIDS policy beyond his short tenure. These were multisectoral activities coordinated by the government, public information and education campaigns, condom promotion, and human rights protections for PLWHA.

Multisectoral Activities Coordinated by Government. AIDS policy was brought under the coordination of the Office of the Prime Minister, with an officially multisectoral National AIDS Prevention and Control Committee, chaired by the Prime Minister. This signaled political commitment at the highest level, but also ushered in the formal participation of NGOs in the policy-making process. The NGOs lobbied strongly for wider-spread public information, protection of human rights, and compassionate care for AIDS patients. Their participation formally opened up the dialogue to those outside the health sector.

While officially this was a multisectoral program with participation by all ministries and was embraced as such by the international community, in reality the main players were the MOPH and the NGO community. The other ministries, even when allocated resources, initially had little expertise with which to implement these programs, which went beyond their sectoral mandates. The National Economic and Social Development Board (NESDB) was eventually given responsibility for planning the national AIDS strategy, and devised the National AIDS Plan of 1992–1996, discussed later.

Public Information and Education. During the Anand administration, a massive public information campaign about AIDS was launched under the leadership of Cabinet member Mechai Viravaidya, a well-known national figure with extensive experience in previous family planning campaigns and strong ties to non-governmental and community groups. Intensive public information on HIV/AIDS prevention, launched through the mass media, included mandatory one-minute AIDS education spots every hour on TV and radio. These messages emphasized preventive behavior change, condom use, and AIDS as not just a health problem but a social problem as well.

All ministries were actively involved in providing education and training to their staff and the population groups they worked with. The Ministry of Education launched peer education programs among students and an annual national competition among schoolchildren at different levels in essay writing on HIV/AIDS, greatly raising their level of awareness. Government efforts were complemented by private initiatives, such as the Thailand Business Coalition on AIDS, formed in 1993 to promote HIV/AIDS policies on education and prevention in the workplace. A program was launched to discourage young girls from entering into prostitution by providing scholarships to continue their education and enhance their employment opportunities.

Condom Promotion. The "100% Condom Use Program" was adopted nationwide to promote the universal use of condoms for FSW. Originally piloted in Ratchaburi Province in 1989, the program was expanded for national replication in 1991–1992. Prostitution was, and still is, illegal. However, the authorities adopted a more pragmatic approach by encouraging widespread condom use to prevent HIV transmission, rather than attempting to suppress commercial sex. The program involved collaboration at the provincial and local levels between public health officials, brothel owners, the local police, and FSW. By ensuring compliance in all sex establishments, those that enforced condom use would not lose business to those that did not.

The mechanisms to monitor compliance already existed—Thailand's extensive network of STI treatment clinics and the public health service's list of sex establishments. Under the program, FSW were screened for STI weekly or biweekly at government STI clinics. They were then treated and provided with a free box of condoms. Male patients presenting at the government STI clinics were considered evidence of non-use of condoms. Compliance could be checked through tracing the STI patients back to the brothels where they were infected. Health workers could then follow up with visits, providing additional information and condoms.

Condom promotion has been extended to cover a broad array of target groups. Social marketing of safe sex and condom use has been conducted to reach both male and female youths in schools and universities, as well as laborers in both the formal and informal sectors, and fishermen. Currently, condoms are available in various outlets—drugstores, supermarkets, convenience stores, and gas stations. Since condoms can be manufactured from Thai rubber products, they are affordable, and accessible in almost any marketplace throughout the country.

Human Rights Concerns for PLWHA. In 1990, activist NGOs succeeded in lobbying

TABLE 1. Government Budget for National AIDS Program and Proportion Allocated to the Ministry of Public Health (MOPH) and Other Ministries from 1991–2002

Fiscal year	Government budget (million Baht)[a]	MOPH (%)	Other ministries (%)
1991	182.662	100.00	0.00
1992	637.492	70.20	29.80
1993	1,121.540	80.64	19.36
1994	1,142.536	87.54	12.46
1995	1,558.350	79.92	20.08
1996	2,057.096	68.96	31.04
1997	1,891.153	73.58	26.42
1998	1,372.304	72.15	27.85
1999	1,439.053	76.70	23.30
2000	1,460.182	74.81	25.19
2001	1,486.878	79.91	20.09
2002	1,472.896	80.03	19.97
2003	1,178.591	85.01	14.99

Source: AIDS Division, Department of Communicable Disease Control, MOPH, Thailand
[a] Baht/US$ = 25 before 1997, 50 in 1997, 45 in 1999–2000, 44 in 2001 and 43 post-2002.

Cabinet members to abolish the mandatory reporting of names and addresses of AIDS patients and in getting the regulations that prohibited immigration of HIV-positive people reversed. Following several public hearings, the AIDS Bill was initiated in 1991. It incorporated the isolation and detainment of people with HIV/AIDS as measures to control the epidemic. However, it made no further progress and was never adopted. The principle of voluntary, anonymous, confidential counseling and testing was established. Central policy has evolved to place increasing emphasis on empowering people with HIV and AIDS. PLWHA have been recognized as an essential resource for prevention and care, rather than a potential reservoir or unfortunate consequence of the epidemic as was often the case in the earlier phases of the response. People with HIV/AIDS have become valuable allies both in formulating the AIDS education messages disseminated through the media, and in curriculum development in schools.

The National AIDS Plan

The National Economic and Social Development Board, the country's authority for national planning, was entrusted with coordinating all sectors to formulate the National AIDS Prevention and Control Plan (NAP), 1992–1996. The NESDB drew up the first five-year AIDS control program and budget, allocating resources to other ministries besides the MOPH, and to NGOs. This was to ensure smooth cooperation among the government agencies, NGOs, and the private sector in formulating and implementing a comprehensive action plan. The plan emphasized mobilization of society and communities to participate in preventing HIV, to care for those who are sick, and to reduce the stigma and discrimination facing those living with HIV/AIDS.

In 1993, all fourteen ministries submitted funding requests in accordance with the programs specified in the NAP, amounting to US$ 44 million. The National AIDS Program budget was subsequently increased to US$ 82.3 million, in 1996. Since 1991, the Royal Thai Government (RTG) has been the major funding source for domestic HIV/AIDS efforts, and financial support for the NAP increased significantly in the years following its inception (Table 1). In addition to the national budget, financial support was received from a total of 19 international organizations and foreign governments, beginning in 1988 and continuing to the present. Even though the authority for coordination of the NAP was transferred back to the AIDS Division of the CDC at the MOPH in 1994, the Prime Minister continues to chair the National AIDS Committee, which still plans and allocates the government budget.

The evolution of Thailand's HIV/AIDS policy may be outlined according to three NAP phases, focusing on orchestrating alliances, guiding community missions, and healthcare reform, respectively.

First Plan to Orchestrate Alliances

The 1992–1996 NAP served as a vehicle for various Thai agencies and departments to become involved in projects in accordance with the policy. The NAP allocated government spending for programs in the areas: prevention (behavioral and social change), health promotion and medical services, counseling, welfare and legal issues, research, and program management.

The budget for HIV prevention was directed at disseminating HIV/AIDS information and supporting education for the public and target groups. The prevention program aimed to promote values that were consistent with non-risk behavior and provide at-risk target groups with the motivation to change risk behaviors. It encouraged community members to accept and realize that AIDS threatened everyone in society.

The program on health promotion and medical services committed a five-year budget to support health and community care for PLWHA. It also invested in the development of guidelines and regimens to improve the standard treatment for AIDS patients. Antiretrovirals (ARV) were purchased to support small-scale clinical trials so that many hospitals in Thailand could be raised to best practice level, and other clinicians in the region could conduct study visits at these facilities. Universal precautions were financially supported under this program so that clinical settings in the country were better equipped to protect both clients and personnel.

Funding for counseling was allocated separately from health care to allow these services to be extended beyond the health care system infrastructure. PLWHA, their family members, service providers, and concerned people had to be able to access counseling in an anonymous manner. Training and refresher courses were offered to expand the service, as well as to ensure its quality. Testing for HIV was provided with pre- and post-test counseling, and with informed consent.

Programming for social and legal issues affecting PLWHA supported the development of guidelines for government attorneys, NGOs, and the community to protect human rights related to AIDS matters. A portion of the budget was allocated to support social welfare and assistance for PLWHA and their families. Efforts were made to reduce stigma and generate positive attitudes toward PLWHA among members of the general public.

Research funding was directed at the promotion and provision of grants for research leading to policy formulation, the practical application of research results, as well as the assessment of AIDS prevention and control efforts in Thailand. The Program provided financial grants through a network of researchers from universities and NGOs to create knowledge that would improve the AIDS program.

The National AIDS Plan had facilitated NGO collaboration with the government by funding their initiatives and related activities. NGOs had demonstrated their capacity to access marginalized populations requiring assistance. Thus, government funding to support NGOs was initiated in 1992, with a budget of US$ 0.46 million, administered by the CDC, MOPH. The amount was increased to US$ 0.6 million in 1993 and was administered by the Office of the Permanent Secretary for Public Health. In 1994, the amount was decreased to US$ 0.4 million and was returned to the CDC, then increased to US$ 3 million and US$ 3.2

million in the years 1995 and 1996, respectively.

Second Plan to Guide Community Missions

By 1996 the AIDS epidemic had spread outward from high-risk groups into other populations. It had reached groups originally considered to be at low risk, namely families, housewives, women of reproductive age in general, and their infants. Thus, the National Plan for Prevention and Alleviation of HIV/AIDS for 1997–2001 was formulated with a more holistic approach to meet the new challenge. HIV/AIDS issues were systematically incorporated into national plans related to economic and social development, such as those for health, education, children and youth, labor and social welfare, and others.

The new strategy sought also to integrate innovative AIDS-related activities into the functions of various sectors and communities. The availability of funding from the National AIDS Budget had clearly mobilized a wide range of stakeholders to join the movement. Furthermore, the community had become a key leverage element in driving and controlling the program.

The National AIDS Alleviation Plan of 1997–2001 focused efforts on mobilizing communities and civil society to initiate their own projects. Unfortunately, the economic crisis strained the funding capacity of the plan, leading to budget cuts and the plan had to be adjusted every year. Despite these budgetary limitations, the Plan included eight main programs, focusing on empowering community and family; developing HIV/AIDS psychosocial care; improving health and medical care for PLWHA; supporting HIV/AIDS research, including vaccine research; and managing integral plans.

Programs were supported to sustain activities relevant to the problems in different geographical areas. A matching fund for the "Villagers' Program," a fund coordinated by the village to help the families of PLWHA, was supported, particularly in the north where most people with HIV/AIDS resided. In other parts of the country, community empowerment was encouraged through the collaboration of the Ministry of the Interior, local government and grass roots civil society. Education in community schools was one of the tools used for empowerment. The provision of social welfare services and policies aimed at assisting PLWHAs, particularly in terms of employment and human rights protections have also become priority issues.

The health care infrastructure in the country was reoriented to be able to better provide HIV/AIDS care. Funding was allocated to build the capability of the health service setting and its human resources so that PLWHA would be able to access appropriate HIV/AIDS care. Home-based care was identified as integral to the continuation of care for PLWHA.

Major research was focused on the development of appropriate clinical practice guidelines in the country, and collaboration with international research groups in HIV vaccine development. Joint plans with UNAIDS were devised to step up HIV vaccine research and development, including plans for a program to conduct phase I and II clinical trials in Thailand. Goals in this area also included strengthening the country's research infrastructure, building capabilities to isolate the virus, integrating GCP and GLP as clinical concepts, improving data management, and the building a repository laboratory. Social and behavioral research results were also needed to strengthen the ongoing prevention program, but there was less investment in this area compared to clinical and vaccine research.

The activities according to the NAP were to be monitored and reported to the National AIDS Committee by the Committee secretary. Inspectors of the Office of the Prime Minister were entrusted with conducting evaluative monitoring of the activities pursued by the provincial authority, then reporting results to the Prime Minister.

However, the economic crisis of 1997–1999, with the political restructuring in 2000–2001 that followed the 1997 constitution, affected implementation of this phase of the National AIDS Program. Adjustments to the operational plan became necessary, and some performance targets were compromised.

Third Plan to Serve Political and Health Reform

In 1997 Thailand's political reform was marked by the establishment of a new revolutionary constitution. Constitutional changes reflected a strong demand for extended societal restructuring, which triggered a paradigm shift in the health system. As a result of this reform, health is now stipulated as a human right, which must be protected by the State. Equal entitlements to health were introduced for a wide range of vulnerable populations, such as the elderly, the disabled, abandoned children, and people with HIV/AIDS. The government's policy of universal healthcare coverage followed in 2001.

Simultaneously, advances in the efficacy HIV/AIDS therapeutics and the prevention of mother-to-child transmission have placed critical pressur on Thai policy makers to increase investment in ARV programs. Since 1998, the government AIDS funding has been increasingly allocated to medical services for AIDS patients and to the prevention of mother-to-child HIV transmission. Currently, the RTG has committed to the allocation of funding for ARV therapy and drugs to treat opportunistic infections (OI) for 50,000 AIDS cases under the universal coverage of the health care regime. This will lead to the inclusion of HIV/AIDS therapy in the health care benefit package of two other main regimes—the Civil Servant Medical Benefit Scheme and the Social Security Scheme for formal labors. With partial support from the Global Fund in 2003–2004, the RTG plans to expand its services to cover holistic care for all PLWHA in the next decade. The key element to this strategy is to manufacture and distribute ARV and essential diagnostic tools domestically. With this capability, it will be feasible for all PLWHA to access necessary medical care. Likewise, NGO coalitions have joined their efforts to empower community and family care, so that continuous care will be sustained.

Decentralization, public sector reform, as well as restructuring of social financing, have occurred in accordance with the ongoing political reform in Thailand. These drastic social shifts have driven health system reforms, which have been coordinated and implemented by the RTG since 2000. The National Health Insurance Act was promulgated in 2002, as an essential tool to support the policy of universal health care coverage. The National AIDS Committee formulated the National AIDS Plan of 2002–2006 to guide policy change for all sectors, particularly in accordance with ongoing restructuring. The plan includes five main programs, addressing HIV/AIDS prevention, HIV/AIDS alleviation, universal health care coverage, and research, including vaccine development.

The third NAP aims to continue support for a broad array of preventive measures for vulnerable populations. The budget has been expanded to support social changes that foster risk reduction among individuals, families, and the community. Addicted patient treatment programs will be supported to cope with increasing numbers of IDU. Small-scale harm reduction community work by NGOs will be initiated and then scaled up. Preventing the transmission of HIV from mother to child has been prioritized as a large-scale operation with nationwide coverage.

Even though preventive strategies have been developed national policy has been inadequate regarding some vulnerable groups, including IDU, MSM, and seamen, who are difficult to reach. Programs for syringe exchange or special education for MSM or seamen have never been well developed. The government's current policy of illicit drug user suppression has pushed this target group farther out of the reach of prevention programs. Thus, the epidemic in this risk group has demonstrated a continuously increasing trend.

Funding for HIV/AIDS alleviation is focused on strengthening clinical and community care services, as well as coordinating financing for universal health care coverage. This program will be supported partly by the Global Fund subsidy in 2004–2005, so that the extension of HIV/AIDS care can be achieved. The Government Pharmaceutical Organization will reorient its mission to produce and maintain some essential drugs and diagnostic devices to guarantee the availability of effective therapeutic measures.

In 2002, 480,063,200 Baht, or 32.6% of the annual national AIDS budget, was transferred to universal health care coverage. This placed responsibility for AIDS care within the national health insurance system. Thus, the National Health Insurance Authority will be accountable for further supporting medical care for Thailand's PLWHA.

The University consortium for HIV/AIDS research will leverage all major research-granting agencies in Thailand to coordinate research, and respond to advances in therapeutic efficacy, new findings on effective socio-behavioral prevention and the alleviation of socioeconomic impacts, so that research results will lead to successful and pragmatic plans. Vaccine research and development programs discussed previously have been renewed for the 2002–2006 plan.

The Impact of the National AIDS Plans on the HIV Epidemic

After initiation of the first NAP in 1992, there was evidence that the dissemination of information on HIV/AIDS had affected profound change in Thai society. The demand for commercial sex declined, condom use in commercial sex rose, STI cases plummeted, and the prevalence of HIV among army conscripts dropped by more than half (Phoolcharoen, 1998). Condom use in brothels rose from about 14% to more than 90% between 1988 and 1998 (Phoolcharoen, 1998). High condom use has been maintained. A 1997 survey of nearly 2,000 sex workers in 24 provinces found that 97% of sex workers always used condoms with casual customers, while 93% always used them with regular customers (Thai Trial Working Group on HIV/AIDS Projection, 2001).

The number of male STI patients reporting to public clinics fell steeply, from about 220,000 per year in 1988, to about 20,000 in 1995 (Thai Trial Working Group on HIV/AIDS Projection, 2001). The number of new STI cases declined from 6.5/1000 in 1989, to 3.2/1000 in 1991, and 1.6/1000 in 1993 (Thai Trial Working Group on HIV/AIDS Projection, 2001). At the same time, two-thirds of the drugstores surveyed in 24 provinces reported a decline in the sale of antibiotics for STI treatment and a sustained increase in the sale of condoms, confirming that patients were not simply diverted to private treatment sources.

Between 1990 and 1993, the percent of men reporting premarital or extramarital sex dropped from 28% to 15%, the percent visiting FSW dropped from 22% to 10%, and the percent consistently using condoms in commercial sex rose from 36% to 71% (Thai Trial Working Group on HIV/AIDS Projection, 2001). HIV prevalence among 21-year old army conscripts, which had risen to 4% in 1993, began a steady decline, to 1.56% in 1999 (Chamratrithirong, 1999).

The decline in HIV prevalence among army conscripts was even more pronounced in the Upper North, falling from more than 12% to less than 2% between 1992–2002 (Phoolcharoen, 1998). The annual incidence of HIV among army conscripts in six northern provinces during their 24-month military service declined from 2.48% in 1991–1993 to 0.55% in 1993–1995 (Phoolcharoen, 1998). Furthermore, there was a very strong association between increased condom use, reduction in visits to sex workers, and reduced incidence of STI and HIV over a relatively short period (Phoolcharoen, 1998). The prevalence of

HIV among young women (age<25) giving birth to their first child at Chiang Rai Hospital, which is an area of high prevalence in the north, rose from 1.3% in 1990 to 6.4% in 1994, then declined to 4.6% and 2.1% in 1997 and 2002, respectively (Phoolcharoen, 1998).

Since 1993, behavior change in Thailand has prevented an estimated 200,000 HIV infections that would otherwise have occurred by 2000 (Thai Trial Working Group on HIV/AIDS Projection, 2001). The most recent estimate of the cumulative number of infections in Thailand in 2000 is 29% less than what was projected to be the case in 1994 (Thai Trial Working Group on HIV/AIDS Projection, 2001). Of this difference of 395,000 infections, about half can be attributed to differences in the models and half to real differences in behavior. The number of new HIV infections in Thailand dropped from about 137,000 per year in 1990 to 29,000 per year in 2000 (Thai Trial Working Group on HIV/AIDS Projection, 2001).

However, PLWHA access to essential health care remains very low. It was expected that the government's policy on universal health care coverage, with pressure from the civil society movement, as well as global price adjustment of ARV drugs, would improve the PLWHA access to treatment and care. Even though comprehensive care, including home-based care, was supported under the National AIDS Program, its impact and cost-effectiveness have not been formally evaluated.

Though Thailand's government uses Performance Based Budgeting and the concept of Result-Based Management has been introduced, HIV/AIDS program planning and implementation are still process-oriented. There has been no official evaluation of Thai NAP since the beginning of the epidemic. Only midterm reviews took place with support from WHO/GPA in the early years. Results monitoring has not been institutionalized. Implementation monitoring has not been conducted systematically.

COST AND EFFECTIVENESS OF HIV/AIDS PREVENTION IN THAILAND

The RTG began to allocate its own budget for AIDS programs in 1988. Prior to 1990 the majority of AIDS-related activities were funded by international and foreign donors. In 1989, with the government slowly becoming more open towards developing HIV/AIDS policy, prominent activists both inside and outside the government joined the anti-AIDS campaign. Armed with the findings of the first round of sentinel sero-surveillance, these individuals, joined by a growing number of NGOs concerned about human rights and the spread of HIV in the communities they served, were able to raise awareness and initiate change. In January 1990, the Prime Minister announced an official campaign to control and prevent HIV/AIDS, making HIV/AIDS control a national policy. Governmental budgetary commitment to combating AIDS also increased significantly, from US$ 437,000 in 1989 to US$ 2.63 million in 1990. A study by the AIDS Division demonstrated that the real expense of programming for all of the ministries was up to 98.7% of the amount allocated in the 1996 fiscal year (Table 2).

The National AIDS Committee directed the National AIDS Plan through budget allocation for broad and integrated activities, according to program design; distribution of funding from 1994 to 1996 is shown in Table 3. Expenditure on Health and Medical Care was the major item, and exhibited an increasing trend. This resulted from the growing number of PLWHA who demanded more services, and from the rise in the cost of evolving therapeutic care. At the end of 1996, a trial to prevent mother-to-child transmission in Thailand demonstrated efficacious results. Thus, funding was allocated for this program in 1997.

Creating a mechanism to coordinate the AIDS programs in every province and community was a predominant focus in 1994. It was crucial to mobilize the NGOs and

TABLE 2. Budget Allocation to Government Sectors in 1996, with Proportion Allocated and Proportion of Real Expense in each Ministry

Ministries	Amount allocated (Baht)	Proportion of budget allocated (%)	Proportion of expense to allocation (%)
Office of the Prime Minister	42,121,500	2.05	89.64
Ministry of Defense	50,183,700	2.44	102.25
Ministry of the Interior	169,747,900	8.25	96.62
Ministry of Education	46,329,800	2.25	95.78
Ministry of University Affairs	243,259,300	11.83	96.46
Ministry of Labor & Welfare	84,232,800	4.09	97.72
Supreme Attorney's Bureau	2,318,400	0.11	119.80
Ministry of Justice	425,500	0.02	100.00
Ministry of Public Health	1,418,477,100	68.96	99.56
Total	2,057,096,000	100.00	98.68

Source: AIDS Division, Thailand

TABLE 3. Budget Allocation Proportions According to 1994, 1995, and 1996 National Budgetary Act, by AIDS Program

AIDS program	1994	1995	1996
Prevention: Behavioral and social change	11.48%	20.98%	14.33%
Health promotion and medical services	57.15%	55.16%	65.67%
Counseling	1.59%	1.85%	1.60%
Welfare and legal issues	3.10%	8.64%	7.51%
Research and evaluation	1.29%	2.88%	2.45%
Program management/administration	25.38%	10.50%	8.44%
Total in US$ (millions)	45.63	62.09	81.96

Source: AIDS Division, Thailand

communities to work as equal partners with the government sector. However, the budget for this program decreased to only 8.4% in 1996. The budget to finance the activities of government officials had tapered off, while support of the community and NGOs continued.

Prevention was always emphasized as a priority in the plan. Yet the expenditure for prevention programs fluctuated between 10% and 20% of the budget. A portion of this budget was allocated to promote AIDS-related information through the mass media. In 1994, the National AIDS Committee attempted to change advertising policy to employ interpersonal media, such as the Fellow's Friendship Support Program, which had been demonstrated to be effective. However, it was found that development of word of mouth communication was more complicated and difficult to sustain. Some research has pointed out that involvement of the community in operational research might be a powerful tool and could overcome diversity among different communities. However, there were very few innovators capable of conducting such work.

The Living with HIV/AIDS Program spent most of its funds on social welfare for people affected by the epidemic. The increasing expenditure resulted from an upsurge in the number of PLWHA and AIDS orphans. The program suggested employing the family and the community to alleviate this epidemic, but a sound methodology for community capacity-building had never been in place. This demanded more research to encourage community empowerment. However, the research budget was very small and the research management was weak, so that research issues were fragmented and scattered. There had never been investment in research to develop appropriate ways to cope with the community or with counseling.

Health and medical care expenditure increased to more than 70% of the total AIDS budget over time, as a result of the increasing burden of clinical care for people with HIV/AIDS. NGOs struggled to include ARV in clinical practice guidelines, since there was increasingly convincing evidence that PLWHA survived longer in western countries where people had access to appropriate care. In 2002, health and medical care for PLWHA were integrated into the national program of universal health care coverage. The budget for development of psychosocial care was increased to 7.42% of the total budget in 1998, and was then integrated into health and medical care, so that the proportion of the allocated budget declined.

The program for empowerment of the family and the community was another component of the AIDS program. After 2001, this program was integrated into local government budget allocations, as a result of the Decentralization Act of 1999. Local authorities became accountable for the governance and administration of their own communities, and 22% of central tax revenue was demanded for allocation to local government. It was expected that local authorities should spend this portion of the budget for community empowerment, to prevent HIV spread, as well as to alleviate the social impact of AIDS.

Financial support for coordination and administration of the plan at the provincial level increased from 1998 to 2001. Collaboration among NGOs and government officials, both at the central level and locally, was supported under this program. After 2000, central control from the National AIDS Committee was weakened by a change in Cabinet, as well as by a policy shift towards an emphasis on illicit drug suppression. In 2002, the program to support administration and integration of the plan was abolished.

Research financing has been generally increasing, with promising signs from HIV vaccine research and clinical trials of findings to extend PLWHA survival. However, HIV/AIDS research in Thailand was reviewed in 2001, and it was found that research management had been very poorly coordinated. Various research institutes conducted numerous studies relevant to HIV/AIDS, but these were still designed within a fragmented context, so that results could not influence modification of either policy or practice. Thus, the organization of better management and coordination of HIV/AIDS research, to meet Thai society's demands, was recommended.

Program Adjustment as a Consequence of the Economic Crisis

In 1997 Thailand was affected strongly by an economic crisis, which was triggered by currency devaluation. The growth of Thailand's gross domestic product (GDP) in 1998 was estimated at minus 5.5%, with inflation of 10.5%. The crisis placed severe constraints on public finances, including the National AIDS Program. The economic crisis caused financial expenditure to be adjusted every third month, so that budgetary allocation was in turmoil. As a result, the government budget was scaled down 18.5%, from the 982 billion Baht that was approved in the 1998 Budget Bill, to 800 billion Baht. In 1998, the AIDS budget dropped to 1,372 million Baht, and slightly increased after that (Table 4). The currency devaluation also caused increases in the prices of imported condoms and drugs.

In 1999, the RTG expended 1.4 billion Baht (US $37.9 million), or about 24 Baht ($0.63) per capita, from its National AIDS Program budget to prevent HIV transmission, to care for and treat AIDS patients, to mitigate the impact of AIDS, and to support AIDS research. The largest share of the AIDS budget (63%) financed treatment and care, including ARV and drugs for opportunistic infections

TABLE 4. Budget Allocation Proportions According to 1998, 1999, 2000 and 2001 National Budgetary Act, by AIDS Program

Program	1998	1999	2000	2001
Empowerment of family and community	10.08%	7.57%	7.41%	8.27%
Psycho-social care development	7.42%	6.22%	6.00%	5.94%
Health and medical care	72.78%	72.92%	74.96%	72.73%
HIV/AIDS research	3.41%	3.80%	3.47%	3.67%
Integral plan administration	6.31%	9.49%	8.15%	9.39%
Total (million Baht)	1,372	1,439	1,460	1,486

Source: AIDS Division, Thailand

(OI) for clinical trials, HIV testing and counseling, blood screening, and universal precautions to prevent HIV infection in medical settings. Of the total 24 Baht per capita spent out of the AIDS budget, 15 Baht (40 cents), or 63% was spent on treatment and care. The next largest share (16%) was spent on services to mitigate the impact of AIDS, including programs to prevent mother-to-child HIV transmission, care of orphans, subsidized living arrangements for people living with HIV/AIDS who are out of work, skills training and legal counsel for PLWHA. Programs to prevent the spread of the epidemic in the population accounted for only 8% of the budget, covering public information, purchase of condoms for free distribution, condom promotion, and other community prevention activities. An additional 6% of the AIDS budget was distributed as grants to NGOs for community-level AIDS prevention and care activities. The remaining 7.2% of the AIDS budget was allocated to management and research.

Total funding for AIDS programs declined by 9% between 1996 and 1997 (from 2,187.5 million to 1,986.1 million Baht) and has declined more dramatically, by 27.8%, since the economic crisis of 1997–1999. The hardest hit has been prevention, with expenditure dropping by half since 1997, and as a share of the total AIDS budget, declining from 11% to 8%. The government is now spending only 2 Baht per capita (5 US cents) to prevent HIV transmission among roughly 40 million adults. Expenditure on treatment and care was also cut by about one third (34.4%). However, most of this decline can be attributed to completion, in 1998, of a program to construct patient wards at five hospitals. If this component is excluded, spending on medical treatment and counseling was relatively protected during and after the crisis, with a 9.3% cut. In fact, the AIDS budget line for treatment is only a share of the total public spending on AIDS treatment, as it covers drugs only for a small group of AIDS patients enrolled in clinical trials. The health care needs of other AIDS patients are financed through the regular budget of the MOPH and cannot be easily disassociated from the health care consumed by other patients.

The cut in prevention expenditure reflects a dramatic decline in financing condoms for free distribution. The number of condoms purchased by the MOPH for free distribution to high-risk groups dropped by 62%, from 53 to 20 million pieces (70 million to 29 million Baht), between 1996 and 1997. These cuts were primarily the result of a decision to transfer more of the costs of condoms to beneficiaries, but coincided with the economic crisis. Some evidence showed that 1996 condom levels represented an oversupply and that a modest reduction in publicly financed condoms might have been in order. Monitoring of the epidemic and of risk behaviors in the population during the crisis years suggested that high levels of condom use in the commercial sex industry were sustained despite these cuts. However, the crisis most likely reduced the demand for commercial sex, reducing the demand for condoms and thus reducing the impact of the cut in the condom budget. Many other high-risk groups still have low condom access and use. The cuts in condom purchases in 1996–1997 have by and large not been reinstated, with projected condom purchases for 2000 (31.5 million condoms) at only 59% of 1996 levels. None of the prevention budget is allocated to preventing HIV transmission by injecting drug use, which accounts for a growing share of total transmission, and where HIV infection levels have risen, not declined.

Public spending on treatment from the AIDS budget is dominated by the purchase of expensive ARV for small numbers of AIDS patients enrolled in clinical trials. With the exception of financing AZT to prevent mother-to-child transmission, the government and most insurance providers in the health system do not subsidize ARV, such as the expensive triple combination therapies used widely in the West. This policy is consistent with that of public funding for other very expensive treatments, such as kidney dialysis, which is not subsidized. However, in the case of AIDS, there is an exception for some 2,100 persons enrolled in clinical trials of dual or triple ARV, whose drug costs are financed by the AIDS budget as part of the clinical trials. The proposed ARV drug budget for 2001 (289.7 million Baht) amounted to 31% of the proposed allocation for medical treatment and roughly one-fifth of the entire AIDS budget. This means that more than twice the amount spent on prevention was being used to finance ART for 2% of all AIDS patients, at an average cost of 138,000 Baht, or US$ 3,449 per patient annually. A share of the regular MOPH budget is also spent on health care for AIDS patients not in these clinical trials, but the MOPH budget does not finance ARV treatment, and in general there is no clear policy on funding drugs for OI. Drugs for the treatment of OI are financed through the regular budgets of the MOPH, through hospitals and other health facilities, and out-of-pocket.

These expenditures have certainly increased over time with the growing number of AIDS patients. Hospitals can allocate some of their non-earmarked drug budgets for OI drugs. In some cases, the same drugs are used to treat AIDS patients and those with other conditions. Thus, it is very difficult to track actual spending on OI drugs (treatment and prevention). The main exception is the tuberculosis (TB) budget, which is funded centrally. Despite the dramatic increase in TB associated with HIV infection, the TB budget declined in nominal terms by 14% between 1997 and1999, from 360.1 million to 310 million Baht.

NGOs have played an important role in the response to AIDS in Thailand. Their critical role in facilitating care for AIDS patients has been well cited. Grant funding for NGO activities remained constant from 1997 to 1999. The two main categories that received increased spending were prevention programs—notably financing programs to reduce HIV transmission from mother to child (41.4% increase since 1997)—and research, which increased by 66%. In 1999, the AIDS Division allocated 87.5 million Baht to 465 projects of 373 organizations, for an average outlay of 188,200 Baht (US $4,704) per project. However, the ongoing decline of HIV infection in FSW, conscripts, and pregnant women in 1999–2000 hinted that the government budget might have catalyzed the use of resources by public and private sectors to sustain prevention. In 2000 and 2001 the allocations for NGOs declined, but this has been partially compensated for by the $2.6 million AIDS component of the World Bank-financed Social Investment Project (SIP). In 2000, the AIDS budget allocated 60 million Baht to nearly 300 NGOs and the SIP project for prevention and care, and an additional 27 million Baht was distributed to six major NGOs to allocate funds to smaller NGO collaborators. The 2000 budget included a modest increase in allocation for prevention (11.7% increase of 12.7 million Baht, still leaving nominal spending on prevention 44% below 1997 levels). The year 2000 budget also emphasized medical treatment (3.8% increase; 33.7 million Baht), and mother-to-child transmission (5.6% increase; 7.9 million Baht).

However, the mix of services provided, program coverage, and likely impact of NGO programs and activities have not been studied. Little information is available about the precise activities of the NGOs, the coverage or effectiveness of their activities, and their potential complement with other public and private programs. In particular, information is not readily available on the extent to which they are involved in prevention activities as opposed to patient care, and whether the prevention activities are focused on those at greatest risk of transmitting AIDS to others, or on the general population. While financing of NGO activities is a small share of the overall expenditures (6.1% in 1999, or about 1 Baht of the 24 Baht per capita), the NGO share is only slightly less than the share spent on prevention (7.6%). The complement of these activities with both the prevention and treatment components of the budget, and their coverage and effectiveness, deserve review.

CURRENT AIDS TREATMENT STANDARDS IN THAILAND

Medical management of the HIV-infected patient includes therapy with ARV, prevention of opportunistic infections and treatment of complications with a holistic approach, including counseling for patients and families, and providing home-based care.

Studies have shown an important role for azidothymidine (AZT) in decreasing the mortality of AIDS patients since 1987, which led to the recommendation of monotherapy from 1987 to 1991 (Fischl, 1987; Volberding, 1990). Later, the Concorde study (1994), ACTG175 and NuCombo trials led to the recommendation of dual therapy in 1991–1995 (Concorde, 1994; Fischl, 1995; Saravolatz, 1996; Delta Coordinating Committee, 1996). Since 1996, many studies have shown that optimal and suitable ARV agents are safe, leading to declines in mortality rates, especially as a result of highly active antiretroviral therapy (HAART) (Palella, 1998; Hammer, 1997). American and Brazilian studies have demonstrated the cost-effectiveness of providing ARV to every AIDS patient requiring treatment; it could reduce the cost of hospital care by 60% (Schechter, 2002; Keiser, 2001).

Based on this knowledge, the RTG has changed its recommendation on the use of ARV therapy over time. The evolution of ARV use according to "The AIDS National Guidelines for the Clinical Management of HIV Infection in Children and Adults", in relation to the recommendation in developed countries, is shown in Figure 1.

The RTG national policy of subsidizing zidovudine monotherapy started in 1992–1993, using the public sector hospital delivery system. After evaluation by the MOPH, the World Bank, and the WHO in 1995, the program was not considered feasible or affordable. Therefore, in 1997 the national policy changed to establish an HIV/AIDS clinical research network, to maintain and increase the expertise of HIV physicians in clinical management. One goal of this network was

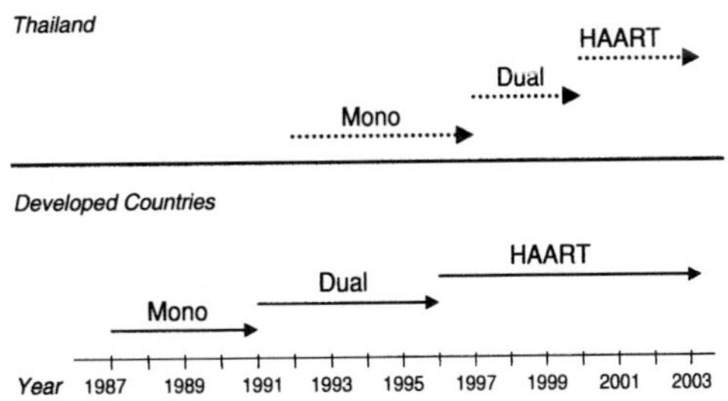

FIGURE 1. Evolution of Thai national guidelines for the clinical management of HIV infection over time (top, dotted lines), compared with those in developed countries (bottom, solid lines).

TABLE 5. NNRTI-Containing Regimens in Thailand and Cost

Regimen[a]	Estimated cost (Baht/month)[b]
d4T/3TC/NVP	1,500 for GPOvir®
AZT/3TC/NVP (Combined AZT/3TC + NVP)	2,500 (generic products)
AZT/3TC/EFV (Combined AZT/3TC + EFV)	5,500 (AZT/3TC = generic products)
AZT/ddI-Ec/EFV	8,500
d4T/3TC/EFV	4,500 (d4T, 3TC = generic products)
ddI-Ec/3TC/EFV	8,000 or more

Source: AIDS Division, Thailand
[a] d4T indicates stavudine; 3TC, lamivudine; NVP, nevirapine; AZT, zidovudine; EFV efavirenz; ddI-Ec, didanosine-enteric coated.
[b] 1USD = 42 Baht.

to develop an ARV core protocol using either dual therapy with AZT + ddl or AZT + ddC and monitoring more than 2,000 patients over a 4-year period. In the year 2000, the Ministry aimed to make HAART available by a triple-drug regimen. The first national guideline on clinical management of HIV infection in children and adults, using triple-drug therapy was published and distributed in late 2000 (UNAIDS, 2000), with the newest revised version in late 2002 (Ministry of Public Health, 2002). These guidelines included criteria for when and how to start combined ARV and guidance for follow-up of patients on HAART. It also included management of HIV/AIDS in infants and children, prevention of mother-to-child transmission, and management after occupational exposure.

For Thailand, ARV is recommended for patients with symptomatic HIV infection, an AIDS-defining illness, or with a CD4 count less than 200–250 cells/μl. The first choice for HAART, used with patients who are treatment-naïve, is two nucleoside reverse transcriptase inhibitors (NRTI) and one non-nucleoside reverse transcriptase inhibitor (NNRTI). Table 5 shows various regimens and prices for ARV, including locally made ARV. The least expensive regimen is a combination of stavudine (d4T), lamivudine (3TC), and nevirapine (NVP), which is locally marketed as GPOvir®.

GPOvir®, an ARV cocktail, was designed by the Government Pharmaceutical Organization (GPO). The drug, a combination of nevirapine, stavudine and lamivudine, is made in two formulations: GPOvir S30 (nevirapine 200 mg, lamivudine 150 mg, and stavudine 30 mg) for patients under 60 kg body weight, and GPOvir S40 (nevirapine 200 mg, lamivudine 150 mg, and stavudine 40 mg) for patients with a body weight of 60 kg or more. The drug costs US $0.40 per tablet, making the monthly cost 1,200 Baht (US $27), which is the cheapest in the world. Under a program launched in 2002 and jointly supported by the government and the Global AIDS Fund, the drugs will be provided to 13,000 HIV/AIDS patients from 400 hospitals nationwide.

The national guidelines also describe clinical approaches to various symptoms of HIV infection, for example, HIV/AIDS-associated skin disease, AIDS with chronic diarrhea, and AIDS with pulmonary problems, with recommendations for the treatment and prophylaxis of OI. Examples of drugs recommended for OI prophylaxis are shown in Table 6.

Various studies in the United States and France since 1994 have shown the use of

TABLE 6. Examples of Drugs Recommended for Primary Prophylaxis of Opportunistic Infections

Infection	Drug recommended[a]
Tuberculosis	Isoniazid 300 mg once daily for one month
Pneumocystis carinii pneumonia	Cotrimoxazole (TMP/SMZ) TMP/SMZ 80/400 (SS) mg, 1 tablet/day; TMP/SMZ 160/800 (DS) mg, 1 tablet/day; or Dapsone 50 mg/day + pyrimethamine (25 mg) 2 tablet/week + folinic acid 25 mg/week
Cryptococcal meningitis	Fluconazole 400 mg weekly
Penicillium marneffei and *Histoplasma*	Itraconazole 200 mg/day

Source: Thai National Guidelines, 2003
[a] TMP/SMZ indicates Trimethoprim/Sulfamethoxazole.

zidovudine (ZDV) to be useful in pregnant women during pregnancy, delivery, and within 6 weeks after birth (Connor, 1994; Lallemant, 2000), reducing the risk of mother-to-child HIV transmission by two thirds (Shaffer, 1999; US Public Health Service, 2000). ZDV began to be provided in 2001 to some HIV-positive pregnant women through a public donation campaign of the Thai Red Cross. The Thai MOPH launched phase III clinical trials to determine the effectiveness of a cheaper and simpler ZDV regimen. A trial in Bangkok demonstrated that short-course antenatal ZDV, from 36 weeks' gestation until delivery, reduced the risk of mother-to-child HIV transmission by half among non-breastfeeding HIV-infected women (Thisayakorn, 1998). A multicenter trial in Thailand, comparing ZDV treatment of various durations, showed that the extent of suppression of *in utero* transmission depended on the duration of ARV during the latter part of pregnancy (Bryson, 1996).

Short-course ZDV regimens have been implemented in pilot projects in two regions, in the northern part of Thailand in 1997, and in the northeast region, starting in 1998 (Kanshana, 2000). Based on the experience and success of these projects, the Department of Health started a nationwide program of voluntary antenatal counseling and testing, short-course ZDV, and infant formula for HIV-infected pregnant women, in 2000.

AVAILABILITY AND AFFORDABILITY OF ANTIRETROVIRAL DRUGS, AND FUTURE GOALS

Over the past ten years, limitations on resources and the high cost of drugs have hampered access to care. The estimated number of AIDS patients needing antiretroviral therapy was about 50,000–60,000 in the year 2002, but currently only 13,000 cases have access to care provided by the government system. The RTG launched a program called "Access for All," in 2003. "Access for All" means everyone in Thailand has access to health care services, including the general population, asymptomatic HIV-positive patients, and symptomatic PLWHA who require ARV treatment. National access to ARV therapy aimed to provide ARV to 23,000 AIDS patients by 2003, and the program will be expanded to cover 50,000 AIDS patients by the end of 2004, supported by a government budget and the Global Fund. To achieve these goals, infrastructure strengthening is needed in terms of ARV delivery and logistical systems, knowledge and experience of physicians to diagnose and treat drug complications, counseling services, follow-up and monitoring systems, to eliminate the risk of treatment failure and the development of resistance (Vanhove, 1996). Other objectives include preventing the occurrence of new infections and preventing mother-to-child transmission by providing 100% AZT to all positive mothers.

Ensuring a continuum of care for PLWHA is an important issue, and includes strengthening community- and home-based care after the patient is discharged from hospital. PLWHA networks have been established in collaboration with NGOs, and have played an important role in providing the following services: HIV/AIDS education, information dissemination to PLWHA, income generation schemes for PLWHA, and home visits. Home visits include health care education, referrals, and monitoring of ARV adherence. Preliminary results from evaluating the follow-up and monitoring program, as part of the continuum of care in the Primary Care Unit (PCU) during the period January to September 2002, identified some difficulties, such as limited resources at the PCU, and dealing with the issue of confidentiality. Confidentiality is of high importance to villagers; HIV/AIDS patients are afraid of others in their neighborhood knowing that they are HIV-infected.

In the upper north of Thailand, the "Access to Care" (ATC) service was launched in 6 provinces: Chiang Mai, Lamphun, Lampang, Chiang Rai, Phayao and Mae Hongson, in 2001. Eight hundred and nineteen PLWHA were provided with ARV, in 54 hospitals. A rapid situation analysis of the project was conducted by the Community Medicine Department of Chiang Mai and supported by the Horizons Program of the Population Council during the period May to June 2002, and the results were disclosed in November 2002 (Thailand Department of Disease Control, 2001). The objectives of this analysis were to assess the ATC delivery system and its integration with other services, the capacity of the logistical systems to provide HAART, the technical capacity of the ATC service providers, adequacy of counseling, follow-up and monitoring system, adherence and the role of community groups e.g., PLWHA groups and NGOs. The results have revealed high levels of support for the program by health providers, PLWHA receiving HAART, their relatives and even those PLWHA who had dropped out of the program. The program provided clear guidelines on how it should be run, especially community participation in the government program, and demonstrated good coordination between the Provincial Health Office and hospitals, with a person in charge of the logistics system at each hospital, which led to improved health among PLWHA receiving HAART. However, from this analysis, 28% were not taking medicine on time, 15% missed a hospital appointment for drugs, and the dropout rate was about 40%. One reason for this was the side effects, in spite of some home visits. The burden of running the program at the district hospital level fell on nurses and pharmacists, as there were no professional counselors in these hospitals and the doctors' workloads caused them to be unable to participate in the program fully.

HIV VACCINE RESEARCH AND DEVELOPMENT PROGRAM

Thailand has been heavily involved in clinical trials of HIV vaccines. It has been estimated that there are between 700,000–1,000,000 Thais infected with HIV and the number is increasing (XV International AIDS Conference, 2004). Changing the population's risk behaviors has proven to be very difficult and slow. Even though the use of condoms is preventative, new cases still appear. Treatment with drugs is very expensive and currently only available to a limited group of PLWHA.

These numbers raise the question of whether to use a first generation vaccine that may have a protective efficacy of only 30% to 50%. Some researchers argue that this may lead to increased risk behavior on the grounds of perceived protection and would therefore lead to more infections. Others argue that the use of such a vaccine in combination with counseling to prevent an increase in risk behavior could save many lives and prevent disabilities (UNAIDS, 2000).

TABLE 7. Summary of Vaccines Being Researched in Thailand

Phase I/II	Candidate vaccine	Subtype	Number of volunteers
1994	Synthetic peptide MN-V3	B	24
1995	Envelope GP120	B	30
	Envelope GP120	B	52
1997	Envelope GP120	B, E, B/E	380
2000	Prime boost Canary pox plus GP120	E + E	130
	Prime boost Canary pox plus GP 120	B, E, B/E	125
Phase III			
1999	Envelope Bivalent GP120	B/E	2,500
2002	Prime boost Canary pox Plus GP120	B, E, B/E	16,000

There are conflicting opinions regarding Thailand's joining the vaccine testing community. One group, mainly scientists, commended the decision to participate in trials and the development of a vaccine. Others argued that Thailand could potentially be harmed by becoming part of the vaccine testing community. It was decided that Thailand would cooperate with vaccine trial efforts provided that: phase I trials for safety and immunogenicity had been conducted in the country of origin of the candidate vaccine; and Thai investigators were responsible for the conduct of the trial with assistance and support from abroad. In 1995–1996 the program began. Thailand would facilitate the trials, provided that good data from animals were available, and that components or genes derived from the local clade of virus, i.e. subtype E would be included in the vaccines to be tested. Although it was unknown whether the eventual vaccine would have to be subtype-specific, assurances were given that, if Thailand needed a specific vaccine (i.e., subtype E), it would be developed. Thailand also required that assistance be given to strengthen its existing capacity for isolating and characterizing HIV viruses; genotyping and phenotyping; maintaining good clinical practice; data management, including analysis, evaluation, and presentation; and maintaining good repositories. Repositories were needed to make use of future technological progress, and also for possible re-testing. Measures were discussed to ensure accessibility of the vaccine to Thais and the populations of neighboring countries.

Between 1996–1998, concerns about vaccine testing were similar to earlier years, but a few new issues were raised. Thai investigators were encouraged to participate in pre-clinical development with the group that wanted to conduct the vaccine trials. Sharing of intellectual property rights was expected. It was emphasized more strongly that serious dialogue on vaccine availability must take place prior to the conduct of any phase III efficacy trial.

One of the many ethical matters concerning the development of an HIV vaccine was the question of how to treat volunteers who developed infection during a trial? The debate here focused on which level of treatment to offer—the best available in the world, or the best available in the country. There is no definitive answer as yet. Currently, treatment of vaccine trial participants who become infected follows national guidelines. HIV prophylactic vaccine trials that have taken place in Thailand are shown in Table 7. The first vaccine that was planned for testing in Thailand was a GP160 vaccine made by Microgenesis. This was tried as a therapeutic vaccine in the

U.S. and was stopped at the phase II trial stage, and the vaccine was dropped from Thailand's trial. The first vaccine to be tested in Thailand, therefore, was the synthetic peptide MN-V3, of United Biomedical. It was tested for safety and immunogenicity on 24 volunteers. The vaccine appeared to be safe, with uncertain immunogenicity (Phanuphak, 1997).

Thailand became involved with phase I and II testing of the GP120 vaccine, used first against clade B and later for clades B and E. The results of phase I/II AIDSVAX® B/E have shown that the vaccine was safe and immunogenic (Pitisuttithum, 2000); this led to the launch of phase III trials in 1999 by Bangkok Vaccine Evaluation Group (Bangkok Metropolitan Administration, Vaccine Trial Centre, Mahidol University, Thai–US Department of Disease Control Collaboration and VaxGen, Inc.) (Pitisuttithum, 2001). The Phase III trial aimed to determine the efficacy of the vaccine in IDU in Bangkok. The primary objective was to determine whether immunization with the vaccine (B/E) protected IDU from HIV-1 infection. Secondarily, the trial purported to determine whether prior immunization with the vaccine prevented persistent viremia.

The study was a randomized, double-blind, placebo-controlled, multi-site efficacy trial. Uninfected IDU at risk of HIV infection were randomly divided into two groups. One group of 1,250 was given the vaccine, while the other 1,250 were given a placebo only. Dose schedule injections would be given 6 times in total (in month 0, 1, 12, 18, 24 and 30). Each dose was 300 μg. Then began a very systematic set-up of the study, with special attention to ethical concerns like whether volunteers understood the trial before enrollment, risk of discrimation or social harm as a result of participating in the trial, especially in the occurrence of vaccine-induced HIV seropositivity, and potential for increased risk behavior as a result of belief in vaccine efficacy. The volunteers underwent intensive screening before and during the trial. The first time a blood test was done, subjects received an informative video and a booklet. A detailed description of the trial and the vaccine was offered. Issues covered included expectations, duties, benefits, confidentiality, privileges, etc. It was also made clear that volunteers could withdraw at any given time. During the second meeting post-test counseling was done and a comprehension test was conducted. Volunteers were required to score 80% twice and know the answers to all important questions. The participants were given diary cards to help monitor the reactogenicity experienced during the three days after each immunization. They were asked to report all adverse events. In addition, participants were counseled to maintain low risk behaviors. Vaccinees who became HIV-positive during the clinical trial would receive triple ARV therapy per national guidelines. Results of this trial, announced in November 2003, showed no efficacy (Vaxgen, 2003). However, risk behavior among IDU participants declined during the study period, with a high follow-up rate (90%).

In parallel, a Phase III trial for VaxGen GP120 was conducted in the United States about one year before Thailand. The trial was designed as a randomized, double-blind, placebo-controlled, multinational efficacy trial. The trial was conducted with MSM only. Results were reported in February 2003. This study showed a reduction of infection among the entire sample, including all racial groups, of 3.8%. There were 78% fewer HIV infections among black volunteers who received the vaccine compared to placebo recipients. There were 67% fewer HIV infections among ethnic minorities, other than Hispanic individuals, who received the vaccine compared to placebo recipients. Trial data indicated that black and Asian volunteers appeared to produce higher levels of antibodies against HIV, while white and Hispanic volunteers appeared to develop consistently lower levels of protective antibodies following vaccination. However, Thailand's results demonstrated that this observation was not statistically significant (VaxGen, 2003).

At present, a prime boost concept vaccine, which had been in phase I/II since the year 2000, is ready to enter phase III trials. The vaccine in the prime immunization of this trial is a canarypox vector made by Aventis. The boost vaccine is VaxGen gp120. The trial is sponsored by the U.S. military's HIV research program, Walter Reed Army Institute of Research, and the U.S. National Institutes of Health (NIH). The study will be launched by the MOPH in collaboration with the Faculty of Tropical Medicine, Mahidol University, and Armed Force Research of Medical Science in the last quarter of 2003. It is going to be one of the largest trials involving 16,000 participants in Cholburi and Rayong provinces (Rerks-Ngarm, 2002).

Currently, a Japanese Thai cooperative project on HIV vaccine development is continuing at the preclinical level. The group is working on two potential candidates for vaccination. They are to be used in a prime boost model. The prime agent is BCG GAG HIV vaccine and the boost agent is Vaccinia HIV vaccine (Falk, 2000).

Thailand has been testing an immune moderator, or therapeutic vaccine, called Remune. The phase II trial was conducted with 397 HIV-positive candidates with CD4 cell counts greater than 300 at enrollment. The trial has lasted four years and the investigators reported good clinical results with elevated CD4 counts (Churdboonchart, 1998; Churdboonchart, 2000). However, other practitioners contested the result.

For the past 8 to 10 years, infrastructure strengthening, capacity building for clinical facilities, quality assurance of laboratories, and data management have been established at institutional levels. Various networks have been set up at the national level to facilitate HIV vaccine development in Thailand, including a laboratory network (supported by WHO/UNAIDS), an epidemiological network, a data management network, and a national repository.

The development of HIV vaccines in Thailand has positive and negative aspects. From the negative perspective, not enough has been achieved in areas of innovative research and data analysis on the part of Thai investigators; the Thai data processing network also needs expansion. Positive features include the strengthening of the HIV laboratory in making diagnoses, and in the application of certain principles for genetic analysis of the virus, and the ability to identify HIV-1 subtypes. Thailand has received assistance from different agencies, such as the WHO/AIDS program (later evolved into an agency of UNAIDS), the U.S. Army, the U.S. NIH, the U.S. CDC, and Japanese and Australian governments. Assistance has helped to push GCP and GLP in clinical investigations, and the data processing system. Now Thailand is in a position to develop an operational framework for HIV vaccine development.

ECONOMIC AND SOCIAL IMPACT OF HIV/AIDS IN THAILAND

In Thailand, HIV/AIDS has caused incalculable human suffering and social disruption as well as huge economic costs. Though life expectancy has never inverted down as a consequence of the HIV/AIDS epidemic, Thailand's mortality rate (per 1,000 population), which had declined from 20 in 1975 to 4.1 in 1986, rebounded to 5.0 in 1997 and 5.1 in 1998 (Rumakom, 2002). The age-specific mortality rate in the labor-aged population has been increasing with HIV/AIDS now the first ranking cause of death in this group.

The HIV/AIDS epidemic, through its depletion of both life expectancy and government funds, poses a threat to economic and development trends in many countries. The World Bank has estimated a 0.4% per year decrease in GDP in the worst affected countries in Africa (Jacqueline, 2003). The extent to which the epidemic has affected Thailand's economy has not been precisely studied. Yet some data exists to help identify how much

HIV/AIDS has affected Thailand's economy during the past decade.

Economic Impact

Health Care Costs

The greatest and most visible economic impact of HIV/AIDS on Thai society has been the growing cost of medical services and health care. Even before the epidemic, the country was already struggling with several existing ill-health conditions. When the epidemic was recognized in the early 1990s, the health care system was not adequately prepared to cope with it. In a developing country with low per capita expenditure on health, like Thailand, the cost of basic HIV/AIDS care and treatment of OI, excluding ARV, can place heavy burdens on both public and private sectors. This burden can be up to 2% to 3% of GDP (Behravesh, 1993). Annual costs for basic medical care for one PLWHA range from US$ 1,000 per person, or about 25 times the government's current per capita health expenditure (United Nations Population Fund/Country Services Technical Team Bangkok, 2000). Including ARV in current treatment regimens, the total costs would be unaffordable to both public and private sectors (Prescott, 1996). Even though the price of ARV drugs has decreased from US$ 12,000 per year to below US$ 300 over the last several years, other supportive and laboratory costs have not been reduced by the same proportion.

After the HIV epidemic leveled off in the mid-1990s, the economic crisis in Asia of the late 1990s threatened further progress in reducing HIV prevalence. At the dawn of economic recovery in the new millennium, health care reform towards universal coverage has added challenges, not only in expanding coverage, but also in maintaining service quality for HIV/AIDS-related illnesses. Financial support from the Global Fund to Fight AIDS, Tuberculosis and Malaria (GFATM) has increased expectations of full coverage among PLWHA, especially after the announcement in 2003 of 100% ARV coverage, beginning in 2004, by the Minister of Health. In brief, while AIDS is steadily claiming more deaths and people are demanding comprehensive management, the Thai health system is overwhelmed with more changes than ever and too preoccupied to build the capacity of Thai society to cope with the economic impacts of HIV/AIDS.

Productivity Loss

HIV/AIDS has direct and indirect effects on labor productivity. WHO data on disease burden in 2001 showed that HIV/AIDS accounted for approximately 3% of DALY (Disability Adjusted Life Years) lost in the South-East Asian Subregion (WHO, 2000). Intermediate data for Thailand during the program review in 1995 indicated an annual 6% quality of life loss due to HIV/AIDS morbidity, probably because of the additional impact of social stigmatization and discrimination.

HIV infection reduces job opportunities but induces out-of-pocket expenditures even before the disease progresses. A prospective follow-up study among 75 people with AIDS, 75 symptomatic, and 75 asymptomatic HIV-infected people seeking care in five public hospitals in different geographic regions in Thailand in 1999, revealed that the proportion of subjects without income increased from 7.6% to 31.6% after they were diagnosed with HIV infection (Chancharoen, 2000). Annual resources utilized among asymptomatic subjects, combining direct and indirect costs, amounted to US$ 3,290, and US$ 2,510 for symptomatic or AIDS cases. When these are added together, the total resource requirement for PLWHA in Thailand this year would be US$ 3,377 billion (Chancharoen, 2000). This would be about 88 times the governmental HIV/AIDS budget. Other important indirect costs are in the form of earning losses to families and communities as a result of the premature death of young adults of working age. In the longer term, these losses will have greater economic implications.

Macro-Level Impact

Measuring any precise economic impact at the macro level requires accurate demographic projections and valid assumptions of disease burden and death toll. Simulation models in other Asian countries indicate that overall, economies would keep growing and surpass the level reached in 2000 (Rhucharoenpornpanich, 2001). For example, in China and India, simulations show that only national prevalence rates of 5% by 2025 would create a noticeable drop in GNP per active person relative to the year 2000 (Eberstadt, 2002). How these simulations would be applicable to a small country like Thailand is questionable. However, every country has an adaptive capacity to absorb and minimize macro-economic impacts, in particular from chronic problems like HIV/AIDS.

Community and Household Impact

The economic impact of HIV/AIDS on Thai society may not be noticeable at the macro or national level, but it is extremely severe at the community and family level, because of its multiplicative effects with poverty. The direct costs of HIV-related illness and death put a direct burden on the families of people infected and affected by HIV/AIDS. In Thailand, the impacts are more noticeable in the northern region, where the epidemic was explosive and went deep among people with limited access to services, such as the poor, FSW, and migrant laborers. A study in Chiang Mai in 1995 demonstrated that households with AIDS deaths had an average annual income of US$ 2,200, compared with US$ 3,370 for households with no AIDS deaths, and US$ 4,200 for households with no deaths (Pitayanon, 1997). It is also common to find families or households with more than one adult and more than one child infected. Private losses are more difficult to quantify, since the financial and material burdens of care shift from the health service system to households, including friends and relatives of the infected and affected people. Economic impacts at the family and community level have profound social impacts, in particular loss of property and lack of educational opportunities. The rapidly expanding epidemic in the northern region has not allowed families and communities time to adapt, thus resources are not well mobilized to alleviate the impact.

Social Impact

The epidemic interferes with development, while developmental factors, especially poverty and migration, fuel the epidemic. Like the economic aspect, the social impact of HIV/AIDS is more visible at the community and household levels than at the national or macro level. The social burden due to HIV/AIDS usually falls on highly vulnerable people, causing even deeper erosion of the family. While PLWHA are discriminated against socially, their family members, in particular women and children, are also affected.

Impact on Women

Like other communicable diseases, HIV/AIDS does not affect males and females at the same rate. Young men showed higher infection rates than young women in the mid-1990s (Ministry of Public Health, 1995). The male to female ratio became almost equal in the late 1990s, and reversed in some villages in the northern provinces because HIV-positive men rapidly progressed to AIDS and death (personal communication, C. Natpratan, 2003). Thai females have had higher infection rates at an earlier age than males for a combination of socioeconomic and biological reasons. While women are in greater need of care, the tendency for families to spend resources on females is less compared with their male counterparts. The rising number of female HIV infections is also a leading cause of mother-to-child HIV transmission.

Impact on Children

A quick survey in Thailand in 1998 estimated that more than 500,000 children were affected by HIV/AIDS nationwide (UNICEF, 2004). The most obvious effects came in terms of higher levels of infant and child mortality among children who had contracted HIV from their mothers. Children have comprised one of the new high-risk AIDS groups in Thailand because of the infection of women by their husbands and the subsequent infection of children during pregnancy or delivery. In 1995 around 15,000 pregnant women were infected with HIV annually. According to the natural history of HIV transmission from mother to child, approximately one-fifth of these cases would result in neo-natal infections (Shaffer, 1999). This implied that large numbers of children would survive and experience the effects of AIDS through the death or disability of their parents. A substantial number of children are likely living in families where HIV affects one or both of their parents, and an increasing number will have one or both of their parents die before they are capable of independent living.

The social impact of the HIV epidemic in term of AIDS orphans has been an issue since the beginning of 1990s. Interventions to support these orphans have been integrated into community development. On June 2, 1998, His Majesty the King expressed his concern for AIDS orphans to the public. His Majesty graciously advised support of AIDS orphans' education in order to assist them to live normal lives in their communities. This solemnly marked a strong national impulse to alleviate the social impact resulting from the HIV/AIDS epidemic. Thus, the Rachapracha Samasai Foundation, under His Majesty's patronage set up a scholarship fund for AIDS orphans in four provinces, and extended it to another five provinces before the end of 1998. Later on, the government pursued the extension of this pilot project to become government policy under the responsibility of the Ministry of Education.

In addition to the sudden loss of household savings, schooling is interrupted for children in families of HIV-positive parents; a study in Chiang Mai found this phenomenon in 15% of families surveyed (Jacqueline, 2003). With support from extended family members, these children could return to school but they were somewhat over-age for the class and thus could not attain normal educational achievement. Those who were not directly economically affected by HIV/AIDS still found it difficult to go back to school, as other school members were afraid of contracting HIV from sitting in the same class with them. Finally, when one or both parents died, they could not live a normal life.

Impact on the Elderly

The HIV/AIDS epidemic has had substantial impact on the elderly. A study published in 2000, using Thai national surveys from 1994 and 1995, estimated that 11% of the Thai population over age 50 in 1995 were likely to lose at least one adult child before their own deaths. The probability of losing an adult child is about 75% greater than if there had been no HIV/AIDS epidemic in the country. Overall, the 1–2% HIV prevalence has affected as many as 12% of older Thais. In the northern region, this figure has been as high as 20%. It was also found that nearly two-thirds of all cases of adults reported to have died of AIDS had lived with or next to a parent who was ill. Both rural and urban informants of the study reported that adult children who have left home for the cities generally move back home after becoming ill (Wachter, 2000).

It is very common for parents to become caregivers for HIV-positive persons. Caregiving always involves some monetary burden, including depletion of savings. Elderly caregivers also frequently have to return to work to generate income for their families. Thai funerals are typically elaborate events incurring unavoidable costs. Moreover, after the deaths of their adult children, older parents sometimes have to foster orphaned grandchildren. These situations can all cause a burden on the health of older people, both physically and mentally. The emotional strain may be greater if the older parents have to deal with social concerns in their community or stigma attached to having one or more HIV-positive children.

Impact on National Program Management

Coordination among governmental agencies and between governmental and non-governmental (including civil society) organizations has been enhanced since the National AIDS Committee was formed in 1991. During the first few years, the public budget was pooled in either the MOPH or the Office of the Prime Minister. Two important phenomena occurred—integration of the budget and workplan for the National AIDS Program, and allocation of a budget to support NGOs working with HIV/AIDS.

Before 1989, HIV infection was perceived as a medical issue. Later, when surveillance and behavioral data were available, HIV/AIDS became both a health and a social concern. The second and third National AIDS Plans have coincided with the National Economic and Social Development Plans (for 1994–1996 and 2000–2004). A total of 42 Departments/government units in nine Ministries have participated in developing and implementing the joint National AIDS Plans, as well as the integrated budget system. Collaboration has enhanced management of HIV/AIDS programs in Thailand.

SUCCESSES, LESSONS LEARNED, AND CHALLENGES

Two Dissociating Trends

Remarkable achievements in reducing HIV transmission through sexual contacts have been well documented (UNAIDS, 2002). The Thailand National HIV/AIDS program has prevented millions of people from getting HIV. The estimated annual number of new HIV infections of 150,000 in 1992 was reduced to 25,000 in 2002 (Thai Trial Working Group on HIV/AIDS Projection, 2001). Prevalence rates among army conscripts decreased substantially from almost 4% in 1993 to less than 2% in 1996. Similar trends were demonstrated among other groups such as pregnant women, blood donors, and FSW (Family Health International, 2001).

However, prevalence rates among IDU, MSM, and young people who do not use condoms in casual sex have been increasing. HIV sentinel surveillance data show a steady increase in HIV prevalence rates among IDU from 30% to 40% in the early 199's to 40% to 50% in the early 2000s, an average increase of 1% per year (Thailand National AIDS Committee, 1999). Behavioral surveillance data have shown an early age at first sex, around 15 years old, and a shift of first sex partner from FSW to casual partners. Condom use among young people has been around 24% in casual sex (Yuntadilok, 2002).

Unfortunately, high achievement in preventing heterosexual transmission of HIV has obscured the ability of the Thai National HIV/AIDS Program to deal with expanding HIV epidemics among IDU, MSM, and young people who engage in casual sex in Thailand. Country reports of the Thai MOPH hardly discuss HIV infection or interventions for MSM. The same phenomenon can be observed in the area of care and support of PLWHA. The focus on expanding access to ARV has distracted the NAP from building a comprehensive continuum of care, as the program has focused on medical supply and improving clinical knowledge among health workers, but not sufficiently on increased knowledge, understanding, and motivation among PLWHA. The perceived sense of success has preoccupied policymakers, and is the most significant barrier to improving the Thai National HIV/AIDS Program.

Significant Achievements

Political commitment and public support have been critical to the effectiveness of Thailand's HIV/AIDS response. This has been developed through a series of interventions such as gathering, analyzing, and disseminating epidemiological surveillance data for increased awareness of the epidemic, formulating policy alternatives, advocating through national AIDS seminars, and building partnerships. Prime Ministers who chaired the National AIDS Committee have facilitated multi-sectoral collaboration. Collaboration, initially supported by international partners evolved into sustainability by national government and non-governmental sectors.

There were three significant preconditions that allowed effective responses to occur. First, there was a sufficient number of epidemiologists in Thailand before the HIV epidemic took place. These epidemiologists have been attached to the Field Epidemiology Training Program (FETP) in MOPH and worked together at the initial phase of HIV/AIDS responses as they also received technical support from the WHO and U.S. CDC. The second precondition was a well-developed health infrastructure along with strong non-governmental partners in health. The third and most important factor was the sharp vision of MOPH, and subsequently the nation's leaders, that Thailand's HIV/AIDS situation would require the highest attention. After a few years of complacency in relation to Thailand tourism campaigns, Mr. Chuan Leekpai, the Minister of Public Health in 1989, disclosed HIV/AIDS information to the public, which created a lot of discussion in Thai society. That was followed by Prime Minister Anand Punyarachun's decision in 1991 to chair the National AIDS Committee.

Program Success

Two important achievements of the national program have been: effective implementation of the 100% Condom Use Program (CUP), which has increased condom use rate and decreased frequency of Thai men visiting FSW, and the development of an integrated national HIV/AIDS budget which has minimized duplication and optimized multisectoral coordination among government and non-government agencies.

Success of the 100% CUP has been built on two existing factors: extensive STI services and familiarity with condoms in Thai society. Well before the HIV epidemic took place, workers in STI clinics of every province in Thailand had conducted annual surveys to enumerate entertainment establishments (EE) in their catchment areas. These surveys and free STI services have provided opportunities for health staff to build relationships with EE managers/owners, resulting in high participation of EE managers/owners in the 100% CUP activities. With respect to condoms, there was almost no need to introduce condoms since many pre-existing family planning campaigns during the previous decades had introduced them already. However, additional effort was needed to build trust in the quality of the free condoms.

An integrated budget system resulted from the consolidated national HIV/AIDS policy. An innovative step in this has been the government's support of NGOs. Analysis of budget requests from both governmental and non-governmental agencies was compared against the National HIV/AIDS Strategic Plan, which helped to avoid duplication and enhance program effectiveness and synergy.

It is clear that program success and national policy are both causes and effects of each other. Supportive policy facilitated effective implementation and scaling up of the 100% CUP and integration of the budget system. Clear evidence of successful implementation of the 100% CUP and effective integrated budget system, in turn, strengthened HIV/AIDS policy.

Clinical Trials and Vaccine Research

The treatment and care component of HIV/AIDS responses in Thailand expanded rapidly in mid 1990s because of an increasing governmental budget. Financial allocation for medical services doubled every year for almost half a decade during the early 1990s (Phoolcharoen, 1998). Subsequent to provision of free AZT andmedical services were expanded to include provision of ARV, treatment of OI, and laboratory tests for CD4 and viral load. A clinical research network including capacity development of health workers involving in HIV/AIDS care has also transformed Thailand's response to the epidemic. HIV vaccine research has been developed in a parallel manner but with a greater proportion of support from international agencies. Clinical research on prevention of mother-to-child transmission was also developed and expanded in the late 1990s. These activities have increased the number not only of clinical researchers but also virologists and immunologists working in the HIV/AIDS area.

International collaboration on clinical and vaccine research has been significantly improved. The HIV-NAT (Netherlands, Australia and Thailand) program of the Thai Red Cross AIDS Research Center has coordinated and conducted clinical trials. Results from these trials have been used in guiding national policy (Kunanusont, 1999). Collaboration among local and international academic institutions has also been developed. In addition, the HIV/AIDS Collaboration, a joint program between MOPH and the U.S. CDC, has been expanded to cover more health issues under the new name, Thai MOPH-US CDC Collaboration. These factors have significantly improved HIV/AIDS clinical research capacity among Thai staff.

CHALLENGES

Keeping the Program Effective

With the support of WHO/GPA, Thailand's NAP initiated HIV sentinel surveillance in 1989 and expanded it to cover all provinces. While discussing whether nationwide coverage follows the principle of sentinel surveillance, NAP integrated HIV sentinel surveillance in MOPH routine work. Data sets obtained in the system have proven extremely effective in elucidating HIV infection trends, but not behavioral (before infection) or survival (after infection) trends. The second generation HIV surveillance system has been initiated recently, after the completion of combined HIV, STI and behavioral surveillance in neighboring countries in South-East Asia. The need to collect data on survival trends has not been sufficiently assessed. With expanding access to ARV, only highly selected groups of PLWHA are included in longitudinal studies. HIV infection trends then have little implication in guiding national policy.

Improving Prevention

As the NAPs were replicated from Thailand's STI program, interventions to prevent heterosexual transmission of HIV were disproportionate to those for IDU and MSM. An epidemiologically-oriented program obscures the role of social science, in particular anthropological approaches aiming to change high-risk behaviors of IDU, MSM and young people. Even for groups at risk of sexual transmission of HIV with additional characteristics like FSW, seafarers, or a mobile population, the current approaches of 100% CUP and public education are not sufficiently effective. Life skills education has been integrated into school curricula, but whether it has a greater or lesser influence on young people in comparison with peer pressure to experience sex or drug use is doubtful. Thailand's HIV prevention program has stagnated since the announcement of its success in 1996 at the XI International Conference on AIDS in Vancouver.

Formulating Plausible Plans for Treatment and Care

The courageous policy of "Access for All" to provide treatment to all PLWHA in Thailand by 2004 keeps the Thailand NAP at the forefront. However, the goals of this policy may be too ambitious given that there are inadequate data on the number of people needing care. The available estimates of new cases do not take into account the fact that positive therapeutic effects directly affect caseload because of the reduction in mortality.

As the health service system in Thailand has been heavily oriented toward acute illnesses and short episodes of treatment, it requires a great deal of effort to prepare for long term, chronic illness care for PLWHA. Follow up and monitoring of treatment outcomes need to be strengthened.

Even though clinical and HIV vaccine trials have been conducted for more than a decade, some Thais are still confused between approved therapeutic regimens and trials. Public knowledge and the ability of Thais to differentiate between therapeutic and research activities should be strengthened. Potential subjects should be capable of making informed decisions regarding whether to participate in clinical research or not.

A master plan for clinical research is needed. It should encompass the whole spectrum of development from clinical research question formulation, clinical research coordination and implementation, quality data management, translation from research findings to policy and identification of future research needs. The ultimate goal should be to rely on internal production of medical equipment and supplies with international quality.

Participation of primary stakeholders (primary beneficiaries, i.e., PLWHA) is fundamental to Thailand's program effectiveness and sustainability. There is a need to involve individuals infected and affected by HIV/AIDS as well as community leaders and civil society partners in planning, implementing, and assessing results. This requires a shift of orientation among health care providers, program planners, and policy makers toward client-oriented approaches.

Acknowledgements. We would like to thank Dr. Sanchai Chasombat and Dr. Cheewanan Lertpiriyasuwat , Bureau of AIDS, TB and STIs, Department of Disease Control, Ministry of Public Health for providing information on preliminary evaluation of the ARV program.

REFERENCES

Behravesh, N. (1993). Measuring the global economic impact of the AIDS epidemic (January 1993), an Insight Report from DRI/McGraw-Hill.

Bryson, Y.J. (1996). Perinatal HIV-1 transmission: Recent advances and therapeutic interventions. *AIDS.* 10 Suppl. 3:533–542.

Chamratrithirong, A., Thongthi, V., Boonchalaksi, W., Guest, P., Kanchanachitra, C., and Varangrat, A. (1999). The success of the 100% Condom Promotion Programme in Thailand: survey results of the evaluation of the 100% Condom Promotion Programme. IPSR Publication No. 238. Institute for Population and Social Research, Mahidol University, Bangkok, Thailand.

Chancharoen, K., Kunanusont, C., and Resource Utilization Group of HIV/AIDS in Thailand. (2000). Dollars and sense: cost of medical care. The XIII International Conference on AIDS, Durban, South Africa, July 2000, Session D23. (Unpublished Abstract WeOrD543).

Churdboonchart, V., Moss, R.B., Sirawarapom, W., Smutharaks, B., Sutthent, R., Jensen, F.C., Vacharak, P., Grimes, J., Theofan, G., and Carlo, D.J. (1998). Effect of HIV-Specific Immune-based Therapy in HIV-1 Positive Subjects Infected with HIV-1 Subtype E in Thailand. *J. AIDS.* 12(12):1521–1527.

Churdboonchart, V., Sakondhavat, C., Kulpradist, S., Na Ayudthya, B., Chanderying, V., Rugpao, S., Boonshuyar, C., Sukeepaisarncharoen, W., Sirawarapom, W., Carlo, D.J., and Moss, R. (2000). A double-blind, adjuvant-controlled trial of human immunodeficiency virus type 1 (HIV-1) immunogen (Remune) monotherapy in asymptomatic, HIV-1-infected Thai subjects with CD4-cell counts of >300. *Clinical and Diagnostic Laboratory Immunology.* 7(5):728–733.

Concorde Coordinating Committee. (1994). MRC/ANRS randomized double-blind controlled trial of immediate and deferred zidovudine in symptom-free HIV infection. *Lancet.* 343:871–881.

Connor, E.M., Sperling, R.S., Gelber, R., Kiselev, P., Scott, G., O'Sullivan, M.J., VanDyke, R., Bey, M., Shearer, W., Robert, L., Jimenez, J.E., O'Neil, E., Bazin, B., Delfraissy, J.F., Culnane, M., Coombs, R., Elkins, M., Moye, J., Stratton, P., Balsley, J., for The Pediatric AIDS Clinical Trials Group Protocol 076 Study Group. (1994). Reduction of maternal-infant transmission of human immunodeficiency virus type 1 with zidovudine treatment. *N Engl J Med.* 331:1173–1180.

Delta Coordinating Committee. (1996). A randomized double-blind controlled trial comparing combinations of zidovudine plus didanosine or zalcitabine with zidovudine alone in HIV-infected individuals. *Lancet.* Erratum. 348:283–291.

Eberstadt, N. (2002). The Future of AIDS. *Foreign Affairs.* November-December 2002.

Family Health International. (2001). Monitoring the AIDS pandemic: the status and trends of HIV/AIDS/STI epidemics in Asia and the Pacific, MAP Symposium, Melbourne (4 October 2001).

Falk, L.A., Goldenthal, K.L., Esparza, J., Aguado, M.T., Osmanov, S., Ballou, W.R., Beddows, S., Bhamarapravati, N., Biberfeld, G., Gerrari, G., Hoft, D., Honda, M., Jackson, A., Lu, Y., Marchal, G., McKinney, J. and Yamazaki, S. (2000). Related Articles, Recombinant bacillus Calmette-Guerin as a potential vector for preventive HIV type 1 vaccines. *AIDS Res Hum Retroviruses.* 16(2):91–98.

Fifteenth International AIDS Conference website. (2004). Available at: www.aidsthai.org. Accessed January 30, 2004.

Fischl, M.A., Richman, D.D., Grieco, M.H., Gottlieb, M.S., Volberding, P.A., Laskin, O.L., Leedom, J.M., Groopman, J.E., Mildvan, D., Schooley, R.T., Jackson, G.G., Durack, D.T., Phil, D., King, D., and the AZT Collaborative working group. (1987). The efficacy of azidothymidine (AZT) in the treatment of patients with AIDS and AIDS-related complex. A double-blind, placebo-controlled trial. *N Engl J Med.* 317:185–191.

Fischl, M.A., Stanley, K., Collier, A.C., Arduino, J.M., Stein, D.S., Feinberg, J.E., Allan J.D., Goldsmith, J.C., and Powderly, W.G., The NIAID AIDS Clinical Trials Group. (1995). Combination and monotherapy with zidovudine and zalcitabine in patients with advanced HIV disease. *Ann Intern Med.* 122:24–32.

Hammer, S.M., Squires, K.E., Hughes, M.D., Grimes, J.M., Demeter, L.M., Currier, J.S., Eron, J.J. J.r., Feinberg, J.E., Balfour, H.H. J.r., Deyton, L.R., Chodakewitz, J.A., and Fischl, M.A., AIDS Clinical Trials Group 320 Study Team. (1997). A controlled trial of two nucleoside analogues plus indinavir in persons with Human Immunodeficiency Virus infection and CD4 cells counts of 200 per cubic millimeter or less. *N Engl J Med.* 337:725–733.

Jacqueline, P. (2003). Child Rights and the Media. In: Conference report of IFJ Asia Regional Workshop; June 24–25. Bangkok, Thailand.

Kanshana, S., Thewanda, D., Teeraratkul, A., Limpakarnjanarat, K., Amornwichet, P., Kullerk, N., Akksilp, S., Sereesittipitak, V., Mastro, T.D., and Simonds, R.J. (2000). Implementing short-course zidovudine to reduce mother-infant HIV transmission in a large pilot program in Thailand. *AIDS.* 14:1617–1623.

Keiser, P., Nassar, N., Kvanli, M.B., Turner, D., Smith, J.W., and Skiest, D. (2001). Long-term impact of highly active antiretroviral therapy on HIV-related health care costs. *Acquir Immun Defic Syndr.* 27:14–19.

Kunanusont C. (1999). Report of the International Conference on HIV Vaccine Development, Thailand, March 15–19, 1999.

Lallemant, M., Jourdain, G., Le Coeur S., Kim, S., Koetsawang, S., Comeau, A.M., Phoolcharoen, W., Essex, M., McIntosh, K., Ithayasai, V., and the Perinatal HIV Prevention Trial (Thailand) Investigators. (2000). A trial of shortened zidovudine regimens to prevent mother-to-child transmission of human immunodeficiency virus type 1. *N Engl J Med.* 343:982–991.

Ministry of Public Health, Thailand (1995). Division of Epidemiology. Epidemiological Surveillance Reports.

Ministry of Public Health, Thailand. (2002). National guidelines for the clinical management of HIV infection in children and adults. 7th ed. Bangkok: Ministry of Public Health, pp.158–163.

Myers, C. and Ashakul, T. (1991). AIDS in Thailand: Some Preliminary Findings. *TDRI Quarterly Review.* 6(1): 8–11.

Palella, F.J. J.r., Delaney, K.M., Moorman, A.C., Loveless, M.O., Fuhrer, J., Satten, G.A., Aschman, D.J., and Holmberg, S.D. (1998). Declining morbidity and mortality among patients with advanced Human Immunodeficiency Virus Infection. *N Engl J Med.* 338:853–860.

Phanuphak, P., Teeratakulpixarn, S., Sarangbin, S., Nookhai, S., Ubolyam, S., Sirivichayakul, S., Leesavan, A., Forrest, B.D., Hanson, C.V., Li M, Wang, C.Y., and Koff, W.C. (1997). Phase I Trial of an HIV-1 synthetic peptide vaccine in Bangkok, Thailand. *Asian Pac J Allergy Immunol.* 15:41–48.

Phoolcharoen, W., Ungchusak, K., Sittritrai, W., and Brown, T. (1998). Thailand: Lessons from a strong national response to HIV/AIDS. *AIDS* 12(SupplB):S123–S135.

Phoolcharoen, W. (1998). Experience from Thailand, Partners in Prevention: International case studies of effective health promotion practice in HIV/AIDS. UNAIDS Best Practice Collection: Joint United Nations Programme on HIV/AIDS.

Pitayanon, S., Kongsin, S., Janjaroen, W.S. (1997). The Economic Impact of HIV/AIDS Mortality on Households in Thailand. In Bloom, D. and Godwin, P. (eds), *The Economics of HIV and AIDS: The Case of South and South-East Asia.* Delhi, Oxford University.

Pitisuttithum, P., Phonrat, B., Suntharasamai, P., Raktham, S., Srisuwanvilai, L., Kitayaporn, D., Kaewkangwal, J., Migasena, S., Chernow, M.,

Berman, P., and Francis, D. (2000). Initial Report of a phase I/II Safety and Immunogenicity trial of AIDSVAX® B/E rgp120 HIV Vaccine-Bangkok, Thailand. The XII International AIDS Conference. June 9–14. Durban, South Africa. (Unpublished Abstract).

Pitisuttithum, P., and The Bangkok Vaccine Evaluation Group. (2001). Thailand's Success in Moving to the First Phase III HIV Vaccine Efficacy Trial in a Developing Country (Abstract). AIDS VACCINE 2001, Philadelphia , USA. September 5–8, 2001. p.144.

Prescott, N., Kunanusont, C., Phoolcharoen, W., Rojanapithayakorn, W., Perriens, J., and Boonyuen, D. (1996). Formulating Rational Use of Antiretrovirals in Thailand. 11th International Conference on AIDS, July 7–12 1996. Vancouver, Canada. (Unpublished Abstract MoB 533).

Rerks-Ngarm, S., Pitisuttithum, P., Kitayaporn, D., Gurunathan, S., Heyward, W., and Brown, A. (2002). Joint Thai-US phase III trial of HIV prime boot vaccines. The XIV International AIDS Conference; (July 7–12, 2002); Barcelona, Spain. (Unpublished Abstract).

Rhucharoenpornpanich, O., and Chamratrithirong, A. (2001). Demographic impact of AIDS on the Thai population. *Asia-Pacific Population Journal.* 16(3):71–88.

Rumakom, P., Prasartful, P., Guest, P., Thongthai, V., and Punpuing, S. (2002). Change to the epidemiological transition in Thailand due to HIV/AIDS: Implications for population and health policy. Paper presented at the 2002 IUSSP Regional Population Conference, Bangkok, (June 10–12, 2002)

Saravolatz, L.D., Winslow, D.L., Collins, G., Hodges, J.S., Pettinelli, C., Stein, D.S., Markowitz, N., Reves, R., Loveless, M.O., Crane, L., Thompson, M., and Abrams, D.(1996). Zidovudine alone or in combination with didanosine or zalcitabine in HIV-infected patients with the Acquired Immunodeficiency Syndrome or fewer than 200 CD4 cells per cubic millimeter. *N Engl J Med.* 335:1099–1106.

Schechter, M. (2002). Universal access to antiretroviral therapy: the Brazilian experience. Powerpoint presentation available at: http://hivinsite.ucsf.edu/InSite.jsp?page=md-rr-06. Accessed January 30, 2004.

Shaffer, N., Chuachoowong, R., Mock, P.A., Bhadrakom, C., Siriwasin, W., Young, N.L., Chotpitayasunondh, T., Chearskul, S., Roongpisuthipong, A., Chinayon, P., Karon, J., Mastro, T.D., Simonds, R.J. and the Bangkok Collaborative Perinatal HIV Transmission Study Group. (1999). Short-course zidovudine for perinatal HIV-1 transmission in Bangkok, Thailand: A randomised controlled trial. *Lancet.* 353:773–780.

Sittitrai, W., Wongsukol, N., Phanuphak, P., and Brown, T. (1992). Female Sexual Behavior: A report on the 1990 Survey of Partner Relations and Risk of HIV Infection in Thailand, Thai Red Cross Society Program on AIDS, Research Report.

The Thai Trial Working Group on HIV/AIDS Projection. (2001). Projections for HIV/AIDS in Thailand: 2000–2020, Karnsana Printing Press, Bangkok.

Thailand Department of Disease Control. (2001). Guidelines for management and monitoring system for provision of HAART in the upper north of Thailand, Disease Control Region 10.

Thailand National AIDS Committee. (1999). Epidemic Status Report.

Thisayakorn, U., Ruxrungtham, K., and Phanuphak, P. (1998). Risk reduction of HIV–1 vertical transmission: Progress and implementation in Thailand. *HIV & AIDS Current Trends.* 4:1–3.

UNAIDS. (2000). Ethical considerations in HIV-1 preventive vaccine trials. Geneva, Switzerland.

UNAIDS. (2002). Thailand Epidemiological Fact Sheets on HIV/AIDS and Sexually Transmitted Infections, Geneva.

United Nations Children's Fund (UNICEF) website. (2004). The Mekong Partnership & Beyond. UNICEF and HIV/AIDS in East Asia and the Pacific. Available at: http://www.unicef.org/eapro-hivaids/home.htm. Accessed: January 30, 2004.

United Nations Population Fund/Country Services Technical Team (UNFPA/CST) Bangkok. (2000). HIV/AIDS and STDs: Causes, Consequences and Preventive Programmes. Occasional Paper Series No. 8. Bangkok, Thailand.

United States Public Health Service. (2000). Task Force recommendations for the use of antiretroviral drugs in pregnant women infected with HIV-1 for maternal health and for reducing perinatal HIV-1 transmission in the United States. *HIV Clin Trials.* 1:39–64.

Vanhove, G.F., Schapiro, J.M., Winters, M.A., Mcrigan, T.C., and Blaschke, T.F. (1996). Patient compliance and drug failure in protease inhibitor monotherapy. *JAMA.* 276:19956.

Vaxgen. (2003). VaxGen Announces Initial Results of its Phase III AIDS Vaccine Trial.Press release available at: http://www.vaxgen.com/pressroom/index.html. Accessed January 30, 2004.

Volberding, P.A., Lagakos, S.W., Koch, M.A., Pettinelli, C., Myers, M.W., Booth, D.K., Balfour, H.H. Jr., Reichman, R.C., Bartlett, J.A., Hirsch, M.S., et al. (1990). Zidovudine in asymptomatic human immunodeficiency virus infection. A controlled trial in persons with fewer than 500 CD4-positive cells per cubic millimeter. The AIDS Clinical Trials Group of the National Institute of Allergy and Infectious Diseases. *N Engl J Med.* 322:941–949.

Volberding, P.A., Lagakos, S.W., Koch, M.A., Pettinelli, C., Myers, M.W., Booth, D.K., Balfour, H.H. Jr., Reichman, R.C., Bartlett, J.A., Hirsch, M.S., Murphy, R.L., Hardy, W.D., Wachter, K.W., Knodel, J.E.,

VanLandingham, M. (2000). AIDS and the Elderly of Thailand: Projecting Familial Impacts. Report No. 00–446. Population Studies Center, Institute for Social Research, University of Michigan.

Wachter, K., Knodel, J., and Vanlandingham, M. (2000). AIDS and the elderly of Thailand: protecting familial impacts. PSC Research Report 00–446, May 2000.

World Health Organization. (2000). The World Health Report 2002: Reducing Risks, Promoting Healthy Life.

Yuntadilok, N. (2002). Keys of effective responses for HIV/AIDS prevention at the border areas (Thai-Myanmar). International AIDS Conference, July 12–14; Barcelona, Spain. Abstract ThPeD-7609.

2

History of HIV in India

Srikanth P. Tripathy

National AIDS Research Institute, Pune, India

HISTORY OF INFECTIOUS DISEASES IN INDIA

Communicable diseases have been major public health problems in India for centuries. As the population increased, morbidity and mortality due to infectious diseases assumed sizable and noticeable proportions. In the first half of the early part of the 20th century, the approach to their management and control was through public health. There have been outbreaks of infectious diseases like cholera, plague, Japanese encephalitis, Dengue fever, jaundice due to Hepatitis viruses, filariasis, malaria, and typhoid. Tuberculosis and leprosy had been endemic in many parts of India. However, there was a good infrastructure for health services, which included personnel from the army medical services, medical college staff, public health staff and some research organizations. There were appropriate control programs for each of the major communicable diseases. Realizing the importance of research, the Indian Research Fund Association was established in 1911, which formed the seed for the current research body, the Indian Council of Medical Research (ICMR). The inputs of this body helped to a considerable extent in the formulation of appropriate control measures for infectious diseases.

Large portions of the resources for medical research were earmarked for research in communicable disease. Plague, cholera and smallpox are good examples of control programs resulting in virtual elimination of the deaths due to these diseases, which had taken heavy toll of human life in earlier years. Morbidity due filariasis has been reduced considerably. Vector control measures against malaria have substantially reduced not only the prevalence of malaria but also that of Kala-azar. Tuberculosis morbidity and mortality have seen a considerable decline through formulation of a national program and through conducting research on epidemiology and chemotherapy of tuberculosis. Indeed, research in India has provided the basis for creating principles of chemotherapy for tuberculosis. This has led to the establishment of National Tuberculosis Programs based on the application of appropriate treatment regimens. India's contribution to the formulation of the Directly Observed Treatment Short-course (DOTS) strategy currently employed by most countries in the world has been substantial. With the strong research background in India, it was possible to immediately establish a network of research units all over the country to tackle the newly emerging threat of the HIV epidemic in 1986.

HISTORY OF HIV INFECTION IN INDIA

It has been 17 years since the first few cases of HIV and AIDS were detected in India. Prior to April 1986, the few HIV positive cases detected in India were among Indians who had contracted the infection abroad or among foreigners who were tourists or were residing in India temporarily. Indeed, most Indians believed that HIV/AIDS was unlikely to be a major problem in India. The first report on indigenously infected HIV positive persons was among commercial sex workers in the state of Tamil Nadu (South India) in 1986 (Simoes *et al.*, 1987). Subsequently, the first clinical case of AIDS in India was reported in 1986 from Mumbai (Lele *et al.*, 1986). Realizing that HIV infection may become a major problem in India, the Indian Council of Medical Research in collaboration with the Directorate General of Health Services and the State Health Authorities initiated a national surveillance for HIV infection in 1986 (ICMR, 1991). Initial studies revealed that commercial sex workers, hemophiliacs, STD clinic patients and professional blood donors were the main groups that were infected with the HIV virus (John *et al.*, 1987; Singh *et al.*, 1991; Banerjee *et al.*, 1989). Blood products were found to be contaminated with HIV (Tripathy *et al.*, 1991). Later, hemophiliacs were found to be infected with HIV (Singh *et al.*, 1991). In 1991, an explosive outbreak of HIV-1 seropositivity was reported among intravenous drug users in the state of Manipur in the northeastern part of India (Naik *et al.*, 1991).

HIV AND AIDS CASES REPORTED IN INDIA

From 1986 to July 1993, a total of 444 cases of AIDS were documented. Of these, 269 cases were documented from the states of Tamil Nadu in the south and Maharashtra in the west (NACO, 1993). At that point in time, it was estimated that the numbers reported represented only a small fraction of the actual number of HIV/AIDS cases in India, due to underreporting, and that the actual number of HIV-infected individuals in India was probably about 400,000 to 1,000,000. Of these, 50,000 to 75,000 were expected to develop AIDS by 1995 (ICMR, 1991; NACO, 1993). By the end of July 1992, 1.5 million individuals had been screened and 12,519 were found to be HIV seropositive; these cumulative figures for HIV seropositives increased to 22,529 by March 1996, and 67,067 by September 1997; at the latter time point, 4980 AIDS cases had been reported (data obtained from the National AIDS Control Organization, Ministry of Health and Family Welfare, Government of India).

The risk factors for transmission of HIV were reported by several investigators (Tripathy *et al.*, 1992; John *et al.*, 1993; Satpathy and Shaukat, 1997); they identified heterosexual transmission as the major risk factor accounting for over 75% of the infections. Until 30th September 2003, a total of 55,764 AIDS cases had been officially reported to NACO. Of these, 85% had been infected through heterosexual sex, 2.7% by blood and blood products, 2.7% through perinatal transmission, 2.4% through intravenous drug use, and in the remaining 7%, the risk factor was not known. From the above data, it is evident that only a fraction of the total number of people living with HIV/AIDS (PLWHA) were aware of their status. Most of the AIDS cases had been detected in advanced stages, and the patients did not survive beyond a year from diagnosis.

HIV Infection in STD Clinics

Since the presence of sexually transmitted diseases is a major risk factor for transmission of HIV, STD clinics have been the focus of studies on the prevalence of HIV in different parts of India. Since 1986, there has been an increase in the HIV seroprevalence in female commercial sex workers and patients attending sexually transmitted diseases clinics in India (Bollinger *et al.*, 1995).

The prevalence of HIV in STD clinic attendees has been investigated extensively in Pune city in Maharashtra state. By 1992, the prevalence of HIV among patients attending STD clinics in Pune was 10% (Tripathy *et al.*, 1993) and reached 23% by 1995 (Rodrigues *et al.*, 1995). A finding of high HIV prevalence (13%) in married monogamous women attending STD clinics in Pune for treatment of STDs (Rodrigues *et al.*, 1995; Gangakhedkar *et al.*, 1997) indicated that the HIV infection had also affected the low risk population as well. Screening of 5321 individuals between May 1993 and October 1995 from two STD clinics in Pune indicated that the overall HIV-1 prevalence was 21.2% (Mehendale *et al.*, 1996 b).

In the Vellore region of South India, only nine of 2215 STD patients investigated during 1986–88 were found positive for HIV antibodies, showing a seroprevalence of 0.4% (Mathai *et al.*, 1990). Subsequent data showed that the HIV seroprevalence in STD patients in Vellore increased from 0.26% in 1986 to 2.64 in 1993 (Jacob *et al.*, 1995). In a study carried out in New Delhi in northern India during the period from 1990 to 1992, the HIV seropositivity was 1.3% with syphilis, 1.0% with chancroid, 0.3% with genital herpes, 0.2% with Donovanosis and 0.3% with lymphogranuloma venereum. For non-ulcerative genital ulcer disease, the HIV seroprevalence was 1.3% with gonorrhea, 1.4% with trichomonas infection, 0.4% with genital warts and 0.3% with non-gonococcal urethritis (Ray *et al.*, 1995).

HIV Infection in FSW

In Pune, the marked increase in HIV seropositivity in STD clinic patients has been associated with a rise in HIV seropositivity in sex workers. Of 424 female sex workers (FSW) attending STD clinic in Pune during the period between May 1993 and October 1995, the HIV seroprevalence was found to be 47.4% (Mehendale *et al.*, 1996b). A similar rise in HIV seropositivity has been shown among sex workers in Mumbai, where the seroprevalence increased from 2% in 1988 to 30% in 1990 and 40% in 1991 (Indian Council of Medical Research, 1991).

In the state of Tamil Nadu in South India until February 1986, ten out of 102 (9.8%) sex workers screened in Chennai were found to be HIV seropositive; in the same year, the HIV seroprevalence among sex workers in other cities was 3.3% in Madurai, 1.8% in Vellore and 0% in Coimbatore and Salem. In Vellore, the HIV seroprevalence in sex workers increased from 1.8% in 1986 to 28.6% in 1990 (Simoes *et al.*, 1990).

HIV Infection Related to Blood Transfusion and Blood Products Administration

Blood transfusion has been a source of HIV infection in a limited number of cases in India. Steps have been taken to minimize the risk of transfusion-associated HIV-infection by screening all donated blood. Routine screening of donors indicated that the proportion of HIV-positive among them was increasing over the years. HIV seropositivity in blood donors in Pune increased from 0% in 1986 to 0.17% in 1990 (Wadia and Karve, 1992). Higher HIV seropositivity has been noted in professional remunerated blood donors in comparison with voluntary donors (Singh *et al.*, 1990) and hence, guidelines were introduced for blood banks to avoid the collection of blood from professional blood donors.

In some parts of India, thalassemic children have been found to be at high risk for HIV infection (Khan, 1992; De *et al.*, 1990). In Delhi, out of 203 thalassemic and multiply transfused children screened for HIV antibodies, 18 (8.9%) were found be HIV seropositive and six of them had clinical features of AIDS

TABLE 1. HIV Serosurveillance in STD Patients in Pune (1991–1996)

Year	Period	No. Tested	Positive No.	(%)	No. HIV-1	No. HIV-2	No. HIV 1&2
1991	Nov–Dec	273	26	(9.5)	22	3	1
1992	May–Jun	351	62	(17.7)	58	4	0
	Nov–Dec	285	58	(20.4)	56	1	1
1993	May–Jun	248	55	(22.2)	53	1	1
	Nov–Dec	190	34	(17.9)	31	1	2
1994	May–Jun	188	48	(25.5)	47	0	1
	Nov–Dec	128	26	(20.3)	26	0	0
1995	May–Jun	208	47	(22.6)	45	1	1
	Nov–Dec	208	54	(26.0)	54	0	0
1996	May–Jun	241	52	(21.6)	52	0	0
	Nov–Dec	171	26	(15.2)	26	0	0
	Total	2491	488	(19.6)	470	11	7

Source: Mehendale *et al.*, 1996

according to the WHO criteria (Sen *et al.*, 1993).

HIV Infection in Injecting Drug Users (IDU)

In the state of Manipur in India, the prevalence of HIV in IDU had increased from 0% to 50% in a period less than six months to reach 89% in 1994 (Sarkar *et al.*, 1991; Sarkar *et al.*, 1995). Injecting drug use has been a problem for the youth of Manipur since this state is located on the border of the Golden Triangle, which consists of Myanmar, Laos and Thailand. More than 20% of the world's opium is grown here and processed to obtain heroin. Between July 1986 and September 1989, a total of 2322 IDU had been screened for HIV and none were found to be HIV seropositive. However, between October 1989 to June 1990, of 1412 IDU screened, 765 (54.2%) were found to be seropositive for HIV antibodies. Over 70% of the IDU were in the 20 to 29 age group and 96.7% of the IDU were male (Naik *et al.*, 1991). Initial studies had shown that 90% of IDU shared needles (Sarkar *et al.*, 1991) and this had reduced to 70% by 1995 (Sarkar *et al.*, 1995).

Subsequent studies have shown that most of the HIV transmission through injection drug use occurs in the northeastern states of Manipur, Nagaland and Mizoram.

HIV-2 Seroprevalence

Most of the virus strains in India are HIV-1, and the prevalence of HIV-2 is low. The presence of HIV-2 infection has been reported from Mumbai and Pune in India (Kulkarni *et al.*, 1992; Rubsamen-Waigmann *et al.*, 1991; Pfutzner *et al.*, 1992). Data from studies ongoing at Pune indicate that HIV-2 seroprevalence in Pune has not increased during 1991–96 (Table 1). Out of 5668 STD patients screened from 1993–1995, 1180 (20.8%) were HIV seropositive. Of these 1180 seropositive individuals, 95% were HIV-1 seropositive, 1.7% were HIV-2 seropositive and 3.3% were dually reactive to both HIV-1 and HIV-2 antibodies (Mehendale *et al.*, 1996a). The annual breakdown of the sentinel surveillance data in Pune from 1991 to 1996 is given in Table 1 and indicates that HIV-2 seroprevalence in the STD clinic population in Pune has remained low. However, there was a marked increase in HIV-1 seroprevalence in the STD clinic population from 1991 to 1992.

Studies done in Mumbai showed a higher HIV-2 seroprevalence (4.5 to 4.8%) as well as a much higher seroprevalence of dual reactive samples (17.5 to 25%) in the STD clinic patients (Hira *et al.*, 1996; Zhang *et al.*, 1996). Apart from Pune and Mumbai, HIV-2 infection has also been detected in Goa in the western part of India (Rubsamen-Waigmann *et al.*, 1994) and in South India (Solomon and Ganapathy, 1991; Babu *et al.*, 1993).

HIV Incidence

For the first time in India, HIV incidence studies done in the STD seronegative cohort in Pune (HIVNET Study) between 1993 and 1995 (Mehendale *et al.*, 1995) showed the overall incidence rates to be 10.2/100 person-years (9.39/100 person-years in men and 14.07/100 person-years in women). The incidence among FSW during the same period in Pune was 26.1/100 person-years.

NATIONAL AIDS CONTROL ORGANIZATION (NACO)

The National AIDS Control Organization (NACO) was established in 1992 by the Ministry of Health and Family Welfare to manage HIV/AIDS program activities; Phase I of the National AIDS Control Program was implemented between 1992 and 1999 with an $84 million loan from the World Bank. NACO collaborated with many agencies like the UN (United Nations), WHO (World Health Organization), DFID (UK Department for International Development) and USAID (U.S. Agency for International Development), which provided financial and technical support at the state level. The various components of Phase I of the NACO program were information, education and communication (IEC), social mobilization, HIV surveillance, increased blood safety, condom promotion, clinical management, treatment, care and support of HIV infected individuals, strengthening of the control of sexually transmitted diseases (STD), and monitoring the development of the HIV/AIDS epidemic in the country. Surveillance capacity was developed in 62 centers and 180 sentinel sites nationwide in India. Decentralization of the HIV control activities and setting up of State AIDS cells in all the states and union territories of India was done to help the States to carry out efforts for HIV prevention and care.

Phase II of the National AIDS Control Program started on 9th November 1999. This scheme is sponsored by the Central Government in India and is implemented through the State AIDS Control Societies in India. Phase II of the National AIDS Control Program is aimed at changing risk behavior patterns through interventions, supporting decentralization of HIV-related service delivery to the states and municipalities, protecting human rights by encouraging voluntary counseling and testing and discouraging mandatory testing, supporting structured and evidence-based annual reviews and ongoing operational research, and encouraging management reforms, such as better managed state level AIDS Control Societies and improved drug and equipment procurement practices.

The objectives of the National AIDS Control Project are to reduce the spread of HIV infection and to strengthen India's capacity to respond to HIV/AIDS on a long-term basis.

Financial Resources for Phase II of the National AIDS Control Program in India

In addition to the funds provided by the Government of India, funding from International Agencies for Phase II of the National AIDS Control Program include the following:

- International Development Agency (IDA): World Bank has provided an assistance of US $ 229.8 million (Rs. 11550.00 million) of which $191 million is a soft loan for the project and the domestic budgetary support is US $ 38.8 million.
- United States Agency for International Development (USAID) has extended its assistance to the Govt. of Maharashtra for implementation of 'AVERT' Project. The funding from USAID for the 'AVERT' project is Rs. 1660 million.
- Department For International Development (DFID) of the UK is supporting

implementation of Sexual Health Projects in the States of Andhra Pradesh, Gujarat, Kerala and Orissa. The funding for this project is Rs. 1040 million.

NACO Approach to AIDS Control

Since its inception in 1992, NACO has established control measures in India in a phased manner, concentrating in initial stages in states with high HIV prevalence and expanding the program to cover the entire country. The program is flexible, dynamic and is evolving continuously, incorporating modifications based on new research findings and success stories within the country and outside. The program has been an unqualified success as seen from the low magnitude of increase in the prevalence of HIV over successive years.

NACO has established a State AIDS Society in each state. The states in turn have established a district AIDS Control Society in every district. International agencies such as WHO, UNAIDS, DFID and others, as well as many international and national non-government organizations have been partners in the development and execution of the program. The states of Maharashtra and Tamil Nadu have been in the forefront in undertaking anti-HIV/AIDS efforts. The control measures are backed by appropriate operational as well as basic and clinical research. The National AIDS Research Institute, located in Pune in Maharashtra state, is an institute under the Indian Council of Medical Research. The Institute works in close collaboration with the National AIDS Control Organization and assists the latter in evaluating the implementation of some components of the program and in planning new approaches.

Core Activities

Most efforts were directed at prevention of transmission of HIV. Since most of the transmission was heterosexual, the program stressed health education of the community and the high risk behavior/core transmitter groups to increase awareness and to educate them on modes of transmission. The program included targeted interventions to bring about behaviour changes, condom promotion, provision of quality STD care to the targeted groups and to provide information to PLWHA to standardize management of opportunistic infections and other complications.

Prevention of Mother-to-Child Transmission of HIV

The risk of transmission of HIV from mother to child can be drastically reduced through the detection of HIV-infected pregnant women in ANC clinics and treating them with a single dose of nevirapine during childbirth. This policy was adopted by NACO after conducting feasibility studies in selected ANC clinics. As a policy, nevirapine is offered free of cost to pregnant HIV-positive women as a part of the MTCT program.

Prevention of HIV among IDU

NGOs supported by NACO and some international agencies have attempted to promote the concepts of use of clean syringes and non-sharing of needles and syringes by intravenous drug users by providing clean syringes in exchange for used ones.

Blood Safety

Prevention of transmission through blood and blood products has been achieved by improving blood banks and ensuring safety of blood products through testing of blood donors for HIV, hepatitis viruses, syphilis and malaria.

Antiretroviral Therapy (ART)

So far, drugs required for ART have been beyond the reach of most PLWHA because of their cost. Beginning April 1, 2004, PLWHA who qualify for treatment with ART will be able to access ART through the 3 by 5 Initiative (see below).

Anti-HIV Vaccine

As yet, there is no available vaccine against HIV. Several candidate vaccines are under development and are undergoing trials in many developing and technically advanced countries. Realizing that the efficacy of a vaccine may be influenced by the subtype of the infecting strain and that most HIV strains prevalent in India belong to Clade C, Indian scientists, in partnership with the International AIDS Vaccine Initiative, have developed a candidate HIV vaccine, using an Indian HIV Clade C strain. The vaccine will be undergoing Phase 1 Clinical Trials in the near future.

Sentinel Surveillance for HIV Infection

NACO has established HIV sentinel surveillance throughout the country for obtaining estimates of HIV prevalence in India. HIV sentinel surveillance was conducted in 320 sites in all the States and Union Territories in India during August–October 2001 and in August–November 2002 in 384 sentinel sites; the sites included 200 antenatal clinics (ANC), (reflecting the prevalence in the general population) and the remaining 184 sites targeted in high risk groups—166 STD clinics, 13 sites for IDU, three for men who have sex with men and two for FSW. A table indicating HIV prevalence by state in various risk groups during 2002 and its comparison since 1998 is available at the NACO website at www.naco.nic.in. (NACO, 2003).

Based on the findings, eight states (Andhra Pradesh, Karnataka, Maharashtra, Manipur, Mizoram, Tamil Nadu, Nagaland and Goa) have been identified as having high HIV prevalence (over 1% in ANC cases) and one state (Rajasthan) with moderately high prevalence (less than 1% in ANC cases but 5% or more in STD and other high risk groups) (Table 2). The remaining states had low HIV prevalence (less than 1% in ANC cases and less than 5% in high risk groups).

HIV Estimates for India

Based on the HIV sentinel surveillance data from the general population and the risk groups surveyed in the different parts of the country, the number of HIV infections is estimated at the national level. The HIV estimates among adults (15–49 year group) for the years 1998, 1999, 2000, 2001 and 2002 were 3.5 million, 3.7 million, 3.86 million, 3.97 million and 4.58 million respectively (Table 3).

Between 2001 and 2002, there was an increase of about 0.6 million infections. This increase has been due to an increase in HIV seroprevalence in ANC clinics in the States of Karnataka, Rajasthan and West Bengal, while in certain other States like that of Andhra Pradesh, Tamil Nadu, Gujarat, Bihar, Madhya Pradesh and Rajasthan, the increase has been noticed in STD clinic sites (NACO, 2003). India continues to be in the category of low HIV prevalence countries, with overall HIV prevalence of less than 1% in the general population. However, due to the large population of over one billion population in India, the overall number of HIV-infected individuals is large.

The distribution of PLWHA in the country is uneven. Many states have low prevalence of HIV. Even in the eight states with high HIV prevalence, only some districts in each state have high prevalence (Table 4). Thus, only about 49 districts out of a total of 158 in the eight states have high prevalence of HIV. Even so, in each of these eight states, the entire state has been targeted for intensive AIDS control activities in addition to the basic package of control measures under the National AIDS Control Program.

Impact of the Program on HIV Transmission

There has been no direct assessment of the impact, but there are indications that the

TABLE 2. States With High or Moderate Levels of HIV Prevalence[a]

S. No	Name of State/UT	Number of sites in 2002	HIV Prev. 1998 (%) (180 sites)	HIV Prev. 1999 (%) (180 sites)	HIV Prev. 2000 (%) (232 sites)	HIV Prev. 2001 (%) (320 sites)	HIV Prev. 2002 (%) (384 sites)
1.	Andhra Pradesh	STI 8	24.90	29.50	30.00	26.60	30.40
		ANC 14	2.25	2.60	2.00	1.50	1.25
2.	Goa	STI 2	19.40	13.50	12.02	15.00	11.29
		ANC 2	1.20	0.80	1.17	0.50	1.38
		FSW 1			53.20	50.79	24.00
3.	Karnataka	STI 7	16.70	15.50	12.80	16.40	13.60
		ANC 10	1.75	1.00	1.68	1.13	1.75
		IDU 1	—	1.30	4.23	2.00	2.26
4a.	Maharashtra	STI 9	16.00	20.00	18.40	9.20	7.60
		ANC 14	2.00	2.10	1.12	1.38	1.25
4b.	Mumbai	STI 3			33.33	21.06	14.84
		ANC 6			2.00	2.25	0.75
		IDU 1			23.68	41.37	39.42
		MSM 1			23.94	23.60	16.80
		FSW 1			58.67	52.26	54.50
5.	Manipur	STI 2	4.15	12.00	11.60	10.50	9.60
		ANC 10	0.75	2.30	0.75	1.75	1.12
		IDU 3	70.70	48.80	64.34	56.26	39.06
6.	Mizoram	STI 2	1.49	0.76	2.00	2.20	2.60
		ANC 3	0.48	0.48	0.37	0.33	1.50
		IDU 1	1.00	1.50	9.61	2.00	1.60
7.	Nagaland	STI1	11.10	4.40	6.90	7.40	2.42
		ANC4	0.70	1.30	1.35	1.25	1.25
		IDU 3	13.20	7.60	7.03	5.50	10.28
8.	Rajasthan	STI 7	5.20	3.20	2.84	4.00	6.00
		ANC 6	0.00	0.30	0.25	0.00	0.50
9.	Tamil Nadu	STI 11	16.30	10.40	16.80	12.60	14.7
		ANC 10	1.00	1.00	1.00	1.13	0.88
		IDU 1			26.70	24.56	33.80
		MSM 2			4.00	2.40	2.40

Source: Website of the National AIDS Control Organization (India) at www.naco.nic.in

[a] HIV prevalence: High (1% or more in ANC group): 8 states; moderate (less than 1% in ANC but 5% or more in STI): 1 state; low (less than 1% in ANC, less than 5% in STI): remaining 27 states (data not shown).

TABLE 3. Estimates of HIV Infection in India

Year	Estimated HIV Positives (in Millions)[a]
1998	3.47
1998	3.68
2000	3.86
2001	3.97
2002	4.58

Source: Website of National AIDS Control Organization at www.naco.nic.in (2003)

[a] Estimates have been made on the basis of sentinel surveillance in the general public and in risk groups.

program has contributed to reduced levels of transmission in the community. Data from sentinel surveillance of HIV among pregnant women attending ANC clinics in the high prevalent states of Maharashtra and Tamil Nadu have shown a flattening of the trend in HIV prevalence in antenatal women.

There is evidence of behavioural change among the core transmitter groups. The AIDS Prevention and Control (APAC) Project in Tamil Nadu has conducted seven rounds of behaviour surveillance surveys (BSS). Their findings are highly encouraging. Condom use among FSW increased from 56% in 1996 to

TABLE 4. Number of Districts With High Prevalence of HIV Among STD, IDU and ANC Attendees: Statewide 2001

S.No	Name of State/UT	Total Districts	# with High Prevalence
1.	Andhra Pradesh	23	7
2.	Goa	2	1
3.	Gujarat	25	3
4.	Karnataka	27	10
5.	Maharashtra	35	14
6.	Manipur	9	4
7.	Nagaland	8	3
8.	Tamil Nadu	29	7
	Total	158	49

Source: Website of National AIDS Control Organization at www.naco.nic.in

88% in 2002. In the same period, condom use during paid sex among transport workers increased from 55% to 92%.

The national estimates of HIV prevalence over successive years have shown only marginal increases each year, indicating that the program has been able to contain the epidemic in six high prevalence states and has prevented any large scale spread to the rest of India.

3 BY 5 INITIATIVE

The 3 by 5 Initiative is a global effort aimed at providing access to antiretroviral therapy to the six million HIV infected persons in the developing world who need the drugs, while currently only about 400,000 of them have this access. Recognizing the urgency, WHO and UNAIDS have formulated a plan to enable three million patients to have access to ART by 2005—3 (million) by 5 (2005)—in developing countries and in countries in transition. This program is highly relevant to India and the Government has affirmed its commitment to provide access to ART to 300,000 patients by 2005. The approaches contemplated are somewhat similar to the DOTS strategy for tuberculosis and include: a) develop simplified, standardised tools to deliver ART b) ensure an effective, reliable supply of medicines and diagnostics c) rapid identification, dissemination, and application of new knowledge and successful strategies d) sustained support by NACO to different states in India and e) advocacy, political commitment, and formation of strong partnerships with national and international agencies and stakeholders.

Five drugs have been chosen for ART. They include three NRTIs- zidovudine (AZT), stavudine (d4T) and lamivudine (3TC) and two NNRTIs—nevirapine (NVP) and efavirenz (EFZ). Each patient will be initiated on a first line regimen of d4T-3TC-NVP or d4T-3TC-EFZ. All PLWHA in WHO clinical stage III (moderate disease) or stage IV (severe disease: AIDS) will be targeted for ART (World Health Organization, 2003). The Government of India is committed to providing ART and the required tests for monitoring for about 100,000 patients in the first year, with a tentative provision of approximately 50 million dollars.

India has several accredited pharmacological concerns that manufacture and supply ART drugs to developing countries at negotiated, affordable and competitive rates, with minimal profit margins; it would therefore be possible to meet the drug requirements for the 300,000 patients in the Indian program from in-country resources. The drugs will be provided to patients free of charge in the states of Tamil Nadu, Maharashtra, Andhra Pradesh, Karnataka, Manipur and Nagaland, from April 2004. The program is likely to continue beyond 2005 on a larger scale, providing access to ART to all HIV/AIDS patients in India.

SUMMARY

India is facing an enormous challenge of containing an HIV/AIDS epidemic with about 4.58 million currently living with HIV, and with threats of the numbers increasing in the coming years, largely through sexual and mother to child transmission, and to a smaller extent, through intravenous drug use. Control efforts by NACO and other partners have been successful in limiting, to a large extent, further spread of HIV in India. An ART chemotherapy program scheduled to start in April 2004 is expected to reduce mortality among PLHWA, improve their quality of life and productivity, enable them to live longer and possibly reduce the risk of HIV transmission to others. The national commitment to HIV/AIDS control is high, including allocation of considerable resources, despite other urgent priorities, such as TB and malaria, competing for limited funds. The determination of the Government of India to spare no efforts in reducing the HIV/AIDS burden bodes well for the National AIDS Control Program and may result in the acceptance of HIV/AIDS as one more chronic infectious disease which can be controlled.

REFERENCES

Babu, P.G., Saraswathi, N.K., Devapriya, F. and John, T.J. (1993). The detection of HIV-2 infection in Southern India. *Indian J Med Res* 97:49–52.

Banerjee, K., Rodrigues, J.J., Israel, Z., Kulkarni, S., and Thakar, M. (1989). Outbreak of HIV seropositivity among commercial plasma donors in Pune, India (letter). *Lancet* 2:166.

Bollinger, R.C., Tripathy, S.P., and Quinn, T.C. (1995). The human immunodeficiency virus epidemic in India: Current magnitude and future projections. *Medicine* 74:97–106.

De, M., Banerjee, D., Chandra, S., and Bhattacharya, D.K. (1990). HBV and HIV seropositivity in multi-transfused haemophilics and thalassaemics in Eastern India. *Indian J Med Res* 91:63–66.

Gangakhedkar, R.R., Bentley, M.E., Divekar, A.D., Gadkari, D.A., Mehendale, S.M., Shepherd, M.E., Bollinger, R.C., and Quinn, T.C. (1997). Spread of HIV infection among married monogamous women attending STD clinics in India. *JAMA* 278:2090–2092.

Hira, S., Oberoi, C., Gharpure, H., and Dupont, H. (1996). Clinical profile of persons with single and dual HIV-1/2 infections in Bombay. XIth International Conference on AIDS, Vancouver. Abstract No. Mo. B. 1210.

Indian Council of Medical Research (ICMR). (1991). HIV infection—current status and future research plans. *Bulletin of the Indian Council of Medical Research* 21(12):126–139.

Jacob, M., John, T.J., George, S., Rao, P.S., and Babu, P.G. (1995). Increasing prevalence of human immunodeficiency infection among patients attending a clinic for sexually transmitted diseases. *Indian J Med Res* 101:6–9.

John, T.J., Babu, P.G., Jayakumari, H., and Simoes, E.A.F. (1987). Prevalence of HIV infection in risk groups in Tamil Nadu, India. *Lancet* 1: 160–161.

John, T.J., Babu, P.G., Saraswathi, N.K. Jayakumari, H., Selvaraj, R., Kaur, A., Chacko, S., Jacob, M., Ramachandran, P., and Tripathy, S.P. (1993). The epidemiology of AIDS in the Vellore region, Southern India. *AIDS* 7:421–424.

Khan, M.A. (1992). Psychosocial aspects of HIV infection and AIDS in multiple transfused thalassemic children. *Indian J of Pediatrics* 59(4):429–434.

Kulkarni, S., Thakar, M., Rodrigues, J.J., and Banerjee, K. (1992). HIV-2 antibodies in serum samples from Maharashtra state. *Indian J Med Res* 95:213–215.

Lele, R.D., Parekh, S.J., and Wadia, N.H. (1986). Transfusion associated AIDS (TA-AIDS) and AIDS dementia. *J Assoc Physicians India* 34:549–553.

Mathai, M., Prasad, P.V.S., Jacob, M., Babu, P.G. and John, T.J. (1990). HIV seropsitivity among patients with sexually transmitted diseases in Vellore *Ind J Med Res* 91:239–241.

Mehendale, S.M., Rodrigues, J.J., Brookmeyer, R.S., Gangakhedkar, R.R., Divekar, A.D., Gokhale, M.R., Risbud, A.R., Paranjape, R.S., Shepherd, M.E., Rompalo, A.E., Sule, R.R., Tolat, S.N., Jadhav, V.D., Quinn, T.C. and Bollinger, R.C. (1995). Incidence and predictors of HIV-1 seroconversion in patients attending sexually transmitted disease clinics. *India J Infect Dis* 172:1486–1491.

Mehendale, S.M., Risbud, A.R., Gangakhedkar, R., Divekar, A., Thilakavathi, S., Paranjape, R., Gadkari, D., Bollinger, R., and Rodrigues, J. (1996a). HIV-2 infection in STD patients in Pune, India. XIth International Conference on AIDS Abstract No. Mo. C. 1666.

Mehendale, S.M., Shepherd, M.E., Divekar, A.D., Gangakhedkar, R.R., Kamble, S.S., Menon, P.A., Yadav, R., Risbud, A.R., Paranjape, R.S., Gadkari, D.A., Quinn, T.C., Bollinger, R.C. and Rodrigues, J.J. (1996b). Evidence for high prevalence and rapid transmission of HIV among individuals attending STD clinics in Pune, India. *Indian J Med Res* 104:327–335.

Naik, T.N., Sarkar, S., Singh, H.L., Bhunia, S.C., Singh, Y.I., Singh, P.K., and Pal, S.C. (1991). Intravenous drug users—a new high risk group for HIV infection in India. *AIDS* 5(1):117–118.

National AIDS Control Organization (NACO). (1993). National AIDS Control Program: India country scenario, an update. pp. 9–12.

National AIDS Control Organization (NACO). (2003). HIV/AIDS Indian Scenario. HIV/AIDS

Surveillance in India (as reported to NACO as of 31st September, 2003). www.naco.nic.in.

Pfutzner, A., Dietrich, V., von Eichel, V., von Briesen, H., Brede, H.D., Maniar, J.K., and Rubsamen-Waigman, H. (1992). HIV-1 and HIV-2 infection in a high risk population in Bombay: Evidence for spread of HIV-2 and presence of a divergent HIV-1 subtype. *J Aquir Immune Defic Syndr* 5(10): 972–977.

Ray, K., Sachdeva, K.G., Jaisal, N.L., Tiwari, V.K. and Misra, R.S. (1995). HIV seropositivity in an STD center in a cosmopolitan city in northern India. *Genito Urinary Medicine* 71(1):58–59.

Rodrigues, J.J., Mehendale, S.M., Shepherd, M.E., Divekar, A.D., Gangakhedkar, R.R., Quinn, T.C., Paranjape, R.S., Risbud, A.R., Brookmeyer, R.S., Gadkari, D.A., Gokhale, M.R., Rompalo, A.M., Deshpande, S.G., Khaladkar, S.G., Mawar, N., and Bollinger, R.C. (1995). Risk factors for HIV infection in people attending clinics for sexually transmitted diseases in India. *BMJ* 311:283–286.

Rubsamen-Waigmann, H., Briesen, H.V., Maniar, J.K., Rao, P.K., Scholz, C., and Pfutzner, A. (1991). Spread of HIV-2 in India. *Lancet* (letter) 337(8740):550–551.

Rubsamen-Waigmann, H., Maniar, J., Gerte, S., Brede, H.D., Dietrich, U., Mahambre, G., and Pfutzner, A. (1994). High proportion of HIV-2 and HIV-1/2 double reactive sera in two Indian states, Maharashtra and Goa: First appearance of an HIV-2 epidemic along with an HIV-1 epidemic outside of Africa. *Int J Med Microbiol Virol Parasitol Infect Dis* 280(3):398–402.

Sarkar, S., Mookerjee, P., Roy, A., Naik, T.N., Singh, J.K., Sharma, A.R., Singh, Y.I., Singh, P.K., Tripathy, S.P., and Pal, S.C. (1991). Descriptive epidemiology of intravenous heroin users- a new risk group for transmission of HIV in India. *J Infect* 23:201–207.

Sarkar, S., Panda, S., Sarkar, K., Hangzo, C.Z., Bijaya, L., Singh, N.Y., Das, N., Agarwal, A., Chatterjee, A., Deb, B.C. and Detels, R. (1995). A cross sectional study of factors including HIV testing and counseling determining unsafe injecting practices among injecting drug users of Manipur. *Indian Journal of Public Health* 39: No.3.

Satpathy, S.K. and Shaukat, M. (1997). HIV/AIDS in India—the present scenario. Publication of the National AIDS Control Organization, India.

Sen, S., Mishra, N.M., Giri, T., Pande, I., Khare, S.D., Kumar, A., Chaudhry, V.P., Chattopadhya, D., Kumari, S., and Malaviya, A.N. (1993). Acquired immunodeficiency syndrome (AIDS) in multitransfused children with thalassemia. *Indian Pediatr* 30(4):455–460.

Simoes, E.A., Babu, P.G., John, T. J., Nirmala, S., Solomon, S., Lakshminarayana, C.S., and Quinn, T.C. (1987). Evidence for HTLV-III infection in prostitutes in Tamil Nadu, India. *Indian J Med Res* 85:335–338.

Simoes, E.A.F., Babu, P.G., Jeyakumari, H.M. and John, T.J. (1990). The initial detection of human immunodeficiency virus and its subsequent spread in prostitutes in Tamil Nadu, India. *J Aquir Immune Defic Syndr* 3:27.

Singh, Y.N., Chand, M., Nanu, A., Bhasin, R., Kapoor, S., and Malaviya, A.N. (1990). HIV infection in blood donors of Delhi, India. *J Aquir Immune Defic Syndr* 3:152–154.

Singh, Y.N., Bhargava, M., Malaviya, A.N., Tripathy, S.P., Kakkar, A., and Khare, S.D. (1991). HIV infection in Asian Indian patients with hemophilia and those who had multiple transfusions. *Indian J Med Res* 93:12–14.

Solomon, S., and Ganapathy, M. (1991). HIV-1 and HIV-2 among HRGs in Madras. 2nd Asia-Pacific Congress on AIDS and STD. New Delhi, India: Abstract No. 89.

Tripathy, S.P., Malaviya, A.N., Singh, Y.N., Chaudhuri, K., Varghese, T., and Seth, P. (1991). HIV antibody screening of commercially available blood products in India. *Indian J Med Res* 93:15–18.

Tripathy, S., Rodrigues, J.J., Sukumaran, K., Thakar, M., Kulkarni, S., Surve, B., and Shinde, V.N. (1992). Risk factors for HIV infection in a group of 168 HIV seropositive individuals at Pune. Proceedings of the First National Conference on AIDS (Bombay 28th–29th Mar. 1992):42.

Tripathy, S., Banerjee, K. , and Rodrigues, J. (1993). Increasing HIV infection in western India. IXth International Conference on AIDS. Berlin, Abstract No. PO CO8-2764.

Wadia, M.R., and Karve, S.R. (1992). Rising trend of HIV infection with special reference to blood donors. *J Assoc Physicians India* 40:No.8.

World Health Organization. (2003). Chronic HIV Care with ARV therapy: Integrated management of adolescent and adult illness: Interim guidelines for first level facility health workers. pp.12–27.

Zhang, J., Maniar, J.K., Saple, D.G., Tsuchie, H., Kageyama, S., Wakamiya, N., and Kurimura, T. (1996). Study of HIV-1/HIV-2 dual infection in Bombay. Int Conf AIDS (Vancouver Jul 7–12) 11:169. Abstract No. Mo.C.1668.

3

The Chinese HIV/AIDS Epidemic and Current Response

Shen Jie[1], Liu Kangmai[1], Han Mengjie[2] and Zhang Fujie[1]

[1]*National Center for STD/AIDS Prevention and Control, Chinese Center for Disease Control, Beijing, China*
[2]*Office of State Council, AIDS Committee, Chinese Ministry of Health, Beijing, China*

THE HIV/AIDS SITUATION IN CHINA

Since the first HIV/AIDS case was reported in 1985, the HIV/AIDS epidemic in China has gone through three phases: The Entry Phase (1985–1988), the Spreading Phase (1989–1994), and the Expansion Phase (1995–Present). By the end of June 2003, the accumulated number of reported HIV cases in the whole country was 45,092, of which 3532 were AIDS patients, with 1800 deaths. According to estimates by experts from the Chinese Centre for Disease Control and Prevention, the accumulated number of HIV infections and AIDS cases has reached 840,000, and 8000, respectively. Because of China's large population, the overall prevalence rate is still less than 0.1%, which signifies a relatively low level HIV/AIDS epidemic. In recent years, the number of people living with HIV/AIDS (PLWHA) has increased quickly, and the affected areas have expanded. The cumulative number of reported HIV/AIDS cases in 1999 increased from that of 1998 by 37.0%. In 2000, there was an increase of 30.0% over the year 1999, 2001 saw an increase of 36.5%, and 2002 saw a further increase of 32.0% (MOH/UNAIDS, 2003). These increases indicate that the situation for HIV/AIDS prevention and control in China is very serious.

The Three Phases of China's HIV/AIDS Epidemic

The first phase of the epidemic was from 1985 to1988: then, there were only 19 reported cases of HIV/AIDS in the whole country, scattered in different regions. Most cases were in the coastal urban areas and were among foreign nationals or Chinese from abroad. Only four haemophilia patients in Zhejiang province were infected with HIV/AIDS by imported contaminated blood products.

The second phase was from 1989 to 1994: 146 people with HIV were found in Ruili city, the southwest border city in Yunnan province in October 1989. Since then the epidemic covered the local areas of a few cities and counties in Dehong Prefecture. Only a few HIV-positive persons were found among injection drug users (IDU) in other provinces. There were also a few cases of sexually transmitted HIV found among sexually transmitted infection (STI) patients, female sex workers (FSW), and repatriated individuals; the numbers among these groups has increased year by year.

The third phase has been from 1995 to the present: reported HIV/AIDS cases have been increasing rapidly. One expansion has occurred among IDU in Yunnan province and spread rapidly to other prefectures, then to Xinjiang, Guangxi, Sichuan, and other provinces. Additionally, since 1995, a large amount of paid blood donors in Central China have been found to be HIV-positive, most of them members of a highly mobile population with a high transmission risk. In addition, cases of HIV/AIDS among STI patients and FSW have increased very quickly.

High HIV Prevalence among IDU

The HIV epidemic among IDU was reported only in Yunnan province from 1989 to 1995. After 1995, other provinces began to report HIV infections among IDU. By the end of 2002, all 31 provinces (municipalities and autonomous regions) reported HIV infections within this population. According to epidemiological research, the HIV infection rate in IDU in some regions of Yunnan province has reached 80%. In 2001, five of the 24 sentinel surveillance sites for IDU reported an infection rate of over 10%. The HIV infection rate is more than 80% in the surveillance site in Yining City, Xinjiang Province. Eight sentinel sites had HIV/AIDS infection rates ranging from 1% to 10%, and another eight sentinel sites with HIV-positive individuals (MOH, 2003).

Data from sentinel surveillance in 2002 indicated that the infection rate reached 78% among IDU in some areas of Xinjiang. The HIV infection rate among IDU in a few areas of Yunnan province is greater than 50%. In certain areas of Sichuan, Guangxi, and Guizhou, the HIV/AIDS infection rate among IDU reached 50.0%, 43.1% and 34.8%, respectively. There were seven provinces with an infection rate higher than 10% among IDU in China (MOH, 2003).

By the end of 2002, nine provinces, municipalities, and autonomous regions, Yunnan, Xinjiang, Guangxi, Guangdong, Sichuan, Hunan, Guizhou, Jiangxi, and Beijing, reported a serious HIV/AIDS epidemic among IDU (with a infection rate exceeding 5%). The syringe-sharing ratio is very high among IDU. Data from surveillance and epidemiological investigations between 2000 and 2002 showed that the infection rate among the high-risk population in the low epidemic areas had reached the level of some high epidemic areas. For example, the HIV/AIDS epidemic among IDU was surveyed in Jiangxi, Hunan, and Guizhou. Data from sentinel sites indicated the infection rate among IDU in Jiangxi reached 17.7% in 2000, 34.8% in some areas of Guizhou province and 13.9% in Hengyang, Hunan province in 2002 (MOH, 2003). Such data indicate that the epidemic situation of HIV/AIDS is very serious among IDU and that the risk of further transmission in this group is high.

Severe HIV Epidemic among Former Plasma Donors (FPD)

In many provinces, especially the central areas of China, farmers were involved in paid blood donation from 1985 to 1995. A large number of former blood donors became infected with HIV/AIDS. According to epidemiological investigations, the HIV infection rate among FPD in Henan, Anhui, and Shanxi, Shaanxi, Hubei, Hebei, Shandong, and Guizhou provinces reached 60% in certain communities. A survey undertaken in 2001 in Henan by the AIDS Prevention and Control Center of the Ministry of Health (MOH) (now called National Center for STD/AIDS Control and Prevention, the Chinese CDC) showed that 21.6% of the

0–60 year old population were paid blood donors and the proportion of paid blood donors in the 20–59 years old population reached 42.8% (MOH, 2003). In certain villages with a concentrated number of former plasma donors, several hundred villagers were infected with HIV.

Mounting AIDS-Related Deaths

The number of AIDS patients is increasing quickly according to case reports from recent years. The reported number of AIDS cases in 2002 increased by 46.4% over that of 2001 and increased by 206.4% in 2001 compared to that of 2000. According to data from the annual HIV/AIDS case reports between 1985 and 2000, the cumulative reported number of AIDS cases was 880, with 466 related deaths, while the reported number of AIDS cases and related deaths from 2001 to 2002 were 1719 and 581, respectively (MOH, 2003).

In some counties in Henan and Anhui, there have been particularly high numbers of HIV/AIDS cases and deaths since 2001. This has not only had a severe impact on individuals and their families, but also on the regions' social stability and development. According to international research in the natural history of HIV/AIDS and China's estimated HIV/AIDS prevalence situation in the past few years, it is estimated that approximately 200,000 people have developed AIDS in recent years, and between 80,000–100,000 of those people might still be alive. HIV/AIDS patients usually live for only 1–2 years without ARV therapy after the onset of symptoms, which indicates that China will have mounting numbers of AIDS-related deaths.

Expansion of the HIV/AIDS Epidemic from High-Risk Populations to the General Population

HIV/AIDS is transmitted via all three possible routes in China: sexual behavior, blood transfusion, and vertical transmission from mother to child all exist in China. Case reporting results indicate that until now the main transmission route in China has been the sharing of contaminated needles and syringes among IDU; until December 2002, 63.7% of the total reported cases were infected through injecting drug use. The proportion of HIV transmitted by sexual behavior increased from 5.5% in 1997 to 11.0% at the end of 2002 (MOH, 2003). Chinese sentinel surveillance results indicate that HIV prevalence among FSW is an increasing trend. The infection rates among FSW in Guangxi in 1995, 1997, 1999, 2000, and 2001 were 0%, 0.4%, 6.3%, 9.9%, 11.1%, and 9.5%, respectively (MOH, 2003). In addition, the investigation showed that the prevalence rate among premarital physical checks was also serious in some areas. In 1997, anonymous, un-linked HIV testing of premarital youth was started in Yining, Xinjiang autonomous region, showing an infection rate of 1.72%. According to another survey in Yining in 2001, the HIV infection rate was 1.14%, and 1.78% among males in this area. In Yunnan and Xinjiang provinces, the HIV infection rate among pregnant women in certain areas reached 1.3% and 1.2%, respectively (MOH, 2003); this is similar to infection rates of pregnant women in high prevalence neighbouring countries. Previous data from HIV/AIDS case reports show that the proportion of HIV-infection transmitted homosexually by men who have sex with men (MSM) has been relatively low. In the cumulative report in 2001, the proportion of HIV infections acquired through homosexual sex accounted for 0.2% (MOH, 2001a). However, in certain areas, results from surveys showed a higher infection rate. According to one investigation in Harbin in 2001, HIV infection rate among MSM was 1–3% (MOH/UNAIDS, 2003). In 2001, surveillance among 400 MSM in Beijing showed the overall infection rate among this group was about 5%. Some groups in China face a high risk of HIV infection, and the HIV/AIDS epidemic is spreading from these high-risk populations into the general population.

ACCOMPLISHMENTS IN HIV/AIDS PREVENTION AND CONTROL IN CHINA

Increased Political Recognition and Commitment by Government

The Central Government and the State Council are focusing serious attention on HIV/AIDS prevention and control. The leaders of the Central Government and the State Council have seriously considered the special reports for HIV/AIDS prevention and control many times, and have made important decisions based on these reports.

At the end of 1992, a Chinese state council committee member, Mr. Li Tieying, presided over the coordination of the national conference. Leaders from related ministries took part in the conference, and responsibilities for HIV/AIDS prevention and control were discussed and delegated. In 1994, the Minister of Health, Chen Minzhang, participated in the AIDS Summit in Paris, France. As the delegate of the Chinese Government, Chen Minzhang signed the "Paris Declaration," and announced China's ongoing political commitment. In 1996, the Chinese state council committee member in charge of public health, Ms. Peng Peiyun, presided over the State Council AIDS Coordination Working Group conference. Delegates from 34 ministries participated. Later that year, the National AIDS Prevention and Control Conference was held, at which Ms. Peng Peiyun gave an important lecture.

Chinese Central Government leaders have also been paying serious attention to HIV/AIDS prevention and control. Li Lanqing, the Vice Prime Minister until 2003, has participated in HIV/AIDS summary reports and made some important directives. Zhu Rongji, the Premier until 2003, paid close attention to the report from the Ministry of Health on HIV/AIDS prevention and control. President Hu Jintao and Premier Wen Jiabao have also made it clear that HIV/AIDS prevention and control is a high priority.

Laws and Guidelines Related to HIV/AIDS Prevention and Control

The Chinese People's Congress, the State Council, the related ministries, and local governments at different levels have released a series of laws, codes, regulations, and standardized documents, which guide HIV/AIDS prevention and control efforts.

In 1989, the "Law on Infectious Disease Prevention and Control" was issued, identifying HIV/AIDS as a "category B infectious disease." In September 1995, "Suggestions for Enhancing the Prevention and Control of HIV/AIDS" was issued by the MOH, with the permission of the State Council. Seven measures were emphasized at the macro level, and the tasks for HIV/AIDS prevention and control were further defined. In April 1999, "Perspectives of Management for People Living with HIV/AIDS" was issued by the Ministry of Health. It has been very helpful to people living with HIV/AIDS (PLWHA) and the further prevention of HIV/AIDS transmission. It is also an important measure for general population transmission prevention, care and support for PLWHA, anti-discrimination, and legal rights protection.

The Ministry of Health, Ministry of Propaganda, Ministry of Education, Ministry of Public Security, Ministry of Justice, Ministry of Culture, Ministry of Broadcasting, Film and Television, and the State Family Planning Commission jointly issued "Disseminating Education Principles for HIV/AIDS Prevention and Control" in January 1998. Concrete suggestions were made concerning content and dissemination of education, including scientific and policy aspects. Later that year, the State Council released "China's Long- and Medium Term Plan for HIV/AIDS Prevention and Control (1998–2010) (MoH, 1998)." All provinces, municipalities, autonomous regions, and related ministries are involved in advocacy, education, and intervention activities to fulfill the plan. Some progress has been made. As of today, nearly all provinces, municipalities, and autonomous regions have established provincial Long and Medium Term Plans, creating a great foundation for implementation of the national plan.

In May 2001, the "China Plan of Action for Containment and Control of HIV/AIDS (2001–2005) (MoH, 2001b)" was issued. The "Action Plan" made the " Medium- and Long-Term Plan" more measurable and detailed. It complements to the Long- and Medium Term Plan, with objectives in 2002 and evaluation in 2005. The Action Plan outlines detailed targets for the end of 2005.

In addition, the Ministry of Health, together with the related Ministries, jointly issued "Regulations for HIV/AIDS Surveillance Management," "Information for Imported Blood Products Control," and "Ordinance on Disinfections." Official guidelines, such as "Information Concerning HIV Antibody Tests in Hospitals, Blood Stations, and Institutions for STI Prevention and Control" and "Criterion for National HIV Surveillance (Draft)" were issued. Also, guidelines for preventing HIV infection through blood transmission, including "Basic Standards for Blood Stations," "The Regulation of Institutions for Blood Donation and Collection and Blood Management," and "The Information for Enhancing Blood management," were released.

The Construction of HIV/AIDS Organizations and Systems

In order to control the HIV/AIDS epidemic, the Central Government established the National Specialists Committee for HIV/AIDS Prevention and Control and the State Council AIDS Coordination Committee. The Ministry of Health HIV/AIDS Coordination Committee was established in 1986, and the team enlarged to become the National Specialists Committee for HIV/AIDS Prevention and Control in September 1990. The Committee was expanded in 1996 to include four sub-committees with the following responsibilities: i) advising the MOH on national laws, regulations, rules, policies, organizations, and technical measures for HIV/AIDS prevention and control; ii) providing suggestions related to scientific research, training schemes, and research projects for HIV/AIDS control and prevention; iii) technical review for national HIV/AIDS prevention and control programs; and iv) providing technical guidance for national HIV/AIDS prevention and control activities.

Reacting to the reality that the HIV/AIDS epidemic was worsening, in 1995, the State Council authorized the establishment of the State Council AIDS Coordination Committee, and its scope was expanded to cover STI and AIDS in 1996. The committee includes 34 ministries and commissions, as well as other relevant departments. The leaders of the State Council lead the committee. The state defined the responsibilities of each ministry and strengthened coordination between different departments. An annual meeting is held to build consensus for HIV/AIDS prevention and control. In order to strengthen coordination of HIV/AIDS control and prevention, the Coordination Committee established a functional standing office in 2001. The purpose of this office is to coordinate the different Ministries and provinces to carry out HIV/AIDS prevention and control activities.

Financial Investment for HIV/AIDS Prevention and Control

Governmental funding has been established as the major resource for HIV/AIDS prevention and control, supplemented by fundraising through various channels for additional resources. It is required that the central government sets up a special fund to carry out activities for HIV/AIDS prevention and control, and for special assistance to difficult areas. Local governments allocate their financing budgets according to local HIV/AIDS prevention and control needs. Investments from philanthropic donations and from other countries are also actively pursued to raise resources. More than half of all 31 provinces have established special funds for HIV/AIDS prevention and control, which will ensure strengthening of national HIV/AIDS control and prevention.

A special fund for HIV/AIDS control and prevention has been in place since 1998. Between 1998 and 2000, the annual contribution was 15 million CNY (Chinese Yuan). In 2001, the allocation was increased to 100 million CNY per year and is pledged at this level until 2005. In 2003, the Ministry of Finance began work on an additional 100 million CNY per year for 2003 to 2005. This will be used to improve HIV/AIDS treatment and comprehensive care in the most affected areas. In 2001, the State Development and Reform Commission transferred 1.25 billion CNY from national bonds, combined with one billion CNY from local governments to improve the basic infrastructure of blood banks in midwest China. Over four hundred and fifty blood banks and stations have been established, reconstructed, and enlarged. This investment plays a significant role in the prevention of HIV/AIDS transmission through blood donation and transfusion. In 2002, the State Development and Reform Commission allocated 0.8 and 2.1 billion CNY from national bonds to support the capacity building of the Centers for Disease Control at the provincial, prefecture, and county level in central and western China. This has greatly benefited the national HIV/AIDS program.

Investment from local governments has also increased. More than half of all provinces have set up special funds for HIV/AIDS prevention and control. The total contribution by local governments is roughly equal to that of the central government. For example, in 2001 and 2002, the government of Henan allocated the highest financial contribution in China, 14 million CNY per year. Since 2002, Guangdong has secured 10 million CNY each year for HIV/AIDS. There are six provinces that allocated more than five million CNY in special funds for HIV/AIDS prevention and control in China in 2002.

The Role of Non-Governmental Organizations (NGOs)

In 1993, the China Association of STI/AIDS Prevention and Control and the Chinese Foundation for the Prevention of STI/AIDS were established. This marks a new phase for mobilizing Chinese society, especially mass organizations, to take part in HIV/AIDS prevention and control. These organizations confer great assistance for coordinating NGOs to carry out activities in raising public awareness, health counseling, academic exchanges, and other activities. Local associations have also been established in some provinces and cities.

Since 1996, the China Association of STD/AIDS Prevention and Control has held the Chinese NGOs' coordination meeting. There, more than 20 NGOs joined together; they have issued the Joint Action Creed for Chinese NGOs taking part in HIV/AIDS prevention and control as the action guideline to fight HIV/AIDS.

Besides mass media education and training, Chinese NGOs also have greatly helped with the care and support of PLWHA, and with interventions in high-risk populations in recent years. The HIV/AIDS epidemic has many contributing social factors and it can only be successfully controlled if all sectors of society are actively involved. During the HIV/AIDS epidemic, the Chinese government has recognized that mass organizations are an important strength, and have provided powerful support and assistance. Some mass organizations related to HIV/AIDS control and prevention have been established in China, such as the China Association of STD/AIDS Prevention and Control, the Chinese Foundation for the Prevention of STD/AIDS, Chinese Drug Abuse Control Association, Chinese Gender Association, and the Chinese Drug Rehabilitation Association. These newer emerging associations have joined together with some previously established organizations, such as the Chinese Medical Association, the China

Preventive Medicine Association, All China Trade Union, All China Women's Federation, and All China Youth League, to form a national network. This network covers all of the target populations and can reach all sections of society. They have actively worked on the front line for in the fight against HIV/AIDS. They have made some significant impacts through interventions among high-risk populations, mass media education, care and treatment for PLWHA, and promotion of HIV/AIDS prevention and control.

Increased Health Education and Public Awareness

It is important to mobilize the whole society to take part in HIV/AIDS control and prevention. The related departments of the State Council have established policies for carrying out widespread health education activities through radio, TV, and newspapers. A series of campaigns are held on and around World AIDS Day on December 1st every year to raise public awareness, increase society's understanding of HIV/AIDS, and promulgate scientific knowledge. Under the unified leadership of the local government, the related departments cooperate actively, according to the local situation, to carry out various HIV/AIDS education activities for the public.

According to incomplete statistics, nearly 1000 exhibitions about HIV/AIDS have been held throughout China since 1998. More than 100 million persons have been educated through thousands of educational programs through TV, radio broadcasting, and other activities nationwide. A large number of HIV/AIDS educational posters, leaflets, and other materials have been created and distributed in different places (National Center for AIDS, CAIDS, unpublished data).

Interventions in High-Risk Populations

Injecting drug use and commercial sex work are the main routes for HIV transmission in China. In order to fight the HIV/AIDS epidemic, the Ministry of Health has cooperated with the Ministry of Public Security closely to control the spread of HIV through drug abuse, drug trafficking, and commercial sex work. These Ministries have carried out some pilot studies, according to international best practice experiences. Many strategies for effective prevention among different high-risk populations, which work in the context of China, have been identified.

Until now, intervention pilot studies have been carried out among 11 high-risk populations in China. In 2002, with the support of WHO, Wuhan and several other places began a pilot study to promote 100% condom use and have achieved a certain success. In 2002, the first pilot project for the social marketing of syringes and needles was conducted in Guangdong Province. IDU can buy sterile injection equipment at designated pharmacies for harm reduction among those potentially infected. Some achievements have been made concerning organizing, training, health education, intervention, and the provision of standardized services. Beneficial experience for further preventing HIV/AIDS among high risk populations have been obtained.

International Cooperation for HIV/AIDS Prevention and Control

China is actively involved in collaborating with both multilateral and bilateral organizations. Through these collaborations, China has gained much support and assistance, both technically and financially. Long and effective partnerships with the World Health Organization (WHO), World Bank, United Nations Development Program (UNDP), United Nations Children's Fund (UNICEF), United Nations Joint Program on AIDS (UNAIDS), and the European Union (EU) have been established. According to incomplete statistics in the National Center for HIV/AIDS Control and Prevention (NCAIDS), more than 30 international organizations, countries, and regions have collaborated with China for HIV/AIDS prevention and control. More than

100 international cooperation projects have been carried out. Many achievements have already been made through completed projects, and many more projects are currently being implemented.

During the last ten years, the Chinese government has collaborated with many organizations and countries for technical assistance. Australia, the United Kingdom, the United States, Germany, Japan, Luxembourg, and South Korea, as well as several other countries are all partners. A significant amount of technical support and assistance have been gained from close cooperation with UN organizations and the World Bank. All these collaborations have benefited Chinese HIV/AIDS prevention and control.

CHINA'S GOALS FOR HIV/AIDS PREVENTION AND CONTROL

China's goals on HIV/AIDS prevention and control have been principally composed into two plans, "the Medium and Long Term Plan of HIV/AIDS Prevention and Control in China (1998–2010)" and "China Action Plan to Contain, Prevent and Control HIV/AIDS (2001–2005)." These medium and long-term goals include objectives to be achieved by 2010.

Medium- and Long-term Goals

The Ministry of Health, together with three other ministries, developed "the Medium and Long Term Plan of HIV/AIDS Prevention and Control in China (1998–2010)" in October 1998, in which China's overall goals on HIV/AIDS prevention and control were described. One goal is to set up a multi-sectoral STI/AIDS prevention and control system with participation by the whole society. Under the leadership of government, the plan aims to disseminate knowledge and information about STI/AIDS control and prevention, and ultimately to prevent HIV transmission. It is explicitly proposed that "STI prevalence be steadily decreased and the number of people living with HIV/AIDS be controlled under 1,500,000 by 2010".

Immediate Goals on HIV/AIDS Prevention and Control in China

China's immediate goals on HIV/AIDS prevention and control are embodied in the "China Action Plan to Contain, Prevent and Control HIV/AIDS (2001–2005) (MoH, 2001b)," developed by the State Council of China. This document quantifies and specifies the chief goals in "the Medium and Long Term Plan of HIV/AIDS Prevention and Control in China (1998–2010) (MoH, 1998)," and complements the stated goals in 2002 and 2005 in the "the Medium and Long Term Plan." It clarifies the specific objectives that the annual increase of HIV infection and STI be brought below 10% and HIV infection through clinical blood transfusion be decreased to a rate of under 1/100,000 in most areas, and under 1/10,000 to 1/50,000 in areas with high HIV prevalence by the end of 2005.

THE SOCIOECONOMIC IMPACTS OF HIV/AIDS

The Macro- and Microeconomic Impacts of HIV/AIDS

In China, a very limited amount of research concerning the socioeconomic impact of HIV/AIDS has been conducted. Even with such limited study, it is clear that the HIV/AIDS epidemic has already had great social and economic impacts in China.

Microeconomic impact can be seen mainly in decreased incomes and high medical costs caused by HIV/AIDS. With respect to medical costs, in 1999, the Chinese Academy of Preventive Medicine conducted a retrospective survey of two hospitals in Beijing where PLWHA were treated. The results showed that the annual medical cost for each case was 54,549 CNY, 87.22% of which was spent on hospitalization. A further analysis of 29 AIDS patients receiving treatment showed that the average hospitalization fee per case was 23,231 CNY annually, and the cost of outpatient treatment was 16,009 CNY. Patients receiving ARV treatment had an extra expenditure of 23,857 CNY. Recently, due to the production and sale of generic ARV drugs, treatment costs for PLWHA have decreased significantly. However, the cost for drugs and testing remains approximately 20,000 CNY (Yip *et al.*, 2002).

According to statistical data on the social and economical impact of the HIV/AIDS epidemic in China, the number of PLWHA who need to be treated will be 200,000 within the next five years. It is estimated that from 2002 to 2006, the number of patients needing treatment will be 10,000 in the first year, 30,000 the second, 70,000 the third, 120,000 the fourth, and 200,000 in the fifth year. The costs of ARV treatment alone will be 8.6 billion CNY in five years.

According to that same research, given that the average age of death for a Chinese PLWHA is 35.22 years, the average age of retirement for Chinese people is 60 years, and the annual wealth generation of each person is 15,000 CNY, the average economic loss due to each case of HIV/AIDS infection and consequent decrease of wealth generation is about 370,000 CNY. If the number of people living with HIV/AIDS reaches one million at the end of 2002, the medical costs and the socioeconomic loss will be 370 billion CNY. If Chinese preventive measures are not effective and the number of HIV/AIDS cases reaches 10 million in 2010, the amount will exceed 3,700 billion.

Economic Effect of HIV/AIDS on Health Services

As the number of HIV/AIDS cases increases worldwide, the epidemic has brought about unprecedented pressure on health departments in all countries. According to incomplete statistics, by the end of 1992, the cumulative expenditure on HIV/AIDS prevention and control in China spent by the central government and international agencies was 30 million CNY. From 1993 to 1998, the MOH budget for HIV/AIDS prevention and control was 54.9 million CNY. In 1998, the central government increased the annual HIV/AIDS budget to 15 million CNY, and in 2001 the annual AIDS budget increased again to 100 million CNY. In order to deal with the rapid increase of HIV/AIDS patients, the government again significantly increased its budget in 2002 (MOH/UNAIDS, 2003).

Alternately, considering some of the present successful prevention projects, interventions for six months in every high risk target population would cost between 200 and 400 CNY. If China provides interventions to 10% of the estimated number of high-risk individuals, taking into account the cost decrease and other factors when interventions are expanded, the annual budget would be 60–120 million CNY. If China is to conduct effective interventions nationally, the interventions need to cover at least 60% of the target population and will require a budget of at least 360–720 million CNY per year.

AIDS-Related Social Problems and Their Influence on Social Stability

Firstly, the HIV/AIDS epidemic can lead to a large number of orphans. According to a survey among 143 PLWHA in selected parts of China, 16.8% of them have children younger than five years old, and these children are likely to become orphans prior to adolescence. According to Chinese statistical data, if a low-level HIV/AIDS epidemic continues, the number of orphans will reach 138,000 by the end of 2010. With a mid-grade HIV/AIDS epidemic, there will be 200,000 orphans. And if China has a full-blown HIV/AIDS epidemic, the number of AIDS orphans may reach 260,000 by the end of 2010 (MOH/UNAIDS, 2003).

Secondly, the HIV/AIDS epidemic will increase both the number of poor people and the disparity between the rich and the poor. Most PLWHA in China live in resource-constrained areas where there are few natural resources and where health and education resources are limited; most people live in poverty. In order to increase incomes, poor people are more likely to be involved in selling blood or sex, both of which increase the risk for the spread of HIV/AIDS. Families affected by HIV/AIDS have a lower income and higher medical expenditures. These factors will exacerbate poverty in areas where prevalence is highest. It was found recently that people in certain areas who have just risen out of poverty and began to have a steady income returned to poverty because of HIV infection. This disease-induced poverty increases the disparity between rich and poor areas.

In addition, various rumors about HIV/AIDS may severely impact the social stability and sense of public safety due to panic. For example, in 2000, a local newspaper in northeast China published an article concerning HIV/AIDS patients who infused their blood into watermelons, stating that "it is possible for people to become infected by AIDS through eating these watermelons," which brought about a great decrease in sales of watermelon and considerable economic loss to producers. At the end of 2001, some self-identified HIV/AIDS patients made disturbances by threatening to puncture others with blood contaminated syringes and needles, creating social confusion in Tianjin, Beijing, and Shijiazhuang. Such information was spread, exaggerated, and distorted, and finally became a stirring rumor. It caused panic in some regions and seriously impacted the stability of local society (South China Morning Post, 2002).

COST-EFFECTIVENESS OF HIV/AIDS PREVENTION AND CONTROL MEASURES

Although the epidemic situation of HIV/AIDS in China is serious, prevalence is still low compared to other countries. Many prevention intervention activities are still in the pilot stage. In China, there are not yet estimates of the cost-efficacy of HIV/AIDS prevention intervention measures at the national level. According to some successful HIV/AIDS intervention programs, if effective intervention is provided to everyone at high risk for six months, and perception rate and condom usage rates are elevated by 30%–50%, and 30%–40%, respectively, 200–400 CNY per person is needed.

As predicted in one study in China, in an area where there are 3000 drug users, among which 1000 are IDU whose HIV prevalence rate was initially 10%, the predicted infections would decrease by more than 100% in five years (MOH, 2003). This result can be achieved if behavioral interventions and other prevention activities reduce the annual increase in incidence rate among IDU from 20% to 10%, and if the frequency of sharing needles among IDU decreases from once every three days to once every seven days. The same result can also be achieved in the activities that are conducted to prevent HIV transmission between FSW and their clients. For example, if there were 2000 FSW and 20,000 clients in a certain area, the prevalence among FSW and their clients is 0.1% at the beginning, and the unprotected sex behaviors of one FSW per month is 40, an intervention which successfully got FSW to use condoms in 50% of their commercial sexual encounters would decrease HIV infections over the following five years by half.

Suppose one five-year intervention activity, "Stop drugs and prevent AIDS," is implemented in one urban community. The target population is 100,000, among which 1000 are drug users and 300 are IDUs. The program is to hold a course every month for drug users, which aims to educate them about the hazards of drug abuse, HIV/AIDS, and HIV prevention methods. In addition, activities such as showing a video four times per year, distributing handbooks on AIDS prevention, and posting pictures concerning HIV/AIDS prevention in target areas, will provide educational opportunities for the general public. It is predicted that 88 HIV infections will be prevented by this intervention plan in the next five years. The total investment required would be 977,100 CNY. If the total economic loss for one HIV/AIDS patient is 250,000 CNY currently in China, the economic loss would be decreased by 22,000,000 CNY. The cost-benefit ratio for such an intervention is 1: 22 (Yip *et al.*, 2002; Liu *et al.*, 1999).

ARV THERAPY IN CHINA

The Criteria for ARV Treatment in China

In order to standardize anti-retroviral (ARV) treatment in China and elevate local clinic doctors' capacity for diagnosis and treatment, the Chinese Center for STI /AIDS Prevention and Control, China CDC, has organized experts to establish "Guidelines for HIV/AIDS Diagnosis and Treatment (draft)." The general symptoms and signs needed to initiate ARV treatment are clarified in the guidelines.

At present, in several areas of middle and western China, where resources are constrained and PLWHA are relatively centralized, CD4 cell counts and viral loads are difficult to obtain. When patients require treatment, the local medical organization must give a basic examination, necessary before ARV treatment is initiated. Basic laboratory examinations include HIV antibody testing, hemoglobin measurement, and blood cell capacity level measurements. The main objective is to validate HIV infection. Based on these results, most patients in the area are given basic examinations: white cell counts and classifications (to evaluate the side-effects of potential neutrophilic granulocyte decrease and lymphocyte count), GPT (glutamic-pyruvic transaminase) and GOT (glutamic-oxaloacetic transaminase) in plasma (to primarily validate coinfection with hepatitis at the same time to monitor the hepatic toxicology of the drugs), creatinine and/or urea nitrogen (to evaluate kidney function), blood sugar and pregnancy examinations for women. ARV treatment is carried out for suitable patients.

The Estimated Number of PLWHA Needing Treatment in China

There are 840,000 PLWHA now, about 80,000 of which have AIDS. Because of the shortage of equipment, experienced doctors, and funds, it is planned that 40–50,000 people will receive ARV treatment in the next five years to reach the WHO's mandate that 60% PLWHA are given ARV treatment.

The Preliminary Results of ARV Therapy in China

At present, about 6000 people are undergoing ARV treatment. A small proportion of them pay for the expense by themselves, another small proportion of treatment is supported by international cooperation projects; others, mainly in Henan, Anhui, Hubei, and Shandong provinces, are being provided with free treatment. The treatment results so far are good. According to the treatment of 3426 PLWHA in a target county in midwest China (726 people were not suitable for ARV treatment, 165 people were not willing to receive ARV treatment, and 2550 patients have taken two months of ARV treatment), 15.9% of patients have had their condition dramatically improve. The proportion of patients whose illness has improved, unchanged, or been aggravated is, 54.2%, 27.1%, and 2.5%, respectively (Zhang, 2003). According to other results, in which 113 people were suitable for ARV treatment, the proportion of patients who have dramatically improved, improved, not obviously changed is 31%, 42.5%, 21.2%, respectively; one patient quit ARV treatment and five died (Zhang, 2003).

The Price of ARV Drugs in China and Their Availability to the Target Population

Before August 2002, the price of ARV drugs in China was quite high because the supply was dependent solely on importation. Through many negotiations, in early December 2001, GlaxoSmithKline, Merck & Co.,

Inc., and Bristol-Myers Squibb Company reduced drug prices by one-half to two-thirds. The average expense for one patient was reduced from 110,000–130,000 CNY to about 35,000 CNY annually. Nevertheless, most Chinese PLWHA still cannot afford the cost. It is an unbearable burden for most, especially those in rural areas. To them, ARV drugs are completely inaccessible.

In order to quickly reduce the price of ARV drugs and to increase the availability of the drugs, under the authority of the State Council, MOH and the State Council Coordinating Committee on HIV/AIDS, active negotiations took place, and the relevant departments in the State Council gave their full support. In early 2003, the State Development Planning Commission approved the reduction and constriction of the retail prices of four kinds of drugs produced by GlaxoSmithKline, Merck & Co., Inc., and Bristol-Myers Squibb Company. The State Drug Administration agreed to expedite the registration for imported ARV drugs at first, approving the clinical trials, simplifying the requests of the packaging, and accelerating the application processes. The Ministry of Finance, State Administration of Taxation and Customs General Administration exempted the customs and the value-added tax for imported ARV drugs. While the tax rate of customs and value-added tax is 4–5% and 17%, respectively, after the exemption, the drug price reached 8,000–10,000 CNY for every person-year, according to a declaration by foreign companies (NCAIDS, unpublished results).

Domestic pharmaceutical companies are also developing generic ARV drugs. In August 2002, AZT, the first domestically manufactured generic ARV drug, was approved. D4T, DDI, and NVP were subsequently approved. At present, the first regimen of domestically manufactured generic drugs is complete and its price is only one-tenth of that of the imported drugs, or 3,000 CNY for every person-year. The Chinese government continues to try to reduce prices even further.

In order to resolve the problems of ARV treatment costs to workers, labor, and social security sections, China has put ARV drugs into the covered drug list within basic medical insurance policies. There are plans to include ARV drugs on the list of the basic medical insurance drugs for more policies in the future.

In order to resolve the problem of ARV treatment for PLWHA in undeveloped rural areas, 100 comprehensive care demonstration sites focused on treatment and care have been set up. The emphasis is to maximize the benefits of treatment and care in high epidemic areas. Subsidies for drug costs and examination fees are given to PLWHA. The subsidies vary according to the poverty situation of the patients. At present, the Chinese government is trying its best to provide ARV treatment for more PLWHA using domestic and international financial support.

REFERENCES

Liu, Kangmai, *et al.* (1999). Behavioral analysis and intervention strategy in main HIV target groups in China. Project Report. (unpublished)

Ministry of Health, China (MoH). (1998). China's Long- and Medium Term Plan for HIV/AIDS Prevention and Control (1998–2010). State Council Office Document. Ministry of Health, Communicable Disease Control Division.

Ministry of Health, China (MoH). (2001a). Annual HIV/AIDS Surveillance Report, 2001. Center for Disease Control, Beijing.

Ministry of Health, China (MoH). (2001b). China's Action Plan for Reducing and Preventing the spread of HIV/AIDS (2001–2005). State Council Office Document 2001–2040. Ministry of Health, Communicable Disease Control Division. (June 2001).

Ministry of Health, China (MoH). (2003) Annual HIV/AIDS Surveillance Report, 2003. Center for Disease Control. Beijing.

Ministry of Health, China/Joint UN Program on HIV/AIDS (MOH/UNAIDS). (2003). A Joint Assessment of HIV/AIDS Prevention, Treatment and Care in China. China Ministry of Health and United nation theme group on HIV/AIDS in China. (December, 2003).

South China Morning Post (SCMP) (2002). AIDS Needle Fear Grips City. January 19, 2002.

Yip, R., Stover, J., Liu, K., Laurence, C., Yuan, J., Xu, Y., Jiang, T., Wang, W., Li, Y., Liu, K., Qu, S., Bai, Y., Wang, L., Bollinger, L., Walker, N., He, J., Ionita, G. (2002). The Socioeconomic Impact of HIV/AIDS in China. Socioeconomic Impact of HIV/AIDS Research Team, August 2002.

Zhang, F. (2003). ARV Treatment Report, in the Division of Treatment and Care Quarterly Report to Ministry of Health. National Center for AIDS Prevention and Control.

4

HIV/AIDS and Public Health Care in the Greater Mekong River Region

Origin, Disease Damage, Control and Regional Collaborative Effort

Huyen Cao[1], Tung Nguyen[2], and Nicholas Daniels[2]

[1] *California Department of Health Services, Richmond, California, USA*
[2] *Department of Medicine, University of California, San Francisco, California, USA*

INTRODUCTION

More than 240 million people live in the Greater Mekong River Region, an area defined by the Mekong River, which flows 4,800 kilometers from the Tibetan plateau through China's Yunnan province, Myanmar, Lao People's Democratic Republic (Lao PDR), Thailand, Cambodia and Vietnam. After decades of wars and political conflicts, relative peace in recent years has fostered economic liberalization, intergovernmental co-operation, and increasing flow of labor and goods across regional borders (U.S. Bureau of Affairs, 1987). The long periods of war and political instability, and the emerging economic growth, have created a variety of challenges to the public health systems in these countries. In the face of the increase in population mobility, illicit drug use and prostitution, many areas of the Mekong River region have become flashpoints in the HIV/AIDS pandemic.

In this chapter, we will focus on the countries of Vietnam, Lao PDR, Cambodia, and Myanmar. We will examine the strengths and weaknesses of the public health infrastructure as well as the HIV/AIDS prevalence and control in these countries. The aim is to describe the scope of the problem of HIV/AIDS and to outline the current capacity of health systems in these countries to respond to the threat of HIV.

VIETNAM

Background

Vietnam shares borders with China to the north, Cambodia to the southwest, and Lao PDR to the northwest. Its coastline borders the

Gulf of Tonkin, the South China Sea, and the Gulf of Thailand. Vietnam had a population of 79 million people in 2001 (Nguyen *et al.*, 2001; World Health Organization, 2001). The largest urban centers are Hanoi, with a population of three million, and Ho Chi Minh City, with a population of five million. The major religions are Buddhism, Christianity, and ancestor worship.

Vietnam was a French colony from 1884 until the end of World War II when the Vietnamese Communists defeated France and controlled North Vietnam. In 1975, the Communist-led North Vietnam defeated the United States-backed South Vietnam and created a unified Socialist Republic of Vietnam. Under the rule of the Communist Party, the country has slowly adopted reforms toward a free market economy but remains under one party rule.

The market system reforms in the early 1990s have led to a remarkable economic growth in Vietnam. It has currently the fastest growing economy in Southeast Asia and one of the fastest in all of Asia. In 2002, the per capita income was US$430 (World Bank, 2003b). The Growth Domestic Product (GDP) per capita was $441 in 2002 with a purchasing power parity of nearly $2000. The average annual growth rate of the GDP was 6.6% from 1990 to 2002 (United Nations Development Program, 2003). Approximately two-thirds of the labor force remains in agriculture while one-third work in industries and services. Despite the impressive growth rate, however, there remains significant poverty, with an unemployment rate approaching 25% and approximately one-third of the population living below poverty level.

Health and Healthcare System

Life expectancy at birth in Vietnam is 69 years (Canh and Do, 1993; World Health Organization, 2001). Infant mortality rate is approximately 30 per 1000 live births. Malaria, tuberculosis, viral hepatitis and diarrheal diseases remain endemic in Vietnam. Despite the years of political conflicts, Vietnam has always had a strong central government and, due to exposure to Western medicine through French, American, and Russian influences, the health care system has been well-organized. The country is divided into 61 governing provinces and municipalities. The health care system consists of four levels: national, provincial, prefecture, and the basic unit of town or village (Matsuda, 1994). At the national level, the Health Department manages health care while the Health and Welfare sections of the People's Committee manage health care at all other levels. Medical services are provided by the National Central Hospital at the national level, by general hospitals at the provincial level, by general hospitals and multi-purpose health clinics at the prefecture level and by health stations at the basic unit levels.

Below the provincial level are districts, consisting of communes and villages. The District Health Centers formulate and implement preventive healthcare services and provide technical support to commune health centers. The commune health center is the first level of health care in the Vietnamese health system and is responsible for primary care in the community. Health services providers at the basic unit level include doctors, nurses, pharmacists, and paramedical staff (Matsuda, 1994).

The transition from a centrally planned economy in the 1980s and the implementation of health policy reforms in 1989 affected the financing and delivery of health care services. Legalization of private medical practice, liberalization of the pharmaceutical industry, and introduction of user charges at public health facilities have effectively transformed Vietnam's near universal, publicly funded health care system into a highly unregulated private-public mixed system, particularly in urban centers. State health budgets decreased, and public hospitals increasingly rely on user charges and insurance premiums to finance services. As a consequence, health care costs are substantial for many low- and middle-income households (Sepehri *et al.*, 2003). In 1998, 80% of health spending in Vietnam was paid out-of-pocket (Naraan *et al.*, 2000). User fees in the public sector are rising, especially for hospital care, where fees have risen by over 1000% in real terms between 1993 and 1998 (World Bank, 2001).

One consequence of the increased cost of care is an increasing reliance on self-treatment or treatment outside of the health care system. Approximately 40–60% of people in Vietnam depend on self-medication (Okumura *et al.*, 2002; Van Duong *et al.*, 1997). This has significant implications on public health. An example is the control of tuberculosis. Vietnam has a well-organized national tuberculosis control program and treatment is provided free of charge. Nonetheless, tuberculosis treatment is increasingly administered through the private sector (Lonnroth *et al.*, 2003), despite the superior quality of case management and treatment outcome provided by the national tuberculosis program.

Vietnam has an organized surveillance system for many diseases. The Department of Preventive Medicine and the National Institute of Hygiene and Epidemiology (NIHE) in Hanoi collects disease reports from all health care facilities throughout the country. The NIHE also serves as the central reference laboratory for Vietnam. The Institute collects national surveillance data from all centers of preventive medicine, public health clinics, and hospitals from around the country and annually summarizes data related to the 26 notifiable conditions in Vietnam. The investigation of disease outbreaks is largely the responsibility of the district and provincial health departments, which rely on the close cooperation between local hospital doctors, hygiene inspectors, epidemiologists, and veterinary officers.

The National Institute of Hygiene and Public Health is a research institute based in Ho Chi Minh City and provides technical support to 21 provinces in southern Vietnam. It does not conduct any epidemiological or laboratory surveillance. The Pasteur Institute in Nha Trang provides technical support for most of the 14 provinces. All of the four national laboratories (which include the three regional Pasteur Institutes and NIHE) have email communications with their provinces and other national institutes except for the Pasteur Institute at Thai Nguyen. The Pasteur Institute of Ho Chi Minh City has an electronically based surveillance system called "PasteurNet." PasteurNet was created in collaboration with a Vietnamese telecommunications company. Through this internet-based system, provinces transmit disease reports of four diagnoses under active surveillance (typhoid, cholera, dengue, and plague) weekly and other reportable diseases monthly. Attempts by the NIHE to establish PasteurNet in northern provinces have previously failed due to lack of trained personnel and sufficient funds for computers and telecommunications necessary to reliably access the internet/email. The efficiency of this public health system was demonstrated in the Severe Acute Respiratory Syndrome (SARS) global outbreak in 2003 (World Health Organization, 2003a). Vietnam was among the first countries to be affected by the severe respiratory illness. Strong political commitment translated into rapid task force and provincial team establishment and eventually proved effective in preventing further spread of this virus. The World Health Organization removed Vietnam from the list of SARS-affected areas in April 2003, making it the first country to successfully contain its SARS outbreak.

HIV/AIDS Surveillance and Control

Since the first reported HIV case in 1990, Vietnam has established an extensive sentinel surveillance system (Sarrel *et al.*, 1996). In 2002, the government reported 55,000 people with HIV/AIDS, although other agencies have provided different estimates. In 2001, the

Joint United Nations Program on HIV/AIDS estimated that 130,000 adults (0.3% of the population) were infected. As many as 50.5% of total HIV cases reported are from people from 20–29 years of age (UNAIDS, 2002).

While HIV prevalence is high among sex workers and clients of sex workers, injecting drug users (IDU) account for the majority of Vietnam's HIV infection (Nguyen *et al.*, 1999; Quan *et al.*, 2000). Molecular epidemiological studies have tracked HIV infection flowing from northern Vietnam, where heroin is purer and cheaper, to southern China (Beyrer *et al.*, 2000; Piyasirisilp *et al.*, 2000; Yu *et al.*, 1999). The number of drug users in Vietnam is reportedly as high as 183,000 and is believed to be the highest in Ho Chi Minh City (MOLISA and UNDCP, 2000; Tran, 2000). A needle exchange program began in 2002 (Cohen, 2003b), but has so far shown limited success without concurrent comprehensive drug treatment programs. Methadone is still considered an illegal drug and the "cold turkey" rehabilitation centers have high relapse rates (Hien *et al.*, 2001). Efforts at mass information, peer education and outreach among high risk groups have been inconsistent among different regions (Khoat *et al.*, 2003). Prior to 2000, governmental policy focused on prevention of transmission by education. However, recent policy changes have used the "social evils" approach of defining prostitution, drug use, and homosexuality as socially deviant behaviors and drug users and sex workers have been committed to detention centers (CDC News, 2002). Population studies on HIV prevalence are comprised of individuals who have been arrested by the police or caught up in a sweep by the authorities and may skew the HIV statistics. The new policy has had a chilling effect on detection and prevention and has done little to promote a sense of trust between the high-risk populations and the authorities. This trust is necessary to implement the harm reduction programs that are so important in reducing the spread of HIV in these same populations (Pisani *et al.*, 2003).

LAO PDR

Background

The Mekong River runs through the Lao People's Democratic Republic (Lao PDR), one of the poorest countries in Southeast Asia. Lao PDR borders China and Myanmar to the north, Thailand and Cambodia to the west and south, and Vietnam to the east. Lao PDR has approximately 5.6 million inhabitants, with 500,000 living in Vientiane, the capital city. The country is divided administratively into 16 provinces and the Municipality of Vientiane. Below the provincial level are districts, which are comprised of villages. The major religions are Buddhism and animism.

Laos was a French colony until 1949 when it returned to monarchy rule. In 1975, the Communist Pathet Lao gained control of the country and has since ruled it as a single-party state. In the late 1980s, the Communist Party slowly began to implement private enterprise reforms.

From 1988 to 1997, the economy grew at a brisk 7% annually, but Southeast Asia's lackluster economic performance has slowed its growth. Most of the populace are farmers. The GNP per capita was US$320 in 2001, and the GDP per capita purchasing power parity was US$1700 in 2000. Nearly half (46%) of the population lives below poverty level. There is no railroad. Electricity is available only in some urban areas, and there is a limited telecommunications system.

Health and Healthcare System

The infant mortality rate in Lao PDR is more than 100–120 per 1000 live births, and the life expectancy at birth is 54 years. Health sector spending as a percentage of GDP is among the lowest in the world (WHO, 2000).

Diarrheal diseases are among the ten leading causes of morbidity and mortality in Lao PDR. Cholera, a rapidly growing public health problem, is endemic in Lao PDR, with transmission occurring throughout the year.

The lack of adequate human waste disposal facilities permits widespread contamination of the environment with fecal material and increased risks for epidemics, and most outbreaks of cholera have occurred in villages with unprotected drinking water. Only half of the population has access to "safe" drinking water (e.g., protected wells, piped water, or gravity systems), while only one-third of the population has access to adequate sanitary facilities. Due to limited funding, monitoring of drinking water for contamination (e.g., fecal coliforms) is not routinely performed in rural areas, and the capacity for monitoring is extremely limited at the provincial level due to the lack of trained personnel. In the cities, sewage is discharged into the environment without treatment. Routine monitoring of the microbiologic quality and chlorine levels of drinking water is only done in water treatment plants of major cities.

The National Center for Laboratory and Epidemiology (NCLE), (formerly known as the National Institute for Hygiene and Epidemiology) monitors infectious diseases through a nationwide, hospital-based, active surveillance system. Provincial surveillance units report the occurrences of infectious diseases in major hospitals and some district hospitals to the Ministry of Health on a weekly basis. None of the national or provincial surveillance units have reliable Internet access or electronic mail and no systemic laboratory-based surveillance system exists in Lao PDR.

HIV/AIDS Surveillance and Control

Lao PDR depends heavily upon its agricultural sector for its livelihood. In a bid to boost its fragile domestic economy, the country is promoting trade with neighboring Cambodia, China, Thailand, and Vietnam. Unfortunately, new trade practices also promote the spread of HIV infection and other sexually transmitted diseases (Zola, 1994). However, available data on HIV/AIDS in Lao PDR are scant. Reported HIV/AIDS prevalence has been low, with estimates of around 0.05% (UNAIDS, 2003b). One explanation for the low HIV infection rate is the isolation of the country in recent decades. Until the mid 1990s, the government restricted movement between provinces and outside the country. The social cost resulting from increased promotion of tourism and trade ties with its neighbors may be high.

Surveillance data in 2000–2001 showed that six of 811 (0.9%) female service workers in entertainment sites were HIV positive, and the sexually transmitted infection (STI) rate in this population is as high as 54% (UNAIDS, 2003b). Among the high risk groups are sex workers and the mobile population. Lao PDR is the third leading producer of heroin in the world (Beyrer *et al.*, 2000). HIV infection is also spreading rapidly among IDU, particularly in the Golden Triangle where Myanmar, Thailand, and Laos converge and where the pure heroin, "China White," is refined. Recent outbreaks of injection drug use and HIV in this area have been associated with Burmese and Laotian overland heroin trafficking routes (Beyrer *et al.*, 2000).

National and international partnerships have fostered a heightened awareness of HIV/AIDS among the general population, especially in urban areas, as evidenced by the increase in condom use. However, with high HIV prevalence rates in neighboring countries, and population mobility increasing within and across borders, it is clear that Lao PDR remains highly vulnerable to the spread of HIV/AIDS (Zola, 1994).

CAMBODIA

Background

Cambodia shares borders with Thailand and Laos to the north and Vietnam to the east and south. Cambodia has approximately 13 million inhabitants, with nearly half of the population under the age of 20 (World Bank, 2002; USAID, 2003). The major religion is Buddhism. The country is divided into 20 provinces and four municipalities. Below the provincial level are operational districts, which are comprised of communes and villages. In 1953, Cambodia declared independence from France and restored monarchical rule. Following many years of fighting, the Communist Khmer Rouge captured control of the country in 1975 and instituted drastic reforms. The Khmer Rouge evacuated all cities and towns. The mass exodus resulted in more than 1 million deaths, including many of the educated class. Vietnam invaded Cambodia in 1978, and the Vietnam-backed government fought and gained advantage over the Khmer Rouge, and in 1993, established democracy with a constitutional monarch.

Economic growth in Cambodia has been slowed by civil unrest and regional economic crises. Growth rate is estimated to be 4% annually. Approximately 80% of the population work in agriculture, but tourism is the fastest growing industry. GNP per capita in 1998 was $260, and GDP per capita adjusted for purchasing power parity was approximately $1300 in 2000. Basic infrastructure is poor, particularly in rural areas.

HEALTH AND HEALTHCARE SYSTEM

The infant mortality rate in Cambodia is 90 per 1000 live births, and the life expectancy at birth is 54 years of age (World Bank, 2002). Given its' recent history, Cambodia has a plethora of disadvantaged groups including internally displaced people and returned refugees, war widows, orphans, and people disabled during the war and by land mines. One out of every 384 Cambodians is an amputee, the highest prevalence of this condition in the world (World Bank, 2002).

After nearly 30 years of civil war, Cambodia is in the process of rebuilding its public health infrastructure. Most government health facilities in Cambodia perform poorly, due to lack of funds, inadequate management, and inefficient use of resources (Soeters and Griffith, 2003). Less than half of Cambodia's population has access to safe drinking water while less than a fourth has access to adequate sanitary facilities (Urbani *et al.*, 2002). Cholera is endemic in Cambodia, with the majority of the cholera outbreaks located in Northwestern Cambodia and areas neighboring the capital city of Phnom Penh. Few detailed epidemiological studies have been conducted in Cambodia during cholera outbreaks because the health care sector lacks training in outbreak response and epidemiological methodology. Cambodia conducts surveillance for diseases such as cholera through a nationwide, hospital-based, passive surveillance system. Since 1992, the National Health Information System (NHIS) has collected disease reports from health care facilities throughout the country. NHIS collects information monthly on the incidence and mortality associated with a variety of diseases such as cholera, dengue fever and acute flaccid paralysis. One component of NHIS is an early warning system, which requests health care facilities to report these diseases weekly. In principle, each hospital completes a weekly report and submits it to the operational district, which sends summarized data to the Provincial Health Department. The Health Department then compiles the data by district and sends information to the Ministry of Health. In practice, there are many communication problems with long delays in reporting, and the early warning system has not been effective in detecting or preventing large disease outbreaks. Instead, communications from non-governmental organizations (NGOs) or provincial health advisors have been the first to report many recent disease outbreaks.

There is no laboratory-based surveillance system for epidemic diseases in Cambodia. The National Laboratory, which has just recently been resurrected, does not routinely process samples because of a lack of funding for supplies. Improved surveillance in the near future is not likely given the lack of trained personnel and limitations in funding.

HIV/AIDS Surveillance and Control

The prevalence of HIV among Cambodian adults is estimated to be 1.6% (UNAIDS, 2003a). The epidemic was initially fueled by a burgeoning heterosexual sex industry (Ryan *et al.*, 1998). Prevention efforts focused on increasing protection in sex work and have been very successful. Cambodia has mounted a "100% condom use program" that, with help from sex workers themselves, aims to persuade everyone to use a condom with each sexual encounter (AIDS Wkly Plus, 1999; Cohen, 2003a). "Consistent condom use" has increased and HIV prevalence in brothel-based sex workers has decreased (Wong *et al.*, 2003; Cohen, 2003a). The proportion of men in mobile occupations buying sex has dropped from 76% to 32% (Gorbach *et al.*, 2002), and condom use has doubled over the five years of the study. In 1997, Cambodia's national HIV/AIDS program reported 75.8% of urban police buying sex but that number had dropped to 32% by 2001 (Cohen, 2003a). In spite of a poor public health infrastructure and lack of adequate funding, Cambodia waged a highly effective battle to control the HIV/AIDS crisis.

MYANMAR

Background

Myanmar (formerly Burma), borders China to the north and east, Lao PDR and Thailand to the east, the Bay of Bengal to the south, and India and Bangladesh to the west. It is estimated that there are 50 million people living in Myanmar, but information on population demographic and public health issues remains limited (Chelala, 1998). Only two-thirds of the population is Burmese. The country is divided into seven divisions and seven states. The major religion is Buddhism.

Myanmar gained independence from the United Kingdom in 1948. Since 1962, it has been governed by a military dictatorship, the State Peace and Development Council (known from 1988–1997 as the State Law and Order Restoration Council, or SLORC). Although a national election for a democratic government was held in 1990, the elected Assembly never convened, and the military dictatorship continues to rule the country.

Myanmar has a mixed economy with the state controlling the energy sector, heavy industries, and the rice trade. Estimated GDP per capita adjusted for purchasing power parity was $1500 in 2000. Two-thirds of the populace are in the agricultural sector.

Health and Healthcare System

In 1996, Myanmar's infant mortality rate was 105 per 1000 live births. The life expectancy at birth is 55 years. The major causes of child mortality and morbidity are intestinal and respiratory infections, malaria, malnutrition, and vaccine-preventable diseases. Low birth weight, iodine and vitamin A deficiency diseases, and iron-deficiency anemia are widespread. Cholera outbreaks occur each year, and there are still reported outbreaks of plague.

Like many developing countries, Myanmar faces an enormous task of bringing modern medical care, sanitation standards, and basic health education to a predominantly poor and rural population. The Universal Child Immunization Program, supported by UNICEF, reaches less than 60% of eligible children. The maternal mortality rate is 580 per 100,000 live births; most are related to unsafe abortion. Basic reproductive health care is available only in select areas of the country, and less than 1/4 of women use modern contraception (Chelala, 1998).

The military dictatorship that rules Myanmar has emphasized military spending at the expense of social welfare. United Nations statistics showed that Myanmar spends over 200% more on its military expenditure than for health and education combined (UNAIDS, 2003c). Since the current military junta reasserted direct army rule in 1988, health services have further deteriorated, and universities remained closed for most of the last thirteen years. The United Nations estimated that government spending on health declined from 0.38% GDP in 1995–1996 to 0.17% of GDP in 1999–2000 (Pinheiro, 2002). In terms of overall health system performance, the World Health Organization ranked Myanmar 190th out of 191 countries surveyed (World Health Organization, 2000).

Forty percent of Myanmar's populace has no access to safe water, and 60% lack basic sanitation. The National Health Laboratory is poorly equipped. Since 1991, a handful of international NGOs have begun work in Myanmar. However, the severe and strict regime's controls over health assistance programs discouraged more systematic outside assistance. The country's poor human rights record and the suspected association of the ruling junta with narcotics production and trafficking have hampered access to much-needed foreign aid.

HIV/AIDS Surveillance and Control

The true extent of the HIV/AIDS epidemic in Myanmar remains unclear and high prevalence rates have been disputed by Myanmar's officials (Beyrer *et al.*, 2003). UNAIDS has estimated that 440,000 Burmese are HIV-infected and that there are 14,000 AIDS orphans (UNAIDS, 2003c).

As in neighboring regions, HIV is spread through intravenous heroin use and sexual transmission (AIDSlink, 1993). HIV prevalence is 26.5% in urban sex workers, 91% among IDU near the Chinese border, and 10.6% among pregnant women in one border town (Chelala, 1998). The junta's ceasefire agreements with some ethnic groups promoted the heroin trade in the country's border areas, as well as the larger cities, Mandalay and Rangoon. Sharing needles is common among addicts. Many young women from Myanmar's poorer regions have been sold or coerced into prostitution in wealthier, neighboring countries (Beyrer, 2001; Swaddiwudhipong *et al.*, 1990). Tragically, a large percentage of them become HIV-positive within a few years. The government has taken little action to halt the trafficking of women, and local military officials have been accused of endorsing the trade. Migrant workers who buy sex, mostly miners and loggers, provide the major mode of HIV transmission into the general population.

Although Myanmar offers treatment for IDU, anyone caught with drugs or drug paraphernalia faces imprisonment. Myanmar's law also commits drug users to inpatient treatment facilities. Needles can be purchased in some regions but in more remote areas, they are not available. No distribution or exchange programs exist, despite the established effectiveness of such programs in the control of HIV transmission. Methadone is considered an illegal narcotic by the government, and as such, cannot be used in the drug rehabilitation process. HIV/AIDS public health and treatment programs have been implemented largely by the United Nations and a few other international NGOs. The Joint Program on HIV/AIDS has recently offered a plan to improve care and treatment for infected people and to significantly expand campaigns to prevent transmission from sex and injecting drugs. The plan also will provide studies on harm-reduction programs for IDU to include substitution drugs such as methadone and easy availability of clean injecting needles. Increased condom accessibility and use is also being promoted.

However, the junta remains largely in denial regarding the scale and urgency of Myanmar's AIDS crisis. The press and media in Myanmar are tightly regulated and heavily censored. Myanmar's military also tightly controls the medical community response to the HIV/AIDS epidemic. In this atmosphere, the scarce health education and information about HIV/AIDS are not widely accessible to Myanmar's general population.

CONCLUSIONS

The countries in the Greater Mekong River Region share many similarities with respect to their HIV/AIDS control programs. All have recent histories filled with major conflicts and, as a result, have infrastructures that are ill-equipped to handle major epidemics. Other health and social welfare concerns compete with HIV/AIDS expenditures. Although estimates of HIV prevalence exist for the region, the quality of the data is compromised by the current surveillance systems. With the exception of Myanmar, the movement toward market economies has introduced increased trade, which may have facilitated the spread of infectious diseases. The high levels of poverty, the rapidly changing social fabric, and the accessibility of illicit intravenous drugs have increased the number of people who are at risk for HIV/AIDS. As in other countries in the world, those who are at risk are often sex workers and their clients, as well as IDU. Due to social mores, the degree of homosexual transmission remains speculative.

Control of HIV/AIDS in these countries remains elusive. With the exception of Cambodia, the other countries in the region are single-party states. Social policies are not often dictated by health concerns. Lao PDR has a policy similar to benign neglect, and Myanmar has generally ignored the problem. Vietnam, which initially took an educational approach, has more recently adopted a "social evil" approach to those who are engaging in risky activities. The combination of these policies and the increasing risk of HIV/AIDS spreading in these countries is a combustible mix that will fuel the pandemic.

The example of Cambodia provides some hope. Cambodia successfully curbed the HIV/AIDS spread despite widespread poverty, poor infrastructure, and social stigmatization of those at risk. With governmental policies re-directed towards improving the public health system and committed international assistance, there is hope that the scourge of HIV/AIDS will not join the other disasters that have befallen the people of the Greater Mekong River Region.

REFERENCES

AIDSlink. (1993). Global update: Burma. 23:15.

AIDS Wkly Plus. (1999). Anti-AIDS program to be expanded throughout Cambodia. March 8, 1999.

Beyrer, C. (2001). Shan women and girls and the sex industry in Southeast Asia; Political causes and human rights implications. *Soc Sci Med.* 53:543–550.

Beyrer, C., Razak, M.H., Lisam, K., Chen, J., Lui, W., and Yu, X.F. (2000). Overland heroin trafficking routes and HIV-1 spread in south and south-east Asia. *AIDS* 14:75–83.

Beyrer, C., Razak, M.H., Labrique, A., and Brookmeyer, R. (2003). Assessing the magnitude of the HIV/AIDS epidemic in Burma. *J AIDS* 32:311–317.

Canh, D.G., and Do, T. (1993). General and diarrhea related mortality rates in Vietnamese children. *J Preventive Med Vietnam* 3:38.

CDC News. (2002). The CDC HIV/STD/TB prevention news update: 04/19/02. Centers for Disease Control and Prevention, Atlanta, Georgia.

Chelala, C. (1998). Burma: A country's health in crisis. *Lancet* 352:556.

Cohen, J. (2003a). Asia—the next frontier for HIV/AIDS. Two hard-hit countries offer rare success stories: Thailand and Cambodia. *Science* 301:1658–1662.

Cohen, J. (2003b). HIV and heroin: A deadly international affair: Vietnam. *Science* 301:1657–1658.

Gorbach, P., Sopheab, H., Leng, H.B., and Vonthanak, S. (2002). Sexual behavior among urban sentinel group: Cambodia 2001. National Center for HIV/AIDS, Dermatology and STDs, Ministry of Health, Phnom Penh.

Hien, N.T., Giang, L.T., Binh, P.N., Deville, W., van Ameijden, E.J., and Wolffers, I. (2001). Risk factors of HIV infection and needle sharing among injecting drug users in Ho Chi Minh city, Vietnam. *A J Subst Abuse* 13: 45–58.

Khoat, D.V., West, G.R., Valdiserri, R.O., and Phan, N.T. (2003). Peer education for HIV prevention in the socialist republic of Vietnam: A national assessment. *J Community Health* 28:1–17.

Lonnroth, K., Thuong, L.M., Lambregts, K., Quy, H.T., and Diwan, V.K. (2003). Private tuberculosis care provision associated with poor treatment outcome: Comparative study of a semi-private lung clinic and the NTP in two urban districts in Ho Chi Minh City,

Vietnam. National tuberculosis program. *Int J Tuberc Lung Dis.* 7:165–171.

Matsuda, S. (1994). Health system of Vietnam. *Nipon Koshu Eisei Zasshi* 41:82–94.

Ministry of Labor, War Invalids, and Social Affairs (MOLISA), and UNDCP. (2000). Report on drug abuse situation in Vietnam. UNDCP, Vietnam.

Naraan, D., Patel, R., Schafft, K., Radeacher, A., and Koch-Schulte, S. (2000). *Voices of the poor: Can anyone hear us?* Oxford University Press, New York.

Nguyen, T.H., Hoang, T.L., Pham, K.C., van Ameijden, E.J., Deville, W., and Wolffers, I. (1999). HIV monitoring in Vietnam: System, methodology, and results of sentinel surveillance. *J AIDS* 21:338–346.

Nguyen, V.M., Nguyen, V.T., Huynh, P.L., Dang, D.T., Nguyen, T.H.T., Phan, V.T., Nguyen, T.L., Le, T.L., Ivanoff, B., Gentsch, J.R., Glass, R.I., and the Vietnam Rotavirus Surveillance Network. (2001). The epidemiology and disease burden of rotavirus in Vietnam: Sentinel surveillance at six hospitals. *J Infect Dis.* 183(12):1707–1712.

Okumura, J., Wakai, S., and Umenai, T. (2002). Drug utilisation and self-medication in rural communities in Vietnam. *Soc Sci Med* 54:1875–1886.

Pinheiro, V. (2002). Report of the UN special rapporteur on Burma. United Nations, New York.

Pisani, E., Lazzari, S., Walker, N., and Schwartlander, B. (2003). HIV surveillance: A global perspective. *J AIDS* 32:S3–S11.

Piyasirisilp, S., McCutchan, F.E., Carr, J.K., Sanders-Buell, E., Liu, W., Chen, J., Wagner, R., Wolf, H., Shao, Y., Lai, S., Beyrer, C., and Yu, X.F. (2000). A recent outbreak of human immunodeficiency virus type 1 infection in southern China was initiated by two highly homogeneous, geographically separated strains, circulating recombinant form AE and a novel BC recombinant. *J Virol.* 74: 11286–11295.

Quan, V.M., Chung, A., Long, H.T., and Dondero, T.J. (2000). HIV in Vietnam: The evolving epidemic and the prevention response, 1996 through 1999. *J. AIDS* 25:360–369.

Ryan, C.A., Vathiny, O.V., Gorbach, P.M., Leng, H.B., Berlioz-Arthaud, A., Whittington, W.L., and Holmes K.K. (1998). Explosive spread of HIV-1 and sexually transmitted diseases in Cambodia. *Lancet* 351:1175.

Sarrel, M., Kloser, P., Correll, P., and Bean-Mayberry, B. (1996). The increase of HIV infection in Vietnam: Describing the epidemic for program planning. In: Int. Conf. AIDS, Vancouver, British Columbia. p. 144.

Sepehri, A., Chernomas, R., and Akram-Lodhi, A.H. (2003). If they get sick, they are in trouble: Health care restructuring, user charges and equity in Vietnam. *Int J Health Serv.* 33:137–161.

Soeters, R., and Griffith, F. (2003). Improving government health services through contract management: A case from Cambodia. *Health Policy Plan.* 18:74–83.

Swaddiwudhipong, W., Chaovakiratipong, C., Siri, S., and Lerdlukanavonge, P. (1990). Sociodemographic characteristics and incidence of gonorrhoea in prostitutes working near the Thai-Burmese border. *Southeast Asian J Trop Med Public Health* 21:45–52.

Tran, C.L. (2000). Harm reduction to prevent HIV/AIDS in injecting drug users in Vietnam: Dificulties and direction. In: Policy Forum on Harm Reduction to prevent HIV/AIDS in infecting drug users, Hanoi.

UNAIDS. (2002). Report on the global HIV/AIDS epidemic 2002, UNAIDS, Geneva.

UNAIDS. (2003a). Cambodia. http://www.unaids.org/eng/geographical+area/by+country/cambodia.asp. accessed 10/09/03.

UNAIDS. (2003b). Lao PDR. http://www.unaids.org/eng/geographical+area/by+country/lao+pdr.asp. accessed 10/09/03.

UNAIDS. (2003c). Myanmar. http://www.unaids.org/eng/geographical+area/by+country/myanmar.asp. accessed 10/09/03.

United Nations Development Program. (2003). Vietnam. UNDP, New York, http://www.undp.org.vn/undp/fact/base.htm. accessed 10/09/03.

United States Department of State. Bureau of Public Affairs, (USDSBPA) 1987. Cambodia. Backgr Notes Ser April: 1–11.

Urbani, C., Sinoun, M., Socheat, D., Pholsena, K., Strandgaard, H., Odermatt, P., and Hatz, C. (2002). Epidemiology and control of mekongi schistosomiasis. *Acta Trop.* 82:157–168.

USAID. (2003). Country profile: Cambodia No. 2003. USAID, Washington, DC.

Van Duong, B., Binns, C.W., and Van Le, T. (1997). Availability of antibioticscs as over-the-counter drugs in pharmacies: A threat to public health in Vietnam. *Trop Med Int Health* 2:1133–1139.

Wong, M.L., Lubek, I., Dy, B.C., Pen, S., Kros, S., and Chhit, M. (2003). Social and behavioural factors associated with condom use among direct sex workers in Siem Reap, Cambodia. *Sex Transm Infect.* 79:163–165.

World Bank. (2001). Vietnam: Growing healthy: A review of Vietnam's health sector, (June 2001), World Bank, Hanoi.

World Bank. (2003a). Cambodia at a Glance (August 20 2003); http://www.worldbank.org/data/countrydata/aag/khm_aag.pdf; updated 8/20/03, accessed (10/09/03).

World Bank. (2003b). World Development Indicators. Database.http://www.worldbank.org/databytopic/GNIPC.pdf. accessed 1/18/04.

World Bank, the World Bank Group. (2002). *Country brief. Cambodia.* World Bank, Cambodia.

World Health Organization. (2000). World health report 2000, World Health Organization, Geneva. http://w3.whosea.org/healthreport/pdf/whr2000 content.htm. accessed 10/09/03.

World Health Organization. (2001). Vietnam. www.who.int/country/vnm/en. accessed 10/09/03.

World Health Organization. (2003a). Severe acute respiratory syndrome: Status of the outbreak and lessons for the immediate future, WHO, Geneva.

World Health Organization. (2003b). WHO Global Salmonella Surveillance 2003. http://www.who.int/salmsurv. accessed 10/09/03.

Yu, X.F., Chen, J., Shao, Y., Beyrer, C., Liu, B., Wang, Z., Liu, W., Yang, J., Liang, S., Viscidi, R.P., Gu, J., Gurri-Glass, G., and Lai, S. (1999). Emerging HIV infections with distinct subtypes of HIV-1 infection among injection drug users from geographically separate locations in Guangxi province, China. *J AIDS*. 22:180–188.

Zola, A.M. (1994). Laos: Rural economy threatened by AIDS. AIDSlink: 5–6.

5

Update on HIV/AIDS in Japan, 2003

Tadashi Nakasone, Takashi Hara, Naoto Yoshino, and Mitsuo Honda

AIDS Research Center, National Institute of Infectious Diseases, Tokyo, Japan

INTRODUCTION

In Japan, the first case of HIV-1 infection was discovered in 1983 (Miyoshi *et al.*, 1983) and incidence continued to increase among Japanese hemophiliacs through 1985 by repeated inoculations of coagulation factor products VIII and IX imported from the United States into Japan. Approximately 2000 hemophiliacs were estimated to be infected with HIV, demonstrating a 40% infectivity rate of HIV among a total of 5000 hemophiliacs treated with the contaminated blood products. Furthermore, 12 non-hemophiliacs were retrospectively defined to be infected with HIV-1 (hereafter referred to simply as HIV) by their treatment with the contaminated products.

Surveillance of HIV/AIDS in Japan began in 1984 on a voluntary basis and become mandatory by the AIDS Prevention Law in 1989. According to this law, all HIV-positive individuals except those infected through the use of coagulation factor products are to be reported to the National AIDS Surveillance Committee, Ministry of Health and Welfare, as the repository of National HIV/AIDS Surveillance in Japan. Six AIDS patients were initially reported in 1985 and 55 HIV-positive individuals were detected in 1987. The number of HIV/AIDS cases has since increased every year. As of October 28, 2003, 5573 HIV infections had been reported, along with 2776 cases of AIDS, for a total of 8349 reported cases. This number translates to 4.05 HIV cases and 2.014 AIDS patients per 100,000 population in Japan (Infectious Disease Surveillance Center, 2003). Since sexual behavior among young people has been changing, there is concern over the prediction that the number of HIV-positive individuals may reach 100,000 by the end of the year 2010 (Kihara, 2003).

INITIAL DETECTION OF HIV IN JAPAN

The first report of HIV infection was detected in a non-hemophiliac co-infected with adult T cell leukemia virus in 1983 (Miyoshi *et al.*, 1983), followed by the identification of two additional AIDS cases and one HIV infection in Japan (Aoki *et al.*, 1984; Kobayashi

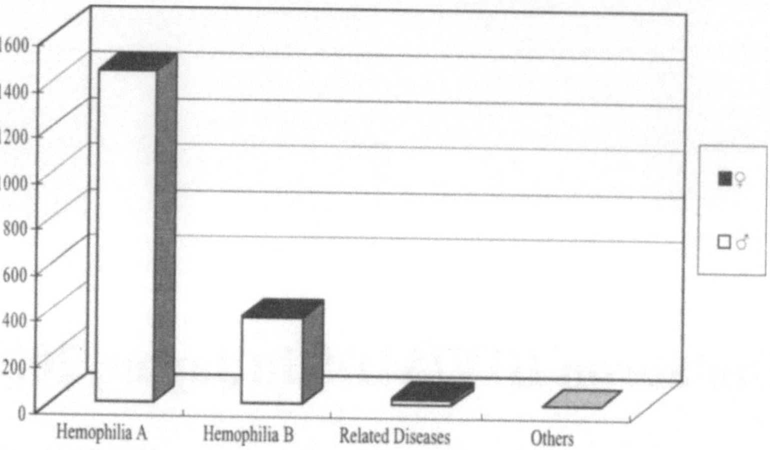

FIGURE 1. Total numbers of HIV-positive hemophiliacs treated with coagulant factor products prior to May 1996 in Japan. HIV-infected individuals treated with coagulant factors were categorized into 4 groups: hemophilia A, hemophilia B, related diseases, and others.

et al., 1984), suggesting that there had already existed an unidentified HIV-1 reservoir among non-hemophiliacs prior to 1983.

Since hemophiliacs seropositive for HIV had been reported in the United States from 1982, Abe *et al.* (1985) screened 50 samples of sera from Japanese hemophiliacs in collaboration with Dr. Robert Gallo of the US National Cancer Institute and the National Institutes of Health in 1985. Surprisingly, 46% (23 hemophiliacs) were seropositive for HIV, including two hemophiliacs who had developed AIDS (Abe *et al.*, 1985). These hemophiliacs had been injected with imported and domestic coagulant factor VIII or IX for over six years. Based on these results, researchers recommended preparation of virus-free blood products for the prevention of HIV infection.

To establish a profile of HIV infection among hemophiliacs in Japan, the National Survey for HIV-positive Hemophiliacs began in 1987 (Yamada, 1996). Through May of 1996, 1862 hemophiliacs had been defined as HIV-positive; 1448 cases were among hemophilia A patients, and 382 cases were among hemophilia B patients (Figure 1). In 1996, 630 cases (33.7%) progressed to AIDS—33.4% of the hemophilia A patients and 35.1% of the hemophilia B patients; approximately 70% of the cases from both groups died until the same year (Figure 2).

The hemophiliac population provided an opportunity to study and identify the risk factors for HIV infection and its disease progression. Interestingly, the rate of long-term non-progressor status (more than 10-years maintenance of $CD4^+$ T-cells above 500 cells/mm^3) was as high as 14% among HIV-infected Japanese hemophiliacs (Yamada, 1996).

SURVEILLANCE OF HIV IN NON-HEMOPHILIACS IN JAPAN

Since HIV was not detected in hemophiliacs treated with coagulant factor products after 1986, due to the increased safety concern of the blood supply, the National AIDS Surveillance Committee examined analyses of reported cases of HIV infection and released its updated HIV/AIDS surveillance information twice per year.

In the most recent report in 2003 (Infectious Disease Surveillance Center, 2003), newly reported HIV infections and AIDS cases numbered 614 and 308, respectively (Figure 3A), and Japanese males dominated

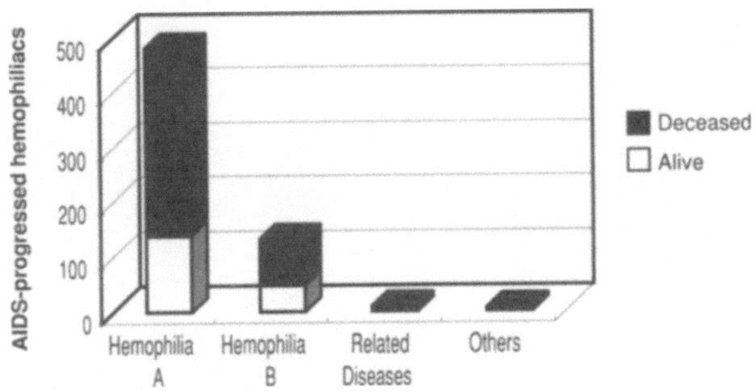

FIGURE 2. Total numbers of AIDS-progressed hemophiliacs treated with coagulant factor products prior to May 1996 in Japan. Deaths are shown in black.

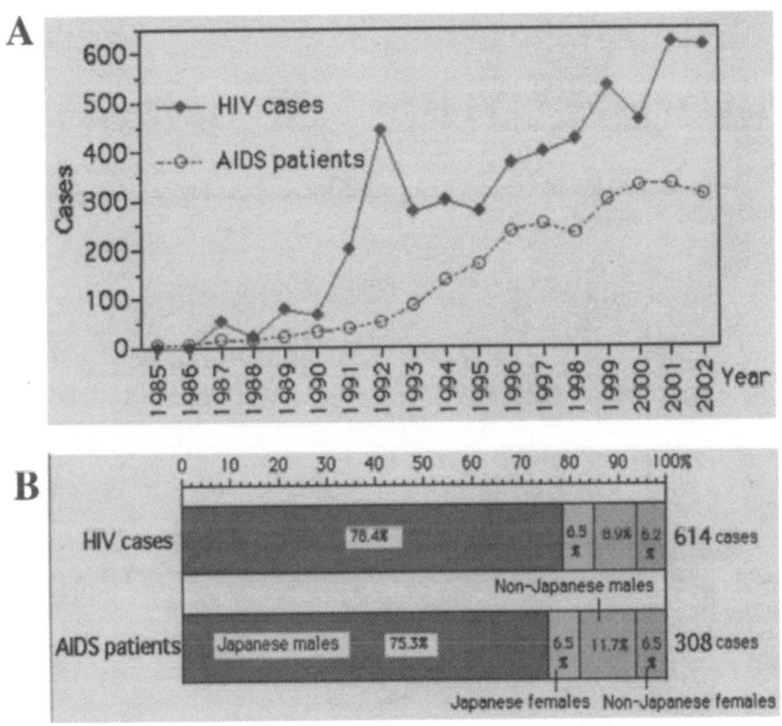

FIGURE 3. Increase of HIV/AIDS incidence in Japan. Increase of annual incidence of HIV/AIDS from 1985 to 2002 **(A)**. HIV and AIDS cases in 2002 by gender and Japanese nationality **(B)**. Japanese males predominated among both HIV-positive individuals and people with AIDS in 2002. Non-Japanese represented 15.1% of HIV-positive non-hemophiliac individuals and 18.7% of people with AIDS in 2002 (MHLW, 2002; NIID, 2003).

both of these groups, 78% and 75%, respectively (Figure 3B).

HIV infections among Japanese males have been continuously increasing; cases among Japanese females are also increasing but the total number has been less than 50 per year (Figure 4). It is important to note that HIV infections among Japanese men who have sex with men (MSM) are rapidly increasing (Figures 4 to 5). Cases among non-Japanese males are gradually increasing, and cases among non-Japanese females peaked

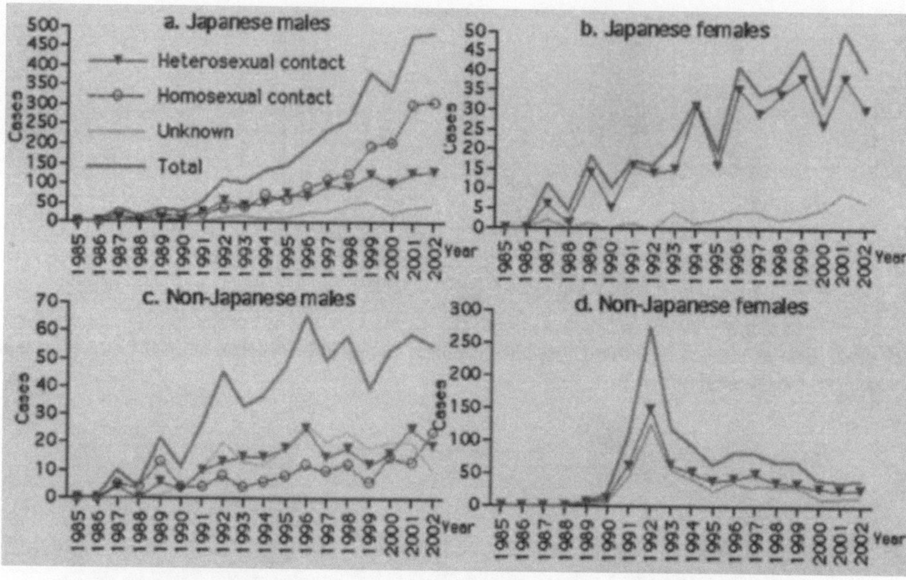

FIGURE 4. Study of the increase of HIV incidence by nationality, gender, and mode of infection from 1985 to 2002 in Japan (MHLW, 2002; NIID, 2003).

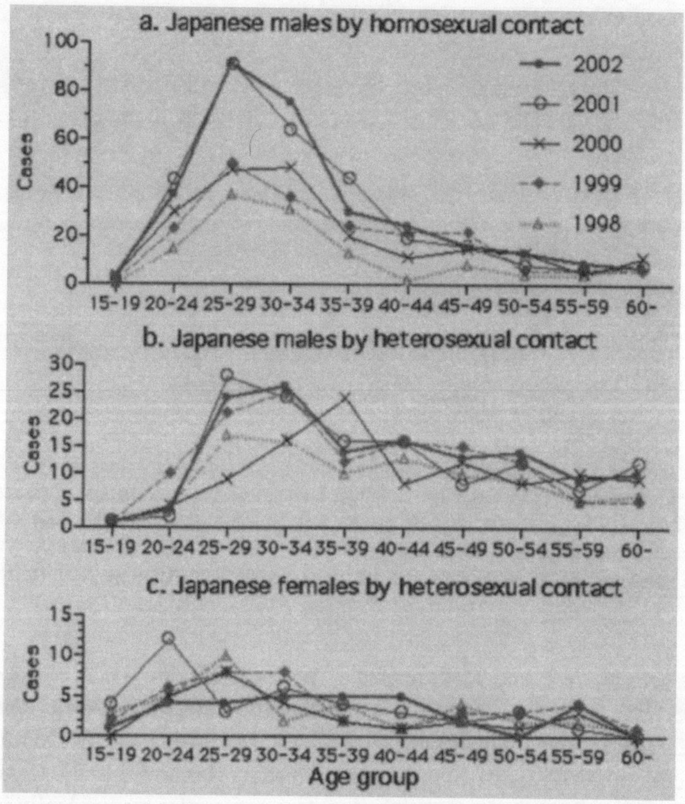

FIGURE 5. Age distribution analysis of HIV incidence by gender and mode of infection from 1998 to 2002 in Japan (MHLW, 2002; NIID, 2003).

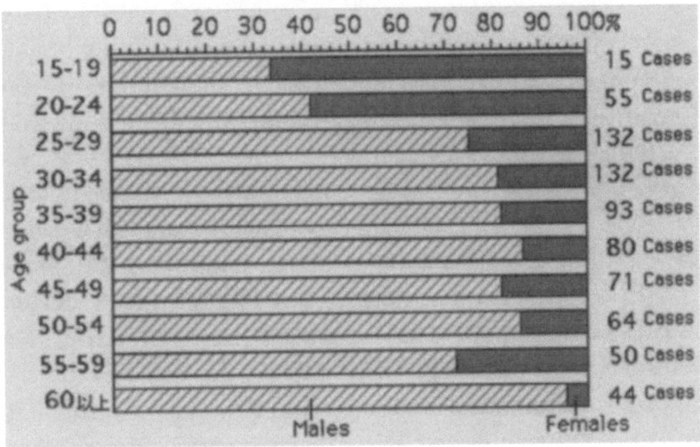

FIGURE 6. Distribution of heterosexual HIV infections by gender and age group, 1998–2002. Japanese females predominated among young HIV-positive Japanese contracting HIV by heterosexual contact from 1998 to 2002. Ten age categories were created to cover ages 15 to over 60 (MHLW, 2002; NIID, 2003).

in 1992, but the percentage of non-Japanese in the total of HIV cases is more than 18%, higher than that of other countries.

HIV infections are considered to be mainly due to sexual transmission among Japanese males in Japan (Figures 5 and 6). Although the prevalence is low as described above, heterosexually acquired HIV has been rapidly increasing since the early 1990s in Japan (Umeda, 1999).

Interestingly, the first HIV-antibody-positive case among blood donors was detected in 1987, and the positive rate per 100,000 donations increased to 1.368 (2.259 in males and 0.043 in females) in 2001, a rate approximately 10–100 times higher than that of European and American countries (Figure 7). Contaminated blood was found in 67, 79, and 82 donors in 2000, 2001, and 2002, respectively; six infections were detected by nucleic acid test with PCR detection. These data suggest the need for careful evaluation of whether HIV-positive blood donors may be more likely to donate blood frequently for the purpose of HIV testing, as speculated, or whether HIV may truly be spreading vigorously in Japan.

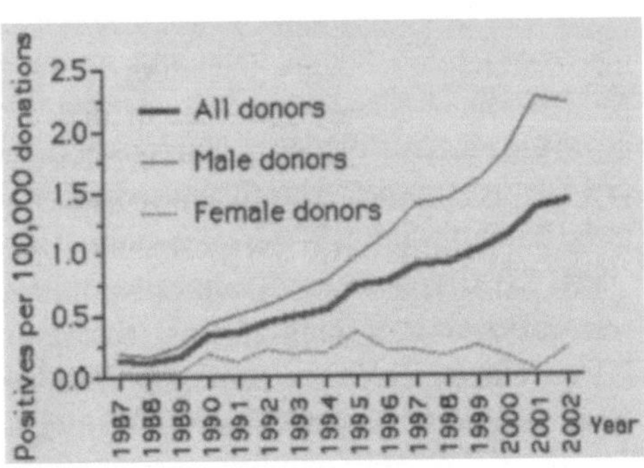

FIGURE 7. Rate of HIV-antibody positives per 100,000 blood donors, 1987–2002. HIV infections among blood donors were rapidly increasing from 1987 to 2002, at a rate much higher than that of European countries. Numbers of HIV-positive blood donors detected in 2000, 2001 and 2002 were 67, 79, and 82, respectively, and only 6 of 228 positives were detected by the nucleic acid amplification test (MHLW, 2002; NIID, 2003).

PHENOTYPIC CHARACTERIZATION OF HIV IN JAPAN

The molecular epidemiology of HIV in Southeast Asian countries has been well characterized by studying this unique geographical hot spot, where extensive recombination events appear to be ongoing. These events suggests the presence of highly exposed individuals and social networks of HIV transmission (Motomura *et al.*, 2003; Takebe *et al.*, 2003; Weniger *et al.*, 1994; Yang *et al.*,

2003). In Japan, hemophiliacs who received frequent transfusions of HIV-contaminated blood products comprised the largest population of HIV-positive cases until 1998 (Kamakura *et al.*, 1998). The HIV-1s detected in the hemophiliacs were all HIV-1 clade B; the major HIV clade circulating in Japan has also been identified as clade B by genotypic analysis of HIV-1 *env* C2-V3 region (Hattori *et al.*, 1991; Yamanaka *et al.* 1997). However, the National Survey of HIV/AIDS in 1999 found sexual transmission to be a major risk factor in the population of HIV-positive individuals in Japan. During the rapid increase in sexually transmitted HIV infections in Japan, which took place from 1996 to 1998, 40% of the HIV-positive individuals infected via MSM contact were grouped into subtype E. Others were subtype B, including Japanese males infected by heterosexual contact with multiple partners both abroad and in Japan (Kitsutani *et al.*, 1998). Furthermore, a replication-competent molecular clone of HIV-1 was isolated from an HIV-1 NH1 isolate in Japan as an CRF01_AE strain, and the infectious molecular clone was designated p93JP-NH1 (Kusagawa *et al.*, 2002). Further epidemiological research of HIV in Japan has detected a gradual shift toward an increase with predominantly heterosexual and MSM contact. (Infectious Disease Surveillance Center, 2003). Apart from subtypes B and E, other HIV-1 subtypes A, C, D, and G, and HIV-2 have also been sporadically found in Japan (Hara *et al.*, 2001; Kusagawa *et al.*, 2003; Nakasone *et al.*, 1998). Efforts to isolate infectious clones of various HIV subtypes continue to define the HIV phenotypes spreading in the field (Mochizuki *et al.*, 1999).

ANTI-HIV CHEMOTHERAPY IN JAPAN

Between 1988 and 1999, HIV was isolated from 614 HIV-positive individuals out of a total of 2785 cases. During those 11 years, annual HIV isolation rates were found to decrease, reflecting the success of anti-HIV chemotherapy with single, double, and triple combinations of antiretroviral drugs (Figure 8) (Nakamura *et al.*, 1987).

In 1997, three protease inhibitors, Saquinavir, Ritonavir, and Indinavir, became available for clinical use in Japan, and highly active antiretroviral therapy (HAART) began being used for treatment of people with HIV/AIDS (PLWHA) in Japan. Among 446 cases, 87 (60.0%) out of 145 naïve cases and 150 (49.8%) out of 301 drug-treatment-experienced cases showed a reduction of plasma viral load to undetectable levels. Successful therapy with HAART was maintained for more than twelve months among 50% of the medicated patients (Oishi *et al.*, 1999). The prevalence of emerging drug resistance-related mutations has been systematically monitored to evaluate the efficacy of HAART in Japan (Sugiura, 2001; Sugiura *et al.*, 1999).

VERTICAL TRANSMISSION OF HIV IN JAPAN

A national collaborative group for studying vertical transmission of HIV in pregnant women and their infants was established by Dr. Ryozo Totani in Japan in 1989. Through this research, 42 infants, including 13 HIV-positive, 25 HIV-negative, four of undetermined status, and 15 control children born to HIV-positive mothers were diagnosed and followed from birth to 1.5 years (Yoshino *et al.*, 1998). All strains from HIV-positive infants were either clade E (eight infants, 61.5%) or B (five infants, 38.5%) according to DNA sequencing specific for the HIV-1 C2-V3 region. The 42 HIV-positive mothers were women with sexual risk behaviors from all regions, but were concentrated in the Kanto District. In this group of HIV-positive children, there was no significant difference between the transmissibility of their mother's clade E and B viruses. Eight (61.5%) of the 13 HIV-positive babies were Japanese and five (62.5%) of the

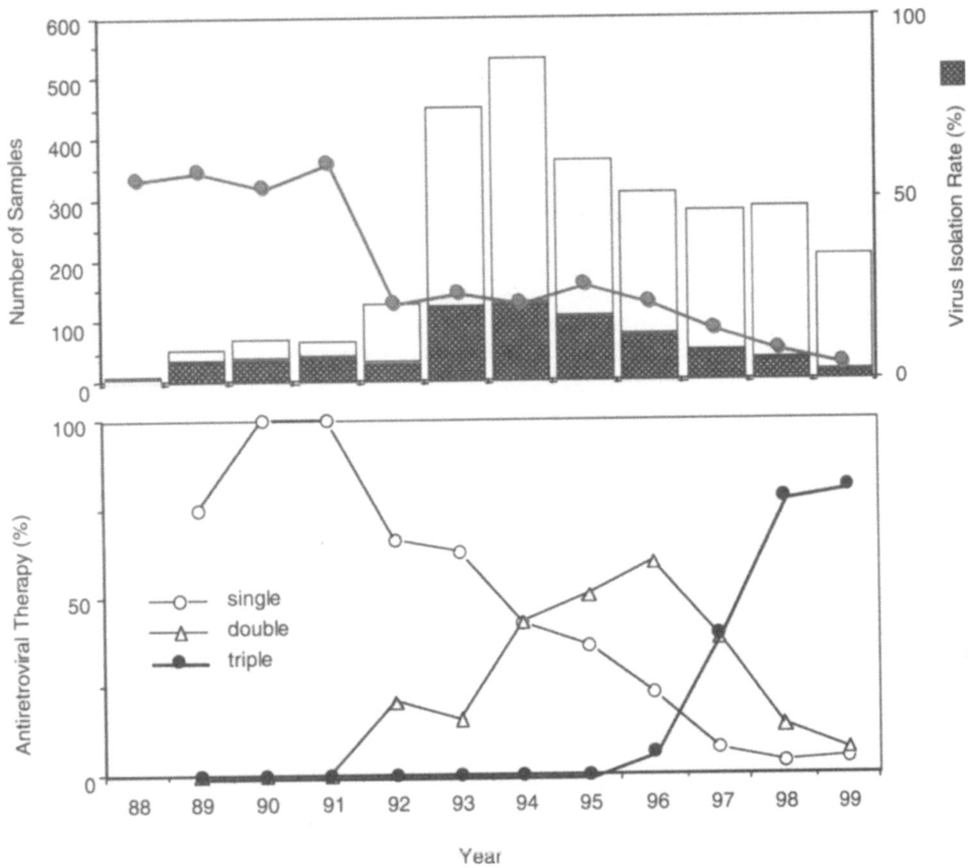

FIGURE 8. Viral isolation rate and antiretroviral therapy coverage, 1988–1999. Decline in the HIV-1 isolation rate in Japan may correspond to anti-HIV chemotherapy. Upper panel: light and dark dotted bars indicate the total number of samples, and sample numbers positive for HIV-1 isolation, respectively. Bold line indicates the kinetics of the rate of HIV-1 isolation. Lower panel: open circle, open triangle and closed circle lines indicate percentage of patients treated with single, double, and triple anti-HIV chemotherapies, respectively.

eight were positive for HIV-1 clade E. The V3 loop region of the clade E virus of the babies was conserved, but approximately 60% of the sequences showed a substitution of aspartic acid by asparagine at position 29. These results suggest that HIV clade E may be predominant in cases of vertical transmission and are phenotypically different from HIV in persons with various other risk behaviors in Japan. Prevention efforts against vertical transmission have been quite successfully undertaken through a combination of Caesarian-section deliveries and chemotherapy during the delivery stage.

REFERENCES

Abe, T., Kinoshita, T., Matsuda, J., Ryu, T., Ting, R.C., Aoki, T., Robert-Guroff, M., Miyakoshi, H., Gallo, R.C. (1985). Detection of antibodies to HTLV-I and -III in sera from Japanese hemophiliacs. *Cancer Res.* 45:4621s–4623s.

Aoki, T., Miyakoshi, H., Usuda, Y., Chermann, J.C., Barre-Sinoussi, F., Ting, R.C., Gallo, R.C. (1984). Antibodies to HTLV I and III in sera from two Japanese patients, one with possible pre-AIDS. *Lancet* 2:936–937.

Hara, T., Yoshino, N., Takayama, N., Minamitani, M., Naganawa, S., Ohkubo, H., Takizawa, M., Izumi, Y., Kantake, M., Suzuki, S., Takano, M., Kita, T., Totani, R., Nagai, Y., Honda, M., Nakasone, T:

(2001). Presence of multiple HIV type 1 subtypes among mothers and children in Japan. *AIDS Res Hum Retroviruses* 17:569–575.

Hattori, T., Shiozaki, K., Eda, Y., Tokiyoshi, S., Matsushita, S., Inaba, H., Fujimaki, M., Meguro, T., Yamada, K., Honda, M., *et al.* (1991). Characteristics of the principal neutralizing determinant of HIV-1 prevalent in Japan. *AIDS Res Hum Retroviruses* 7:825–830.

National Institute of Infectious Diseases (NIID). (2003). HIV/AIDS in Japan, 2002. Infectious Agent Surveillance Report 24:203–204. Infectious Disease Surveillance Center, Tokyo.

Kamakura, M., Soda, K., Hashimoto, S., Morio, S., Kitamura, T. (1998). A consideration on the current epidemic of HIV infection in Japan and the problems in the prediction of its future. Proceedings of Japan-U.S. Cooperative Medical Science Program 9:21–22.

Kihara, M. (2003, October 1). Epidemiological surveillance in Japan and enlightenment for HIV prevention. Proceedings of UNAIDS; Dr. Peter Piot welcoming symposium. Tokyo, Japan.

Kitsutani, P.T., Naganawa, S., Shiino, T., Matsuda, M., Honda, M., Yamada, K., Taki, M., Sugiura, W. (1998). HIV type 1 subtypes of nonhemophiliac patients in Japan. *AIDS Res Hum Retroviruses* 14:1099–1103.

Kobayashi, M., Yoshimoto, S., Fujishita, M., Yano, S., Niiya, K., Kubonishi, I., Taguchi, H., Miyoshi, I. (1984). HTLV-positive T-cell lymphoma/leukaemia in an AIDS patient. *Lancet* 1:1361–1362.

Kusagawa, S., Imamura, A., Yasuoka, A., Hoshino, H., Oka, S., Takebe, Y. (2003). Identification of HIV type 2 subtype B transmission in East Asia. *AIDS Res Hum Retroviruses* 19:1045–1049.

Kusagawa, S., Sato, H., Tomita, Y., Tatsumi, M., Kato, K., Motomura, K., Yang, R., Takebe, Y. (2002). Isolation and characterization of replication-competent molecular DNA clones of HIV type 1 CRF01_AE with different coreceptor usages. *AIDS Res Hum Retroviruses* 18:115–122.

Ministry of Health, Labor and Welfare (MHLW) Japan. (2002). Annual Report on HIV/AIDS Surveillance in Japan, the National Surveillance Committee.

Miyoshi, I., Kobayashi, M., Yoshimoto, S., Fujishita, M., Taguchi, H., Kubonishi, I., Ohtsuki, Y. (1983). ATLV in Japanese patient with AIDS. *Lancet* 2:275.

Mochizuki, N., Otsuka, N., Matsuo, K., Shiino, T., Kojima, A., Kurata, T., Sakai, K., Yamamoto, N., Isomura, S., Dhole, T.N., Takebe, Y., Matsuda, M., Tatsumi, M. (1999). An infectious DNA clone of HIV type 1 subtype C. *AIDS Res Hum Retroviruses* 15:1321–1324.

Motomura, K., Kusagawa, S., Lwin, H.H., Thwe, M., Kato, K., Oishi, K., Yamamoto, N., Zaw, M., Nagatake, T., Takebe, Y. (2003). Different subtype distributions in two cities in Myanmar: Evidence for independent clusters of HIV-1 transmission. *AIDS* 17:633–636.

Nakamura, K., Yoshida, Y., Ando, T., Yamazaki, K., Ohnuki, N., Ito, T., Yano, K., Sekine, S., Hayashi, Y., Sinkai, T., *et al.* (1987). A serological survey for human immunodeficiency virus types 1 and 2 of individuals who visited health centers in Tokyo. *Jpn J Med Sci Biol.* 40:159–164.

Nakasone, T., Totani, R., Yamazki, S., Honda, M. (1998). HIV-1 subtype A in Japan. *AIDS* 12:950–952.

National Institute of Infectious Diseases (NIID) Japan (year). Infectious Agents Surveillance Report (IASR).

Oishi, T., Sugiura, W., Matsuda, M., Abumi, H., Okano, A., Yamada, K., Koike, M., Taki, M., Ishikawa, M., Miura, T., Fukutake, K., Gouchi, K., Ajisawa, A., Iwamoto, A., Hanabusa, H., Mimaya, J., Takamatsu, J., Takata, N., Kakishita, E., Higasa, S., Yoshioka, A., Kashiwagi, S., Shirahata, A., Nagai, Y. (1999). Status of anti-HIV-1 chemotherapy in Japan. *Jpn J Infect Dis.* 52:51–52.

Sugiura, W. (2001). Effect of introduction of highly active antiretroviral treatment and the changes in patterns of drug-resistant HIV-1 in Japan. *J Infect Chemother.* 7:127–132.

Sugiura, W., Matsuda, M., Abumi, H., Yamada, K., Taki, M., Ishikawa, M., Miura, T., Fukutake, K., Gouchi, K., Ajisawa, A., Iwamoto, A., Hanabusa, H., Mimaya, J., Takamatsu, J., Takada, N., Kakishita, E., Yoshioka, A., Kashiwagi, S., Shirahata, A., Nagai, Y. (1999). Prevalence of drug resistance-related mutations among HIV-1s in Japan. *Jpn J Infect Dis.* 52:21–22.

Takebe, Y., Motomura, K., Tatsumi, M., Lwin, H.H., Zaw, M., Kusagawa, S. (2003). High prevalence of diverse forms of HIV-1 intersubtype recombinants in Central Myanmar: Geographical hot spot of extensive recombination. *AIDS* 17:2077–2087.

Takeda, A., Igarashi, H., Nakamura, H., Kano, M., Iida, A., Hirata, T., Hasegawa, M., Nagai, Y., Matano, T. (2003). Protective efficacy of an AIDS vaccine, a single DNA priming followed by a single booster with a recombinant replication-defective Sendai virus vector, in a macaque AIDS model. *J Virol.* 77:9710–9715.

Umeda, T. (1999). Increase in heterosexually acquired AIDS among Japanese, 1986 to 1996. *Jpn J Infect Dis.* 52:167–168.

Weniger, B.G., Takebe, Y., Ou, C.Y., Yamazaki, S. (1994). The molecular epidemiology of HIV in Asia. *AIDS* 8 Suppl 2:S13–S28.

Yamada, K. (1996). Annual report on AIDS prevention and clinical control. *Proceedings of HIV/AIDS Prevention and Therapy* 10:1–360.

Yamanaka, T., Fujimura, Y., Ishimoto, S., Yoshioka, A., Konishi, M., Narita, N., Mimaya, J., Meguro, T., Nakasone, T., Okamoto, Y., Yoshizaki, H., Yamada, K., Honda, M. (1997). Correlation of titer of antibody to principal neutralizing domain of HIVMN strain with disease progression in Japanese hemophiliacs seropositive for HIV type 1. *AIDS Res Hum Retroviruses* 13:317–326.

Yang, R., Kusagawa, S., Zhang, C., Xia, X., Ben, K., Takebe, Y. (2003). Identification and characterization of a new class of human immunodeficiency virus type 1 recombinants comprised of two circulating recombinant forms, CRF07_BC and CRF08_BC, in China. *J. Virol.* 77:685–695.

Yoshino, N., Naganawa, S., Nakasone, T., Imura, S., Kita, T., Honda, M. (1998). Vertical transmission of human immunodeficiency virus type 1 in Japan, 1989–1997: Presence of two subtypes B and E with subtype E predominance. National Cooperative Study Investigators on Vertical Transmission of HIV-1. *Acta Paediatr Jpn.* 40: 503–509.

6

HIV/AIDS in Malaysia

Marina Mahathir

Malaysian AIDS Council, Kuala Lumpur, Malaysia

INTRODUCTION

Malaysia recorded its first case of HIV in 1985 and responded immediately by forming an InterMinisterial Committee on HIV/AIDS, aided by a Technical Committee and a National Coordinating Committee on HIV/AIDS. Since then, largely through mandatory testing of drug users in rehabilitation centers, prisoners, and blood donors, the number of infections reported to the Ministry of Health (MoH) has risen steadily. (All confirmed cases are reported to the MoH) In 2002, 6,978 new cases of HIV infection were recorded, the highest annual figure ever, bringing a cumulative total of 51,256 cases by the end of December 2002 (Ministry of Health, Malaysia, 2002). These statistics are based on reported cases, not estimates. The MoH, however, estimates that actual numbers are twice the numbers of reported cases. It is not clear how this is derived.

Young people at their prime age (20–39 years) make up 80.1% of HIV infections in the country. 76.3% of the transmission continues to be through sharing needles while injecting drugs, followed by unprotected sex (13.8%). Only 0.7% and 0.05% of the infections are attributed to vertical transmission and blood transfusion, respectively. Women with HIV are still relatively few in number. However, in the last ten years, there has been a worrisome, steady rise in the number of women infected from none in 1991 to 698 in 2001.

The government's antenatal testing program detected 306 HIV-positive pregnant women since 1998 (Ministry of Health, Malaysia, 2002), which indicates that most women detected did not come from this program. Since the MoH antenatal screening program began in 1998, 1,066,507 pregnant women have been tested for HIV, out of which 306 (0.03%) were found HIV-positive and provided with zidovudine treatment to prevent transmission to their babies. In 2002, out of 359,411 pregnant mothers, or 92.2% of all mothers attending government antenatal clinics, 141 (.039%) were found to be HIV-positive. From these, only five babies born to 110 mothers in the program were HIV-positive.

The use of mandatory testing in government-run drug rehabilitation centers and in prisons creates a bias in the statistics towards drug users, men and ethnic Malays (Malaysian National Drug Agency, Ministry

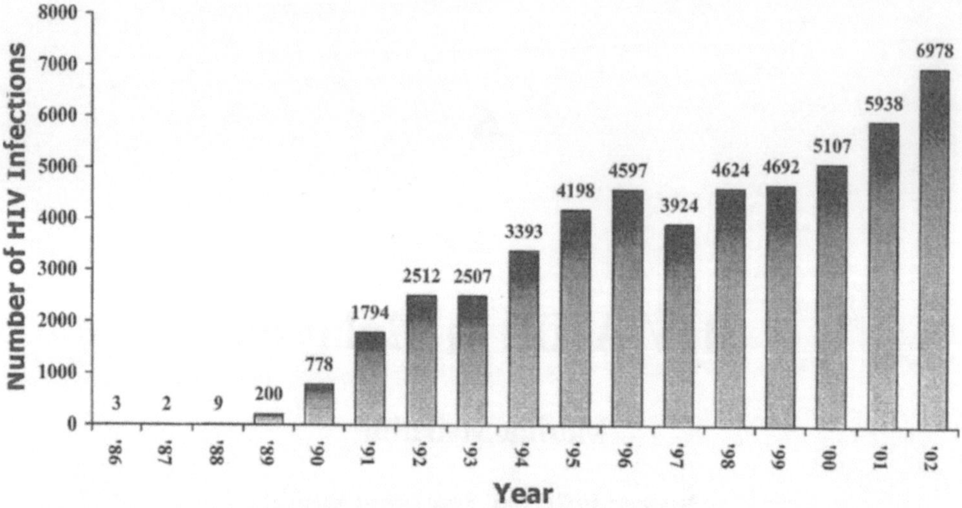

FIGURE 1. Number of Reported HIV Infections in Malaysia (1986–2002). (Ministry of Health, Malaysia)

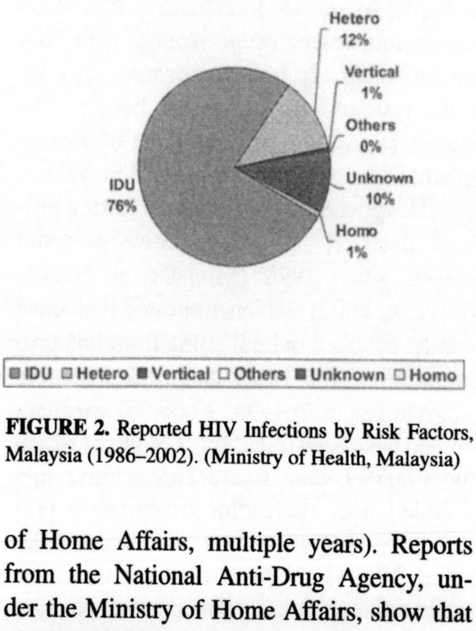

FIGURE 2. Reported HIV Infections by Risk Factors, Malaysia (1986–2002). (Ministry of Health, Malaysia)

of Home Affairs, multiple years). Reports from the National Anti-Drug Agency, under the Ministry of Home Affairs, show that an overwhelming majority of drug users in Malaysia are male and of ethnic Malay origin. Reasons for this are unclear.

Mandatory screening of drug users in government rehabilitation centres results not only in bias towards Malay males but also early detection of HIV. However, among AIDS cases, not only is there a higher proportion of those infected through sexual transmission, but ethnic distribution matches almost exactly the proportions of the major ethnic groups of Malays, Chinese and Indians in the general Malaysian population. This indicates that no particular ethnic group is more vulnerable to HIV infection than others although Malays who take drugs seem to be at higher risk.

Sexual transmission is an important route, as shown by the number of late-presenting cases being seen by doctors. The government has recently instituted a nationwide anonymous testing program after a pilot project in Johor state and it is hoped that this will give a better indication of the epidemic. The Ministry of Health is also carrying out behavioral studies among drug users and sex workers with the assistance of the World Health Organization (WHO) in order to ascertain risk factors among vulnerable groups.

In terms of treatment, Malaysia is providing more than most countries in the region. All People Living with HIV/AIDS (PLWHA) are entitled to one free drug in government hospitals, either zidovudine (AZT) or stavudine (D4T), but they would have to pay for the other needed drugs. Treatments for opportunistic infections are free or of minimal cost at government hospitals. Certain

TABLE 1. Screening of Inmates in Drug Rehabilitation Centers (*Pusat Serenti*) and Prisons, 2001 and 2002

	Pusat Serenti		Prisons		Total	
Year	2001	2002	2001	2002	2001	2002
No. Drug Users Screened for HIV	8,823	12,170	27,591	46,980	36,414	59,150
No. of HIV-Positive	1,448	2,004	3,275	4,342	4,728	6,346
Rate of Positivity (%)	16.4	16.5	11.9	9.2	12.8	10.7

Source: Ministry of Home Affairs, Malaysia

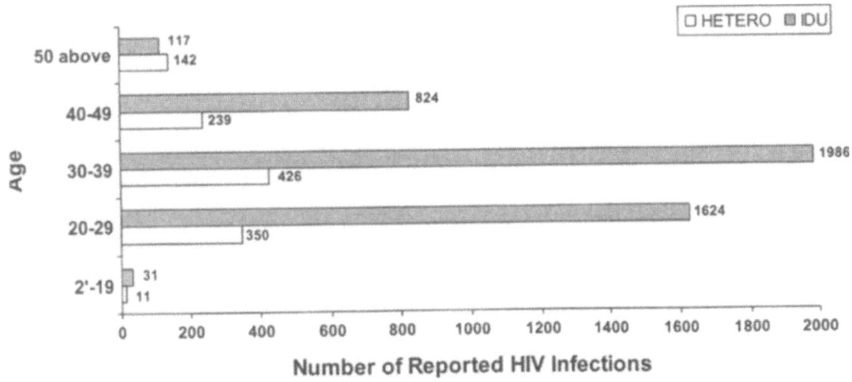

FIGURE 3. Number of Reported HIV Infections by Age Groups and Risk Factors (2001/2002). (Ministry of Health, Malaysia)

categories of people are entitled to free highly active antiretroviral therapy (HAART) treatment, including all infected babies and children, people infected through tainted blood and blood products, women tested positive through the government's antenatal screening program, government servants, and healthcare workers infected occupationally.

However, most PLWHA have to pay for treatment, and despite the 60% reduction in ARV drug prices over the last few years, only about 1500 of the estimated 4000 people who need ARVs are on treatment. In order to increase access to treatment, the government has taken several measures to reduce drug prices, including amending the Patents Act to allow for generic drugs and negotiating with multinational pharmaceutical companies to reduce prices. While more can be done, these measures have demonstrated the government's commitment to reducing drug prices and have benefited PLWHA.

PREVENTION

Prevention remains the key to effective management of HIV in Malaysia. Thus far, despite generous allocations to HIV/AIDS (approximately US$10.3m per year over the last two years and US$1.5m in the 2004 Budget for NGOs working in HIV/AIDS), there is little indication that the rate of infection is slowing down. In fact, the rate over the past two years has increased from 13 new reported infections per day in 2000 to 19 per day in 2002.

Much of this can be attributed to the lack of realistic and targeted interventions among vulnerable groups, particularly among injecting drug users (IDU). IDU make up about 72% of infections, but there is no commensurate response on a scale large enough to make a difference. Small NGOs carry out outreach work among drug-using communities in the major cities, but this is not enough to halt or slow down the rate of infection. Harm reduction measures, such as methadone replacement therapy and needle-exchange programs, have long been politically unfeasible. However, recent advocacy by NGOs and medical professionals has enabled pilot methadone programs to be initiated. Legal barriers to needle-exchange programs remain, though advocacy by NGOs has at least begun to educate policymakers on their benefits.

Both the government and NGOs run several programs targeted towards young people. The Ministry of Health's Anti-AIDS Program among Youth (PROSTAR) seeks to train young leaders on HIV/AIDS in order to educate their peers. No evaluation, however, has been done to gauge its effectiveness. Most recently, in 2003, the Federation of Family Planning Associations of Malaysia was given a US$500,000 grant by the government to run a sexual and reproductive health information program for young people through the Internet. Questions remain as to what information can be given to young people, and sex education in schools remains a sensitive issue.

Programs for the prevention of HIV among women are still lacking. The government antenatal screening program, begun in 1998, aims to reduce transmission of HIV from HIV-positive pregnant women to their babies, and with only a 4.92% transmission rate, is highly successful. However, it does not address the prevention of infection of women themselves. It has become clear in the past few years that women are increasingly becoming infected, mostly through sexual contact with their husbands or partners. Difficulties in addressing this issue are no different from other developing countries where the status of women is unequal to that of men. Programs that seek to prevent infection among women tend to be patriarchal and protective rather than empowering. For example, in November 2001, despite opposition from the Federal Ministry of Health, the Malaysian AIDS Council, the Malaysian Medical Association, amongst others and the Johor State Islamic Affairs Department, in collaboration with the Johor State Health Department, instituted a requirement that all Muslim couples intending marriage undergo a mandatory HIV test with the objective of protecting women from becoming infected by men with risky sexual behavior. Preliminary reports showed the expected very low incidence of HIV among a very low-risk sector of the population. Surprisingly, however, of those found to be HIV-positive, women make up a significant proportion. Given that this is a policy of the Islamic Affairs Department, there could be significant consequences for such women. Those couples found to be HIV-positive who still wish to marry have not been prevented from doing so, although it is not clear whether they receive counselling on safe sex thereafter.

The Ministry of Women and Family Development is allocating money to conduct research on women's vulnerability to HIV, while the women's wing of the second-largest political party, the Malaysian Chinese Association, has embarked on Project Iceberg, a program to educate sexually-active young people on HIV/AIDS and to train counselors to deal with HIV/AIDS-related issues.

The multisectoral response to HIV in Malaysia is slowly building although without any clear strategic plan. In 2001, the Ministry of Human Resources, taking the cue from the International Labor Organization's Code of Practice on HIV/AIDS, embarked on a project to establish a Code of Practice for HIV/AIDS in the Workplace, which was launched in 2002. Working with the Malaysian AIDS Council, the Ministry is conducting workshops around the country to explain the Code to companies and encourage them to adopt their own HIV/AIDS policies based on the Code. Some multinational companies, such as Standard Chartered Bank, have their own HIV/AIDS employee education programs that are proving very successful.

By and large, most community-based programs and programs for vulnerable groups are carried out by NGOs. Of these, thirty-seven are grouped under the umbrella of the Malaysian AIDS Council (MAC), which coordinates the work of its affiliates, builds their capacity and carries out advocacy work on behalf of the NGO sector and People Living with HIV/AIDS. The MAC has been at the forefront, particularly in advocating for the reduction of drug prices and for encouraging the participation of religious bodies in the national response. In collaboration with the Islamic Development Department of the Prime Minister's Department (JAKIM), the MAC organized the 2nd International Muslim Leaders' Consultation on HIV/AIDS in May 2003 and is conducting training of Muslim religious officials using a manual developed with JAKIM. It is hoped that this will reduce some of the religious-based stigma and discrimination attached to HIV/AIDS.

Funding for NGOs under the MAC is largely sourced from the government. In 2003, the Ministry of Finance allocated RM40 million (approximately US$10 million) to be given to NGOs via the MAC over a period of 10 years. This will go to prevention, care and support programs. For core funding of the MAC, fundraising is done by the Malaysian AIDS Foundation, a related organization. In addition, the Malaysian AIDS Foundation manages several funds to address the needs of Malaysians Living with HIV/AIDS. These include the PLWHA Drug Assistance Scheme, which provides some of the ARVs needed by low-income PLWHA as well as three viral load tests per year, the Pediatric AIDS Fund, which provides financial, non-medical support to children with HIV (treatment is free in government hospitals) and other affected children, and the Business Assistance Scheme which provides microcredit loans to PLWHA or affected persons to start small businesses in order to maintain income levels for themselves and their families.

These three schemes have yielded several interesting outcomes. For example, the PLWHA Drug Assistance Scheme was begun in 1999 to provide access to HAART treatment to low-income patients (earning below RM2000 per month) who have CD4 counts below 200. As the MoH provides one drug free, of the other two drugs that are required, the patient pays for one while the scheme pays for the more expensive of the two drugs as well as three viral load tests per year. The Drug Assistance Scheme has given the MAF leverage to negotiate with multinational drug companies on price reductions for ARVs, and has provided data on how PLWHA fare on treatment. From only 30 patients registered on the scheme in 1999, it now benefits 100 patients (The Malaysian AIDS Foundation, 2003).

The Pediatric AIDS Fund has highlighted the growing problem of AIDS orphans in Malaysia. Most of the 300+ children aged 0–14 being assisted by the scheme are affected children (i.e., they are not infected themselves but are the children of PLWHA, some of whom have died). Relatives are caring for most of them. Although they qualify for assistance from the Welfare Department of the Ministry of National Unity and Community Development, many of these children do not access these funds due to the fear of stigma and discrimination. The MAF has initiated discussions with the Welfare Department on a special track for such children. UNAIDS estimates that there are some 14,000 AIDS orphans in Malaysia, although most are untraceable (UNAIDS, 2002).

The Business Assistance Scheme was begun in 2003 to meet the needs of PLWHA and their families whose incomes are limited due to the cost of treatment. A RM1000 (US$250) loan is given to persons recommended by affiliates of the MAC for a specific business activity. A repayment scheme is agreed upon and the affiliate stands as guarantor to the borrower. Thus far, six people have benefited from this scheme, borrowing money to start small businesses such as a pet grooming service and a clothes folding service for garment manufacturers. All loans

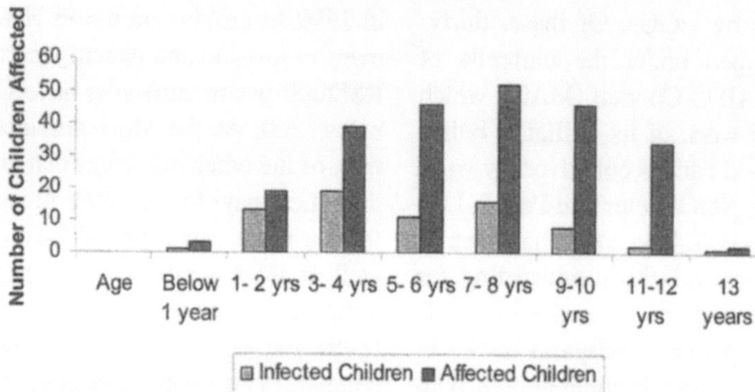

FIGURE 4. Pediatric AIDS Fund Recipient Profile (HIV Status & Age). "Affected Children" are defined as children who are NOT infected by HIV but are nevertheless affected because their parents have HIV/AIDS.

have been repaid, mostly on time. There is also a plan to hold small business planning workshops for potential borrowers.

OUTCOMES

Despite the level of spending on HIV/AIDS programs by the Government over the past 15 years, the continuing rise in infections points to a lack of overall effectiveness of current prevention efforts. This can be attributed to several factors:

1. The level of research on behaviors and vulnerability of the Malaysian population has been poor, although the Ministry of Health is attempting to redress that now. Research, however, tends to focus on limited groups and socio-behavioral factors. Furthermore, research by other agencies, such as the National Family Development Board, now under the Ministry of Women and Family Development, which has conducted surveys on the sexual and reproductive health of adolescents, has not been used to guide HIV/AIDS policy. In addition, the results of existing research conducted by government agencies tends to be classified as secret, making it impossible for outside agencies and NGOs to use them to design programs.

2. The capacity of NGOs to meet all the needs of communities has been limited by lack of funding and reach. Although the government acknowledges that NGOs can be far more effective in reaching vulnerable communities such as drug users and sex workers, the capacity to do this has thus far been restricted by lack of funding and human resources to do the work. Most such work is concentrated in Kuala Lumpur and other major cities, while smaller towns and rural areas are badly served. Recently, the government increased funding for NGOs in these fields, but scaling-up has not yet occurred. The Malaysian AIDS Council is addressing this problem as a priority issue.

3. Various laws, especially anti-drug laws, have inhibited effective prevention programs. Malaysia has had tough anti-drug trafficking laws for over 20 years. Drug traffickers face mandatory death sentences and drug users are sent to government-run rehabilitation centres. These laws have not curbed the drug problem and have actually exacerbated the HIV rates among drug users. Tough police action to curb the supply of drugs led to the practice of injecting; difficulties in obtaining needles and syringes led to the sharing of injecting equipment, thus facilitating the rapid spread of HIV. (When the supply of drugs became limited due to police action, drug users started to inject rather than smoke because it is far more economical. Also, the drugs became adulterated, so in order to get the same high, they took to injecting because this got the drugs into the bloodstream more quickly and directly.)

Political considerations make harm reduction programs, especially needle-exchange programs, unfeasible at the moment. However, due to NGO advocacy and better education of drug policymakers, certain harm reduction methods such as methadone replacement therapy are being allowed and other methods are being discussed.

But full implementation of these methods would require changes in some anti-drug laws that are not currently foreseeable. Recently, the MoH asked NGOs for input into amending the Prevention and Control of Infectious Diseases Act, which provides the opportunity to clarify and streamline some laws that have inhibited effective prevention.

4. There is a lack of understanding of the multisectoral nature of the HIV/AIDS epidemic and the need for better collaboration among different agencies. HIV/AIDS in Malaysia still remains largely a Ministry of Health responsibility and all policies tend to be seen through medical and public health eyes. This does not always prove useful in prevention for women or in understanding the role of various laws and religions in both prevention and care. NGOs have played an important role in pushing for the multisectoral response to HIV/AIDS, and this is slowly building among government agencies. The most successful multisectoral effort thus far is in the issue of drug pricing where, after a Cabinet directive, the Ministry of Health, the Ministry of International Trade and Industry, which conducts WTO negotiations, and the Ministry of Domestic Trade and Consumer Affairs, which handles patent issues, have worked together to try and reduce drug prices either through negotiations with multinational drug companies or through the importation or manufacture of generic drugs. The collaboration between Muslim religious agencies, the Ministry of Health and the Malaysian AIDS Council on the training of religious officials on HIV/AIDS is another example of multisectional collaboration.

5. Stigma and discrimination remain major barriers in ensuring the effectiveness of prevention, treatment, care, and support programs. While much of the population is aware of the existence of HIV/AIDS within Malaysian borders, stereotypes as to who may be infected abound. Mostly, it is assumed that only male drug users, gay men, sex workers and migrant workers can become infected. Thus, many PLWHA suffer discrimination at home, at work, in hospitals and in schools. Stigma and discrimination are being addressed through better education programs, particularly of religious and community leaders. The involvement of PLWHA in these programs, particularly in giving talks in schools, has proven effective in dispelling myths and stereotypes. However, this is not occurring at a large enough scale, due to the fear of many PLWHA themselves of disclosure. Videos and books produced by the MAC have helped to circumvent this problem to some extent, as well as programs to empower community groups, including PLWHA, to speak out for themselves.

FUTURE

Malaysia has many opportunities to succeed in controlling HIV/AIDS. It has a committed Government that has taken the lead on HIV/AIDS issues both nationally and regionally. Domestically, funding of HIV/AIDS programs, particularly for NGOs, has grown in recognition of their crucial role in prevention, care, and support. In 1999, at the 5th International Congress on AIDS in Asia-Pacific (ICAAP) in Kuala Lumpur, the Prime Minister suggested a meeting of Asian Heads of Government on HIV/AIDS. This resulted in the Association of Southeast Asian Nations (ASEAN) Heads of Government Summit meeting on HIV/AIDS in Brunei Darussalam in 2001 that produced the ASEAN Declaration on HIV/AIDS and the ASEAN Work Plan on HIV/AIDS.

Malaysia is also far ahead of many countries in the treatment it is able to provide its infected citizens, much of it free through Government hospitals. Although it can be further improved, the infrastructure exists to deliver treatment effectively to PLWHA, as long as costs and stigma are not deterrents.

However, prevention remains problematic if many difficult and sensitive issues are not addressed. This particularly involves the conflict between anti-drug policies and the need to respond to the rapid HIV transmission rates among drug users. Sensitivity towards the provision of frank information to young people also remains a barrier, as well as the limited understanding among both government agencies and women's groups of the link between women's issues and HIV among women.

As in many countries, what would move the way forward in Malaysia would be the creation of a new agency that would have powers over all the multisectoral players in the national response, as well as a national HIV/AIDS strategic plan that takes into account the multisectoral dimension of HIV/AIDS. Until this is done, Malaysia's capacity to meet the targets set in the United Nations Declaration of Commitment and Platform for Action of 2001 will be limited.

REFERENCES

Malaysian AIDS Foundation. (2003). Drug Assistance Scheme Patient Progress Report 2003.

Malaysian National Drug Agency, Ministry of Home Affairs (multiple years). Buletin Dadah (Drugs Bulletin).

Ministry of Health, Malaysia. (2002). HIV/AIDS Statistics, HIV/AIDS Update 2002.

UNAIDS. (2002). UNAIDS Global HIV/AIDS Report. (December 2002).

7

HIV/AIDS in Indonesia

Dynamics and Challenges in the Emergence of the National Response

Jane S. Wilson

Joint United Nations Program on HIV/AIDS (UNAIDS), Jakarta, Indonesia

NATIONAL HISTORY AND CURRENT STATUS OF INFECTIOUS DISEASES

With a population of nearly 210 million people, Indonesia is the fourth largest country globally, and the largest Islamic country. It has over 250 ethnic groups most of whom are Muslim (Indonesian National AIDS Commission, Republic of Indonesia, 2001). As the fourth largest country in the world as well as being the largest Islamic nation, the evolution of the Indonesian response to HIV/AIDS deserves special attention and analysis. This analysis provides a consideration of some of the factors in the Indonesian response but should not be seen as a comprehensive overview.

Of particular significance is the General Election in 1999 that marked the start of a democratic approach to government, including greater freedom of the press and more opportunities for civil society.

Commercial sex is widespread with an estimated 190,000–270,000 female sex workers in Indonesia and approximately seven to ten million clients of sex workers (National AIDS Commission, 2002). In addition less than 10% of clients use condoms to avoid STI and HIV infection. There are an estimated 8–15,000 transvestites and 2500 male sex workers in Indonesia. Studies of men who have sex with men indicate unsafe sexual behaviour, with transvestites having a high rate of STIs. Rates of STIs among sex workers reported in 2000 indicate that Gonorrhea is a consistent problem, with rates of 30% in Kupang, 25% in Surabaya and 13.9% in Manado (Department of Health, 2002). The Chlamydia rate follows a similar pattern. Women visiting family planning centers in Bali, West Java, Surabaya, South Kalimantan and Riau had rates of Trichomoniasis from 1.2–6.2%, Gonorrhea from 0.8 to 1.8%, Chlamdydia 4.2 to 8.2% and higher rates Syphilis from 0.7 to 0.8%. In contrast, clients had higher rates of Trichomoniasis,

5%, Gonorrhea 0.5%–4.3%, and Syphilis, 4.6%.

NATIONAL HEALTHCARE HISTORY, PRACTICES, AND SPENDING

Rapid economic growth from the 1970s–1990s resulted in significant improvements in the health sector and in sanitation. Access to health care systems in particular improved with the establishment of a network of government health centers prioritizing mother and child health, disease prevention, and basic medical services (World Bank, 2003). As a result, life expectancy increased by around ten years during the 1980s to 1990s. Infant mortality also declined sharply, dropping from 124 per 1000 live births in 1967 to 41.44 per 1000 births 30 years later in 1997. Despite this, maternal and neonatal mortality rates, particularly in rural areas, are among the highest in the region.

Infectious diseases have declined but have not been eliminated. Respiratory infections, malaria, diarrhea and intestinal parasites, gastroenteritis, skin and eye diseases, and tuberculosis are still common, particularly among children. The economic crisis of the late 1990s severely stretched the country's limited health resources and raised the price of drugs by as much as 200–300%.

High birth rates in the 1950s and 1960s prompted the Indonesian Government to introduce what has been cited as being one of the most successful birth control programs in the developing world. More recently, in 2001, the government started implementing a policy of decentralized government which delegates decision-making, managing, and financing for health care to local governments.

At the Health Dialogue preceding the 13th Meeting of the Consultative group in Indonesia, Professor Azwar noted that Indonesia spends only US $3–4 per capita on health annually, 50% of which is public funding (World Bank, 2003).

NATIONAL AND REGIONAL HISTORY AND CURRENT STATUS OF HIV/AIDS

HIV infections and cases of AIDS to the end of December 2003 total 4094 people but this figure is widely regarded as being the tip of the iceberg (Green, 2004). During the 1990s Indonesia had a low prevalence of HIV with an official estimate of 52,000 people (Sujudi, 2001). The estimates were revised in 2002 to a range of 90,000 to 130,000 people (National AIDS Commission, 2002). Some experts predicted that most of the new infections in 2003 would result from injecting drug use, which is fast becoming the preponderant mode of transmission, a trend that started during the economic and political crisis of the late 1990s. Rates of HIV among injecting drug users in treatment in Jakarta were 48% and among prisoners linked with injecting drug use also increasing sharply at a similar rate (National AIDS Commission, 2002). It is estimated that there are an additional 13–20 million people who are vulnerable to HIV infection, including injecting drug users, female sex workers and their clients, men who have sex with men, transvestites and their clients (National AIDS Commission, 2002).

IMPACT OF AND RESPONSES TO HIV/AIDS

The evolution of the Indonesian response deserves special attention and analysis because Indonesia is the world's largest Muslim nation. Initial responses were by civil society, including non governmental organizations, and the Ministry of Health, supported by the UN Global Programme on AIDS (GPA). Government action was broadened in 1993–1994 with the establishment of the National AIDS Strategy and Presidential Decree Number 36 that called for AIDS control commissions at national, provincial and district levels. The United Nations Development Program (UNDP), AusAID and USAID provided strategic assistance during this time and bilateral assistance from Australian, American and German was negotiated during this period, with bilateral assistance initiatives starting in 1996.

From 1995 on, the Indonesian response was mobilized more systematically, although with very limited central government resources, and only in those provinces where bilateral donors were active such as Bali, South Sulawesi, East Nusa Tengarrah, East Java, Jakarta and North Sumatra. The Global Programme on AIDS then the newly established UN Joint and Cosponsored Programme on HIV/AIDS (UNAIDS) also played key roles, with the World Health Oganization (WHO), UNDP and the United Nations Population Fund (UNFPA) being very active. The Secretariat of the National AIDS Commission was established and efforts were made to mainstream HIV/AIDS in the national planning cycles of the sectoral relevant ministries under the aegis of the Coordinating Ministry of People's Welfare whose Minister was the Chair of the National AIDS Commission. The World Bank started implementation of a large-scale project in Jakarta and Riau.

The onset of the Indonesian economic and political crisis or *krismon* in late 1997 led to the first democratic General Election in 1999, but precipitated a sharp decrease in government budget available for HIV/AIDS.

The first Indonesian Human Development Report (2001) concludes that an emphasis on economic growth in the 1980s and 1990s neglected social support systems and structures so that the community was hard hit during the *krismon*. Unemployment and poverty increased sharply and some observers linked increased risk and vulnerability to HIV infection to these factors, although definitive analysis is not yet available. During this period, the government dissolved the Coordinating Ministry of People's Welfare in an effort to streamline the number of ministries. Responsibility for HIV/AIDS was placed with the Vice President, Megawati Sukarnoputri, returning to the re-established Coordinating Ministry of People's Welfare when the Vice President became the President of the Republic of Indonesia.

The UN General Assembly Special Session on HIV/AIDS (UNGASS) was held 25–27 June 2001. Preparation for the event from December 2000 to June 2001 coincided with the start of the economic and political recovery in Indonesia and provided the impetus for a renewed official response to HIV/AIDS in Indonesia (Wilson, 2003). The Minister for Health, Dr. Achmad Sujudi MHA, led Indonesia's involvement in UNGASS and many Indonesians participated in the preparatory process. Drafts of a declaration of commitment were circulated among all participating nations and organizations. Indonesia reached its position on the issue involved through a mix of internal discussion, consultation with partners and inputs from the community through meetings and written submissions (Murni, 2001). The Declaration of Commitment represents global consensus on issues involved with HIV/AIDS prevention and control, as well as specifying time bound goals and targets against which all country responses are to be measured. Senior Indonesians officials attended the May 2001 pre-UNGASS consultations in New York where delegates were intensely involved in the negotiation of the Declaration of Commitment. This process was protracted and complex as delegates globally tried to reach consensus about a wide range of controversial issues related to the HIV/AIDS pandemic for the first time ever.

The official UNGASS delegation consisted of nine Indonesians: the Ministries of Health, Women's Empowerment, Family Planning and Reproductive Health, the National AIDS Commission, Members of Parliament and the Ministry of Foreign Affairs. Suzana Murni, Aty Uleng and Dr. Nasser attended representing Indonesian NGOs. There was a considerable sense of anticipation about what the Declaration of Commitment would mean in practice (Wilson, 2003).

During UNGASS the Minister for Health made the first official reference to the new higher official estimate of HIV/AIDS in Indonesia. At the same time, officials were reported in the media (Jakarta Post, 2001) stating that harm reduction strategies would be tested in Indonesia and, if successful, would be adopted as government policy. In February 2003, harm reduction for injection drug users (IDU) was included as a part of the new strategic plan developed by the Ministry of Health (Ministry of Health, 2002).

The Minister of Health initiated two valuable post-UNGASS strategic press conferences to brief civil society, in particular NGOs, the sectoral ministries and donors. Returning delegates reported back directly about their experiences, the positions taken by Indonesia in the negotiations and the implications of the Declaration of Commitment. This process marks the start of the resurgence of the Indonesian response, concurrently with the upsurge in IDU infections, with participants at the press conferences initiating the establishment of the working group that updated the Ministry of Health strategic plan (Wilson, 2003).

Delegates were open about the need for change and in particular about the limitations of government resources: only 1.6% of the government budget being currently allocated for health and 2.0% for education (personal notes, 16 August, 2001). The newly established Global Fund to fight AIDS, TB and Malaria was seen by Indonesia as an important source of future funding. The UNGASS Declaration of Commitment was translated into the Indonesian language and circulated widely to make the public familiar with it as a framework for action.

Another factor in the Indonesian response was the country's participation in the International Congress on AIDS in Asian and the Pacific in Melbourne (ICAAP), October 2001. Suzana Murni represented positive people from South East Asia at the Opening Ceremony and stressed the urgent need for affordable and accessible ARV treatment for positive people.

Also significant was the agreement by the Ministerial Meeting during ICAAP to form a new leadership initiative, the Asia Pacific Leadership Forum (APLF), aimed at improving leadership related to HIV/AIDS in the region. APLF is developing as Indonesian owned and an integral part of the Indonesian national response.

Following the establishment of the Ad Hoc Committee the new strategy was developed over the following six months. The Ad Hoc Committee was a creative solution to the uncertain status of the National AIDS Commission since the temporary abolition of the coordinating ministry in which it was situated. By March 2002, the Ministry of Health completed its Strategic Plan to Control HIV/AIDS in Indonesia 2003–2007, a precondition for Indonesia's successful first round proposal to the Global Fund to fight HIV/AIDS, TB, and Malaria on 10 March 2002 (Wilson, 2003). The application resulted in an allocation of 15 million USD for Indonesia in four provinces. The National AIDS Commission then initiated the revision of the multi-sectoral National AIDS Strategy, 1994 that took approximately nine months.

On 28 March 2002, the Indonesian Cabinet held a Special Cabinet Meeting on HIV/AIDS. It was jointly led by the Minister for Health, Dr. Achmad Sujudi, who has been deeply committed to the Indonesian response throughout, and the Coordinating Minister for People's Welfare, Jusuf Kalla, a well-known and successful Indonesian businessman (Wilson, 2003). The Indonesian Cabinet endorsed a national commitment to HIV/AIDS (2002–2010) in the form of a National AIDS Movement that prioritizes HIV/AIDS in annual development planning, specifying the need for 20 million USD for HIV/AIDS in the budget annually and mainstreaming HIV/AIDS into the planning of all involved ministries (National AIDS Commission, 2002). The Cabinet endorsed a range of technical strategies consistent with the UNGASS Declaration of Commitment including the importance of the provision of ARV treatment.

A second Special Cabinet Meeting on HIV/AIDS took place on 5 July 2003. At this meeting Cabinet Ministers officially endorsed the new national HIV/AIDS strategy and announced the six priority provinces, Riau, Jakarta, East Java, East Java, Bali, and Papua, and reiterated the importance of the provision of ARV treatment. The leadership of Dr. Achmad Sujudi, the Minister for Health, and Jusuf Kalla, the Coordinating Minister for People's Welfare has been outstanding and is deserving of global recognition (Wilson, 2003). Similarly, the extraordinary dedication and creativity of Indonesians living with HIV/AIDS, such as Suzana Murni, must also be recognized.

Following the first Special Cabinet Meeting, the National AIDS Commission held a Country Consultation, 23 April 2002, to introduce the cabinet meeting's outcomes to all those involved in the national response. With hundreds of participants from across the country, government, Persons Living with HIV and AIDS (PLWHA), Civil Society, donors, the new National AIDS Movement (NAM) was launched. Indonesians from five provinces, living with and affected by HIV/AIDS, addressed the meeting and spoke of their experience of discrimination and called for the Government to support them. This was the strongest demonstration of Indonesian Government commitment to the GIPA principle (the Greater Involvement of People living with AIDS), consistent with Indonesia's participation in the Paris Summit in 1994. Ministers Achmad Sujudi and Jusuf Kalla briefed the meeting about the Special Cabinet Meeting on HIV/AIDS, again reinforcing the importance of Civil Society in the National AIDS Movement. In May 2003, the revised National HIV/AIDS Strategy 2003–2007 (National AIDS Commission, 2003) was launched by Minister Kalla, with UNAIDS Executive Director Dr. Peter Piot who was in Indonesia for the first time, to acknowledge the importance of the Indonesian response.

In December 2001, The President participated in the Association of South East Asian Nations (ASEAN) Heads of State Summit at Brunei Darussalam, at which the ten Member Countries held the first ever session on HIV/AIDS. The Heads of State endorsed the *ASEAN Declaration on HIV/AIDS*, a demonstration of their commitment to implement the ASEAN Work Plan on HIV/AIDS (Permanent Representative of Brunei Darussalam, 2001). Paralleling UNGASS, a review of HIV/AIDS activities will be an annual event at each summit. Each ASEAN Summit now reviews progress made toward the commitments in the *Declaration*. This regional framework is consistent with the UNGASS *Declaration of Commitment* and reflects increased political will and leadership in the South East Asian Region.

President Megawati Sukarnoputri has given stirring addresses at the Presidential Palace on World AIDS Day (December 2002), calling on the nation to reach out and support people with HIV/AIDS. President Megawati has repeatedly stressed the need to support people living with HIV/AIDS. Scrapping a prepared speech in 2002, the President spoke passionately of her experience when meeting Indonesians living with HIV/AIDS, noting that fear of discrimination is one of the reasons for the rapid spread of HIV and speaking out strongly for the need for understanding and acceptance (Wilson, 2003).

In February 2003, a photographic exhibition featuring 35 large-sized photographs of people living with HIV/AIDS was held at the House of Representatives. The exhibition attracted hundreds of legislators, celebrities and other public figures to the opening (Jakarta Post, 2003). The event was dedicated to the memory of the late Suzana Murni who died on 6 July 2002. The exhibition was organized by, among others, the Spiritia Foundation, a non-governmental organization set up by Suzana, who was among the first Indonesians to speak publicly about living with HIV/AIDS. The participants, who had been photographed by Rio Helmi, members of the All Indonesia Network of People Living with HIV/AIDS, said it was Suzana's vision that had encouraged them to join.

Despite such breakthroughs, people living with HIV/AIDS continue to experience stigma and discrimination, especially in health care settings, as documented in the qualitative research of Yayasan Pelita Ilmu and Spiritia Foundation (Spiritia Foundation, 2002). Both studies, carried out during 2001–2002 show that most discrimination was experienced in health care settings, that there was a general perception that there were no drugs available to treat HIV-related illness or HIV itself.

In the Spiritia study (2002) 31% of the respondents had been refused treatment by a hospital or doctor. 55% were given no information before they were tested. 57% said there was a third person (family member, friend or other) in the room when they were tested, 63% indicating that this was not with their agreement. Government officials attending the dissemination of the data welcomed this groundbreaking research, acknowledging that new anti-discrimination policy was needed, as well as extensive training of health care workers, advocacy with decision-makers and emphasizing the importance of supporting people living with HIV/SAIDS (Wilson, 2003).

Over the two years from 2002 to 2003, Spiritia teams have carried out visits to 36 cities in 20 provinces to assess assistance available to people living with HIV/AIDS (PLWHA) (Spiritia, 2003). The overall impression is that the AIDS epidemic is escalating rapidly but that the response is lagging far behind. Recommendations include a need for more active AIDS commissions, involvement of members of parliament and NGOs, training of health care workers, provision of Voluntary Counselling and Testing (VCT), greater involvement of PLWHA, and coordinating donor activities.

In May 2003, following the revision of the National HIV/AIDS Strategy, the United Nations Theme Group on HIV/AIDS, led by Alan Boulton, ILO Country Director and Theme Group Chair, started the development of the United Nations Joint Action Programme (UN JAP), to ensure that UN system support is coordinated and that it has a strategic response based on needs identified by the National AIDS Commission. The UN JAP (UN, 2003) was completed in December 2003 and focuses on strategic support support for policy development as well as support to assist the Government to scale up its efforts. The Resident Coordinator in Indonesia, Bo Asplund played a key role in the design of the JAP. The UN JAP details current commitments by the UN system involving 10 agencies and over six million US $. UNAIDS has allocated two fixed term national program officers to the UNAIDS Secretariat in acknowledgment of the importance of strong support for the Indonesian response and in response to the strong leadership and commitment shown by the UN Theme Group on HIV/AIDS in Indonesia. Joint action based on WHO's 3×5 Initiative will become one of the cornerstone's of the UN JAP and will enable the UN to maximize support to the Government so that 10,000 people can be reached with ARV treatment by the end of 2005.

On 22 September 2003, Minister Achmad Sujudi reported to the United Nations at a one day meeting convened before the World Health Assembly in New York (National AIDS Commission, 2003). Principle achievements noted in the report are the Composite Policy Index of 65% as well as overall expenditure on HIV/AIDS by the Government of USD 3.25 million in 2002 and USD 5.6 million in 2003 (National AIDS Commission, 2003). However, despite these advances in policy, coverage of risk populations across Indonesia remains extremely limited; for example, fewer than 5% of the estimated 160,000 IDU are being reached. The same can be said for sex work outreach. Coupled with these trends, the consistently low rate of condom use by clients of sex workers is very concerning. In addition, Indonesia is yet to mount an effective and sustained national campaign to educate the community about the basic facts about transmission and prevention as well as anti stigma and discrimination messages.

In June 2001, Indonesian NGO activists wrote to the President of the UN General Assembly (Murni, 2001) advocating for the *Declaration of Commitment*. "We believe that the adoption of a strongly worded and rational *Declaration of Commitment by* the UN member states can lend impetus to a more concerted and effective effort in addressing the epidemic . . . and should emphasize a human rights-based approach in the response to the epidemic."

The events following Indonesia's participation in UNGASS are having a significant cumulative effect (Wilson, 2003). The annual Special Cabinet Meetings on HIV/AIDS have strongly demonstrated the presence and legitimacy of a central Government that decides new policy. This has significance at national, regional and global levels.

There is increased momentum and commitment for the development of more effective partnerships. The repeated call for greater involvement of Civil Society is resulting in a new stage in Government and Civil Society relations and a greater commitment to partnerships with religious leaders, the private sector, and civil society. The Government is also providing space for positive Indonesians to be involved, the essence of the Greater Involvement of People with HIV/AIDS.

The three major bilateral partners, America, Australia and Germany, have been integral players and strong supporters in the sequence of events described in this article. UN involvement, initially represented by a few agencies, has now evolved into a broad UN system response. Strong commitment by the Ford Foundation, Church World Service, Medecins Sans Frontiers, and many other organizations, is playing a vital role.

The sustainability of the response to HIV/AIDS is potentially greatly enhanced by the renewed leadership of the Indonesian government and the leadership from Bali, East Java, North Sumatra and other provinces. There remain, however, some provinces where progress has been slower and leadership limited. At the district level, levels of progress vary greatly and as yet no monitoring and evaluation system in place.

The new National HIV/AIDS Strategy 2003–2007 gives donors a clear framework within which to make decisions about development assistance. The scale-up of the capacity of the Secretariat of the National AIDS Commission is a promising sign of increased commitment to HIV/AIDS by the government. In December 2003, Dai Bachtiar, National Chief of Police and Minister Jusuf Kalla, Head of the National AIDS Commission, signed an historic Memorandum of Understanding that formally states Indonesia's commitment to a policy of harm reduction for IDU (National AIDS Commission and National Narcotics Board, 2003).

Despite the many achievements at national level since 2001, the Indonesian response remains very limited at the local level in coverage of prevention and care activities. Decision-making has been decentralized to local governments, which means that priorities and budgets are decided locally and much advocacy and action is needed at this level. The UNAIDS/WHO AIDS Epidemic Update (2003) points out the warning signals in Indonesia are not lessening. Condom use remains consistently low and a large part of the epidemic is driven by injecting drug use. With many injecting drug users regularly spending time in jail, there is great potential for rapid transmission of HIV to other vulnerable populations as well as the general population.

At times, the government's response to HIV has almost seemed to drive the development of political culture in Indonesia. Nevertheless, while progress has been astonishing on many levels, preventing a devastating epidemic will demand more and more of the Indonesian government and people.

REFERENCES

Department of Health, Republic of Indonesia. (2003). National Estimates of HIV Infection in Indonesian Adults, 2003, Report of the Estimation in Poplations Vulnerable to HIV Infection, Director General of Communicable Diseasees and Environmental Health.

Green, C. (2004). Report of the Cases of HIV/AIDS until 31 December, 2003, email communication.

Jakarta Post. (2001). Government to boost campaign on HIV/AIDS. (July 14, 2001).

Jakarta Post. (2003). HIV/AIDS photo event major break through. (January 28, 2003).

Media Indonesia. (2003). HIV/AIDS Prevention and Control, Special Supplement. (in Indonesian language)

Ministry of Health, Republic of Indonesia. (2002). Strategic Plan to Control HIV/AIDS in Indonesia 2003–7, Directorate of CDC and Environmental Health.

Murni, S. (2001). Indonesian National Forum of NGOs and Organizations Concerned about AIDS (FK-LOPA) to His Excellency Mr. Harri Holkeri President of the General Assembly of the United Nations. (unpublished letter).

National AIDS Commission, Republic of Indonesia. (2001). HIV/AIDS and Other Sexually Transmitted Infections in Indonesia: Challenges and opportunities for action 2001. (unpublished document).

National AIDS Commission, Republic of Indonesia. (2002). The Threat of HIV/AIDS in Indonesia is Increasingly Evident and Calls for More Concrete Measures of Prevention. (unpublished report to the Indonesian Cabinet).

National AIDS Commission, Republic of Indonesia. (2003a). National HIV/AIDS Strategy 2003–2007, Office of the Coordinating Minister for People's Welfare, National AIDS Commission. (unpublished).

National AIDS Commission, Republic of Indonesia. (2003b). Country Report on Follow-up to the Declaration of Commitment on HIV/AIDS (UNGASS), Reporting period 2001–2003, (unpublished document).

National AIDS Commission and National Narcotics Board. (2003). Agreement between the Coordinating Minister of People's Welfare on behalf of the National AIDS Commission and the Chief of Police on behalf of the National Narcotics Board, Number 20, Decision, Coordinating Ministry of People's Welfare. Number B, 01, 12, 2003, National Narcotics Board. The Establishment of the National Team for Integrated Efforts on Prevention of HIV/AIDS Transmission and the Eradication of Misuse of Injecting Narcotics, Psychotropic and Addictive Drugs. (unpublished Ministerial Decree/ unofficial translation).

Permanent representative of Brunei Darussalam to the United Nations. (2001). The ASEAN Summit of HIV/AIDS (November 7, 2001).

Spiritia Foundation. (2002). Documentation of Human Rights Violations against People Living with HIV/AIDS in Indonesia: A peer group Documentation Project. (unpublished).

Spiritia Foundation. (2003). Report on Local Strengthening Visits November 2001–August 2003. (unpublished).

Sujudi, A. (2001). Ministerial remarks of the Ministry of Health of Indonesia: Impact of HIV/AIDS in Indonesia. Presentation made at the ICAAP in Melbourne. (unpublished transcript).

United Nations (2003). UN Joint Action Programme. (17 December, 2003). Geneva. (unpublished program).

UNAIDS/WHO. (2003). AIDS epidemic update, December 2003, Geneva.

United Nations Development Program (2001). Human Development Report. Geneva.

Wilson, J. (2003). A Post UNGASS Analysis: The Indonesian Response (9 September 2003). (unpublished paper).

World Bank. (2003). Meeting notes from the Pre CGI Health Dialogue, December 2003. (unpublished).

8

HIV/AIDS in the Philippines

Maria Consorcia Lim-Quizon

Infectious Disease Surveillance and Control Project,
National Epidemiology Center, Manila, Philippines

GEOGRAPHY AND POPULATION

The Philippines is an archipelago of 7,100 islands with a total land area of about 300,000 square kilometers. It lies in the Pacific Ocean off the coast of Southeast Asia. The two largest islands are Luzon in the north and Mindanao in the south. There is a cluster of islands in between them, collectively called the Visayas. The country is divided into 16 regions: Regions I–XII, the National Capital Region (NCR), the Cordillera Administrative Region (CAR), the Autonomous Region of Muslim Mindanao (ARMM), and Caraga (Region XIII). These regions are composed of 78 provinces, 82 cities, 1525 municipalities, and 41,940 villages or *barangays*. Manila is the capital city located near the south of Luzon, and is part of the NCR. This is the biggest urban center in the country.

The estimated population in 1999 is 74,723,373, projected to increase to 82,636,689 in 2004 with the annual growth rate of 2.32%. The Philippines is one of the world's most populous countries with a population density of 249/km^2. It is also a relatively young country, with an estimated 51% of the population under 20 years old. There is an almost equal ratio of males to females (101:100). More than half (56%) of the population lives in urban areas (UNDP 1999). The simple literacy rate is high (93%), and the rates for males and females do not vary significantly. Urban areas, however, have higher literacy rates with more people reaching higher levels of education compared to rural areas. The Philippines is the only predominantly Christian country in Asia; the majority of Christians in the Philippines are Roman Catholics (83%). There are 110 ethnolinguistic groups and about 70 languages spoken in the country, English and Tagalog being the most widely spoken.

HEALTH SERVICES

The state ensures the constitutional right of every Filipino to health and health care. The Department of Health (DOH) is the lead agency and maintains specialty hospitals and tertiary care hospitals in all regions. Public health and provincial as well as district hospitals were devolved to the local government unit in 1992 with the passage of the local health code into law. The private sector plays a large role in providing health care through hospitals, hospital insurance, the pharmaceutical industry, vaccines, medical supplies and equipment, research and development and other health-related services. Health care is distributed unevenly in the country and is largely concentrated in NCR.

In 1997, only 3.5% of the gross national product (GNP) went to health (NSCB, 1998); this is below the 5% spending that the WHO prescribes for developing countries. Of this, 46% was paid out of pocket exacting a heavy toll on the average Filipino family, which has an annual income of less than $3000 (FIES, 2000). Although the National Health Insurance Program is moving quickly towards its goal of providing health financing for most Filipinos, it still has a long way to go: presently, less than half the population has coverage. Health spending is still heavy on hospital or curative care compared to preventive health services.

GENERAL HEALTH INDICES

Standard health indices show that life expectancy improved from 61.6 years in 1980 to 68.6 years in 1999; life expectancy for females was higher (71.28 years) than for males (66.03 years) (NSO,199). The crude birth rate (CBR) stands at 28.4 per 1000 population, while the crude death rate (CDR) stands at 6.1 per 1000 population (UNPOP). Although the infant mortality rate (IMR) and maternal mortality rate (MMR) showed decreasing trends over the years, they are still high compared to neighboring countries, with the IMR at 35 per 1000 live births and MMR at 179.7 per 100,000 live births in 1998 (NDHS 1998).

The leading causes of morbidity are still communicable diseases, specifically diarrheal diseases, pneumonia, upper respiratory tract infections, and tuberculosis. While the prevalence of communicable diseases is high, of the prevalence of chronic degenerative diseases is increasing and has actually overtaken the former as leading causes of mortality, as shown in Table 1 (Philippine Health Statistics, 1997).

THE AIDS SITUATION IN THE PHILIPPINES

The first case of HIV/AIDS was reported in 1984, with the death of a foreign national from pneumonia brought about by AIDS. The Philippines knew that the epidemic had reached its shores and it had to act fast in order to prevent its spread. In 1986, the DOH classified HIV as a reportable disease. The following year, the HIV/AIDS Registry, a passive form of surveillance, was institutionalized in the DOH, requiring all licensed hospitals, laboratories and testing clinics to report serologically confirmed cases to the DOH. From January 1987 to June 2003, there were 1892 HIV antibody seropositive cases reported. At the time of the report, 1280 (68%) were asymptomatic and 612 (32%) were AIDS cases, of which 254 had died from AIDS-related complications (Figure 1). Most of the cases (62%) were males, and the age group with the highest number of cases was the 20–39 years age group (Figure 2). The most common mode of transmission was sexual transmission (93%); of these, 72% were from heterosexual contact, 18% were from homosexual contact, and 6% from bisexual contact. Fewer than 1% reported the infection through blood and blood products, all of these were contracted abroad.

Considering the limitations inherent in passive surveillance, such as underreporting and delay in reporting, the DOH, in 1993, established the National HIV Sentinel Surveillance System (NHSSS) through the support of the U.S. Agency for International Development (USAID), the Japan International Coordination Agency (JICA), and the World Health Organization (WHO). The objective was to monitor the trend of HIV prevalence among high risk groups (HRG) which included male and female sex workers (MSW, FSW), men who have sex with men (MSM),

TABLE 1. Trend of Leading Causes of Mortality in the Philippines, 1975–1995

Rank	1975	1980	1985	1990	1995
1	Pneumonia	Pneumonia	Pneumonia	Heart diseases	Heart diseases
2	TB, all forms	Heart diseases	Heart diseases	Pneumonia	Vascular diseases
3	Heart diseases	TB, all forms	TB, all forms	Vascular diseases	Pneumonia
4	Vascular diseases	Vascular diseases	Vascular diseases	TB, all forms	Malignant neoplasms
5	Malignant neoplasms	Malignant neoplasms	Malignant neoplasms	Malignant neoplasms	TB, all forms
6	Gastroenteritis/colitis	Diarrhea	Diarrhea	Diarrhea	Accidents
7	Nutritional deficiencies	Accidents	Accidents	Septicemia	COPD
8	Accidents	Nutritional deficiencies	Measles	Nephritis, nephrotic syndrome, and nephrosis	Other respiratory diseases
9	Bronchitis	Measles	Nutritional deficiencies	Accidents	Diabetes Mellitus
10	Tetanus	Nephritis, nephrotic syndrome, and nephrosis	Nephritis, nephrotic syndrome, and nephrosis	Measles	Diarrhea

Source: Philippine Health Statistics, 1995

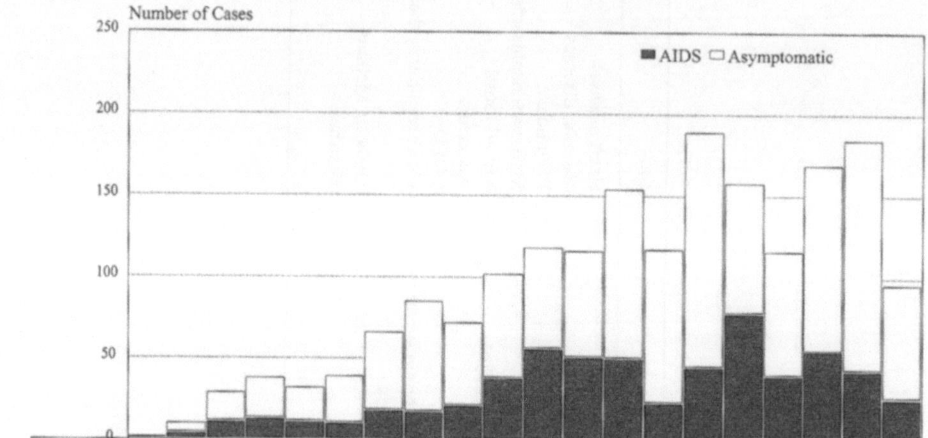

Year	84	85	86	87	88	89	90	91	92	93	94	95	96	97	98	99	00	01	02	03
TOTAL	2	10	29	38	32	39	66	85	72	102	118	116	154	117	189	158	116	169	184	96
Asymptomatic	0	6	18	25	21	29	48	68	51	64	62	65	104	94	144	80	76	114	141	70
AIDS	2	4	11	13	11	10	18	17	21	38	56	51	50	23	45	78	40	55	43	26
Death	2	4	10	12	9	8	15	13	13	11	19	24	27	10	16	16	9	20	11	5

FIGURE 1. HIV Ab Seropositive Cases by Year, Philippines HIV/AIDS Registry, January 1984–June 2003 (n = 1892).

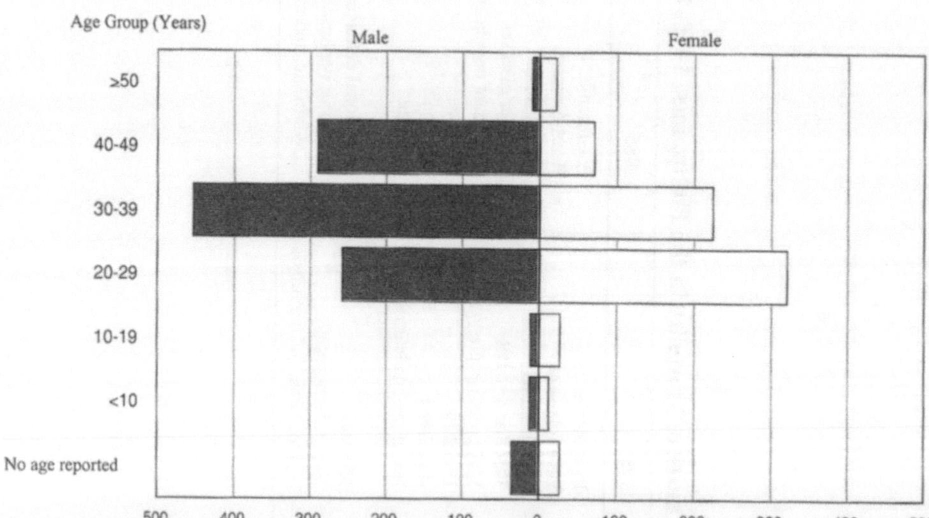

	≥50	40-49	30-39	20-29	10-19	<10	No age reported
Male ■	10	291	454	258	12	13	35
Female □	23	72	225	322	28	14	29

FIGURE 2. HIV Ab Seropositive Cases by Gender and Age Group, Philippines HIV/AIDS Registry, January 1984–June 2003 (n = 1892).

injecting drug users (IDU), and males with other sexually transmitted infections (MSTI). This serologic surveillance was done twice a year, until 1997, when an external evaluation team recommended that it be done annually as there was no expected change that could be appreciated in six months. Ten major urban cities constituted the sentinel sites: Baguio, Angeles, Quezon, Pasay, Cebu, Iloilo, Cagayan de Oro, Davao, General Santos, and Zamboanga.

After eight years of surveillance, the estimated prevalence among the FSWs in these ten cities is between 1–2%; among MSMs in the cities of Cebu and Quezon, prevelance may be as high as 4%, but this finding is not consistent through the years (NHSSS Technical Report, 2001).

In 1995, NHSS included military recruits from the Armed Forces of the Philippines as surrogates for the general male population. To date, none has tested positive for HIV among of military recruits. This does not mean that there is no HIV transmission, but rather that transmission may be so low that it is not detected by the HIV sentinel surveillance methodology.

In 1997, behavioral sentinel surveillance (BSS) was started in the same sites already implementing serologic surveillance to monitor the level of risk behaviors among HRGs that predispose them to acquiring HIV. Knowledge about HIV prevention, health seeking behavior, and sources of information about HIV/AIDS were included in this surveillance. After six years of annual monitoring, it looked like the high awareness and knowledge among HRGs was still not translated into a change in behavior, particularly condom use. Only one in every three respondents consistently and correctly used condoms; IDUs continued to share injecting equipment although there was an increasing trend of IDUs who cleaned their injecting equipment with soap and water or bleach before sharing it; and many of the HRGs who had symptoms of sexually transmitted infection continued to self-medicate. The BSS also showed that more and more MSM practiced anal sex.

LOW AND SLOW TRANSMISSION

Analysis of passive and active surveillance shows that the Philippines still has a very low prevalence of HIV, even in the most vulnerable groups. There are those who argue that the surveillance system methodology is not sensitive enough and is not able to detect HIV effectively. This issue has been addressed by two consensus workshops where stakeholders from other agencies, academe, NGOs, and international organizations have gathered to review HIV epidemiology in the Philippines. All have agreed that the Philippines has a good surveillance system. Though the possibility of underreporting is present, there could not be many missed cases, without a higher number of AIDS admissions in hospitals. In addition, several independent surveys have been done, and none have shown prevalence greater than 1% in any of the groups surveyed.

In the early 1990s, AIDS authorities in the Philippines used the EPI model to project that there would be 100–200,000 HIV-infected people by 2000. They compared the situation in the Philippines with Thailand and assumed that the Philippines would follow the same path Thailand had. These experts were proven wrong when there were only a little more than 1000 HIV-infected people at the end of that year, and there was no evidence that there could be more than what we were seeing. Using population disaggregation, we estimated from available data that there could be no less than 6,000 and no more than 15,000 HIV-positive people, with the official number rounded out to 10,000. This figure will not remain so low indefinitely. Many agree that it may just be a matter of time until a critical number of HIV-infections is reached, and the number of infections explodes exponentially. There is no room for complacency.

WHAT SEEMS TO PROTECT THE PHILIPPINES FROM HIV/AIDS?

Considering that risk behavior has not improved, the following factors are hypothesized to be protective or to have contributed to the low and slow transmission:

1. Low partner turn-out for FSW. BSS consistently showed an average of

1–2 partners per week for establishment-based female sex workers, and five per week for freelance female sex workers. Since establishment-based FSW already earn wages from working as waitresses, models, promotion girls, or masseurs, they can afford to have only few partners and still be assured of an income.

2. Only about 15% of Filipino males admitted to have exposure to sex workers in the last 12 months prior to interview (WHO/DOH, 2002).
3. The estimated prevalence rates of sexually transmitted infections such as syphilis and gonorrhea are high (5–7% and 15–30% respectively among HRGs and <4% and <2% respectively among low risk females), but STI lesions such as herpes, warts, and syphilitic lesions are rare (WHO/DOH, 2002).
4. The Philippines has a drug problem but very few people inject drugs. In fact, IDUs had to be dropped in 9 of 10 sentinel sites because the sites could not provide the required sample size of 100 respondents for the surveillance. Cebu is the only city reporting IDUs, and the estimated prevalence of HIV there is about 1% or up to 3% in a worst case scenario (2001 NHSSS Technical report).
5. Almost all Filipino males are circumcised. A study done in Bangkok showed that circumcision may be protective (Mastro *et al.*, 1994)). Circumcision among male Filipinos is not religious or cultural, but rather a file of passage to manhood. It is socially unacceptable and embarrassing for an adolescent male to be branded as uncircumcised.
6. Social Hygiene Clinics (SHC) were established more than 50 years ago. SHCs provide regular screening for gonorrhea and syphilis for FSW; if a FSW is found positive for either of the two diseases, she is not allowed to work in the establishment until after she is treated and tests negative. The Philippines is the only country in Southeast Asia which has this kind of screening service for FSW, as was observed by the STI office of the WHO Western Pacific Regional Office.

THE PHILIPPINES: STILL AT RISK

There are, however, subpopulations outside of the classical HRGs that can still drive the epidemic in the Philippines. This includes returning overseas Filipino workers (OFW), MSM, and youth, who collectively, comprise about a third of the whole population.

Overseas Filipino Workers (OFW)

About a third of HIV/AIDS cases recorded in the AIDS Registry are returning overseas contract workers; specifically, seamen (Figure 3). Most of them may not practice any risk behavior while in the country, but when they go abroad, they become vulnerable. Their vulnerability stems from several factors: that they are away from their regular partners, they have excess money to spend, they experience peer pressure and loneliness, and sexual entertainment is available in the ports where they dock. A study done in 1998 by KALAYAAN (League of Women for Freedom)/CARAM(Coordination for Action Research on AIDS and Mobility) among those who worked abroad for the first time showed poor knowledge of HIV/AIDS, low condom use, poor health-seeking behavior, and an attitude of invincibility where HIV/AIDS is concerned. OFW are the bridge population which may bring the infection to their unsuspecting wives or regular partners (Marin, 2000). The Philippine Overseas Employment Agency (POEA) reported less than a million documented OFWs in 2002. There are estimates that the number may rise up to 2–5 million. In light of this, this group should be prioritized or at least included in the surveillance system. Unfortunately, they are not tested when they come back to the Philippines, as there is no mandatory AIDS testing according to the Philippine AIDS Law. They may be tested when they leave the Philippines as a requirement of the receiving country, and they usually test negative. But they are not tested when they come back, and it is when they

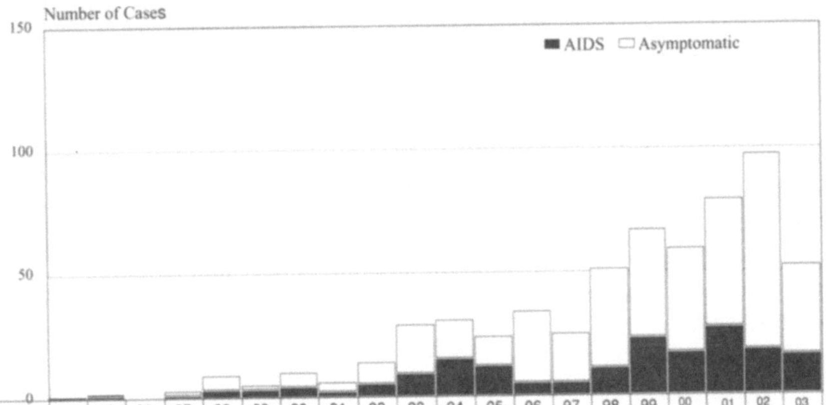

Year	84	85	86	87	88	89	90	91	92	93	94	95	96	97	98	99	00	01	02	03
TOTAL	1	2	0	3	9	5	10	6	14	29	31	24	34	25	51	67	59	79	97	52
Asymptomatic	0	1	0	2	6	2	6	4	9	20	16	12	29	20	40	44	42	52	79	36
AIDS	1	1	0	1	3	3	4	2	5	9	15	12	5	5	11	23	17	27	18	16
Death	1	1	0	1	3	1	3	2	4	3	6	7	3	2	5	4	2	10	5	3

FIGURE 3. HIV Ab Seropositive Cases among Oversease Filipino Workers (OFWs), Philippines HIV/AIDS Registry, January 1984–June 2003 (n = 600).

are abroad that they may have been exposed. There were many instances wherein the returning OFW infected their partners at home and both never knew of their infection until they were already symptomatic.

MSM

A national male sexuality survey done by De La Salle University (Lee, 1990) showed that 15% of respondents had sex with another male. Several other studies among the youth gave similar findings. If this number is correct, that would be 15% of 20 million, or 300,000 males.

The AIDS Registry consistently reports more males than females; they report that the mode of transmission of their infection was through heterosexual contact. Considering that it is not likely that these males will admit their sexuality or sexual preference to complete strangers such as the laboratory personnel, then this particular item in the AIDS Registry report may not be true. Even though MSM are included in HSS and BSS, most of the respondents are usually openly gay men or transvestites. There are subsets of this group (MSM) such as those who remain confidential, bisexuals, or those who engage in sex with other men infrequently, which are not included in the surveillance system because it is almost impossible to do so. The implication is that the health authorities may be focusing their AIDS prevention program to the wrong groups, or at least not on the populations that would need it most.

Youth

Youth are at risk, particularly adolescents up to age 24, who comprise 38% of the population. Surveys show that sexual debut for both males and females occur when they are about 18 years old (range of 15–20 years). Most are not aware of the risk of sexually transmitted infections or unwanted pregnancy as evidenced by the increasing number of abortion cases reported by hospitals. College students living away from home are most vulnerable because of their "freedom" from parental supervision. Some turn to sex work to be able to afford material goods such as cellular phones, clothes and shoes, or even for more practical expenses, such as payment for tuition fee. These young people are the most difficult to reach, even more difficult than sex workers, because they are in denial. They do not want information or advice because they feel they are not at risk.

If the health authorities do not exert more effort in including these subpopulations for the surveillance system and planning interventions that target them, it will be only a matter of time before the Philippines finds itself in the same situation as its high prevalence neighbors.

FACTORS INFLUENCING THE HIV/AIDS EPIDEMIC

Poverty

The Philippines has a high poverty index, with more than a third of the population living below the poverty line . This may be the reason only a small percentage of males have excess cash to spend for sex workers. But this is also a reason more men and women turn to sex work as a main or supplementary source of income.

Conservatism

Generally, Filipinos are sexually conservative. It may be the influence of Catholicism or the socio-cultural environment that influence over 90% of the males to be monogamous. Even the small percentage of males who professed to have more than one sexual partner do not have these partners all at the same time, but rather in successive monogamous relationships. Sexual practices of the general male population, the sexual network of MSM, and commercial sex work are "tame" compared, for example, to what has been documented in Thailand and the United States (specifically San Francisco).

This conservatism hampers sex education and information initiatives because sex is considered "taboo" and is not discussed openly, especially not with the youth. It also prevents people from seeking sexual advice or health care because of the embarrassment of having to do so. This leads to self-medication at best, or at worst, not seeking care at all.

Injecting Drug Use (IDU)

This is not the preferred method of drug use in the Philippines because it is more expensive and less accessible than metamphetamines and marijuana, and because males generally resist injections. The injectable drugs of choice are nalbuphine, which is an analgesic, or local anaesthetics. Since these drugs are common and not illegal, they are harder to monitor and may not be prioritized by drug enforcement agents. For this reason, there may be undetected IDUs, and it may be too late before this threat is recognized.

THE PHILIPPINES: RESPONSE AND CHALLENGES

The Philippines responded quickly to the threat of HIV/AIDS by including it in the list of reportable diseases, establishing a surveillance system, establishing the National AIDS/STD Prevention and Control Program (NASPCP) under the DOH in 1987, creating the Philippine National AIDS Council in 1992 (by virtue of Executive Order No. 39 issued by then President Fidel V. Ramos), and passing the Philippine AIDS Law in 1998. The academe, non-governmental organizations, private individuals, and the business sector were also quick to respond. Technical support from the WHO, USAID, JICA, AusAID, and the European Union helped prepare the country to fight the epidemic.

A Medium Term Plan (MTP) was formulated by NASPCP in 1987, which aimed to reduce HIV transmission, morbidity and mortality associated with HIV infection, and minimize the impact of HIV infection and AIDS on the individual, the family, and the community. Unfortunately, there were not sufficient mechanisms put in place for the plan to be effectively carried out. A second MTP was developed to strengthen the implementation of the strategies while retaining the objectives of the first MTP. Unfortunately, the multi-sectoral involvement in the MTP became an impediment, as some stakeholder activities were inconsistent with the policies or were even in direct conflict with the position of the DOH. The national and local responses were not unified, even when there was a plan.

The Philippines prided itself on being the first country in the Asia to enact an AIDS Law in 1998. The law ensures the rights and privileges, especially privacy and confidentiality, of HIV/AIDS patients, provides a mechanism for their care and treatment, institutionalizes HIV prevention education programs in government agencies, and formalizes the monitoring and surveillance system through AIDSWATCH. However, after four years, it cannot be claimed that this law has been fully implemented. Lack of political will, insufficient funds, and lack of commitment from government agencies in all levels contribute to the poor implementation.

Most of the projects supported by international agencies have had a 3–5 year project life. These projects began in the early 1990s, so all had ended by 2000. Though some were continued at the national and local level, there are many gaps that can only be filled with funding and technical support from the international community. Unfortunately, interest in the prevention of the HIV/AIDS in the Philippines is waning because of the perception that HIV is not a problem here. Global support is being channeled to Africa and other countries devastated by high morbidity and mortality from HIV/AIDS.

It had been almost twenty years since the first HIV case was reported in the Philippines. Although much has been accomplished, there is more that needs to be done in order to prevent a full-blown epidemic from occurring. Program implementation is hampered to a great extent by religious, cultural, social, and economic concerns, not to mention lack of political will, ignorance, and stigmatization of and discrimination against persons living with AIDS. But these are barriers that can be overcome if the Philippines seizes the opportunity while it is ahead of the epidemic. And this can only be done with the full commitment and political will of a nation united in the fight to prevent and contain the epidemic.

REFERENCES

FIES (2000). Family Incomes and Expenditures Survey, www.census.gov.ph/data (accessed Jan. 25, 2004)

Lee, R. (1990). Psychosocial Determinants of Risk Taking and Preventive Behavior Related to HIV and AIDS Among Male Homosexuals. SDRC Completed project, De La Salle University. Manila.

Marin, M.L. (2002). HIV/AIDS Knows No Borders: Addressing HIV Vulnerability of Overseas Filipino Workers (OFWs). KALAYAAN/CARAM-Asia, www.phssa.org/pubs/nchss1/hiv.htm (accessed January 30, 2004).

Mastro, T.D., Satten, G.A., Nopkesorn, T., Sangkharomya, S., and Longini, I.M. Jr. (1994). Probability of female-to-male transmission of HIV-1 in Thailand. *Lancet*. 343:204–207.

National Demographic and Health Survey (NDHS). www.census.gov.ph/hhld/ndhs9803.html.

NHSSS (2001). www.usaid-ph.gov/documents/2001 (accessed Jan. 25, 2004).

National Statistical Coordination Board (NSCB). (1998). www.nscb.gov.ph (accessed Jan. 25, 2004).

National Statistical Office (NSO). (1999). www.census.gov.ph (accessed Jan. 25, 2004).

Philippine Health Statistics (1997). www.nationamaster.com/country/rp/health/ (accessed Jan. 25, 2004).

WHO/DOH (2002). Consensus Report on STI, HIV, and AIDS Epidemiology. World Health Organization and Department of Health, Philippines. *www.wpro.who.int/document/sti_phl2002/* (accessed Jan. 27, 2004).

9

Evolving HIV Epidemic in Pakistan

Sharaf Ali Shah[1] and Syed Abdul Mujeeb[2]

[1] *Sindh AIDS Control Program, Karachi, Pakistan*
[2] *HIV/AIDS Surveillance Centre, Jinnah Postgraduate Medical Centre, Karachi, Pakistan*

COUNTRY PROFILE

Pakistan is one of the most populous countries in the world, with a current population of 145.5 million, an annual growth rate of 2.1%, an infant mortality rate of 85/1000 births, and a maternal mortality rate of 350/100,000 (Government of Pakistan, 2001). Situated in the western part of South Asia, Pakistan is bordered by Iran and Afghanistan to the west, China to the north, India to the east, and the Arabian Sea to the south.

One-third (34%) of the population, around 48 million people, currently live below the poverty line. Per capita GNP is US$429. Pakistan's education and health indicators are depressed relative to other countries of similar per capita income or growth rate, and reveal large regional, urban/rural, and gender disparities. For example, the male literacy rate is 56.6%, while the female literacy rate is only 32.6%. Rural poverty rates are much higher than poverty rates in the urban areas (World Bank Pakistan, 2002).

INFECTIOUS DISEASES AND THEIR PUBLIC HEALTH SIGNIFICANCE

Infectious diseases including tuberculosis, viral hepatitis, malaria, respiratory tract infections and diarrheal diseases are major causes of morbidity and mortality in Pakistan, and are problems of great public health significance. In spite of its efforts, Pakistan is among the few countries in the world which has not yet been declared free of polio.

Tuberculosis

Pakistan ranks sixth among the countries with highest burden of tuberculosis in the world. It accounts for about 44% of total tuberculosis cases in the Eastern Mediterranean region. According to the WHO (2001), the incidence of sputum-positive tuberculosis in Pakistan is 80/100,000 per year, and incidence for all forms of tuberculosis is 177/100,000 about two-thirds (2/3) of which belong to the 15–45 age group. Tuberculosis is responsible for 5.1% of the total national disease burden in Pakistan (Government of Pakistan, 2003).

Hepatitis A to E

Hepatitis, viral infections types A to E, are a major public health concern. They are a significant cause of mortality and morbidity in all age groups and segments of the society. Unsafe drinking water is responsible for most of the hepatitis A infections among children and hepatitis E infections among adults. Unsafe injection practices, blood transfusion and poor immunization against hepatitis B infection are responsible for the high prevalence of hepatitis B and C infection among the general population (Luby *et al.*,1997; Mujeeb,1998; Zuberi, 1996).

Sexually Transmitted Infections (STIs)

Information about STI and RTI (reproductive tract infection) prevalence in Pakistan is scarce. Diagnosis and treatment services at the primary and secondary health care levels are almost non-existent. Dermatologists and gynecologists provide clinical care to STI and RTI patients at the tertiary health care level. In the non-formal health care sector, a large number of sex clinics provide treatment services exclusively to male clients.

Studies conducted in 2001 among antenatal clinic attendees and gynecological patients revealed that 78% of women had pathological vaginal discharge, 29% had pelvic tenderness, 17% had cervical ulcers and 3.7% had vesicles on genitalia (National AIDS Control Program, 2002b).

A multi-center study among women attending public sector hospitals in Sindh with the complaint of vaginal discharge showed *Neisseria gonorrhea* infections in 6.5%. *Chlamydia trachomatis* was found in 2.2% of these women and *Trichomonas vaginalis* in 5.6% (National AIDS Control Program, 2002c; Shah *et al.*, 2001; Baqi *et al.*, 1999).

HEALTH CARE DELIVERY SYSTEM IN PAKISTAN

History

National public health is a recent development in Pakistan. Before partition, during British rule, people of the subcontinent relied mostly on alternative medicine for their healthcare needs. In the early 1970s, a decentralized system was developed in which basic health units (BHU) and rural health centers (RHC) were established.

Practices

Currently, in addition to public and private sector biomedicine, there are indigenous forms of treatment such as Unani Tibb (Arabic or Greek medicine). Practitioners of Unani Tibb are called Hakims. Homeopathy is another commonly practiced alternative medicine (1 up info, 1994) .

Allocation of Resources

The total allocation for health in the public sector for 2001–2002 was 25,405 million Pakistan Rupees (Rs), or US$444 million. Rs18,717 million (US$327 million) have been allocated as recurrent and Rs 6,688 million (US$117million) as development budget, including Rs 4405 million (US$77 million) as the federal component. This total allocation (Rs 25,405 million or US$444 million) is 0.7% of GDP (Government of Pakistan, 2003).

Accessibility, Acceptability and Affordability of Health Care Services

In the public sector, there is a nationwide network of healthcare facilities. On January 1, 2002 there were 906 hospitals with 80,655 beds, 4590 dispensaries with 2815 beds, 285 tuberculosis clinics with 212 beds, 550 rural health centers with 8840 beds, and an additional 254 beds in maternal-child health centers. There is also a growing number of health care facilities in the private sector, mostly concentrated in urban areas. The public sector is accessible to almost 70% of the population. It offers services almost free of charges, but quality of services is variable. Mostly people of low socioeconomic groups tend to use the public sector healthcare facilities. Quality of health care services in the private sector is also variable but there exist some state-of-the-art institutions (Government of Pakistan, 2003).

Preventative versus Curative Care

Currently, the health care system in Pakistan is predominantly curative, and a large portion of the public health funding allocation is spent on tertiary care. However, a recent shift to a preventive approach is visible, and the government has established several preventive programs to address issues of public health significance (Government of Pakistan, 2003).

HIV/AIDS

History

The first case of AIDS in Pakistan was reported in 1986, in the city of Karachi, province of Sindh. The HIV-infected person was an African sailor (not a Pakistani national). The first case of AIDS in a Pakistani citizen, who was believed to have become infected with HIV while traveling outside of Pakistan, was reported in 1987 in the city of Lahore, province of Punjab. In 1988, a Pakistani family, including husband, wife and child, with no history of travel abroad were found infected with HIV, and two recipients of multiple blood transfusions from local paid donors were also diagnosed as being HIV-positive. In 1993, the first recognized transmission of HIV infection through breastfeeding in Pakistan was reported in the city of Rawalpindi (Kazi,1998; Ministry of Health and UNAIDS, 2000). Since the early 1990's, the majority of HIV/AIDS cases reported in the country were Pakistani citizens deported from Gulf Countries and their spouses. A similar pattern was observed in all provinces / regions of Pakistan (Shah *et al.*, 1999).

Current Status of the Epidemic

The current HIV/AIDS situation in Pakistan, as in some other Asian countries, is at a precarious and dangerous crossroads. Pakistan is currently considered a low prevalence / high-risk country, due to low numbers of reported cases—1998 by December 2002 (National AIDS Control Program, 2002a). Based on WHO /UNAIDS epidemiological forecast models, calculated estimates of HIV is 50,000 to 70,000 infections, which is a relatively low prevalence for a nation of 145 million persons (0.05% of adult population). Seroprevalence studies conducted among the high risk groups such as female sex workers, hijras (transsexuals and transvestites), injecting drug users (IDU), long distance truckers, and prison inmates have revealed a low prevalence of HIV infection but a high prevalence of other sexually transmitted infections such as syphilis (Ministry of Health and UNAIDS, 2000; Ministry of Health and UNAIDS, 2001; Baqi *et al.*, 1999).

Risk Factors

With low HIV prevalence, Pakistan is still in a good position to halt a major epidemic. However, the current epidemic stage could rapidly change from low prevalence to a generalized epidemic, as has happened in other countries due to the following risk factors:

- increasing levels of poverty with high population growth rate,
- low levels of literacy, particularly in women,
- legal and illegal cross-border mobility with a huge Afghan refugee population (2.2 million),

- risky sexual practices and very low use of condoms,
- large drug user population shifting away from inhalation to injecting drug use,
- irrational use of injections and reuse of used syringes and needles,
- unsafe blood transfusion and lack of proper screening, and
- high prevalence of other sexually transmitted infections and blood borne infections.

(Kazi, 1998; Khuwaja, *et al.*, 1997, Luby *et al.*, 1997; Mujeeb *et al.*, 1998; Baqi *et al.*, 1999; Shah *et al.*, 1999).

Threats and Challenges

Vulnerable populations and high risk groups are difficult to approach for HIV/AIDS prevention interventions in Pakistan due to their illegal status, marginal social status and/or limited education. Due to social and cultural constraints, specific HIV/AIDS prevention messages on print and electronic media are difficult to present.

A considerable challenge to Pakistan's HIV/AIDS prevention efforts is the existence of a lobby which considers HIV/AIDS a foreign problem rather than an issue of public health significance and opposes the allocation of resources towards HIV/AIDS instead of towards Pakistan's numerous, more urgent public health problems.

Opportunities and Lessons Learned

The current low prevalence of HIV presents our greatest opportunity to control the disease in this country. There are increasing numbers of NGOs and CBOs (community-based organizations) working in HIV/AIDS-related fields. There is a wide stakeholder commitment to the control of the HIV/AIDS pandemic. An enhanced HIV/AIDS control program, which was launched in 2003 in Pakistan with the support of the World Bank, holds the promise of strengthening the AIDS control program at national and provincial levels. Media, particularly electronic media have increased awareness of HIV/AIDS among difficult to reach populations. There is better acceptance of HIV/AIDS prevention messages when they are incorporated with prevention information about other prevalent infections which are spread through blood or sexual contact. A recent outbreak of HIV/AIDS among IDU in Larkana in which 22 injecting drug users tested positive for HIV during June, July and August this year (Shah, *et al.*, 2003), has further emphasized that Pakistan is a high-risk country.

IMPACT OF AND RESPONSE TO HIV/AIDS

Impact

Until now, Pakistan has seen little measurable impact of HIV/AIDS. Deportation of HIV-positive Pakistani workers working in Gulf countries (Shah *et al.*, 1999) has the potential to produce some economic loss in terms of remittances but this population is only a fraction of the total Pakistani workforce currently working overseas. Since the number of HIV-infected individuals in the country is still very low, there has been no visible strain on healthcare facilities and resources, or on the overall economy. More clearly visible have been the positive steps taken so far in response to the threat of HIV/AIDS: an increased level of political commitment for HIV/AIDS prevention, and efforts by the media, civil society (NGOs), UN agencies, and donors.

Governmental Response

Soon after the diagnosis of the first HIV/AIDS case in the country, the Ministry of Health of the Government of Pakistan established the National AIDS Control Program in Islamabad. In 1994–1995, this federal program was decentralized and provincial programs were established. In

1999, the Government of Pakistan, with the assistance of development partners in collaboration with all stakeholders developed the National HIV/AIDS strategic framework.

Beginning in 2003, and for the next five years, the Enhanced HIV/AIDS Control Program is being implemented nationwide with the assistance of a loan of US$ 27.83 million and a grant of US$9.28 million from the World Bank/International Development Association (IDA) (Hyder *et al.*, 1999; Kazi, 1998; Ministry of Health and UNAIDS, 2000; Ministry of Health and UNAIDS, 2001; World Bank, 2002).

NGO Response

Currently as many as 86 NGOs and CBOs are working on HIV/AIDS issues (UNAIDS, 2002) throughout country through consortia formed in all four provinces, and with the assistance of UNAIDS and provincial programs. Nonetheless due to poor infrastructure, limited financial resources, and weak cooperation and coordination among themselves, their meaningful contribution to the overall HIV/AIDS response has been very limited.

MINIMIZING THE FUTURE IMPACTS OF HIV/AIDS IN PAKISTAN

Multi-Sectoral Efforts

Considering the dynamics of HIV infection and learning from global experiences, multi-sectoral, coordinated efforts are urgently required. Pakistan still has a window of opportunity: since HIV infection is still confined to certain populations, timely prevention efforts could halt its spread.

Expanded Role of NGOs/CBOs

NGOs/CBOs working at the grassroots level, particularly those who are working with vulnerable and marginalized populations such as sex workers, drug users, and prisoners, should be encouraged to play a role in reducing the vulnerabilities of such groups.

The majority of NGOs/CBOs, which work with vulnerable and marginalized populations in Pakistan, need to further build their capacities.

Safe Blood Transfusion Services

Although the safety of blood has been included in the National Program from its inception, only 20% of total blood transfused in the country is properly screened (including both public and private sector transfusions). Voluntary blood donation needs to be increased though education, motivation and recruitment of regular voluntary blood donors (Mujeeb *et al.*, 2002).

Improved Care and Support for People Living With HIV/AIDS (PLWHA)

At present, there are limited resources available for the care and management of PLWHA. Under the Enhanced HIV/AIDS Control Program, provisions have been made for treatment of opportunistic infections, but there is no provision for antiretroviral drugs in the government program. Healthcare providers need to be motivated and trained in necessary skills, antiretroviral drugs must be registered and made available along with good diagnositcs at subsidized rates, and PLWHA need to be involved in decision-making at all levels (Mujeeb and Altaf, 2003).

REFERENCES

1 up info. (1994). Country study and Country guide-Pakistan. Health care policies and development in Pakistan. Pakistan information resources. http://www.1 upinfo.com.

Baqi, S., Shah, S.A., Baig, M.A., Mujeeb, S.A. and Memon, A. (1999). Seroprevalence of HIV, HBV and syphilis and associated risk behaviors in male transvestites (Hijra) in Karachi, Pakistan. *Int J STD AIDS*.10, 300–304.

Government of Pakistan. (2003). Annual Report of Director General Health 2001–2002. Bio-Statistics Section Primary Health Care Ministry of Health. Islamabad. pp. 27–30.

Government of Pakistan. (2001). Economic Survey 2000–2001. Economic Advisors Wing, Finance Division, Islamabad. pp. 1–9 appendix.

Hyder, A.A., Khan, O.A., Shah, S.A., Memon, M.A., Khanani, M.R., Ali, S. (1999). Sub-national Response in HIV/AIDS: a case study in AIDS prevention and control from Sindh Province, Pakistan. *Public Health*. 113(1): 39–43.

Kazi, B.M. (1998). A review of the HIV/AIDS situation and National AIDS program of Pakistan. *Pak J Med Res*. 37: s13–s17.

Khuwaja, Z.A., Gilbney, L., Ahmed, A.J., Vermund, S.H. (1997). HIV/AIDS and its risk factors in Pakistan. *AIDS* 11:843; 8–10.

Luby, S.P., Qamruddin, C., Shah, A., Omar, P., Pasha, O., Khan, A.J., Hoodbhouy, F., McCormick, J. and Fisherhock, S. (1997). The relationship between therapeutic injections and high prevalence of hepatitis C in Hafizabad, Pakistan. *Epidemiology and Infection*; 119 (3): 349–356.

Ministry of Health and UNAIDS (2001). National HIV/AIDS Strategic Framework, 2001–2006, Pakistan. UNAIDS, Islamabad. pp. 1–46.

Ministry of Health and UNAIDS (2000). HIV/AIDS in Pakistan: a situation and response analysis. Government of Pakistan. Islamabad. pp. 1–27.

Mujeeb, S.A. (1998). Seroprevalence and pattern of viral hepatitis in Pakistan-review. *J Inf Dis* 5; 19–20.

Mujeeb, S.A., Akram, A., Ahmed, M., and Ahmed, S. (2002). State of blood transfusion services in Karachi: a review in the context of blood transmitted infections. *J Inf Dis* 9; 129–130.

Mujeeb, S.A. and Altaf, A. (2003). The AIDS Pandemic. *N Eng J Med*. 349; 814–815.

National AIDS Control Program. (2002a). HIV/AIDS surveillance report December 2002 National Institute of Health, Islamabad.

National AIDS Control Program. (2002b). Pakistan: Expanded response to HIV/AIDS, Enhanced HIV/AIDS Control Program, Project implementation plan draft, Islamabad.

National AIDS Control Program. (2002c). Proposed research strategy and study design. National study of reproductive tract infection and sexually transmitted infections. Ministry of Health, Government of Pakistan, Islamabad. pp. 1–9.

Shah, S.A., Altaf, A., Mujeeb, S.A. and Memon, A. (2003). An out break of HIV infection among IDUs in small town of Pakistan; potential for national implications. *Int J STD AIDS* (in press).

Shah, S.A., Khan, O.A., Kristensen, S. and Vermund, S.H. (1999). HIV-infected workers deported from the Gulf states: impact on southern Pakistan. *Int J STD AIDS*. 10, 812–214.

Shah, S.A., Memon, M.A., Ghauri, A.K., Suhani, S., Kristensen, S., Vermund, S.H., and Khan, U. (2001). Pathogens causing vaginal discharge among women attending clinics in Sindh-Pakistan. 6th ICAAP, Melbourne, Australia.

UNAIDS and Ministry of Health. (2002). NGOs involved in HIV/AIDS prevention in Pakistan. UNAIDS and Government of Pakistan, 2002.

World Bank. (2002). The World Bank Project Appraisal Document Report No. 25109-PAK Human Development Unit South Asia Regional Office.

World Bank Pakistan. (2002). Pakistan Poverty Assessment, poverty in Pakistan: Vulnerabilities, Social Gaps and Rural Dynamics Report no. 24296-Pak (2002), pp. i–xviii

Zuberi, S.J. (1996). Sero-epidemiology of HBV, HCV infections in Pakistan. *Int Hema Commun*. 5; 19–26.

10

HIV/AIDS in Nepal

Context, Current Situation, Response

Ganesh Gurung[1] and B. K. Suvedi[2]

[1] *Nepal Institute of Development Studies, Kathmandu, Nepal*
[2] *Ministry of Health, Kathmandu, Nepal*

BACKGROUND

Nepal is one of the least developed countries in Asia, having a population of 23.1 million with an annual growth rate of 2.2% (CBS, 2001). Even though Nepal allocates five to six percent of its total national budget to the health sector every year, indicators demonstrate the relatively poor health of the Nepali population. The infant mortality rate is as high as 64.2 deaths/1000 live births, and the maternal mortality rate is 415/100,000. In addition, the fertility rate is 4.1%, with the contraceptive-using rate being 39.3%; the average life expectancy is 61.9 years (NPC/CBS, 2001).

In the first half of the 20th century, few formal health services were available in Nepal. Most of these services were preventive, offered through traditional practitioners. As a result, the vast majority of the population did not enjoy a formal health care system. In 1933, the Department of Health Services was established with the objective of providing health services to the Nepali population. Today, the formal health sector is organized through the Ministry of Health, (MoH), with central offices in Kathmandu. The MoH is by far the largest single provider of formal health services. MoH expenditures comprise nearly 50% of total government expenditure on health care.

Besides the MoH, there are international, non-governmental organizations (NGOs) and private institutions that provide health services in Nepal.

NATIONAL HISTORY AND CURRENT STATUS OF INFECTIOUS DISEASES

The Nepalese people have known infectious diseases like smallpox, cholera, malaria, leprosy, and tuberculosis since antiquity. Available ancient documents in Sanskrit mention these diseases, along with herbal treatments for them (Suvedi, 1990). As the diseases were thought to be due to the scourge of the devil, many temples were erected to pacify or cure these diseases. Some examples

TABLE 1. Top Ten Causes of Morbidity, Nepal, 2001

Condition	% of total morbidity
Skin Diseases	5.76
Acute Respiratory Infections	3.44
Diarrheal Diseases	3.38
Intestinal worms	2.76
Fever	2.30
Gastritis	2.20
Ear Infection	1.56
Chronic Bronchitis	1.20
Abdominal Pain	1.05
Sore Eyes	1.02

Source: (MoH, 2002a)

are the Sitala Mai temple in Kathmandu (for smallpox), Kandeutasthan (for ear ailments), Santaneshwor Mahadev (for infertility), and Kilagal (for toothache) (Dixit, 1999). Over time, the practice of worshipping became accompanied by the use of herbal medicines. At present, at least three different forms of treatment exist in Nepal: allopathic, Ayurvedic/homeopathic, and traditional (Dhami/Jhankris/Lamaism) (Suvedi, 1990).

Currently, except for smallpox, which was eradicated about 25 years ago, and poliomyelitis, on the verge of eradication, other infectious and deficiency diseases are still prevalent and contribute to about 48% of the total morbidity in Nepal. The ten leading causes of morbidity among Nepalese outpatients (numbering 8,642,852) for the year 2001 evidences the high prevalence of infectious diseases (MoH, 2002a).

Other infectious diseases like tuberculosis (0.7% of total yearly morbidity), malaria (0.29%), typhoid (0.81%), leprosy (0.03%), and sexually transmitted infections (STI) (0.07%) are also important in the total morbidity.

HIV/AIDS IN NEPAL

The first case of HIV/AIDS in Nepal was reported in July 1988, seven years after the first diagnosis of HIV/AIDS in the U.S.

TABLE 2. Reported HIV/AIDS Cases in Nepal, 1988–2003

Year	Male	Female	Total
1988 (July–Dec)	3	1	4
1989	—	2	2
1990	2	3	5
1991	12	14	26
1992	39	38	77
1993	41	40	81
1994	18	22	40
1995	71	39	110
1996	50	92	135
1997	394	85	489
1998	166	95	220
1999	174	54	222
2000	301	48	396
2001	264	95	324
2002	360	60	467
2003 (Jan–Oct)	428	178	606
Total	2323	881	3204

Source: National Center for AIDS and STD Control, October 2003.

The trend of HIV/AIDS over the last 15 years shows a gradual increase in the reported incidence as well as the estimated incidence (Suvedi, 1994; 1997). As seen in Table 2, the reported number of cases of HIV infection is increasing rather rapidly in Nepal. It has been reported that "almost all" districts in Nepal have cases of HIV/AIDS (Suvedi, 1997; Suvedi and Gurubacharya, 1992).

A study on sexual behavior patterns in Nepal in1992 revealed that pre-marital and extra-marital sexual relationships are not as uncommon in Nepal as was previously thought. This led to a realization of the possibility of widespread HIV/AIDS infections in the country (Suvedi and Gurubacharya, 1992).

Of the total 3204 cases of HIV reported to the National Center for AIDS and STD Control (NCASC) by the end of October 2003, 60.7% are clients of female sex workers (FSW), 15.7% are FSW, and 12.6% are injecting drug users (IDU). HIV infections are most often reported among the sexually active age groups (ages 15–39 years), contributing about 89.9% of total reported infections (Table 3).

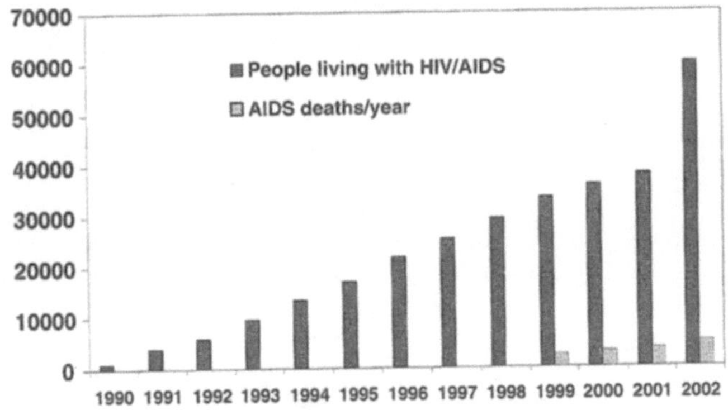

FIGURE 1. Number of PLWHA in Nepal and numbers of AIDS-related deaths per year (UNAIDS/NCASC, 2003).

TABLE 3. HIV Infection in Nepal by Age Group

Age group	Male	Female	Total	%
0–4 years	19	15	34	1.1
5–9 years	13	8	21	0.6
10–14 years	9	6	15	0.5
15–19 years	137	158	295	9.2
20–24 years	497	247	744	23.2
25–29 years	624	213	837	26.1
30–39 years	814	193	1007	31.4
40–49 years	180	36	216	6.7
50+ years	30	5	35	1.1
Total	2323	881	3204	99.9

Source: National Center for AIDS and STD Control, October 2003.

Of the total number of HIV cases, persons below 40 years of age comprise 92.2%. The 15–24 year age group accounts for 32.4% of all reported infections, indicating a rapid spread of HIV/AIDS in the younger population. Of the total number of HIV-positive persons, 20.9% have been reported to have symptoms of AIDS. However, only 182 HIV/AIDS deaths have been reported by the end of October 2003. The low number of deaths might be predominantly due to deaths occurring at home and not being included in hospital death statistics.

An estimate done by UNAIDS and the National Centre for AIDS and STD Control (NCASC) in 2002 shows that there may be 60,000 people living with HIV/AIDS (PLWHA) in Nepal. This translates into an overall prevalence of 0.5%, with an estimated 3000 deaths per year (UNAIDS/NCASC, 2003).

The following factors are considered significant for the rapid spread of HIV in Nepal (Suvedi and Gurubacharya, 1992):

1. Poverty
2. High mobility of young people in search of temporary jobs
3. Trafficking of FSW (luring of village girls into brothels abroad)
4. Low levels of awareness of HIV/STI
5. Discrimination/Stigmatization
6. Poor understanding of the epidemic, consequences of HIV/STI
7. Gender disparities

CURRENT SITUATION OF HIV/AIDS IN NEPAL

There are an estimated 60,000 PLWHA in Nepal. Prevalence is highest among IDU (40–68%), while among FSW it ranges from 3–17%, among blood donors from 0.28–0.48%, and among pregnant women prevalence is 0.2%. The primary mode of transmission is currently sexual (UNAIDS/NCASC, 2003).

Sexually Transmitted Infections

The trend of HIV infection among persons with STI in Nepal is mixed across the country (Figure 2). While the epidemic

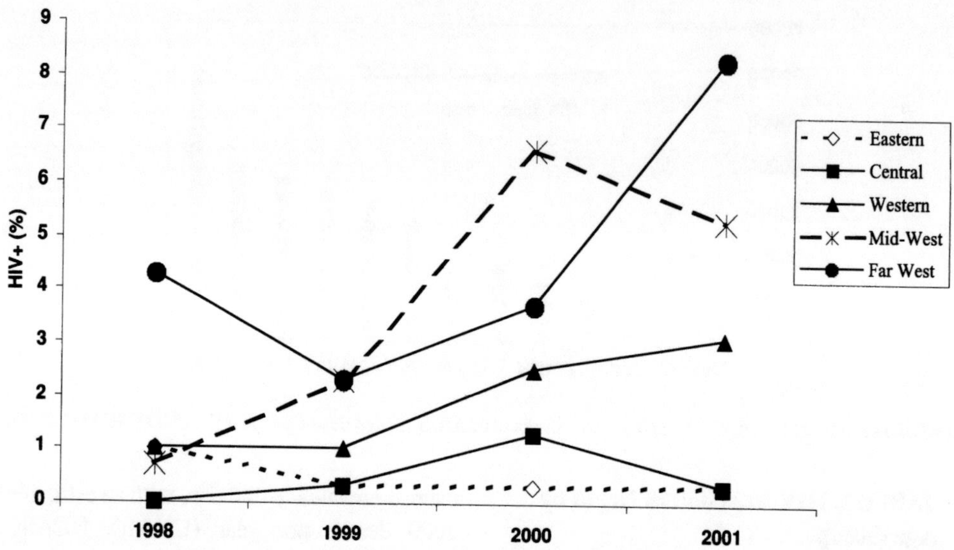

FIGURE 2. HIV prevalence rates among STI patients in several geographic areas of Nepal (Suvedi, 1997). Data from sentinel surveillance sites.

was concentrated in the central region in the first few years (1988–1993) and gradually spread to Eastern and Western regions of Nepal, the surveillance trend over the last five years shows a high incidence in the Far-West and Mid-Western Regions of Nepal (Suvedi, 1997).

STI are not uncommon in Nepal. However, persons with STI usually seek care with private medical practitioners. So, the available reports compiled at the central level do not show the true picture and the prevalence of infections. Unofficial estimates speculate that there may be as many as 200,000–600,000 sexually transmitted infections per year in the country. Limited research carried out in the areas with high migration show that there is a high prevalence of STI: 13% of the samples had one or more STIs. Herpes topped the list with 8.9% of people surveyed testing positive, while 2.3% had HIV, 1.3% had syphilis in the past, 1.1% had chlamydia, 0.7% had gonorrhea, and 0.5% had current cases of syphilis (Suvedi, 1994).

Migration

Seasonal migration in search of temporary jobs is an age-old tradition in the kingdom of Nepal. Many young people migrate to neighboring countries, especially during the winter. Causes of seasonal migration include low agricultural production, insufficient for feeding a family for a whole year; no alternative income activities beside agriculture; demand for unskilled and/or manual laborers elsewhere; lack of education or low-level of education/skills; and free time available during winter and spring. Financial pressures also motivate some to search for opportunities abroad. Family and peer pressure can also encourage Nepalese to migrate (UNAIDS/NCASC, 2003).

The "seasonal migration" takes place during winter and often lasts seven months. A significant majority (84%) of Nepalese migrants fall into the 15–29 year age group, and over two-thirds (68%) of them are married (UNAIDS/NCASC, 2003). During this period of absence from home many migrants have unprotected sexual contact with FSW, especially when outside the country. Infections contracted from FSW may therefore be transmitted to their wives at home after their return.

Studies indicate that the prevalence of HIV among the migrant population might be around 4–10%, which will possibly have a major influence on the future epidemic in

Nepal. Research has also indicated a high HIV prevalence among international migrants (3.7%), compared to 3% in internal migrants, and 0.7% in non-migrants (Poudel *et al.*, 2001; New ERA and SACTS, 2002).

At present, population mobility has increased to a significant level due to various factors including insurgency in the country. It is estimated that some 600,000 to 1,300,000 young people migrate every year in search of work. This has a tremendous socio-economic effect on Nepalese society, and will greatly impact the state of the HIV/AIDS epidemic in Nepal.

IMPACTS OF HIV/AIDS IN NEPAL

The impact of the HIV/AIDS epidemic in Nepal at a macro-level is yet to be seen, but at the family and community level, effects are already visible. Family level impacts include stigmatization and discrimination, including the marginalization of HIV-positive people from families or communities, discouraging them from getting necessary support and care.

The mean age of death in HIV/AIDS cases is reported to be 28.8 years; members of this age bracket are often the breadwinners for their family. Thus, younger age groups are affected, having a tremendous impact in the socio-cultural and economic spheres of Nepal.

NATIONAL RESPONSE

Nepal started HIV/AIDS prevention activities in 1988 with the implementation of a short-term plan. This was followed by a three-year strategy, concentrating on IEC (information, education, and communication) activities, strengthening of laboratory services, and orientation and training. The subsequent development of a medium-term plan for 1993–1997 was accompanied by the development of a policy on HIV/AIDS, and the establishment of an institution for the execution of HIV/AIDS prevention activities-the National Center for AIDS and STD Control (NCASC) under the Ministry of Health. A high level National AIDS Coordination Committee (NACC) under the authority of the Health Minister and with representation from various ministries and civil society was also established. During this period, the Ministry of Education incorporated HIV/AIDS and STI awareness into the curriculum of secondary schools, a policy for universal screening of donated blood was established, and public-private partnerships were initiated.

Condoms are currently provided free of charge through various outlets in Nepal. Both public and private sectors are promoting condoms for HIV prevention. Voluntary Counseling and Testing (VCT) services are so far very limited and need expansion. Support and care to HIV-positive Nepalese is minimal and antiretroviral (ARV) drugs are available only within the private sector. However, major hospitals are providing services to PLWHA.

A five-year Strategy for HIV/AIDS Prevention (1997–2001) was initiated in 1997. This strategy tried to operationalize the HIV/AIDS prevention policies developed earlier. Major activities were identified and targeted for implementation in this strategy. However, during this period, Nepal experienced the following:

1. The epidemiological situation changed, especially in high-risk behavior groups.
2. Nepal committed to the Millennium Development Goals.
3. Nepal also committed to the UNGASS' (United Nations General Assembly Special Session on HIV/AIDS) Declaration of Commitment on HIV/AIDS in 2001.
4. The Tenth Five Year Development Plan has identified HIV/AIDS as an issue affecting national development.

Two studies (Situation Analysis and Response Analysis of HIV/AIDS) were carried out in 2000 to evaluate the epidemic situation and response in Nepal. This research concluded the following:

- Groups already affected by HIV/AIDS (FSW and IDU) must be considered as a priority for immediate targeted interventions.
- Other groups such as mobile populations and young people are vulnerable to HIV/AIDS/STI and appropriate interventions should be designed and implemented to prevent HIV/AIDS/STI in these groups.
- The capacity of the institutions involved in Nepal's HIV/AIDS response is weak and interventions have been limited.
- There is a clear need to develop a national strategy.
- Political commitment is needed to fight HIV/AIDS.
- The capacity of NCASC needs to be strengthened for providing leadership and expertise for an expanded response.
- There is a need for providing care and support to PLWHA.

Keeping in mind that the increasing incidence of HIV/AIDS among high-risk behavior groups is leading to a "concentrated epidemic," Nepal initiated a special program in 2001 called the "Nepal Initiative." It focused on creating awareness and garnering a high level of commitment, which resulted in the formation of the National AIDS Council under the Prime Minister. Multi-sectoral representation and representation from civil society is the major feature of this council, which provides policy directives to the National AIDS Coordination committee.

The Nepal Demographic and Health Survey of 2001 showed that knowledge of HIV/AIDS among men was 71.7%, compared to 49.6% among women of reproductive age (MoH, 2002b). However, knowledge about HIV/AIDS prevention was low in both groups: 46.8% among men, and 32.4% among women. This clearly indicates that there is a wide gap between understanding the epidemic and prevention methods. This also indicates the necessity for more aggressive interventions to raise the awareness level of the Nepalese people regarding prevention.

In 2002, the National HIV/AIDS prevention strategy was developed for the period of 2002–2006. This strategy concentrates its activity on vulnerable populations and promotes care and support activities for those who are infected/affected by HIV/AIDS. The strategy identifies the following vulnerable groups for expanded response during 2002–2006: FSW and their clients, IDU, migrant laborers, men who have sex with men (MSM), and prisoners. Additionally, interventions targeting young people will be developed. The expanded response strategies also include strengthening treatment, care, and support programs; the assessment and monitoring of programs; and improving management of the expanded response projects (MoH/NCASC, 2002).

For the purpose of the effective implementation of HIV/AIDS control, an operational plan along with financial estimates has been carried out recently, which incorporates every intervention currently in vogue. Estimates suggest that US $95 million may be necessary to carry out the activities for a period of five years to curb the epidemic (MoH/NCASC, 2003).

The AIDS Program Effort Index (2003) has shown that Nepal has improved slightly over the last few years; with an index of 61 (out of 100) Nepal exceeds the regional average (API, 2003). However, it is speculated that the future of the HIV/AIDS epidemic in Nepal will be largely determined by the following factors:

- The return of girls trafficked as FSW, infected with HIV.
- Prevalence of HIV infection among the migrant population.
- Provision of comprehensive care and support for PLWHA.
- Greater effort and ownership of the HIV/AIDS program.

The effects of these determining factors are only beginning to be recognized in the emerging state of HIV/AIDS in Nepal.

REFERENCES

AIDS Program Effort Index (API). (2003). USAID, UNAIDS, WHO, and the Policy Project. (December 2003).

Central Bureau of Statistics (CBS). (2001). Population Census of 2001. In Collaboration with United Nations Population Fund (UNFPA). Kathmandu.

Dixit, H. (1999). *The Quest for Health*. Educational Enterprise Ltd, Kathmandu.

Ministry of Health (MoH). (2002a). Annual Report of Department of Health Services, Nepal. Kathmandu.

Ministry of Health (MoH). (2002b). Nepal Demographic and Health Survey 2001. Department of Health Services, Family Health Division. (unpublished)

Ministry of Health, Nepal (MoH) and National Centre for HIV/AIDS and STDs (NCASC). (2002). National HIV/AIDS Strategy (2002–2006). Kathmandu.

Ministry of Health, Nepal (MoH) and National Centre for HIV/AIDS and STDs (NCASC). (2003). National Operational Plan for HIV/AIDS Control (2003–2004). Kathmandu.

National Planning Commission (NPC)/ Central Bereau of Statististic (CBS). (2001). Stastistical Year Book of Nepal. Kathmandu.

Poudel, K.C., Okulura, J., Wasai, M., Sherchand, J.B., Zimba, M., Murakami, M. (2001). HIV/STI Survey in Nepal, Preliminary Findings. Kathmandu. (unpublished paper).

Suvedi, B.K. (1990). On the Road to Primary Health Care: Health Aspects of Baitadi. Kathmandu. (unpublished paper).

Suvedi, B.K. (1994). HIV/AIDS Manual. STD/AIDS Counseling and Training Services. Kathmandu.

Suvedi, B.K. (1997). Mapping the Trend of HIV/AIDS in Nepal. *J Nepal Med Assoc*. Kathmandu.

Suvedi, B.K., Gurubacharya, V.L. (1992). Sexual behavior patterns in Nepal. *J. Inst. Med.* 14(4):298–305.

Suvedi, B.K., Gurubacharya, V.L. and Thapa, K. (1994). Seasonal Migration in Western Nepal and its Relation to HIV Transmission. *J Nepal Med Assoc*. Kathmandu.

New ERA and STD/AIDS Counselling and Framing Series (SACTS). (2002). HIV/STD Prevalence and Risk Factors Among Migrants and Non Migrant Males of Achham District of Far Western Nepal. Family Health International Nepal. Kathmandu.

UNAIDS and National Centre for AIDS and STD Control (NCASC). (2003). The HIV/AIDS/STD Situation and National Response in Nepal: A Profile. Kathmandu.

11

Sri Lanka's Response to an Emerging HIV/AIDS Epidemic

Iyanthi Abeyewickreme[1], H.M.S.S.D.Herath[2], and Hamamal Jayawardena[3]

[1]*National STD/AIDS Control Programme, Ministry of Health Colombo, Sri Lanka*
[2]*National HIV/AIDS Prevention Project, Ministry of Health Colombo, Sri Lanka*
[3]*World Health Organization Dhaka, Bangladesh*

INTRODUCTION

The island of Sri Lanka, situated off the southern coast of India, has a total area of 65,610 square kilometers, of which approximately 62,705 square kilometers is land and 2905 square kilometers is water. In 2001, the population was 18.7 million, with a composition of 74% Sinhalese, 18% Tamils (including those of recent Indian origin residing mainly in the plantation districts), and 7% Muslims; the remaining 1% of the population are members of other ethnic groups (Department of Census and Statistics, 2003). Intensive family planning programs implemented by both the government and non-governmental organizations from the 1950s, when the population growth rate was 2.8%, caused a significant decline in the growth rate, reducing it to a current rate of 1.1%. The population of Sri Lanka is expected to stabilize by about 2025 at about 23 million. Recent years have seen a change in the population structure with a reduction in the child population, an increase in the adolescent and economically active population, and a gradual increase in the elderly population. In addition, there has been a decline in the male to female sex ratio from 103:100 in 1981 to 98:100 in 2001 (Department of Health Services Sri Lanka, 2002). These changes are likely to affect the patterns of disease in future years and consequently the health care needs of the country.

HISTORICAL BACKGROUND

The Early Period

Sri Lanka has had a system of curative and preventive medicine since ancient times, as evidenced by numerous references in the chronicles and ancient inscriptions, as well as evidence from archeological remains of health care facilities and elaborate systems of sanitation (Geiger, 1923; Uragoda, 1987).

The allopathic system of medicine was introduced into the country by the successive occupations by the Portuguese (1505), the Dutch (1656), and the British (1796). The Dutch built hospitals in the Maritime Provinces of the island and manned them with their physicians and surgeons. In 1708, they built a leprosy asylum (which continues as the Leprosy Hospital today) for the segregation of persons suffering from leprosy, which was considered an important public health problem at that time.

The British occupied the Maritime Provinces in 1796 and gained full control of the island in 1815. From 1800, the British established military hospitals and dispensaries in many parts of the island to cater to the needs of the military establishment. Military doctors provided medical care to the civilian population until 1858, when the Civil Medical Department was established with a Principal Civil Medical Officer as head. Provincial Surgeons were given authority over the administration of the provinces. By 1886, the Civil Medical Department had established 26 Civil Hospitals, eight District Hospitals, six Immigration Hospitals (for the care of immigrant Indian laborers who fell ill during their long trek by foot to the plantations) and 14 District Outdoor Dispensaries (De Silva, 1936).

With the realization that environmental factors were responsible for the transmission of many communicable diseases, a special Sanitary Branch was established in the Civil Medical Department, under the aegis of a Senior Sanitary Officer, in 1913. Sanitary Officers, later to be designated Medical Officers of Health, were appointed and stationed mainly in the larger towns. These officers were assisted by Sanitary Inspectors and were responsible for environmental sanitation and the control of communicable diseases (De Silva, 1936).

In 1925, in recognition of the growing importance of preventive health, all curative and preventive services were brought under the control of *one* Director of Medical and Sanitary Services: the Principal Civil Medical Officer. He was assisted by a Deputy Director of Medical and Sanitary Services and two Assistant Directors, one for medical services and the other for sanitary services.

One of the early progressive steps taken after the establishment of the Department of Medical and Sanitary Services was the inauguration of the *Health Unit system* with the establishment, in 1926, of the first *Health Unit* in Kalutara, a coastal town in southwestern Sri Lanka. Over time the Health Unit system was extended to cover the entire country, providing a most efficient system for the delivery of preventive health care at the grassroots level. These units undertook all public health work on an intensive scale in well-demarcated areas, each covering populations of 40,000–80,000 under the administration of a Medical Officer of Health. It has remained the basis for the implementation of public health activities over the years, with little modification. This system was instrumental in changing the whole outlook of public health in the island (Chellappah, 1938).

Contemporary Health Care Delivery in Sri Lanka

Today in Sri Lanka, health care is provided through a network of public and private institutions, by practitioners of the allopathic system of medicine as well as the more traditional systems of medicine such as Ayurveda, Unani, and Siddha, and other systems such as homeopathy. In Sri Lanka, health care is provided free to all who access government health services.

The allopathic system of medicine caters to the needs of the vast majority of people, providing services through both the public and private sectors. A major share of these services is provided by the Ministry of Health (MoH), which is responsible for providing preventive, curative and rehabilitative services through its Department of Health Services headed by the Director General of Health Services (DGHS). In 1987, Provincial Councils were established in the eight provinces, consequent to an amendment to the constitution. This led to the decentralization of administrative powers to the provinces. Provincial health services, previously under the direct administration of the DGHS, became part of the administration of eight Provincial Directors of Health Services (PDHS). The Provincial Directors are supported by 25 Deputy Provincial Directors of Health Services responsible for the administration of the 25 districts of the island. Each district is subdivided into several divisions, which are under the authority of Divisional Directors of Health Services, or Medical Officers of Health. There are 265 such divisions, which have taken the place of the old Health Units (see above) and are responsible for the delivery of primary health care at grassroots level.

State sector curative care services are provided through a network of health care institutions ranging from teaching and provincial hospitals to peripheral health units and central dispensaries. There are 15 teaching hospitals providing tertiary care services, 42 provincial and base hospitals providing secondary care services, and 898 district hospitals, peripheral units, rural hospitals, central dispensaries, and maternity homes providing primary care services. The large number of health care institutions scattered across the island ensures that health care services are available within 1.4 km of a patient's home, on average (Department of Health Services Sri Lanka, 2002). The health expenditure for the year 2001 was 22,899 million rupees, which was 4.9% of the national expenditure and 1.6% of the GNP. A major proportion of the health expenditure—66%—was utilized by patient care services, whilst the preventive health services utilized only 8%. The balance was utilized for administration and staff services and training (Department of Health Services Sri Lanka, 2002).

Despite its low socio-economic status, Sri Lanka has been able to achieve a better health status than most countries in the region, as evidenced by relatively better health indices. Statistics include a low infant mortality rate of 12 per 1000 live births, a low maternal mortality rate of 2.3 per 10,000 live births, a relatively high life expectancy at birth of 73 years, and a Human Development Index of 0.716 (Department of Health Services Sri Lanka, 2002). Certain far-reaching welfare measures introduced since independence from colonial rule in 1948 have contributed to this remarkable achievement, notably free and easily accessible health services, free education up to university level resulting in a total literacy rate of 90% with a male literacy rate of 93% and a female literacy rate of 88%, and provision of food subsidies.

Major Communicable Diseases in Early Times

Smallpox and cholera were major communicable diseases prevalent at the beginning of the British occupation. One of the earliest epidemics that the British had to deal with was a serious outbreak of smallpox, which occurred in 1798. A cholera epidemic in Mannar, in 1820, is reported to have killed one-sixth of the population in that area (De Silva, 1936).

The British replaced a mainly subsistence based economy with an export oriented economy by introducing the three major cash crops of coffee, tea, and rubber. The expansion of the plantation industry necessitated the recruitment of immigrant labor from neighboring India. The free entry of immigrant labor from South India in the 1820s introduced smallpox and cholera, which were endemic in South India, into Sri Lanka (Vidyasagara, 2001). Two detention quarantine camps established in South India in 1899 and 1915 effectively prevented smallpox and cholera from becoming endemic in Ceylon (Uragoda, 1987; Vidyasagara 2001).

Hookworm disease was a major public health problem on the island during the early part of the twentieth century; it was believed that the immigrant Indian laborers employed in the plantations were infecting the Sinhalese in the neighboring villages. In 1915, a campaign for the control of hookworm disease was inaugurated with the assistance of the International Health Division of the Rockefeller Foundation. Treatment of infected persons and the provision of sanitary facilities, particularly for the estate and rural areas, were the chief strategies adopted in the campaign (De Silva, 1936).

Malaria has, from ancient times, affected the population in the dry zone of Sri Lanka causing much morbidity and mortality and periodic epidemics. A major epidemic which occurred in 1934–1935 caused some 80,000 deaths (Uragoda, 1987). The first organized efforts to control malaria started in 1911 at Kurunegala in the Northwestern Province, followed by the opening of additional anti-malaria centers in other parts of the island (De Silva, 1936).

Disease Control Programs

Special disease control programs have been set up, over the years, for the prevention and control of important communicable diseases prevalent in the country-malaria (1911), filariasis (1947), sexually transmitted infections (STIs) (1952) (now includes HIV/AIDS), leprosy (1954), tuberculosis (1945), and rabies. Of these diseases, malaria and to a lesser extent filariasis continue as important public health problems. Leprosy, which was considered a major problem by the Dutch has now reached elimination status mainly through the effective use of multi-drug therapy; and rabies still poses a problem mainly due to the proliferation of stray dogs, who continue to transmit the disease (College of Community Physicians of Sri Lanka, 2001).

Sri Lanka has a history of immunization against vaccine-preventable diseases that dates back to 1886 when vaccination against smallpox was introduced. When the intensified global program for the eradication of smallpox commenced in 1967, Sri Lanka had already achieved eradication status. More recently the introduction of BCG (Bacillus Calmette-Guerin) Vaccine (1949), DPT (diphtheria, pertussis, tetanus) Vaccine (1961), Oral Polio Vaccine (1962), Neonatal BCG Vaccination (1969), and Measles Vaccine (1984), with the achievement of more than 80% coverage with all vaccines enabled Sri Lanka to declare Universal Child Immunization (UCI), in December 1989. The Measles-Rubella Vaccine was introduced in 2000. Today, 90% of children are immunized against tuberculosis, diphtheria, pertussis, tetanus, polio and measles (Kulatilaka and Jayakuru, 2001).

With the control of many communicable diseases, non-communicable diseases such as cardiovascular diseases, diabetes mellitus, traumatic injuries, poisonings, mental disease and cancers are assuming greater importance.

The advent of HIV/AIDS now poses a major challenge to the National STD/AIDS Control Programme (NSACP).

HIV/AIDS IN SRI LANKA

As with many of its South Asian neighbors, HIV came relatively late to Sri Lanka. The earliest detection of HIV infection in Sri Lanka was in 1986 when a tourist convicted of a narcotic offense was found to be HIV positive. The first Sri Lankan with HIV/AIDS was reported in 1987. By the end of June 2003, the reported number of seropositives had risen to 484, including 151 AIDS patients (Table 1). Estimates of persons living with HIV at the end of 2001, however, range from 4700 to 7200 (Sri Lanka Working Group on HIV Estimates, 2002). Poor reporting by private medical institutions and general practitioners, delays in reporting, and under-diagnosis may account for the discrepancy between the reported and estimated HIV infections. Globally, Sri Lanka is classified as a country with a low prevalence of HIV infection. According to UNAIDS estimates, the adult HIV prevalence in Sri Lanka was 0.06% by the end of 2001 (UNAIDS, 2002). Apart from the paucity of data, the low prevalence rate may be due to the fact that the HIV epidemic in Sri Lanka is relatively young and HIV/AIDS related illnesses are only just beginning to surface.

TABLE 1. Number of HIV/AIDS Cases Reported to the NSACP, 1987–June, 2003

	HIV			AIDS[a]		
Year	Male	Female	Total	Male	Female	Total
1987	2	0	2	2	0	2
1988	3	0	3	2	0	2
1989	8	3	11	1	2	3
1990	6	1	7	2	0	2
1991	10	3	13	2	1	3
1992	19	8	27	8	2	10
1993	26	11	37	8	3	11
1994	15	8	23	13	1	14
1995	12	10	22	9	2	11
1996	20	10	30	9	2	11
1997	16	16	32	3	6	9
1998	29	26	55	11	4	15
1999	24	18	42	7	5	12
2000	34	20	54	9	5	14
2001	28	19	47	11	2	13
2002	26	24	50	6	1	7
06/2003	11	18	29	8	4	12
Total	289	195	484	111	40	151

Source: NSACP, Ministry of Health, Sri Lanka
[a] The number of AIDS cases are included within the number of HIV infections.

TABLE 2. Cumulative HIV Cases by Age and Sex by End June, 2003

Age	Male	Female	Total No.	%
0–9	7	3	10	2.1
10–14	1	0	1	0.2
15–19	0	0	0	0.0
20–24	14	15	29	6.0
25–29	35	25	60	12.4
30–34	59	43	102	21.1
35–39	47	39	86	17.8
40–44	46	23	72	14.9
45–49	28	20	49	10.1
50+	22	11	33	6.8
Unknown	26	16	42	8.7
Total	289	195	484	100.0

Source: NSACP, Ministry of Health, Sri Lanka

Age and Sex Distribution

Of the 442 HIV-positive persons whose age is known, 84% are in the sexually active age group of 15–49 years. Of these, as many as 102 persons are in the 30–34 year age group. Through June 2003, HIV infection has not been reported among the 15–19 year age group. The single reported case of HIV in the 10–14 year age group was acquired following repeated blood transfusions given abroad for hemophilia in a 14-year-old boy who was diagnosed as having AIDS on his return to Sri Lanka (Table 2).

As the epidemic has evolved in Sri Lanka, increasing numbers of women have become infected with HIV. In the first five years of the epidemic (1987–1991), the male to female ratio was 4.1:1; this decreased to 2:1 over the next five years. By the end of June 2003, women accounted for 40% of reported HIV cases. The increased vulnerability of women to HIV transmission has implications for the vulnerability of children, who have a significant chance of becoming infected at birth from their infected mothers. It is significant that nearly 45% of the HIV-positive women have been employed as domestic workers abroad. Most countries that employ these workers (mostly Middle Eastern countries) insist that they be subjected to compulsory HIV testing as a prerequisite for obtaining their visas. However, data from this testing needs to be interpreted cautiously, as other population groups are not subjected to compulsory testing in Sri Lanka; therefore, findings may not necessarily indicate true HIV prevalence.

Transmission

The principal mode of HIV transmission during the initial phase of the epidemic was through men having sex with men (MSM), but subsequently it has become clear that heterosexual transmission is the predominant mode of transmission. Of the 376 reported HIV infections where the mode of transmission is known, 86% were heterosexuals, 10% MSM, 1% were infected through transfusion of HIV-positive blood, and 3% had acquired HIV from their mothers. In 22% of cases, the route of transmission remains unknown, but it is suspected that most of these were also acquired heterosexually. Although HIV/AIDS cases have been reported since 1987, transmission through injection drug use has yet to be reported. Unconfirmed reports indicate that Sri Lankan HIV-positive injection drug users (IDU) seek treatment from detoxification centers in South India. It is estimated that only 1% of the 40,000 heroin users in Sri Lanka are IDU (National Dangerous Drugs Control Board, 2002).

Indigenous transmission of HIV was first detected in 1989. Since then, the percentage of reported cases attributed to indigenous transmission has varied between 9% and 51%. In 2002, indigenous transmission accounted for 43% of new HIV infections. The percentage of reported HIV infections attributed to indigenous transmission underscores the fact that most Sri Lankans continue to acquire HIV outside Sri Lanka.

Blood Safety

Sri Lanka was one of the first South Asian countries to reform its blood transfusion services to prevent HIV transmission within the health system. Screening of donor blood for HIV antibodies began in 1987 by the NSACP in collaboration with the National Blood Transfusion Service (NBTS). Today, screening of all donor blood and blood products is mandatory. The Central Blood Bank in Colombo and 54 regional blood banks spread throughout the country screen donor blood on site for HIV, hepatitis B, syphilis, and malaria before transfusion. Screening for hepatitis C was started in 2003 in Colombo and some regional blood banks.

Over 1.6 million blood units have been screened from 1987 to 2002. The HIV seropositivity rate of donor blood was 1.4 per 100,000 in 2002. All donors are interviewed individually and are required to sign a donor declaration form prior to blood collection. The donor declaration form allows for self-deferral. The NBTS adopts a policy of confidential after-donation reporting of HIV-positives with subsequent destruction of blood units. Voluntary donation is encouraged and currently around 65% of all NBTS supplies are from voluntary blood donations. In Colombo, 80% of donations are voluntary. The rest are replacement donations. Given this scenario the possibility of paid donors entering the system has to be acknowledged. During the past 16 years, HIV transmission through blood transfusion has been reported only in two patients.

Guidelines on the appropriate use of blood have been circulated to all healthcare institutions in the public and private sector. The National Blood Policy has been approved by the Cabinet of Ministers and a draft Blood Transfusion Act has been finalized. A Private Medical Institutions Bill that cedes legislative powers to the Ministry of Health to regulate public and private sector blood banks has also been finalized.

Mother-to-Child Transmission

Pregnant women are not routinely screened for HIV, but routine antenatal screening for syphilis has been in existence since 1952. Though the available data indicate a low prevalence of syphilis (1%) among pregnant women screened, congenital syphilis continues to be reported. Twenty- two cases of congenital syphilis (both early and late) were reported to the NSACP in 2002 compared to 14 cases in 1995. The continued occurrence of congenital syphilis in a country where an estimated 95% of pregnant women have access to antenatal services and 97% of deliveries take place in health care institutions is a reflection of the unsatisfactory coverage of antenatal screening for syphilis.

Eleven children aged 0–9 years with HIV/AIDS due to mother-to-child transmission have so far been reported. Seven had AIDS at initial diagnosis. The age at diagnosis ranged from 4 days to 5 years. Common clinical presentations among children with AIDS were recurrent upper respiratory tract infections, recurrent bacterial pneumonia, and tuberculosis.

TABLE 3. Reported Incidence[a] of Sexually Transmitted Infections in Sri Lanka

STI	1993	1994	1995	1996	1997	1998	1999	2000	2001	2002
Infectious Syphilis	3.7	3.7	2.3	2.2	2.7	1.4	1.3	1.4	1	1.1
Gonorrhoea	4.7	3.4	3.2	3.9	3.6	3.2	3.4	3.5	2.8	3.9
Non-Gonococcal Infections	7.5	6.2	5.3	4	3.7	4.3	4.5	4.9	6.5	9.1
Genital Herpes	5.5	5.1	5.1	3.4	4.9	5.8	6.0	6.9	7.2	7.8
Genital Warts	1.9	1.7	2	1.7	1.8	1.9	2.2	2.6	3.2	3.2
Trichomoniasis	2.1	1.8	1.4	1.3	1.2	1.2	0.9	1.0	1.0	1.0

Source: NSACP, Ministry of Health, Sri Lanka
[a] per 100,000 population.

Sexually Transmitted Infections

One of the key factors promoting the spread of HIV is the prevalence of STIs. Provision of comprehensive care in the management of STIs is, therefore, a major strategy adopted for the prevention of HIV through sexual transmission. The NSACP has developed national guidelines on clinical management of STIs. Syndromic management of STIs has been introduced at primary health care level to facilitate treatment of STIs at first point of contact with health services.

STI services are delivered at the Central STD Clinic in Colombo and through a network of 26 clinics at provincial hospitals and base hospitals. The central complex in Colombo also houses the National Reference Laboratory for STI/HIV/AIDS.

STIs, including HIV/AIDS are not notifiable in Sri Lanka. However, the epidemiological patterns of these diseases can be inferred from data reported by the STI clinics of the NSACP. STIs reported to the NSACP during a 10-year period from 1993 to 2002 are given in Table 3. It is estimated that between 60,000 and 200,000 new infections of STIs occur annually. Due to the nature of STIs and the stigma attached to them, most persons with STIs prefer to seek treatment in the private sector. STI data from the private sector are not reported to the NSACP.

Despite the limitations of available data, it is evident that the pattern and prevalence of STIs have changed over the past decade. Non-gonococcal infections and genital herpes are more frequently reported than syphilis and gonorrhea. It is significant that a rising incidence of genital herpes has been noted in the last five years. Genital herpes has emerged as the leading cause of genital ulceration in Sri Lanka, replacing syphilis. The Herpes simplex virus type 2 is almost always sexually transmitted and as such has been shown to be a good marker for sexual behavior in populations. A recent sero-epidemiological study of Herpes simplex virus types 1 and 2 carried out in Sri Lanka showed crude HSV 2 antibodies rates among antenatal clinic attendees to be 8.3% and to be 33% and 43% among male and female STI clinic attendees, respectively (Cowan *et al*, 2003).

Condom Use

A community survey carried out by the NSACP in 1997/98 confirmed that condom use among the sexually active population was very low (National STD/AIDS Control Programme, 1997). The results showed that 89 – 97% of sexually active persons surveyed were aware of HIV/AIDS. However, only around half the respondents were aware of the protective role of the condom. Condom availability at the peripheral level was also found to be unsatisfactory. Given the fact that heterosexual transmission is the predominant mode of HIV transmission in Sri Lanka, the survey has clearly indicated a need to more actively promote condoms. Condoms are currently provided free of charge in STI clinics. A social marketing program actively promoting condoms for disease prevention is to be implemented with World Bank assistance in 2004.

Care and Treatment for Those Living with HIV/AIDS

In keeping with government policy, all persons living with HIV/AIDS (PLWHA) requiring institutional care are admitted to general hospital wards. PLWHA are also managed as out-patients whenever possible. Home health care is encouraged as well. National guidelines on the clinical management of HIV/AIDS have been developed to facilitate uniform and improved management of patients. Counseling services to patients and their families are provided, and large numbers of medical and nursing staff have been trained in counseling. Facilities for HIV testing are available in every province. Although a large number of NGOs are active in the field of HIV prevention, only a few assist the government in providing care for patients with HIV/AIDS. Even fewer NGOs offer voluntary counseling and testing.

Antiretroviral Therapy

In mounting an effective response to HIV/AIDS, in addition to primary prevention for those who are not infected, treatment for individuals who are already infected must be considered.

There is now a demand for anti-retroviral treatment (ART) from PLWHA as well as their support groups. MoH has recognized and accepted the need to provide ART to HIV-positive Sri Lankans and is currently reviewing the logistics involved in introducing ART as part of the national response. MoH plans to begin the process of providing antiretroviral therapy free of charge to AIDS patients during 2004 in a phased manner using its own resources. A country preparedness assessment conducted by the South East Asia Regional Office of the World Health Organization (WHO SEARO) for scaling-up ART by exploring policy guidelines, training, availability of antiretroviral drugs, and essential services showed that Sri Lanka is in a position to begin providing ART. Presently, around 22 PLWHA are on ART and pay for their treatment. However, anti-retroviral drugs for the prevention of mother-to-child transmission and for post-exposure prophylaxis following accidental exposure in the health care setting are provided by the MoH.

SRI LANKA'S RESPONSE TO HIV/AIDS: GOVERNMENT, NON GOVERNMENT AND PRIVATE SECTOR

Sri Lanka responded to the HIV epidemic even before the first case was reported: the establishment of the National Task Force for Prevention and Control of HIV/AIDS in 1986 preceded the detection of the first patient with AIDS in Sri Lanka (World Bank, 2002). In 1988 the National AIDS Committee coordinated the formulation of a Medium Term Plan I (MTP I). By the early 1990s, HIV sentinel serological surveillance was in place. With WHO assistance, Sri Lanka formulated the Medium Term Plan II (MTP II) in 1994. The establishment of the UNAIDS Theme Group and the re-constitution of the National AIDS Committee in 1997, the formulation of the National Integrated Work Plan funded by the United Nations Development Program (UNDP) in 1998, the development of a policy on blood safety, and the development of the National Strategic Plan of 2002–2006 can be considered important milestones in Sri Lanka's response to HIV/AIDS.

Collaborative programming by all cosponsors of UNAIDS with active government participation has been a feature in Sri Lanka's efforts to prevent an epidemic. For example, Sri Lanka's integrated work plan of 1998 was co-sponsored by all UNAIDS agencies. The external review that led to the development of the current National Strategic Plan was co-sponsored by the WHO, the World Bank, and the UNDP in response to a request made by the National AIDS Committee and the NSACP in 1999.

Recognizing Sri Lanka's commitment to HIV/AIDS prevention, the World Bank has provided a substantial grant of US$ 12.6 million to fund a National HIV/AIDS Prevention Project to be implemented from 2003 to 2008. Sri Lanka is the first country to receive such a grant from the World Bank. This is an encouraging indication of the commitment of the World Bank to assist countries in implementing HIV/AIDS prevention programs without contributing to their debt burden. The World Bank-funded National HIV/AIDS Prevention Project (NHAPP) would support the National STD/AIDS Control Program to implement a comprehensive multi-sectoral program. Activities are designed to expand preventive programs for highly vulnerable populations, including young people, through the participation of both government agencies and NGOs. NGOs are expected to play a major role in the project. The response from most NGOs to HIV/AIDS until recently has been rudimentary. Most were involved mainly in information, education and communication (IEC) activities for general population groups. A few NGOs have aimed their efforts at identified risk groups such as female sex workers (FSW) and MSM, and even provided care for people living with HIV/AIDS (PLWHA) and their families. Yet most NGOs were minimally involved in difficult areas such as HIV care, interventions with sex workers, MSM, IDU, and other vulnerable groups. The NHAPP will support NGOs willing to implement innovative projects for identified vulnerable groups by providing necessary resources. The NHAPP also plans to strengthen the commitment of political leaders and reduce stigma and discrimination associated with marginalized populations including PLWHA (National STD/AIDS Control Programme, 2000).

ECONOMIC, SOCIAL, AND HUMAN RIGHTS IMPACT

A precise estimate of the cost of the HIV/AIDS problem has as yet not been made. According to a study titled "AIDS Impact from an Economic Perspective in Thailand and Sri Lanka, and in Pacific Nations," the direct costs of HIV/AIDS per infected person stands between US$ 250 and US$ 985 per year, depending on treatment regimen (UNAIDS Library, 2003). In addition, the indirect costs could be as high as US$ 17,695 during his or her lifespan. While part of the direct costs would be borne by the public sector, indirect costs would be a personal burden on PLWHA and their families. However, considering the low prevalence of HIV in Sri Lanka this high unit cost would not accumulate to be a significant resource constraint on the overall health budget.

Even if it is concluded that the economic impact of HIV would be minimal in the near future, the social impact could be significant. This would especially be related to the stigma, discrimination, and other human rights violations. Such violations affect not only PLWHA, but also other marginalized populations such as FSW and MSM.

Recently, progressive steps have been taken by the MoH to ensure that all HIV patients are admitted to any government hospital. However, in practice there are still occasions where PLWHA are referred to the Infections Diseases Hospital, more for the convenience of the attending physician than for the benefit of the patient.

The media has also contributed to violations of the rights of PLWHA. According to a study on newspaper reporting carried out by an NGO, "a recurring issue in local coverage on issues in HIV/ AIDS relates to infringements on the right to confidentiality. Coverage provided to people living with HIV/ AIDS has breached this right by providing details which allow identification of individuals" (UNDP, 2001).

Education is the key not only to HIV prevention but also for changing attitudes towards sex. Education also helps to dispel myths related to HIV/AIDS that lead to stigma and discrimination. However, there are many barriers to education of target populations. One such barrier is the adults themselves. For example, researchers often experience resistance from school principals to carry out research on issues related to HIV and sex (Abeyratna *et al.*, 2001).

The National Strategy also dictates that an environment should be created where FSW are not harassed, and are able to utilize the reproductive health services offered to the rest of the population.

DRAFT NATIONAL AIDS POLICY

Following on the interest generated by the United Nations Special Sessions on HIV/AIDS (UNGASS) in 2001, the Government of the Sri Lanka, on the advice of the Law and Ethics Subcommittee of the National AIDS Committee decided to formulate a policy on HIV/AIDS and STI related issues. This draft document reflects the policy of the government of Sri Lanka related to the issues that have to be addressed to prevent the spread of HIV/AIDS in Sri Lanka. It is based on the premise that the effective management of HIV/AIDS requires policies and guiding principles that not only address prevention and care, but other factors such as the violations of human rights of individuals, gender-based violence, and the social stigma associated with sex and condoms.

CONCLUSION

Though the prevalence of HIV in Sri Lanka is low, the existence of several risk factors poses a serious threat toward the development of an epidemic. These include an expanding population in the productive age group with high rates of unemployment in the 15–29 age group, and postponement of marriage by young people—the age of marriage has increased to 25.5 years in females and 27.5 years in males. Additionally, a 23-year-old conflict has given rise to the presence of about 150,000 armed services personnel and 600,000 displaced civilians. About 185,000 displaced persons are living in refugee camps, and there has been an influx of a large number of displaced persons who had sought refuge in Southern India, a high HIV prevalence area, following a recent cessation of hostilities. The employment of over 100,000 workers, mainly youth, in ten Industrial Promotion Zones away from their homes, enjoying newly found social and economic freedom has threatened prevalence levels. The annual emigration of some 200,000 persons seeking employment as skilled and unskilled workers can also spread HIV into Sri Lanka—45% of Sri Lankan women testing positive for HIV had been employed in Middle Eastern countries (Central Bank of Sri Lanka, 2001). Low condom use among the general population and those engaged in high-risk behaviors is another threat.

Sri Lanka still has time to prevent a generalized epidemic. With its deep historical commitment to human development, a highly literate population, especially among women, and a well-developed heath infrastructure, the country is in a strong position to confront and control the spread of HIV infection. The National Strategic Plan draws on these strengths to address the priority areas in the prevention and control of HIV/AIDS.

REFERENCES

Abeyaratna, K.P., Moller, A.B., and Ranjanee, S. (2001). Knowledge, attitudes and practice: A survey of adolescent students in two contrasting areas of Sri Lanka. Presented at 6th ICCAP, 5–10 October, 2001. (unpublished paper).

Central Bank of Sri Lanka. (2001). Report of the Central Bank of Sri Lanka 2000, Sri Lanka.

Chellappah, S.F. (1938). Progress of public health in Ceylon. *Journal of the Ceylon Branch of the British Medical Association* 35:303.

College of Community Physicians of Sri Lanka. (2001). Millennium Supplement of the Journal of the Ceylon College of Community Physicians. Sri Lanka.

Cowan, F.M., French, R.S., Maynaud, P., Gopal, R., and Robinson, N.J. (2003). Sero-epidemiological study of herpes simplex virus types 1 and 2 in Brazil, Estonia, India, Morocco, and Sri Lanka. *Sex Trans Infect* 79:286–290.

Department of Census and Statistics. (2003). Sri Lanka demographic and health survey 2001. Ministry of Finance, Colombo.

Department of Health Services Sri Lanka. (2002). Annual Health Bulletin 2001, pp. 1–10.

De Silva, D.M. (1936). *Health progress in Ceylon: A survey*. Government Press, Colombo.

Geiger, W. (1923). *Mahavamsa (translation).* Pali Text Society, London.

Kulatilaka, T.A., and Jayakuru, W.S. (2001). Development of epidemiological services in Sri Lanka and future challenges. In: Herath, H.M.S.S.D., Seneveratne, R. de A., Fernando, H.T.E.I. (eds.) Public health development in Sri Lanka. *Millennium Supplement- Journal of the College of Community Physicians of Sri Lanka*, pp. 21–27.

National Dangerous Drugs Control Board. (2002). Hand book of drug abuse information 1997–2001. Research and Publication Division, National Dangerous Drugs Control Board, Sri Lanka.

National STD/AIDS Control Programme. (1997). Sri Lanka Priority Prevention Indicator Survey. National STD/AIDS Control Programme and WHO, Sri Lanka.

National STD/AIDS Control Programme. (2000). External Review of the National AIDS Programme Sri Lanka. Ministry of Health, Sri Lanka.

Sri Lanka Working Group on HIV Estimates. (2002). Report on HIV Estimates. (limited circulation).

UNAIDS (2002). Report on the global HIV/AIDS epidemic. UNAIDS, Geneva.

UNAIDS Library. (2003). Report from a Consultation on the Socio-Economic Impact of HIV/AIDS on Households (1999; 13 p.) as published in UNAIDS Library CD ROM, Version 2, July 2003.

UNDP. (2001). Alliance Lanka Media Situation Assessment, Policy Advocacy and Outreach Project, UNDP/ RAS/97/602, HIV and Development Project for South and Southwest Asia. New Delhi, 2001.

Uragoda, C.G. (1987). *A History of Medicine in Sri Lanka*. Sri Lanka Medical Association, Colombo.

Vidyasagara, N.W. (2001). Health care in the plantation sector. In: Herath, H.M.S.S.D., Seneviratne, R. de A., Fernanco, H.T.E.I. (eds.) Public health development in Sri Lanka. *Millennium Supplement- Journal of the College of Community Physicians of Sri Lanka*, pp 29–41.

World Bank. (2002). Project proposal document on a proposed grant in the amount of SDR 9.6 million to the Democratic Socialist Republic of Sri Lanka for a National HIV/AIDS Prevention Project. World Bank, Human Development Unit South Asia Region.

12

HIV/AIDS in Taiwan

Yi-Ming Arthur Chen

AIDS Prevention and Research Center, Institute of Public Health, National Yang-Ming University, Taipei City, Taiwan

HISTORY AND CURRENT STATUS OF INFECTIOUS DISEASES IN TAIWAN

Taiwan is located in the middle of East Asia. Since Taiwan is a frontier island, it experienced a complicated transformation in ethnicity during the 17th, 18th, and 19th centuries. Taiwan had been occupied by both the Dutch and Japanese. The main population of Taiwan now includes descendants from four ethnic groups: aborigines, Fukienese, Hakka, and mainland Chinese. The native aborigines consist of nine different tribes. The Fukienese and Hakka are early settlers who immigrated from Fukien and Guangdong provinces of China several hundred years ago. The mainland Chinese are people who came to Taiwan from the mainland after World War II. In the past few years, due to a new openness in society following the relaxation of regulations, many immigrants from mainland China and southeastern Asia have come to Taiwan through marriage arrangements. At present, Taiwan's population is about 23 million.

Tuberculosis

As shown in Table 1, several important infectious diseases in Taiwan have been eradicated or have been under control since 1948. Every five years since 1957, the Department of Health (DOH) of Taiwan has conducted a survey on pulmonary tuberculosis (TB). The surveys showed that in 1957, 5.15% of persons aged >20 had pulmonary TB, among them, 20% had infectious TB. By 1993, the rates of pulmonary TB and infectious TB had decreased to 0.65% and 0.06%. Currently, there are about 15,000 new TB cases every year in Taiwan (Center for Disease Control, Taiwan, 2003a). It is worth noting that the incidence of TB in the aborigines in 1998, 239/100,000, was much higher than that in other populations.

Hand-Foot-and-Mouth Disease

In 1998, an epidemic of enterovirus 71 infection caused hand-foot-and-mouth disease (characterized by vesicular lesions on the hands, feet, and oral mucosa) and herpangina

TABLE 1. The Chronicle of the Control of Infectious Diseases in Taiwan

Year	Event
1948	Eradication of plague
1948	Initiation of vaccination program
1955	Eradication of small pox
1959	Eradication of rabies
1965	Eradication of malaria
1984	Initiation of HBV vaccination program
1990	AIDS control law was launched
1995	Initiation of HAV vaccination program
1997	Free HAART was provided
1998	Initiation of influenza vaccination program, especially among elders
1998	Eradication of poliomyelitis was recognized
1999	Infectious disease control law was launched
1999	Establishment of Taiwan CDC by merging three governmental organizations
2001	Formation of AIDS Advisory Committee at the Executive Yuan

in thousands of people in Taiwan, some of whom died. The sentinel physicians reported nearly 130,000 cases of hand-foot-and-mouth disease or herpangina in two waves of the epidemic, which probably represents less than 10% of the estimated total number of cases. There were 405 (0.3% of the total) patients with severe disease. Most of them were five years old or younger, and most of those who died were young. The majority died of pulmonary edema and pulmonary hemorrhage. Enterovirus 71 infection was associated with most of the serious cases and with nearly all the deaths. A laboratory-network was established linking 10 hospitals island-wide together with the Center for Disease Control (CDC) of Taiwan for laboratory diagnosis. This network has been active since then and more laboratories were added to the network when severe acute respiratory syndrome (SARS) attacked Taiwan in 2003 (Ho *et al.*, 1999).

Severe Acute Respiratory Syndrome (SARS)

The outbreak of SARS, originally referred to as atypical pneumonia, was first identified in Guangdong Province, China in November 2002. By August 7, 2003, SARS had spread to more than 30 countries, affected 8422 people and resulted in 916 deaths worldwide (World Health Organization, 2003). In Taiwan, the first SARS case was diagnosed on March 14, 2003. This index case had traveled to Guangdong, China in February. On April 24, the Taipei city government announced that it was closing down Ho-Ping Hospital for two weeks. Although the government imposed mandatory 14-day quarantine on all air travelers from China, Hong Kong, Singapore, Macau, and Toronto on April 28, the SARS epidemic spread in Taiwan island-wide and more than 29 hospitals reported nosocomial infection. According to the Center for Disease Control of Taiwan, of the 664 probable SARS cases reported to the World Health Organization, there were 346 SARS cases confirmed by either RT-PCR or serological test (Figure 1) (Center for Disease Control, Taiwan, 2003b).

HISTORY AND CURRENT STATUS OF HIV-1 INFECTION IN TAIWAN

The first indigenous AIDS case in Taiwan was found in 1986, and as of Oct 2003, 5464 people living with HIV-1 (hereafter referred to simply as HIV) and AIDS (PLWHA) had been reported to the Department of Health of Taiwan. This number included 5042 Taiwan citizens and 422 foreigners. The numbers of PLWHA increased rapidly, with a rate of increase of more than 15% every year (Figure 2). The male-to-female ratio of the reported cases was 13 to 1. According to risk factor analysis, 40.6% of the cases were heterosexuals, 36.5% were men who have sex with men (MSM), 12.2% were bisexuals, 2.0% were intravenous drug users (IDU), and 0.24% were infected by blood transfusion; 53 cases were among hemophiliacs, and nine cases were due to vertical transmission (Center for Disease Control, Taiwan , 2003c). It has been speculated that the true number

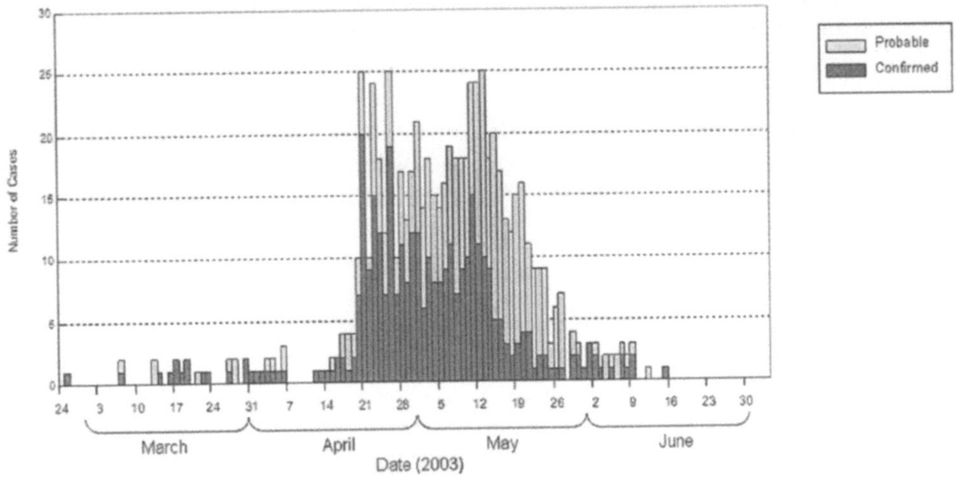

FIGURE 1. Epidemiological curve of the probable and confirmed SARS cases in Taiwan. The confirmed cases were proved by either RT-PCR or serological test. (CDC Taiwan, 2003b)

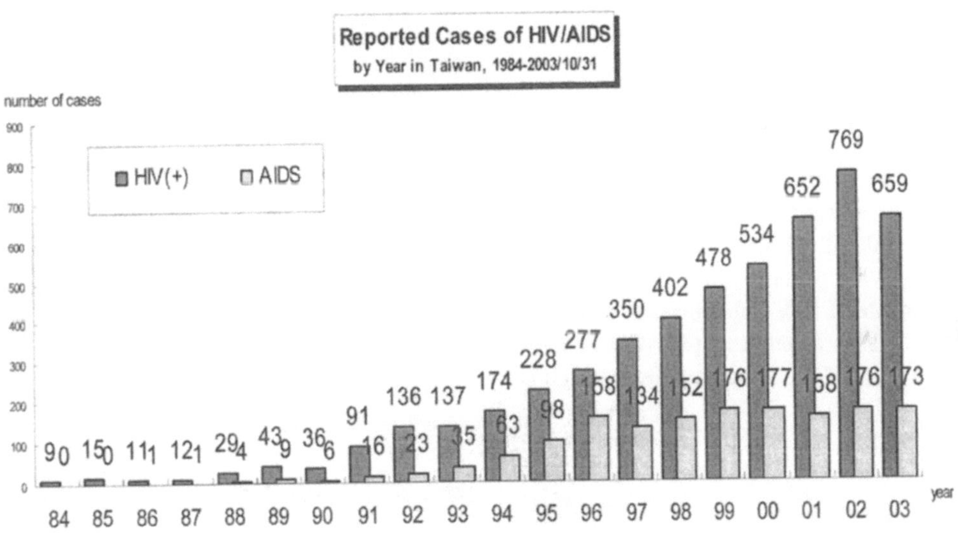

FIGURE 2. The cumulative numbers of HIV/AIDS cases reported to CDC of Taiwan by the end of October 2003. (CDC Taiwan, 2003c)

of PLWHA in Taiwan is about 2–3 times the reported cases.

There are several important characteristics of the HIV/AIDS epidemic in Taiwan: more than 80% of infections have been due to sexual transmission, less than 2% of infections have been as a result of needle sharing, and mother-infant transmission has been very rare. When the trends over time on the distribution of different age groups in the HIV/AIDS patient cohort were analyzed, the results showed that the percentage of patients aged 19 or younger increased from 2% in 1995–1996 to 6% in 1997–1998. In addition, since 1997–1998, the number of patients in their 20s has surpassed the number of those

TABLE 2. The Prevalence Rates of HIV Infection among Different Groups in Taiwan, 2001.

Group	Prevalence Rate
Conscripts	5.3/100,000
First-time blood donors	6.3/100,000
Pregnant women	14.5/100,000
IDU	89.7/100,000
Prisoners	112.0/100,000
FSW[a]	200.0/100,000
STI patients	1,900.0/100,000
MSM in gay saunas	6,700.0/100, 000

[a] 1996 data.

in their 30s and has become the largest age group (Chen *et al.*, 2001b). This is an alarming sign that HIV/AIDS education among Taiwan's youth needs to be strengthened.

The Prevalence of HIV Infection in Different Groups in Taiwan

Men Who Have Sex with Men

As shown in Table 2, judging by the HIV prevalence rates in the populations of conscripts, first-time blood donors, and pregnant women, the general public in Taiwan had a lower rate of HIV infection than other countries in Asia (Monitoring the AIDS Pandemic Network, 2001). Among different high-risk groups in Taiwan, MSM in gay saunas had the highest rate of HIV infection. According to our surveys, the rates of HIV-1 infections among MSM in gay saunas in different cities were: 15.8% (22/139) in Kaohsiung in 1999, 9.5% (33/348) in Taipei in 2000, 5.2% (16/307) in Taipei in 2001, and 6% (6/100) in Taichung in 2002. Besides HIV, this population also had quite high rates of syphilis infection, ranging from 8.1 to 13.8% (Center for Disease Control, Taiwan, 2003c).

Sexually Transmitted Infections (STI)

Both the male homosexual and bisexual HIV/AIDS patients had significantly higher rates of syphilis infection than the heterosexual men in Taiwan. In contrast to the high rate of sexual contact with sex workers in the male heterosexual subgroup, only 16.6% of the HIV-positive MSM had sexual contact with sex workers (Chen *et al.*, 1998a; Chen *et al.*, 2001b). Therefore, the high rate of syphilis infection among HIV-positive MSM may reflect the prevalence rate of syphilis infection in the MSM population in Taiwan. In Taiwan, the HIV-positive MSM were much younger than the HIV-positive heterosexual men were. According to the Yang-Ming AIDS Center database, about 55% of the HIV- positive MSM were aged below 30, while about 30% of HIV-positive heterosexual men were aged below 30 (Chen *et al.*, 2001b). In addition, the group of MSM patients had a higher percentage of persons aged below 20 than the heterosexual group, 3.0% vs. 1.7% (Chen *et al.*, 2001b). This suggests that MSM might be engaging in high-risk behaviors at a younger age than heterosexual men in Taiwan. The synergistic relationship between HIV and certain STIs, especially genital ulcerative diseases, has been reported previously (Plummer, 1998). The lack of sex education and the existing stigmatization of homosexuality both considerably increase the risk for MSM of contracting HIV and other STIs in Taiwan. Therefore, it is important to develop an effective HIV and STI prevention program targeting MSM in Taiwan.

Heterosexual Population and HIV Subtypes

Changes over time in the distribution of different HIV subtypes in the heterosexual population are very striking. According to our analysis, more than half of heterosexual males had HIV subtype B infection, but CRF01_AE surpassed subtype B and became the major subtype between 1997 and 1998 (Figure 3) (Chen *et al.*, 2001b).

According to risk factor analysis, nearly half of the HIV-positive heterosexual males admitted that they had sexual contact with sex workers when they went to Southeast Asia.

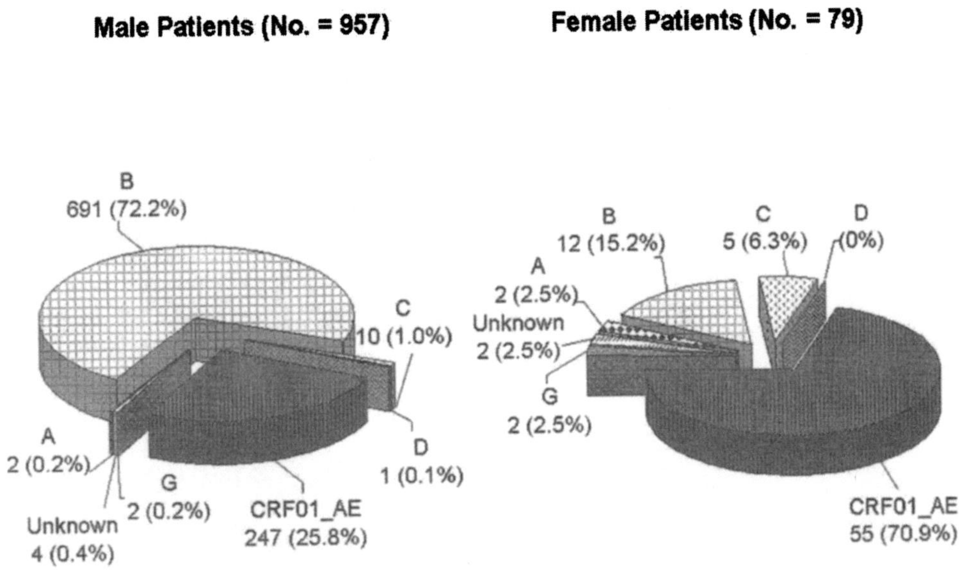

FIGURE 3. Proportions of HIV-1 subtypes in the male and female HIV/AIDS patients recruited by the Yang-Ming AIDS Center from 1988 to 2000 in Taiwan.

This is consistent with the results of the phylogenetic analysis which showed that most of the Taiwanese CRF01_AE clustered with isolates from Thailand (Figure 4).

Women with HIV/AIDS

As shown in Figure 3, about 85% of the female HIV/AIDS patients were infected with non-B clades, with CRF01_AE as the predominant subtype. In Taiwan, the most important risk factor for women was that their husbands were seropositive. Previously, we have reported the results of a study that found 17 of 52 (32.7%) married couples were seroconcordant. When the HIV subtypes of the couples were analyzed, 14 of 33 (42.4%) husbands infected with CRF01_AE had transmitted HIV to their wives, while only 1 of 17 (5.9%) men with subtype B had transmitted the disease to their spouses ($p < 0.01$). Both of the two husbands infected with subtype C had also transmitted HIV to their wives (Chen *et al.*, 2001b). Other recent studies in Thailand have also shown subtype differences, both in level of viral replication during seroconversion and in transmissibility in cohorts of IDU (Hu *et al.*, 2001; Hudgens *et al.*, 2002). Studies on the virological characteristics of both HIV subtype C and CRF01_AE have revealed that they may have adapted better to transmission through the human population (Ping *et al.*, 1999; Montano *et al.*, 1998).

Female Sex Workers (FSW)

In Taiwan, most FSW are infected with HIV CRF01_AE (Chen *et al.*, 2001b). There is a risk of an increasing spread of HIV E in the heterosexual population in Taiwan. In a survey of HIV and STI prevalence among FSW in the Taipei metropolitan area from 1993 to 1996, 0.2% (2/1036) of FSW from karaoke bars were found to have HIV, while none of the 725 FSW from massage parlors and 484 FSW from brothels were infected with HIV (Chen *et al.*, 1998b). Due to the lack of subsequent follow-up study, the current prevalence of HIV infection in this population is unknown.

Injecting Drug Users (IDU)

The prevalence of HIV infection among Taiwanese IDU has never been reported.

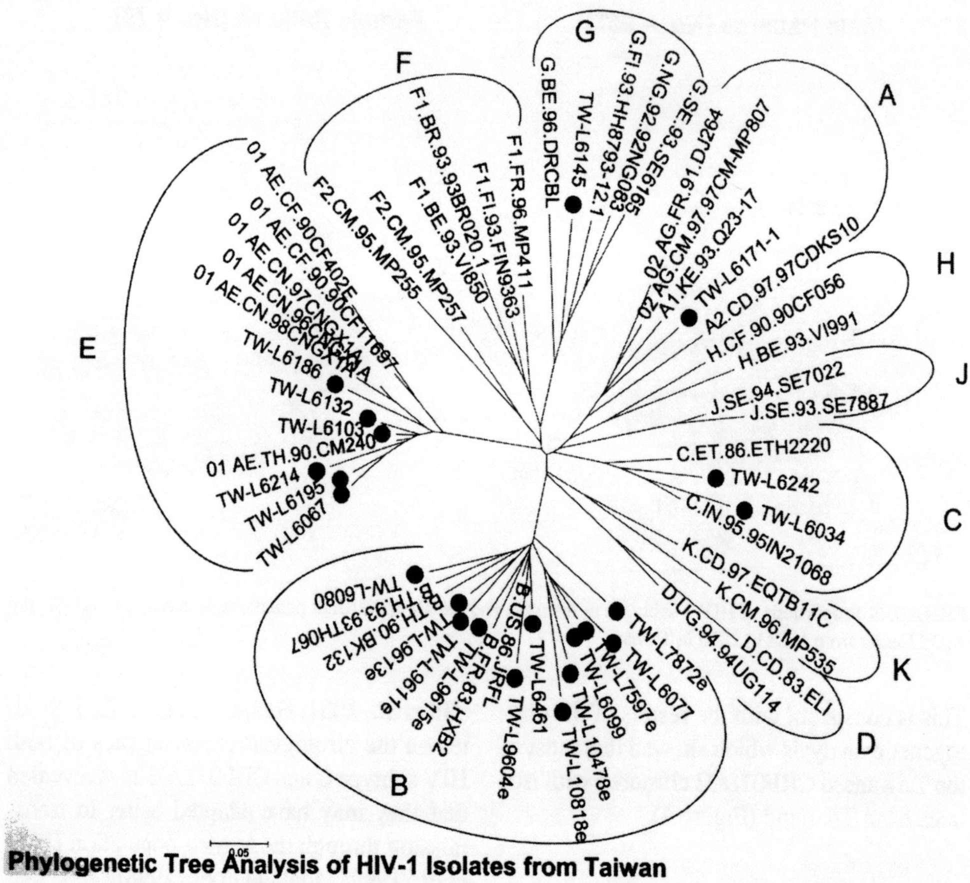

FIGURE 4. Phylogenetic analysis of Taiwanese (TW-) HIV-1 isolates. The neighbor-joining tree was obtained from 100 bootstrap samples of aligned *env* sequences corresponding to the nucleotide residues 7062–7379 of HXB2 from different HIV-1 isolates.

There is relatively little control of the medical supplies market in Taiwan, and syringes are easy to obtain. Because of this, there appears to be a much lower rate of needle-sharing in Taiwan, with the possible exception of the prison inmate population. Although less than 2% of the total number of reported cases of HIV/AIDS were among IDU, it is important to note that according to a survey conducted by a social worker visiting prisons island-wide, the numbers of HIV-positive inmates tripled between 2001 and 2003 (Sr. Teresa Hsieh, Director, Lourdes Home of Taiwan, personal communication, October, 2003). In terms of subtypes, according to our previous study on 22 IDU, 12 heterosexual men and one MSM were infected with HIV B subtype, six heterosexual men and one MSM were infected with HIV CRF01_AE, and two female IDU were infected with HIV B subtypes. Among heterosexual male IDU, five out of six (83.3%) men were infected with HIV CRF01_AE, and only one out of 12 (8.3%) men infected with HIV B had sexual contact history with FSW ($p < 0.01$) (Chen *et al.*, 2001b). Therefore, sexual transmission is a major risk factor of male IDU infected with HIV CRF01_AE in Taiwan.

ISSUES RELATED TO TREATMENT AND CARE

In Taiwan, the AIDS Control Law was launched in 1990 and has been modified five

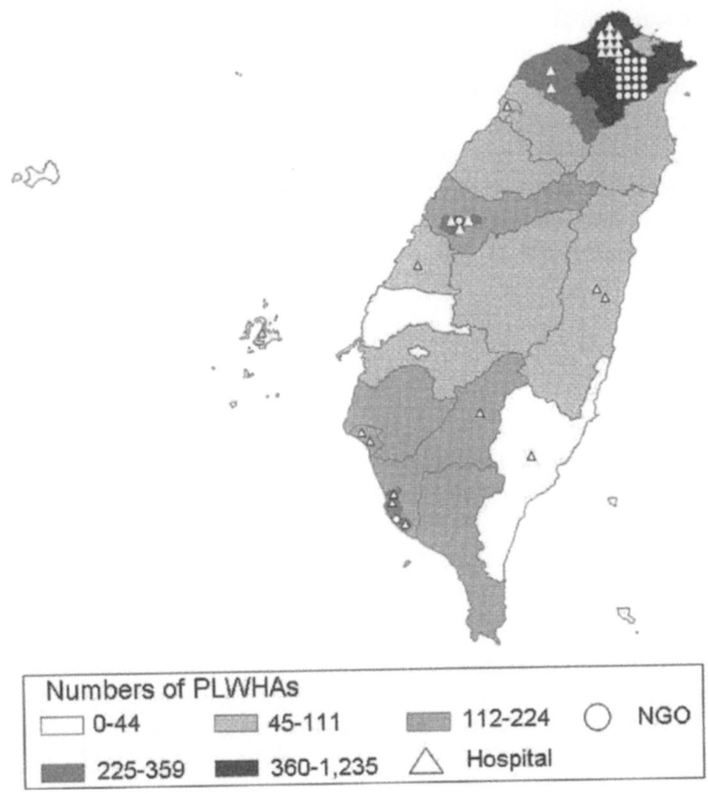

FIGURE 5. The distributions of AIDS designated hospitals and non-governmental organizations against the density of PLWHA in different prefectures and cities in Taiwan.

times since then. Under this law, the government has to provide free treatment to all Taiwanese PLWHA. Currently, there are 27 designated AIDS hospitals in Taiwan. As shown in Figure 5, the distribution of the hospitals is not even and some prefectures and cities do not have an AIDS hospital. The designated AIDS hospital system should be expanded to meet the medical needs of patients.

Highly Active Anti-Retroviral Therapy

Since April 1997, the Taiwanese government has provided protease inhibitors in conjunction with NRTIs (Nucleoside Reverse Transcriptase Inhibitors) and NNRTIs (Non-Nucleoside Reverse Transcriptase Inhibitors). The cost of the highly active anti-retroviral therapy (HAART) is about US$ 1000 per person per month. According to the Bureau of the National Health Insurance (BNHI), by the end of 2002, 2660 of 3425 (77.7%) PLWHA had begun receiving HAART. The implementation of the free HAART program in Taiwan has caused dramatic decreases of both morbidity and mortality of HIV/AIDS in Taiwan. A five-year prospective study on a cohort of 309 PLWHA (83% with AIDS) admitted to a teaching hospital in Taipei City showed that the mortality rate declined significantly from 110.5–148.4 per 100 patient-years in 1995 to 5.5–7.4 per 100 patient-years in 1999 (Hung *et al.*, 2000). The five leading HIV-associated opportunistic infections (OI) in the cohort were oroesophageal candidiasis, Pneumocystis carinii pneumonia, tuberculosis, mucocutaneous herpes simplex infection and cytomegalovirus diseases (Hung *et al.*, 2000).

The clinical spectrum of HIV/AIDS patients in Taiwan was very similar to that in the Western countries, but the incidence of OI differed, e.g. the incidence of tuberculosis in patients with advanced illness (24.6%) was relatively high, and the rate of an endemic fungal infection (*Penicillium marneffei* infection) was increasing (Hsieh *et al.*, 1996; Hsueh *et al.*, 2000).

HIV Drug Resistance

Although the BNHI provided free viral load and CD4 cell counts tests, the cost for genotyping of HIV drug resistance was not covered. Recently, we investigated the prevalence of HIV genotypic mutations in retrospective samples collected between 1997 and 2000. The results showed that among 136 treatment naïve PLWHA, none of the 31 MSM, 32 bisexual males, seven females, or four IDU had any primary mutation, while two of 62 (3.2%) MSM had M184V mutation for RT inhibitors (Elbeik *et al.*, 2002).

Non-Governmental Organizations and Social Movement

In response to the challenge of HIV/AIDS, since 1992, there have been 15 non-governmental organizations (NGOs) established in Taiwan to provide shelter, counseling, anonymous testing, social care, and education for PLWHA, vulnerable groups, and the general public. As shown in Figure 5, there is only one NGO in the middle region of the country and one in the southern part of Taiwan. It is worth mentioning that although there is no PLWHA NGO in Taiwan, a PWA Rights' Advocacy Association (PRAA) was established in 1997.

Issues on the Human Rights of PLWHA

In 1999, a survey was conducted to understand the human rights issues of PLWHA in Taiwan. Social workers from four NGOs-the Living with Hope Organization, Taiwan Hemophiliac PWA Association, PRAA, and Lourdes Home-were trained to be interviewers. In total, 50 PLWHA (45 men and five women) participated in the survey. The results showed that 16% had suffered from discrimination by medical staff and 30% had been refused or delayed when they sought medical care. In terms of education rights, our 1999 survey showed that two PLWHA were expelled and three were refused admission by school authorities. Because of their HIV status, three had lost their jobs, three had been offered early retirement, five had lost their prospects for promotion, and 22 had experienced harassment from their employers. Three patients stated that their children had been taken away from them when they revealed their status. At present, Taiwanese PLWHA are still restricted from taking tests to become government employees and professional technologists.

In 2002, a survey of 1292 medical personnel from 42 hospitals island-wide showed that 42.9% are not willing to care for PLWHA and 97.6% think there should be a law forcing PLWHA to disclose their seropositive status to medical personnel (Taiwan Root Medical Peace Corps, 2002).

To change the attitude of the general public toward PLWHA, family members of PLWHA and volunteers were invited to participate in a floating lantern ceremony at a riverside in Taipei City on World AIDS day in 1994. This memorial has become an annual event since then. In 1995, Taiwan invited the Names Project to bring 576 AIDS quilts for a special exhibition at the Chiang Kai-Sheik memorial plaza on World AIDS day. The Taiwan AIDS Memorial Quilt Project was established under the Living with Hope Organization in 1995. In 2001, Taiwan invited the Photographer Network to show the "Positive lives" of PLWHA from different Asian countries. The images created, of pink and white lanterns floating on a river, and colorful quilts displayed in front of traditional Chinese theaters, have shocked and moved many people in Taiwan.

CONCLUSION

In conclusion, the HIV/AIDS epidemic in Taiwan is evolving. There are several issues that need to be addressed immediately: sentinel surveillance of HIV infection among different high-risk groups should be implemented; prenatal counseling for the HIV antibody test and chemoprevention of mother-to-child transmission should be instituted immediately; and NGOs should receive more financial support from both the Taiwanese government and international agencies.

ACKNOWLEDGEMENTS. The author would like to thank Yu-Ching Lan and Jennifer Chang for their help in preparing the figures, and Dr. Timothy Meagher for his help in editing the manuscript.

REFERENCES

Center for Disease Control, Taiwan. (2003a). Tuberculosis in Taiwan: TB epidemiology. http:203.65.72.83/ch/dt/upload/qc/epi/epi-face.html. Taipei, Taiwan.

Center for Disease Control, Taiwan. (2003b). SARS Data Analysis-Taiwan. http://www.cdc.gov.tw/sars.en. Taipei, Taiwan.

Center for Disease Control, Taiwan. (2003c). Issues of AIDS: reported cases of HIV/AIDS. http://www.doh.gov.tw/focus/aids/. Taipei, Taiwan.

Chen, Y.M.A., Lee, C.M., Lin, R.Y., and Chang, H.J. (1998a). Molecular epidemiology and trends of HIV-1 Subtypes in Taiwan. *J Acquir Immun Defic Syndr Hum Retrovirol.* 19:393–402.

Chen, Y.M.A., Yu, P.S., Lin, C.C., and Jen, I. (1998b). Surveys of HIV-1, HTLV-I and other sexually transmitted diseases among female sex workers in Taipei city and prefectures, Taiwan from 1993 to 1996. *J Acquir Immun Defic Syndr Hum Retrovirol.* 18:299–303.

Chen, Y.M.A., Chung, C.L., Jen, I., Lan, Y.C., Wu, S.I., and Hsu, H. (2001a). Surveys on the HIV-1, syphilis and sexual behavior among men attending gay saunas in Taipei City. The 6th ICAAP in Melbourne, Australia. (Unpublished surveys).

Chen, Y.M.A., Huang, K.L., Jen, I., Chen, S.C., Liu, Y.C., Chuang, Y.C., Wong, J.C., Tsai, J.J., and Lan, Y.C. (2001b). Temporal trends and molecular epidemiology of HIV-1 infection in Taiwan from 1988 to 1998. *J AIDS* 26:274–282.

Elbeik, E., Lan, Y.C., Dileanis, J.A., Marlowe, N., Ng, V., and Chen, Y.M.A. (2002). Prevalence of HIV-1 genotypic mutations in the protease and reverse transcriptase genes from infected individuals in Taiwan: Treatment challenges. The XIV International AIDS Conference, Barcelona, Spain, July 7–12, 2002. (Unpublished paper).

Ho, M., Chen, E.R., Hsu, K.H., Twu, S.J., Chen, K.T., Tsai, S.F., Wang, J.R., and Shih, S.R. (1999). An epidemic of enterovirus 71 infection in Taiwan. *N Engl J Med.* 341:929–935.

Hsieh, S.M., Hung, C.C., Chen, M.Y., Hsueh, P.R., Chang, S.C., and Luh, K.T. (1996). Clinical manifestations of tuberculosis in patients with advanced HIV-1 infection in Taiwan. *J Formos Med Assoc.* 95:923–928.

Hsueh, P.R., Teng, L.J., Hung, C.C., Chen, Y.G., Luh, K.T., and Ho, S.W. (2000). Molecular evidence on strain dissemination of *Penicillium marneffei*: An emerging pathogen in Taiwan. *J Infect Dis.* 181:1706–1712.

Hu, D.J., Vanichseni, S., Mastro, T.D., Raktham, S., Young, K.L., Mock, P.A., Subbarao, S., Parekh, B.S., Srisuwanvilai, L., Sutthent, R., Wasi, C., Heneine, W., and Choopanya, K. (2001). Viral load differences in early infection with two HIV-1 subtypes. *AIDS* 15:683–691.

Hudgens, M.G., Longini, I.M. Jr, Vanichseni, S., Hu, D.J., Kitayaporn, D., Mock, P.A., Halloran, M.E., Satten, G.A., Choopanya, K., and Mastro, T.D. (2002). Subtype-specific transmission probabilities for human immunodeficiency virus type 1 among injecting drug users in Bangkok, Thailand. *Am J Epidemiol.* 155:159–168.

Hung, C.C., Chen, M.Y., Hsieh, S.M., Sheng, W.H., and Chang, S.C. (2000). Clinical spectrum, morbidity and mortality of acquired immunodeficiency syndrome in Taiwan: A 5-year prospective study. *J Acquir Immun Defic Syndr Hum Retrovirol.* 24:378-385.

Monitoring the AIDS Pandemic Network. (2001). Report on the status and trends of HIV/AIDS/STI epidemics in Asia and the Pacific. (http://www.fhi.org).

Montano, M.A., Nixon, C.P., and Essex, M. (1998). Dysregulation through the NF-kappaB enhancer and TATA box of the human immunodeficiency virus type 1 subtype E promoter. *J Virol.* 72:8446–8452.

Ping, L.H., Nelson, J.A., Hoffman, I.F., Schock, J., Lamers, S.L., Goodman, M., Vernazza, P., Kazembe, P., Maida, M., Zimba, D., Goodenow, M.M., Eron,

J.J. Jr., Fiscus, S.A., Cohen, M.S., and Swanstrom, R. (1999). Characterization of V3 sequence heterogeneity in subtype C human immunodeficiency virus type 1 isolates from Malawi: Underrepresentation of X4 variants. *J Virol.* 73:6271–6281.

Plummer, F.A. (1998). Heterosexual transmission of human immunodeficiency virus type 1 (HIV): Interaction of conventional sexually transmitted diseases, hormonal contraception and HIV-1. *AIDS Res Human Retroviruses* 1:S5–S10.

Taiwan Root Medical Peace Corps. (2002). Report on the professional training and attitude towards AIDS patients among medical personnel in Taiwan. (www.taiwanroot.org)

World Health Organization. (2003). Summary table of SARS cases by country, 1 November 2002–7 August 2003. http://www.who.int/csr/sars/country/2003_08_15/en/.

13

HIV/AIDS in Hong Kong

The Emergence and Impact of an Epidemic

Oi-chu Lin, William H.F. Kam, and Suk-yan Chan

Hong Kong AIDS Foundation, Hong Kong

HIV/AIDS SITUATION IN HONG KONG

In Hong Kong, a cumulative total of 2116 HIV infections were reported as of the end of June 2003. On a yearly basis, about 200 cases have been reported under the voluntary reporting mechanism to the Department of Health. Through an analysis of the available epidemiological information, it was estimated that in 1999, HIV infections in Hong Kong ranged between 2000 and 3000, (based on revised projections of HIV infection and AIDS cases in Hong Kong by Professor James Chin, www.aids.gov.hk), a figure supported by results of seroprevalence studies.

Over the years, sexual transmission has remained the single most important route of HIV spread in Hong Kong. Not surprisingly, the HIV prevalence is highest in the 25 to 34 age group. From the reported figures, there has been a notable change from a predominantly homosexual to a heterosexual infection. Between 1985 and 1990, heterosexuals accounted for less than 30% of the reported sexually acquired infections. In 2000, this percentage rose to 82%. However, these figures must be interpreted with care because of the different denominators involved. The importance of homosexually-acquired HIV infections should not be ignored. If we assume that 10% of men in Hong Kong are homosexuals, then the HIV prevalence in homosexual men is at least three to five times that in heterosexual men. (This calculation is made by dividing the male population by 10, then dividing this number by the known number of infections transmitted by male homosexual contact to obtain the prevalence rate among homosexual men. This number can then be compared to the prevalence of heterosexual infections among the general public.) At the same time, the ratio of male to female infection has changed from 8:1 in 1992 to about 3:1 in 1998 (Choi and Lee, 2000).

In 2000, less than 5% of the reported infections were attributable to injection drug use, and the cumulative figure at the end of June 2003 was 2.6%. There are, however, indications that HIV infection among drug users has been on the rise. Unlinked anonymous screening of methadone users revealed a yearly positive rate of less than 0.1% up to 1997, rising gradually in the last few years and reaching 0.27% in 2000 (Hong Kong Advisory Council on AIDS, 2001). The number of newly reported cases has also risen from not more than three per year before 1998, to six in 1999, nine in 2000, 11 in 2001, and 10 in 2002 (Hong Kong Advisory Council on AIDS, 2002a).

Transfusion of contaminated blood or blood products is a known risk factor for HIV infection. In Hong Kong, a total of 64 hemophilia patients and three transfusion recipients contracted HIV before 1985 through the use of contaminated blood or blood product as a result of a lack of blood screening and safer alternatives. Over the years, about a quarter of hemophiliacs had tested positive for HIV. With the risk of infection from blood transfusion seemingly past, we were again reminded of the remote chance of infection from blood collected during the window period, when a patient actually became infected in 1997. There is no absolute safety despite the implementation of donor deferral, donor screening for HIV antibody, and the introduction of nucleic acid test procedures (NAT) by the Hong Kong Red Cross Blood Transfusion Service. An infinitesimal residual risk of infection remains.

HIV can also be vertically transmitted from an infected mother to her newborn baby. In Hong Kong, the HIV prevalence of neonates derived from an unlinked anonymous screening program was about 0.03%. A study conducted at Kwong Wah Hospital in 1999 revealed a positive rate of 0.06% (three out of 5067) (Tse *et al.*, 2001). These figures translate into 15 to 30 HIV-positive pregnancies yearly in Hong Kong. Assuming that the rate of mother-to-child infection is 20%, about three to six HIV-positive babies are born each year if intervention is not instituted. With the implementation of universal antenatal HIV testing and the provision of antiretroviral therapy from September 2001, perinatal HIV infection has become extremely uncommon (Hong Kong Advisory Council on AIDS, 2002b).

HISTORICAL DEVELOPMENT OF AIDS PROGRAMS

The development of Hong Kong's AIDS programs can be divided into the following phases (Hong Kong Advisory Council on AIDS, 2001).

Phase I—The Initial Response (1984–1986)

In November 1984, an Expert Committee on AIDS was set up within the then Medical and Health Department to discuss and review the medical aspects of AIDS and to work out a plan for monitoring and managing the disease. Subsequently, in 1985, a Scientific Working Group on AIDS (SWG) was formed to initiate and to implement medical, surveillance and public health activities in Hong Kong. Key outputs during this period included: establishing an AIDS counseling clinic and a hotline, ensuring supply of safe heat-treated blood products, safeguarding the blood supply through blood-screening by the Hong Kong Red Cross Blood Transfusion Service (HKRCBTS), initiating an HIV/AIDS surveillance system, and providing HIV antibody tests to people at risk of infection.

Phase II—Enhanced Public Education (1987–1989)

Public education was systematically introduced during the second phase, in line with the strategy of the World Health Organization (WHO). The Committee on Education & Publicity on AIDS (CEPAIDS) and a publicity working group was formed by the then Medical and Health Department to initiate, implement, and co-ordinate publicity and educational programs. Support was given by various government departments and community organizations. Media publicity was launched and television Announcements of Public Interest (API) were produced by the

Government Information Service to raise public awareness.

The AIDS Counseling and Health Education Service of the Medical and Health Department was expanded to become an operational arm of the committee which organized activities targeting various community groups.

Phase III—Consolidation (1990–1993)

A central Advisory Council on AIDS (ACA), appointed by the governor, was established in March 1990. The Council has been charged with recommending AIDS strategy and streamlining the operations of Hong Kong's AIDS prevention, care, and control program. Community participation was encouraged and AIDS non-governmental organizations (NGOs) were formed during this period. AIDS Concern and the Hong Kong AIDS Foundation, which were formed respectively in 1990 and 1991, both established their status as organizations providing community education as well as counseling and support services to people living with HIV/AIDS.

In early 1993, the AIDS Trust Fund was set up by the government to provide *ex-gratia* payment to HIV infected hemophiliacs and transfusion recipients, following the public outcry in response to the rejection of an HIV-infected hemophiliac boy from school. The same fund also finances education and AIDS care projects.

The HIV/AIDS surveillance system was strengthened through the conduct of epidemiological serosurveillance, e.g., unlinked anonymous screening (UAS), and the original counseling service evolved to become the AIDS Unit of the Department of Health.

Phase IV—Wider Community Participation (1994–1997)

In 1994, ACA published its first official strategy document, entitled *Strategies for AIDS Prevention, Care & Control in Hong Kong,* which formed the blueprint for policy formulation in the Government as well as community organizations.

There was wider community participation during this period and various new organizations were founded, including Action for REACH OUT, Society for AIDS Care, AIDS Memorial Quilt Project, HIV Information & Drop-In Center of the St. John's Cathedral, and the Teen AIDS. AIDS NGOs, with funding support from the AIDS Trust Fund, have contributed significantly. More pre-existing organizations also started to incorporate AIDS in their conventional activities through new initiatives such as the Community Charter on AIDS by the Lions Club International District 303 Hong Kong and Macau.

During this period, education programs on awareness and prevention were expanded with the participation of more NGOs and the re-organized CEPAIDS.

Phase V—Expanded Response (1998 and onward)

A fundamental review, including an internal assessment and an external review, was conducted in 1998, with the results and recommendations submitted to ACA in July 1998. Based on findings of the review, ACA formulated its medium term strategy through the publication of *AIDS Strategies for Hong Kong 1999–2001* in the same year. To tie in with the strategies formulated, a total of ten targets, ranging from early, through-period, and end-of period targets were identified for prevention work through the years 1999–2001. The key foci of these strategies were:

Focus on Prevention

Special emphasis was put on targeting these groups with risk-taking behavior, involving the community's participation in HIV/AIDS prevention and care activities, and promoting acceptance of people living with HIV/AIDS.

Ensuring Quality Care

Attention was drawn to supporting quality treatment, meeting the needs of people with HIV/AIDS, and promoting HIV testing.

Strengthening Partnership

The need to set a common program direction, to expand responses through Community Planning, to conduct evaluations of progress, and to strengthen surveillance to monitor the HIV situation was established.

HIV/AIDS IN HONG KONG: IMPACT AND RESPONSES

What have we learned from the Hong Kong experience? An equally significant question is: after more than a decade of developments, what should be our next step? We attempt to offer several observations for readers' consideration. The Hong Kong Government has on the whole adopted a proactive attitude towards the issue. Organizational structures were set up in a timely way and financial resources were made available to facilitate the implementation of prevention and related programs. These actions have been important factors accounting for the relatively low prevalence of HIV infection in Hong Kong. As long as AIDS remains an incurable disease, it is essential for us to be proactive instead of reactive. Compared with other developed countries in the West, the Hong Kong case has shown a sharp contrast. In these countries, the governments had been slow to develop AIDS programs (Mann *et al.*, 1992; Theodoulous, 1996), and had lost time as they "reacted by inactivity, a wait-and-see attitude"(Pollak, 1992). In this respect, the Hong Kong Government is commendable for its early intervention efforts by taking prompt actions and making quick determinations.

Taking this proactive attitude one step further, we see the urgent need to prepare for possible challenges that lie ahead (Yeung, 1995; Yeung, 1996). Hong Kong has returned to its motherland, China, and there have been increasing contacts, particularly heterosexual contacts, between people from Hong Kong and the mainland. In the absence of comprehensive empirical data, we are not certain how the flourishing commercial sex industry in some cities in China, and the emerging popularity of phenomena like the "second wife" arrangement, may affect HIV transmission in Hong Kong. Nevertheless, this is a "time bomb" which we cannot afford to ignore. A review of the present AIDS initiatives in Hong Kong reveals the apparent lack of sufficient efforts directed at the situation in China, which indeed warrants more effort from relevant government departments and NGOs. In short, we have to further amplify the established proactive attitude by taking swift actions to defuse the "time bomb."

With the support of the government, NGOs in Hong Kong have been actively participating in the fight against AIDS. AIDS is unique among public health issues in that, at least in the early stages, it has been closely connected with two marginalized groups (in the West, although not in Africa): male homosexuals and bisexuals, and injecting drug users. Prevention of HIV transmission hinges on sensitive and controversial topics like human sexuality and condom education. There is still rampant discrimination against persons with HIV/AIDS. These issues cannot be easily resolved and it often requires the implementation of pilot projects to find solutions to these problems. Under such circumstances, NGOs, being community-based and having wider social connections, have a competitive edge over the government to launch such projects with flexibility, innovation, and effectiveness.

In the case of Hong Kong, the government has rightly introduced measures to involve NGOs at an early stage in the development of AIDS programs by inviting them to join various AIDS committees, or granting financial support to their projects. From 1990 onwards, several AIDS-specific NGOs gradually emerged and have since been playing an increasingly active and significant role in the local AIDS arena. Some have built up close connections with specific groups vulnerable to HIV infection and others have developed various educational projects targeting the general public as well as certain community groups. Still others devote their efforts to reducing discrimination against people living with HIV/AIDS. In short, NGOs in Hong Kong have shown active involvement in and commitment to the fight against AIDS. As a word of caution, active NGO participation does not necessarily mean that the government can relegate its leadership in the fight against AIDS. Community involvement is vital. Therefore, further enhancement of government/NGO partnerships will be desirable (UNDP, 1996).

Hong Kong has generally adopted a flexible approach in the development of AIDS programs and has responded to the changing situation by reviewing and restructuring its response. Indeed, as AIDS is a unique public health issue, we are all uncertain of the most "appropriate" policy or strategy. Under such circumstances, constant self-review, learning from other countries, and updating according to global trends are essential to meeting the changing needs of the society. To this end, Hong Kong has devoted efforts to constantly reviewing policy development and has shown willingness to adopt timely improvements.

It can be generally concluded that local AIDS programs, especially those in the public sector, are initiated, sustained, and developed by the medical and health sector. This has included the former Health and Welfare Branch, the former Medical and Health Department, and later the Department of Health, the Hospital Authority, and the Health, Welfare and Food Bureau. In the first few years, the Director of Health also acted as the chairperson of the Advisory Council on AIDS. In retrospect, the fact that AIDS programs have been generated principally from within the medical and health sector is understandable, particularly given that in the initial stage there were still scientific uncertainties surrounding HIV/AIDS.

However, it has since become clear that HIV/AIDS prevention and treatment should be based on social as much as—if not more than—medical programs. In essence, HIV/AIDS is an encompassing social problem which has triggered endless social controversies, most of which naturally fall outside the scope of the medical sector. As a result of increased understanding of the infection, a multi-sectoral approach with the involvement of more and more varied government departments has been adopted.

To conclude, after more than a decade's development, local AIDS programs are becoming more mature and structured. Hong Kong is now heading towards standardization of its AIDS response, with AIDS becoming a normalized part of the government's public health policy response. With this trend, AIDS must be viewed as a chronic disease that society must live with. In this respect, active participation from civil society to partner with government in the fight against AIDS will be of great importance.

RELATIONSHIPS WITH MAINLAND CHINA

Since the identification of the first AIDS case in China in 1985, HIV infections have been reported in all the provinces, autonomous regions, and municipalities in China. At the end of 2002, the official figure was 40,560 reported HIV-infections with 2639 AIDS cases. It should be noted that the number of reported infections has been escalating in recent years. Experts estimate the actual number of infected individuals to be one million to 1.2 million, with the epidemic spreading rapidly.

The following transmission routes are believed to pose significant threats to China: (1) injection drug use, (2) sexual transmission, and (3) iatrogenic transmission. Among all these, more than 65% of the infections were caused by injection drug use, although the number of infections caused by sexual transmission has increased rapidly.

Hong Kong and China have the same historical and ethnic background. We share the same cultural and traditional heritage. The open policy adopted by China in the last decade has greatly increased exchange in trade and cultural activities as well as tourism. This, coupled with the return of Hong Kong back to China, has intensified the link between the two. The increase in the number of infections in both places and the understanding that effective intervention can only be achieved through collaboration with counterparts across the border have created a very favorable environment for sharing experiences and working together in the fight against the HIV/AIDS.

At the government level, there are systems established for exchange of data and information. On the NGO side, collaboration in the form of joint activities such as training courses, exchange meetings, and sharing of resources is not uncommon. Although Hong Kong is a small city, its early development of HIV/AIDS programs has made it possible for Hong Kong to serve as a role model and a source of technical support for different cities in the mainland. However, in spite of these favorable factors, there are still barriers to overcome to make collaboration effective. Hong Kong is adopting a system entirely different from the mainland, and the "one country, two systems" approach has affected the strengthening of collaboration.

THE WAY FORWARD

With advances in medical treatment, the life span of people infected with HIV has been significantly extended, and HIV infection can be viewed as a chronic disease. However, stigma and discrimination continue to be attached to HIV/AIDS. To meet the challenges posed by the epidemic, we have to work on both education and treatment. Through education, we can help prevent the spread of the infection and reduce the unnecessary fear which leads to discrimination. By working on the treatment side, we can help alleviate the pain and suffering of people living with HIV/AIDS. Relative to some other places, Hong Kong is a supportive place for people living with HIV/AIDS, despite the remaining discrimination. We provide antiretroviral therapy at a very affordable cost and we have anti-discrimination laws to protect the rights of people living with HIV/AIDS. At the same time, we have many community-based organizations providing a wide variety of AIDS education and services for people living with HIV/AIDS. However, there is no room for complacency: HIV prevalence will certainly increase if we fail to keep our efforts up. The latest statistics from UNAIDS have told us that China's situation is very critical in terms of controlling the spread of the virus. Helping our colleagues to turn the tide to their favor at this very important moment will eventually benefit our community. We therefore have to consider allocating some of our resources for HIV prevention work in the mainland.

REFERENCES

Choi, T., and Lee, S.S. (2000). Tracking infection: Hong Kong. *AIDS Reader* 10:29–34.

Hong Kong Advisory Council on AIDS, AIDS Prevention and Care Committee. (2001). *Preventing HIV Transmission Among Drug Users in Hong Kong—Principles of Strategy.* Hong Kong Advisory Council on AIDS, Hong Kong.

Hong Kong Advisory Council on AIDS. (2002a). A Report, August 2001 to July 2002. Hong Kong Advisory Council on AIDS, Hong Kong.

Hong Kong Advisory Council on AIDS. (2002b). *Recommended HIV/AIDS Strategies for Hong Kong 2002 to 2006.* Hong Kong Advisory Council on AIDS, Hong Kong.

Mann, J., Tarantola, D., and Netler, T. (eds.). (1992). *AIDS in the World.* Harvard University Press, Cambridge.

Pollak, M. (1992). *AIDS: A Problem for Sociological Research.* SAGE Publications, London, p. 36.

Theodoulous, S. (1996). Responding to AIDS: Governmental Policy Responses. In: Theodoulous S. (ed.), *AIDS: The Politics and Policy of Disease,* Prentice Hall, New Jersey, pp.108–12.

Tse, H.Y., Lai, F.K., Wong, J., Chan, A.S.M., and Tang, L.C.H. (2001). Universal voluntary screening of HIV in pregnant women in Hong Kong: A prospective study. *Hong Kong Med J.* 7:246–250.

United Nations Development Programme (UNDP). (1996). Enhancing government-NGO collaboration in AIDS policy and services-the case of Hong Kong. UNDP and Hong Kong Polytechnic University Collaborative Center. (April 1996).

Yeung, F.Y. (1995). China as an important factor for further development of AIDS Programs in Hong Kong. Sing Tao Daily (December 30, 1995), in Chinese.

Yeung, V.F.Y. (1996). AIDS Programs in Hong Kong—Past, Present, and Future. In: Proceedings of the 27th International Council on Social Welfare International Conference: Societies in Change—Development in a Political, Economic and Social Context, Vol 2a. International Council on Social Welfare and the Hong Kong Council of Social Service, Hong Kong, pp. 396–403.

14

HIV/AIDS in Hawaii and the Pacific Islands

Arwind R. Diwan[1] and Stephen G. Karel[2,3]

[1]*Department of Tropical Medicine & Medical Microbiology, John A. Burns School of Medicine, University of Hawaii, Honolulu, Hawaii, USA*
[2]*Former WHO staff member, Western Pacific Regional Office*
[3]*Former Executive Director, Pacific Island Health Officers Association, Honolulu, Hawaii, USA*

HISTORICAL BACKGROUND

The Hawaiian Islands, as well as other less populated islands in the Pacific, were, until recent times, the most isolated, inhabitable places, and difficult to reach by sea. The Hawaiian Islands are more than 2000 miles away from the West Coast of the United States. Most of the other islands in the Pacific are also far from populated countries in the region. These islands were inhabited by native populations belonging to Polynesian, Micronesian and Melanesian backgrounds. Fishing and subsistence farming were practiced before contact with Europeans and people from other seafaring nations.

With the discovery of the Hawaiian Islands by Captain James Cook in 1778, the situation changed considerably, in that the European and American populations came to these islands as spheres of colonial influence. The British were the first to arrive, subsequent to the annexation of the Hawaiian Islands in the early 1900s by the United States during the Spanish American War in the Pacific. Missionaries from the East Coast of the United States of America arrived in the Hawaiian Islands after the British. Some of the other islands in the Pacific also came under the jurisdiction of the U.S., subsequent to their reoccupation from the Japanese after the end of the Second World War, under the trusteeship of the United Nations. Hawaii became the 50th state of U.S. in 1959, and other Pacific Islands under U.S. jurisdiction were organized as separate units, such as Federated States of Micronesia, and independent states allied with the U.S., such as the Republic of Marshall Islands and the Republic of Palau.

Since the discovery and occupation of these islands by foreigners, their commercial interests, such as agriculture and tourism, have required them to import immigrant populations from Asian countries and other islands in the Pacific, first to cultivate crops such as sugar and pineapple, and later to work in the tourism industry. Today, Hawaii has a multiethnic population that consists of the native Hawaiian and part Hawaiian populations and people of other ethnic backgrounds such as Japanese, Chinese, Caucasians, Filipinos, Korean, as well as the Samoan, Tongan, and Micronesian populations of the Pacific Islands.

Introduction of people from the foreign lands and the disease they brought to the Hawaiian Islands had tremendous impact on the native Hawaiian population. This impact was so extreme that the native Hawaiian population declined rapidly and very few pure native Hawaiian are alive today in Hawaii. Diseases introduced to the native Hawaiian population included venereal disease, tuberculosis, leprosy, bubonic plague, Asiatic cholera, and measles. These events have been well described by Dr. O.A. Bushnell (1993) in his book, *The Gifts of Civilization: Germs and Genocide in Hawaii.*

RECENT STUDIES OF VIRAL INFECTIONS IN HAWAII

Rubella

In 1969, studies showed that 70–80% of women of childbearing age born in Hawaii lacked antibody to the Rubella (German measles) virus (Halstead *et al.*, 1969). Having found a large susceptible population for rubella, studies were undertaken to evaluate live attenuated Rubella vaccine candidates in the susceptible population. Susceptible women were vaccinated with candidate vaccines and were subsequently monitored for side effects, transmission to close contacts, and development of antibodies. These studies were important in the licensure of Rubella vaccines by the Food and Drug Administration and allowed us to screen women of childbearing age for antibodies and vaccinate them. Further studies were undertaken to vaccinate children ages 5–11 on the outer islands with Rubella vaccine and monitor them for development of antibody and persistence of antibody over 10 to 20 years after immunization.

Human T Lymphotropic Virus—HTLV-1

Discovery of HTLV-1 virus by Robert Gallo in 1980 linked the first human virus to lymphoid cancer, adult T-cell leukemia lymphoma (ATL), an important discovery because it found the first human virus associated with cancer (Poiesz *et al.*, 1980). Studies done by Takatsuki *et al.* in 1977 showed high prevalence of ATL, a new disease clustered epidemiologically in the southern island of Japan (1977). Studies undertaken in Hawaii amongst the blood donors at the Blood Bank of Hawaii showed that all donors positive for antibody to HTLV-1 were in the Japanese ethnic group (Julia Frohlich, personal communication, 1985). This was not surprising in that most of the Japanese immigrant population to Hawaii came from southern islands of Japan, such as Kyushi and Okinawa, where prevalence of HTLV-1 is high. Further studies showed that the prevalence of HTLV-1 antibody was high amongst the first generation (Issei) Japanese population and decreased in second (Neissei) and third generation (Sansei) of Japanese population. Few cases of ATL associated with HTLV-1 and neuropathy HTLV-1 associated with myelopathy/tropical spastic paraparesis (HAM/TSP) are found in Hawaii.

HIV/AIDS IN HAWAII

HIV Infection in Hawaii

HIV infections were not reported from the beginning of the epidemic (1983) because no diagnostic tests were available at that time. With the availability of the test and the opening of HIV testing and counseling centers in 1985–86, it was possible to identify individuals who were HIV antibody-positive. However, they were not reported because of the confidentiality requirement of the testing and counseling centers. In 1996, it was estimated that 2300–3200 HIV infections had occurred in Hawaii (Hawaii Department of Health, 1996). Since August 2001, mandatory reporting of new HIV infections has been required, so it will be possible to more accurately track the epidemic.

AIDS

Hawaii's first AIDS case was diagnosed in Honolulu in 1983, based upon the detection of opportunistic infection by *Pneumocystis carinii* and the pneumonia associated with it in a male homosexual. As of June 2003, 2767 cases of AIDS were reported in Hawaii. Of the 2767 cases, 1977 (71%) occurred in the City and County of Honolulu, 374 (14%) occurred on the Big Island of Hawaii, 295 (11%) occurred in Maui County, which includes the island of Maui and two other islands, Molokai and Lanai, and 121 (4%) occurred on the island of Kauai (Hawaii Department of Health, 2003).

The majority of cases, 2571 (93%), occurred in males, while only 196 (7%) occurred in females. Further analysis of these cases showed the following:

Age

Twenty-five AIDS cases (<1%) occurred in age groups <13 and 13–19, and 342 cases (12%) occurred in age group 20–29. The majority of cases, 1204 (44%), occurred in age groups 30–39, another 850 cases (31%) occurred in age group 40–49, and 346 cases (31%) occurred in age group >49. Thus, it appears that 2742 out of the total of 2767 (or 99% of cases) occurred among adults aged 20 and older.

Ethnicity

One thousand seven hundred thirty-seven (63%) of AIDS cases occurred in Caucasians, 300 (11%) occurred in Hawaiian and part-Hawaiians, 118 (4%) occurred in African Americans, 143 (5%) occurred in Hispanics, and 12 (<1%) of the cases occurred in American Indians.

In the Asian and Pacific Islands group, 145 cases (5%) occurred in Filipinos, 119 (4%) occurred in Japanese, 58 (2%) in Chinese, 128 (5%) from the Pacific Islands and other Asian countries, and seven (<1%) of the cases occurred in ethnically mixed individuals. These observations show that AIDS cases occurred in people of all ethnic backgrounds in Hawaii.

Risk Category

The majority of AIDS cases, 2060 or 75%, occurred in men who have sex with men (MSM), 184 (7%) occurred in MSM who were also injecting drug users (IDU), another 184 (7%) occurred in IDU (non-MSM). Ninety-seven (4% of the cases) occurred in female heterosexuals and 48 (2%) occurred in male heterosexuals. Blood transfusion was the route of transmission in 26 (<1%) of the cases. Similarly, 14 cases (<1%) were acquired perinatally and 20 (<1%) occurred in hemophiliacs through the administration of HIV-contaminated Factor VIII. No risk category could be established in 120 (4%) of the reported AIDS cases.

The total number of reported AIDS cases in Hawaii from 1983 to June 30, 2003 is 2767, of which 1537 (56%) have died.

HIV/AIDS PREVENTION AND CONTROL IN HAWAII

Screening of Blood Donors for HIV infection

As soon as the ELISA test for detection of antibodies to HIV was licensed by FDA in 1985, the Blood Bank of Hawaii started testing blood donors for HIV. HIV ELISA antibody-positive donors were retested using the Western Blot by the Department of Tropical Medicine to confirm the HIV diagnosis. As soon as commercially licensed Western Blot tests became available, this test was used. Forty thousand donors per year are screened for antibody to HIV. Blood collected from HIV-positive donors is not used for transfusion and is discarded after appropriate treatment. Any HIV-positive donor is informed of the results in a confidential manner and advised to seek the help of a physician. During the early part of the HIV epidemic, 21 transfusion-associated cases of HIV were reported. Currently, there are very few transfusion-associated cases, due to regular screening of blood donors for HIV antibody.

Testing and Counseling Centers

This program started concurrently with the testing of blood donors for antibodies to HIV. Tests for antibody to HIV are offered at no cost to individuals who seek testing. Confidentiality is strictly maintained regarding the identity of the individuals and the results of the test. HIV antibody-positive individuals are counseled to seek a physician's help in medical management.

Since 1985, the number of HIV-positive individuals has declined. For example, over the seven-year period from 1985–1991, of the 46,577 individuals tested, 1587 (3.4%) of the samples were positive for antibody to HIV, with an annual average of 227 HIV antibody-positive samples. During the next seven years, from 1992–1998, 99,142 samples were tested; of these, only 320 samples tested positive, a rate of 0.99%. Between 1999 and June 2003, 41,036 samples were tested and 187 (0.46%) were positive. Thus, over the 19-year period of testing, HIV antibody positivity rates have declined from 3.4% to 0.46% (Roy Ohye, personal communication, September 2003).

Hawaii State-Wide Syringe Exchange Program (SEP)

This program, titled the Chow project, started as a Community Health Outreach Work to prevent AIDS in 1990. Highlights of the program can be summarized as follows:

1. Hawaii was the first state to start such a proactive HIV prevention program to reduce the transmission of HIV.
2. Nationally, 35% of AIDS cases occur among IDU. In Hawaii, only 17% of AIDS cases are attributable to IDU. Local and national experts credit this low rate in Hawaii to SEP.
3. SEP is a comprehensive, coordinated, state-wide program. Each year, 10,000 anonymous visits are made to the program by IDU. The number of syringes exchanged continues to grow each year. In 2002, 468,379 syringes were exchanged.
4. The SEP serves as an effective bridge to drug treatment, referring 150 SEP participants into the treatment program per year.
5. The Hawaii SEP is extremely cost effective, saving state money if it prevents just five cases per year.

Hawaii Sero-Positivity and Medical Management (HSPAMM) Program

This program was initiated in 1989. The purpose of this program was to:

1. Encourage those who are HIV-infected or at risk of infection to consult a physician before they become symptomatic.
2. Provide ongoing clinical assistance to those who are already infected.
3. Maintain anonymous clinical and laboratory records on HIV-positive individuals.
4. Classify groups of HIV-positive individuals with certain specified criteria, who may be available for experimental treatments.

Program Structure

HSPAMM participants, through their physicians, get subsidized, limited care from their own physicians. HIV-positive volunteers are recruited through community physicians, social service agencies, HIV testing sites and AIDS service organizations.

After enrolling in the program, participants are seen by a physician twice a year at six-month intervals. Physical examination and a panel of laboratory tests are performed during each visit. Tests include the HIV antibody test; Hepatitis B tests such as Hepatitis B surface antigen (HBsAg), Hepatitis B core antibody (HBcAb), and antibody to Hepatitis B surface antigen (HbsAg); as well as Hepatitis C core antibody; Lymphocyte CD4 and CD8 count; and plasma RNA viral load tests. Besides these tests, other tests such as liver function tests, lipid and urinalysis tests, and differential CBC tests are also done. With regard to tests for opportunistic infections, serological tests for toxoplasmosis and microscopic tests for ova and parasites are done. Physicians are reimbursed for two visits per year and all laboratory tests are paid for.

HSPAMM Participant Demographics

Since the inception of the program, 2625 HIV-positive people have been enrolled. Of the 2407 (92%) males, 34% are still-active program participants, while 66% have died or been lost to follow-up. Of the 218 (8%) females in the program, 49% are still active and 51% have died or been lost to follow-up. With regard to ethnicity, 62% of program participants were Caucasian, 21% were Asian or Pacific Islanders, 6.6% were Hispanic, 4.2% were African American, 1.2% were American Indian, and 4.8% were of mixed race. At enrollment, 46% of the participants had an annual income less than $10,000, while 4% had an annual income over $40,000 (Suzanne M. Richmond-Crum, personal communication, September 2003).

Availability of Drug Treatment for People with HIV and AIDS in Hawaii

The state of Hawaii is the only state in the United States where there is a law mandating that all employees and their families are covered by the private medical insurance. This law allowed medical insurance coverage for treatment and provision of drugs to the patients in majority of cases.

Those patients who have low income and no medical insurance are covered by the HIV Drug Assistance Program (HDAP). This program is funded by state and federal funds. The COBRA (Consolidated Omnibus Budget Reconciliation Act) program provides continuation of private group health insurance benefits to those who are forced to leave their jobs due to asymptomatic HIV infection. This program is funded by the federal government through the Ryan White CARE Act (Title 11).

In 1988, the AIDS Clinical Trial Unit (ACTU) was established under the Research Center for Minority Institutions (RCMI), which is funded by NIH. Experimental drugs against HIV are available for participants in the drug trials undertaken by the unit.

Treatment and Prevention of Pediatric AIDS in Hawaii

Since 1986, it has been important to identify children infected by various routes of transmission. This included children who received transfusions of contaminated blood, hemophiliacs who received injection of HIV-contaminated factor VIII, and children born to HIV-infected mothers. The Pediatric Immunology Program was initiated at Kapiolani Women's and Children's Hospital in Honolulu. The purpose of the program was to provide medical care and assistance to infected children. In the earlier part of the epidemic, HIV-infected children were identified by selecting mothers at risk for HIV, such as those with a history of injecting drug use or those who had sexual partners who were IDU. Since HIV serological tests became available, transfusion-associated cases in Hawaii have been almost eliminated in both adults and children. A new HIV-free factor VIII to treat hemophiliac children has also eliminated this risk of HIV infection. During the late eighties and early nineties, as part of the AIDS Seroprevalance Program of the State Health Department, the majority of neonates were tested for HIV using serological tests. A total of 98,893 samples were tested, and only 38 (0.038%) of the samples were positive for HIV antibody (Joe Elm, Jr., personal communication, September 2003). Pregnant women enrolled in the Pediatric Immunology Program are monitored, and the newborns from these women are tested for HIV and observed for development of AIDS. Since new treatment became available for HIV-infected mothers, the incidence of mother to child transmission has been reduced considerably. At the present time, it is estimated that 87% of pregnant women are screened in the private and public sector for HIV antibodies. With newly available saliva tests for rapid diagnosis of HIV, it may now be possible to test more pregnant women in outpatient clinics as well as during or prior to delivery and to treat mother and child to reduce perinatal transmission of HIV.

HIV/AIDS Prevention Education Programs in Hawaii

In 1986–87, the University of Hawaii Student Health Service organization started a peer HIV/AIDS education training program. The object of this program was to train a cadre of interested university students in HIV/AIDS prevention education. These trained individuals would then act as peers in training other students in various colleges of the university system, including community colleges as well as public and private high schools. This program was well received and has continued to prevent HIV infection in this group. Risk reduction for HIV includes condom use and education to reduce risk for HIV and other sexually transmitted diseases (STDs).

In 1988, the Department of Psychiatry of the University of Hawaii School of Medicine was awarded the AIDS Education Project for Hawaii from the National Institute of Mental Health to provide education in HIV/AIDS to direct health care providers, such as doctors and nurses who care for AIDS patients.

More recently, this program has continued to provide all health care workers information about HIV risk reduction and all other aspects of HIV/AIDS. This program is now funded by a grant from the Health Research Service Administration (HRSA) under the Ryan White Act. The program's annual budget is $350,000, and includes the U.S. Affiliated Pacific Islands. The State of Hawaii also supports HIV/AIDS education and training to the AIDS service organization within the State of Hawaii.

AIDS Service Organizations

Since the beginning of the epidemic of AIDS in Hawaii, it was very important to protect the identity of the individuals in the MSM population. This was done because of the social stigma with regard to homosexuality and also HIV/AIDS, and the discrimination they would encounter when seeking services such as health insurance, housing, and employment. A non-governmental support group named Life Foundation was started in 1985 in Honolulu. This support group has continued to operate with grants from state and private funds. Other islands in the State of Hawaii also have their own support group which helps HIV-positive individuals obtain necessary services in their daily life.

HIV/AIDS IN THE PACIFIC ISLANDS

The Pacific Islands are often divided into the Northern and Southern Pacific Regions for historical, cultural, and socio-economic reasons.

Northern Pacific

The Northern Pacific Islands are often referred to as the U.S.-Affiliated Pacific Islands and include the island states of Micronesia, the Commonwealth of Guam, the Republic of the Marshall Islands, the Republic of Palau, and several others. Seroprevalence is low in this region and limited data has been collected among the populations of blood donors, pregnant women, STD clinic patients, and immigrant groups. It is likely that the HIV prevalence is less than 0.1% and is not expected to increase dramatically. The majority of cases have occurred among men, with sexual contact with other men being the most frequent reported mode of transmission. However, the proportion of heterosexual cases has been increasing over the last few years.

The Commonwealth of the Northern Mariana Islands (CNMI)

The World Health Organization (WHO) had reported cumulative totals of 14 AIDS cases and 29 HIV infections through September of 2000 (WHO, 2000) in this area. Government health officials estimate there are at least 300 positive individuals, most of whom are not receiving treatment. More than 70% of these individuals are male.

The U.S. Centers for Disease Control has provided CNMI with US $293,974 for community-based organizations to finance counseling and testing programs, public information and health education/risk reduction activities, and monitoring/surveillance programs (NASTAD, 2003).

The Commonwealth of the Northern Mariana Islands has received US $51,323 from Title II of the Ryan White CARE Act to support educational and outreach services to help disproportionately impacted communities. The CNMI also has received US $50,000 from Title IV for the operation and development of primary care systems and social services for women and youth (Health Resources and Services Administration, 2003).

The Territory of Guam

The World Health Organization has reported cumulative totals of 64 AIDS cases and 137 HIV infections in Guam through September 2000 (WHO, 2000). The seroprevalence is low, less than 0.1%. The likelihood of an epidemic of heterosexual transmission is low since the necessary factors are not apparent in Guam.

The Federated States of Micronesia

By 2002, the four states of the Federated States of Micronesia (FSM) had reported 76 total AIDS cases (AIDS Action, 2003). The seroprevalence is less than 0.1% and most of the cases have been male.

The U.S. Centers for Disease Control has provided FSM with US $224,710 for community-based organizations. The FSM have also received US $50,000 from Title II of the Ryan White CARE Act for outreach services.

The Republic of the Marshall Islands

By 2002, the Republic of the Marshall Islands had reported 9 cases of AIDS (AIDS Action, 2003). The seroprevalence is believed to be less than 0.1%.

The U.S. Centers for Disease Control has provided the Marshall Islands with $130,330 for community-based organizations. The Marshall Islands have received $51,323 from Title II of the Ryan White CARE Act for outreach services and an additional $50,000 from Title III for early intervention services for low-income, uninsured, and underinsured HIV-infected individuals.

The Republic of Palau

The World Health Organization had reported cumulative totals of two AIDS cases and two HIV infections in the Republic of Palau through September of 2000 (WHO, 2000).

The Republic of Kiribati

The World Health Organization has reported cumulative totals of 16 AIDS cases and 33 HIV infections in the Republic of Kiribati through September of 2000 (WHO, 2000).

Southern Pacific

The number of HIV infections and AIDS cases are significantly higher in the states of the Southern Pacific Region. Papua New Guinea, French Polynesia, and New Caledonia have substantially more HIV infections than the other states of the region. It is important to point out that surveys conducted in some of the countries and territories in the Southern Pacific show that STDs are common. For example, in 2000, studies of women attending antenatal care clinics in Samoa and Vanuatu showed that one in three had an STD. The highest rates of infection (up to 50%) were found in women below 25 years of age. HIV and AIDS programs in the South Pacific will need to concentrate their efforts on the prevention and control of treatable STDs, especially syphilis and gonorrhea, and to develop HIV surveillance mechanisms among persons with the highest prevalence of sexual risk behaviors (WHO, 2001).

The Republic of Samoa

The World Health Organization has reported cumulative totals of 6 AIDS cases and 10 HIV infections in the Republic of Samoa through August 1999 (WHO, 2000).

New Caledonia

The World Health Organization has reported cumulative totals of 77 AIDS cases and 219 HIV infections in New Caledonia through July 2000 (WHO, 2000).

French Polynesia

The World Health Organization has reported cumulative totals of 74 AIDS cases and 202 HIV infections in French Polynesia through September 2000 (WHO, 2000).

Tonga

The World Health Organization has reported cumulative totals of 8 AIDS cases and 11 HIV infections in Tonga through July 1999 (WHO, 2000).

The Republic of Fiji

The World Health Organization has reported totals of 8 AIDS cases and 62 HIV infections in Fiji (WHO, 2000). The most recent Fiji government figures indicate a total of 104 HIV-infected persons. More than 80% of those with HIV were infected through sexual contact, 63% were male, 77% were ethnic Fijians, and 75% were in the age category 20–49 (Fiji Government, 2002).

Papua New Guinea

The first HIV infections in Papua New Guinea (PNG) were reported in 1987, with HIV prevalence increasing annually every year since then. Reported cases are equally distributed among men and women, and infection appears to be concentrated in the capital of Port Moresby. Prevalence remains low among blood donors (0.015% in 1997) and pregnant women (0.37% in 1998). Much higher levels of infection were found in female sex workers (17% in Port Moresby in 1999) and among patients attending STD clinics (7% in 1999). The estimated HIV prevalence in PNG is about 15,000 to 17,000 or 0.6% of the total 15–49 year old population. Prevalence continues to increase due primarily to heterosexual transmission. By 2001, there had been almost 900 AIDS deaths in PNG (WHO, 2001).

It has been reported that 94% of PNG HIV infections were acquired through unprotected sexual intercourse and that 60% of married men in Port Moresby engaged in commercial sex activities (UNIFEM, 2002).

A wide range of social, economic, and cultural factors in PNG have contributed to an environment in which sexual risk behaviors are widespread. PNG has been highly vulnerable to HIV infections due to its poverty, high illiteracy rate, poor health care system, low status of women, and traditional cultural practices involving forced sex and sexual coercion of women and girls. There are low levels of condom use and health centers frequently run out of their supply. Casual sexual partnerships are widespread.

The low level of condom use has been linked to limited supply and availability as well as resistance to use them by the clients of female sex workers. Among sex workers, the proportion reporting consistent condom use is around 15%. The mean number of clients per sex worker was from 3–5 per week. Sexual behavior surveys among sex workers indicate a predominate practice of vaginal intercourse, but 30% also report anal sex. A similar proportion reports forced sex and group sex (WHO, 2001).

Some sexual behavioral research in PNG suggests that sexual networking may resemble the sexual cultures in Africa and therefore the HIV epidemic may eventually spread in a pattern and extent similar to those in some African countries (Jenkins *et al.*, 1994).

STD prevalence surveys in PNG show a high STD prevalence among both high-risk and low-risk groups. A 15% prevalence of gonorrhea among the Highland's populations and 36% among sex workers were found. Chlamydia prevalence was up to 26% in the Highland's populations, and 31% in sex workers. Prevalence of syphilis was 4% in the Highland's populations and 32% in sex workers (WHO, 2001).

Other States in the Pacific

No cases of HIV infection or AIDS have been reported from American Samoa, Cook Islands, Niue, Tokelau or Vanuatu. Only a handful of infections have been reported in Nauru, the Solomon Islands, and Wallis and Futuna.

SUMMARY

During the last 19 years, the State of Hawaii has responded admirably to the AIDS epidemic. The State Government, University of Hawaii, Blood Bank of Hawaii, all hospitals, and social work agencies have participated in the process of responding to the AIDS epidemic. This has resulted in less than 40 new cases of HIV infection being reported to the State Health Department from 1999 to 2002. The availability of drugs for the treatment of almost all HIV-infected individuals is possible because of the liberal medical health insurance program, as well as state and federal funding. This has reduced the mortality rate considerably and most HIV-infected individuals, with the help of drugs, are living productive and relatively healthy lives. The syringe exchange program has reduced transmission among the IDU population. The blood donor screening program, as well as the non-HIV infected factor VIII now used in treatment of hemophiliacs have reduced transmission in these groups. Identifying HIV-positive pregnant women and treating them with drugs has also reduced transmission from mother to child. Peer education programs, education of health care workers, and increased awareness of the public have made significant impacts on the spread of HIV/AIDS. Confidential, no-cost HIV antibody tests are available to all who are at risk. All of these measures have reduced the impact of HIV and AIDS in the State of Hawaii and hopefully this will continue in the future.

In most of the other Pacific Islands, rates of HIV and AIDS remain very low. However, Papua New Guinea is currently vulnerable to the spread of HIV infection, especially via heterosexual transmission, due to widespread sexual risk behaviors evidenced by the high prevalence of sexually transmitted infections there.

ACKNOWLEDGEMENTS. The authors wish to thank the following individuals in Hawaii for providing information about HIV and AIDS: Ms. Pritty B. Borthakur, Mr. Roy Ohye and Ms. Suzanne M. Richmond-Crum of the STD/AIDS prevention branch of the State Department of Health; Dr. Marian Melish, Professor, Department of Pediatrics and Dr. Jane Waldren of the Department of Psychiatry, University of Hawaii School of Medicine; Mr. Joe Elm, Jr. of the Epidemiology Branch of the State Health Department; Ms. Suzzette Smetka of the Chow Project; Dr. Donald Char, former director of University of Hawaii Student Health Services; and Dr. Julie Frohlich, former President, Blood Bank of Hawaii.

REFERENCES

AIDS ACTION. (2003). State Facts, HIV/AIDS in the U.S. Pacific Islands, Washington, DC.

Bushnell, O.A. (1993). *The Gifts of Civilization: Germs and Genocide in Hawaii.* University of Hawaii Press, Honolulu.

Fiji Government. (2002). Education Main Weapon to Fight HIV/AIDS, Press Release (September 11, 2002).

Halstead, S.B., Diwan, A.R. and Oda, A.I. (1969). Susceptibility to rubella among adolescents and adults in Hawaii. *JAMA* 210:1881–1883.

Hawaii Department of Health. (1996). Hawaii Administrative Rules, Title 11, Chapter 156, Section 156:8–9 (January 23, 2004); http://www.state.hi.us/health/rules/index.html.

Hawaii Department of Health. (2003). HIV/AIDS Surveillance Semi Annual Report. (June 2003).

Health Resources and Services Administration, US Department of Health and Human Services. (2003). Special report, Titles III and IV: FY 2002 (March 2003). Washington, DC.

Jenkins, C., and The National Sex and Reproduction Research Team. (1994). National Study of Sexual and Reproductive Knowledge and Behaviour in Papua New Guinea. Papua New Guinea Institute of Medical Research, Port Moresby.

National Alliance of State and Territorial AIDS Directors (NASTAD). (2003). CDC HIV prevention funding for state and local health departments. (January 26, 2004); http://www.nastad.org/PDF/CDCFUNDI.PDF.

Poiesz, B.J., Ruscetti, F.W., Gazdar, A.F., Bunn, P.A., Minna, J.D., and Gallo, R.C. (1980). Detection and isolation of type C retrovirus particles from fresh and cultured lymphocytes of a patient with cutaneous T-cell lymphoma. *Proc Natl Acad Sci USA*. 77:7415–7419.

Takatsuki, K., Uchiyama, T., Sagawa, K., and Yodoi, J. (1977). Adult T-cell leukemia in Japan. In: Seno, S., and Takaku, F. (eds.), *Topics in Hematology.* Exerpta Medica, Amsterdam, p. 73.

World Health Organization. (2000). STI/HIV/AIDS Surveillance Report, No. 16 (November 2000), WPRO, Manila, Philippines.

World Health Organization. (2001). HIV/AIDS in Asia and the Pacific Region, WPRO, Manila, Philippines.

United Nations Development Fund for Women (UNIFEM). (2002). Women, Gender and HIV/AIDS in East and Southeast Asia. UNIFEM Report. East and South East Asia Regional Office, Bangkok, Thailand.

15

HIV/AIDS Preparedness in the CIS, Baltic, East and Southeast Europe, and the Balkans

A Situation Report

Tony Barnett

Development Studies Institute, London School of Economics and Political Science, London, UK

INTRODUCTION: A REGIONAL EPIDEMIC

From an epidemiological perspective the Eurasian landmass, from the Atlantic to the Pacific, must be considered a unified surface, or "region." The area spans from Eastern Europe, the Baltic, and Balkans to the countries of Central Asia and Russia, which lie at its heart. Epidemic events in this central area are important for the whole of Eurasia.

Epidemics do not respect national boundaries, and meeting the challenge of the HIV/AIDS epidemic in this region will necessarily require a high degree of interdependence, synergy, and cross-border cooperation between countries. This paper will look at the region's preparedness for the epidemic. We divide preparedness into the following components: (a) awareness of the epidemic as it develops, (b) administrative infrastructure and resource allocation, and (c) evidence that national authorities appreciate the epidemic's potential social and economic impacts and costs.

In some countries, the epidemic may remain small and concentrated in specific population groups. However, there are already indications that in others a generalized epidemic exists or may be about to emerge. This must give great cause for concern to all politicians, policy-makers, and opinion-formers in the region.

The HIV/AIDS Epidemic in the Commonwealth of Independent States (CIS), Baltic, East and Southeast Europe, and the Balkans

In the Russian Federation, the very steep rise in HIV infections of recent years continues. Reported cases have almost doubled

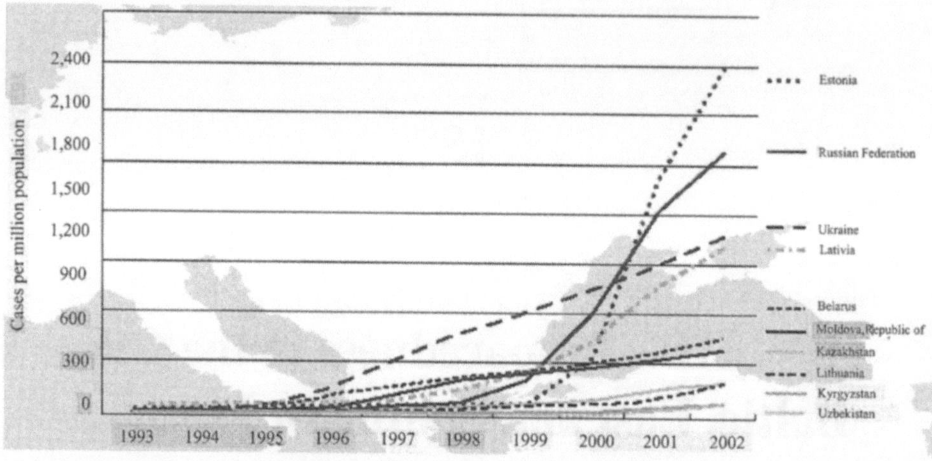

FIGURE 1. Cumulative reported HIV infections per million population in Eastern European countries: 1993–2002. Source: National AIDS Programmes (2002). HIV/AIDS surveillance in Europe. End-of-year report. Data compiled by the European Centre for the Epidemiological Monitoring of AIDS.

annually since 1998. The number of reported infections since the epidemic began reached 177,354 at the end of 2001. A very conservative estimate would put the number of people now living with HIV in the Russian Federation at least four times higher than the reported figures, approaching a prevalence rate of 1% in the adult population. In Estonia, newly reported infections rose from 12 in 1999 to 1474 by the end of 2001, and in Latvia, the incidence jumped from 25 cases in 1997 to 807 cases in 2001. Kazakhstan, where the first case was reported in 1997, reported 1175 HIV infections in 2001. Rapid spread is also apparent in Kyrgyzstan, Tajikistan, Uzbekistan, Azerbaijan, and Georgia. With an adult HIV prevalence rate of 1%, Ukraine remains the most seriously affected country (Henning Mikkelsen, UNAIDS, personal communication, 2003).

Is This A Regional Epidemic?

The answer to this question is not straightforward. It is affected by the politics of interpretation of the epidemiological data. The situation appears fairly clear:

- One country out of 23 (Russia) accounts for close to 70% of all infections.
- Two countries (Russia and Ukraine) make up some 95% of all infections.
- Adult infection rates are around 1% in three countries: Russia, Ukraine, and Estonia.
- Infection rates between 0.2% and 0.4% are found in three countries: Belarus, Moldova, and Latvia.
- Prevalence rates at or lower than 0.1% are found in 17 out the 23 countries.
- Poland has a considerable number of infections, but a low adult infection rate because of the size of its population.
- Taken together, Russia and Ukraine shift the region-wide average adult infection rate to eight times the average of the other countries.

Is this then a Russian, a Ukrainian, or an Estonian problem? Experience elsewhere shows that such thinking is unconstructive and is symptomatic of general denial. Such responses were common in Africa in the late 1980s and early 1990s, and are still heard in India and China today. In Africa, public denials of this kind are now less frequent as politicians appreciate the epidemic's rate of growth and its long-term effects.

Today, the situation seems worse in Russia, Ukraine, and Estonia than elsewhere.

But we must remember that what we know about the epidemic is an artifact of the reporting system in each country. Reporting systems vary. Given that this is a contiguous landmass with a high level of political, social, and economic instability, conditions are ripe for a large and destructive regional epidemic.

SURVEY METHOD

Data were gathered by means of a survey from October 2001 to February 2002. (The survey was carried out through the UNDP offices. UNDP bears no responsibility for the presentation of these data or for their interpretation, which are solely the responsibility of the author.) A detailed questionnaire was used as an interview guide by senior and experienced interviewers in each country. Key informants were interviewed as appropriate in their own language or in Russian in 24 countries: Albania, Armenia, Azerbaijan, Belarus, Bosnia-Herzegovina, Czech Republic, Georgia, Kazakhstan, Kosovo, Kyrgyzstan, Latvia, Lithuania, Moldova, Poland, Romania, Russia, Slovakia, Tajikistan, Turkey, Turkmenistan, Ukraine, Uzbekistan, and Yugoslavia.

The survey questionnaire sought the same set of information for each country:

1. Basic epidemiological and demographic data.
2. Structure and capability of the national sero-surveillance system.
3. National AIDS program structure, organisation and policies, including the participation and involvement of private- and third-sector agencies, and the role of civil-society organizations.
4. Legislative, prevention and treatment framework.
5. Financial information concerning governments' national AIDS programs.
6. Preparedness to engage with the effects of HIV/AIDS on socio-economic development.
7. Known activities concerned with confronting the effects of HIV/AIDS on socio-economic development.

The results of this survey provide a perspective on the following issues:

- Differences in regional "official" knowledge about the epidemic.
- A picture of the "shape" of the epidemic as it appeared to the responsible authorities in each country.
- The range of national financial, legislative, and policy environments.
- The range of prevention and treatment regimes.
- The relative degree of preparedness to meet the challenges of HIV/AIDS for socio-economic development—in other words the degree of preparedness to engage with the question of "impact" beyond the obvious clinical and medical impacts.

Thus, the survey results provide a baseline against which progress in preparedness and engagement with the epidemic may be regularly measured over the coming years. Here we discuss only a selection of key findings from the larger data set.

KNOWING THE EPIDEMIC

Any battle requires intelligence about the enemy. What do the authorities in this region know about this enemy? We asked key informants from the epidemiological services to provide the best information they had about the state of the epidemic in their country. Table 1 indicates the year each country recorded its first AIDS case, as well as which year the national authorities believe the epidemic began.

An HIV/AIDS epidemic is a long-wave event (Barnett and Blaikie, 1992; Barnett and Whiteside, 2002). A component of the amplitude of the wave is the length of time it takes for national authorities to respond to both the epidemic and its potential social and economic effects.

TABLE 1. Years of First Reported AIDS Case and Assumed Start of Epidemic

Country	Year first AIDS case recorded	Assumed start year of epidemic
Albania	1993	1991
Armenia	1988	1988
Azerbaijan	1994	1997
Belarus	1991	1996
Bosnia-Herzegovina	1989	Unknown
Czech Republic	1985	1983
Georgia	1989	[a]
Kazakhstan	1987	1985
Kosovo	1986	2000
Kyrgyzstan	2000	2001
Latvia	1990	1998
Lithuania	1988	[b]
Moldova	1989	1996
Poland	1986	1985
Romania	1987	1990
Russia	1987	1987
Slovakia	1984	Unknown
Tajikistan	1991	2001
Turkey	1985	1983
Turkmenistan	1990	Unknown
Ukraine	1988	1994
Uzbekistan	1987	Unknown
Yugoslavia	1985	1985

[a] It was reported that "the situation in Georgia is pre-epidemic."
[b] Informants believed that "there is no (HIV/AIDS) epidemic in Lithuania."

The first identification of an AIDS case is significant for any country. This is the first time that the epidemic impinges upon the country's medical and clinical services. It is the first time that the epidemic manifests itself as a potential competitor for resources between care and treatment of an individual or individuals and some other use of those resources—first within the national health budget and then in relation to other claims on resources. The first case in the region was recorded in 1984 in Slovakia. The first case in Kyrgyzstan was not officially recorded until the year 2000. The gap between these years may indicate a real difference in the progress of the epidemic—or it may be only a reflection of differences between reporting systems.

We may assume the period of progression from HIV to AIDS to be approximately five years. On this assumption, AIDS cases are an indication of HIV infections which occurred five or more years ago. These reported first cases show that in Slovakia, the Czech Republic, Yugoslavia, Poland, Kosovo, Uzbekistan, Kazakhstan, Russia, Romania, Lithuania, Armenia, and Ukraine initial infections took place between the late 1970s and the very early 1980s.

Epidemics differ from each other in terms of their reported social location as between gay men, recipients of blood donations, and in injecting drug users (IDU). Whatever the differences, it is clear that some parts of the region are now in the second or even third decade of their epidemic. Politicians and policy-makers must take this fact into consideration. However, this also raises the danger of a possible misconception that could obstruct effective regional cooperation.

Countries such as Kyrgyzstan, which have only recently seen an AIDS case, may not share the urgency felt by countries such as Slovakia, the Czech Republic, and Poland. The latter group of countries appears to be managing the situation. In contrast, in Russia and Ukraine, there is substantial overlap between young IDU and heterosexual transmission, and thus a clear danger that a heterosexual epidemic has already begun to develop. Serious engagement by the national authorities in these two countries demands urgent and different priority setting from what is required in the countries bordering the European Union. This inter-country variation, though, should not obscure the fact that this is a regional problem.

Table 1 shows that six countries do not appear to have any official knowledge of the probable start date for their epidemic. This may result from inadequate data or from administrative beliefs that HIV prevalence is currently so low that it is inappropriate to make such estimates at all. For those countries reporting a start date, the epidemic is assumed to have commenced as long ago as 1983 in the Czech Republic, and as recently as 2001 in Kyrgyzstan and Tajikistan. These are only

TABLE 2. Countries by Reported/Assumed Female-to-Male Ratio of HIV Infections[a]

Country	Estimate of females HIV+ as percentage of total HIV+	Estimate of males HIV+ as percentage of total HIV+
Albania	30	70
Armenia	22	78
Azerbaijan	30	63
Belarus	28	72
Bosnia-Herzegovina	Unknown	Unknown
Czech Republic	22	78
Georgia	12	88
Kazakhstan	35	65
Kosovo	68	32
Kyrgyzstan	4	98
Latvia	25	75
Lithuania	19	81
Moldova	27	74
Poland	23	78
Romania	43.5	56.5
Russia	23	77
Slovakia	15	85
Tajikistan	31	69
Turkey	30	70
Turkmenistan	Unknown	Unknown
Ukraine	38	62
Uzbekistan	30	70
Yugoslavia	30	70

[a] Note that percentages in this table do not necessarily sum to 100. This is how the figures were reported. However, this absence of arithmetic accuracy is less important than the overall ratio between the two values.

estimates. They are, however, important, because they indicate something about the policy perspective in each country. "Latecomers" may think they have plenty of time to respond, while the countries reporting an earlier start date may believe that they have the epidemic under control. Both groups will be woefully wrong to believe that there is no urgency.

Where Are the Countries of the Region on the Epidemic Curve?

Table 2 shows the reported ratio of female-to-male infections, as far as these data were available. It is important that policy-makers and politicians understand the significance of this ratio and what it tells about the probable stage and thus future development of the epidemic. That is to say in most settings heterosexual epidemics are characterized by a larger male-to-female ratio in the early period, followed by progressive equalization as the epidemic progresses, and finally a larger female-to-male ratio. Thus, policy-makers need to understand that the gender ratio is a simple indicator of the stage of the epidemic they are confronting. This in turn is a guide to establishing a desirable balance between the urgent needs for prevention and impact mitigation responses, workplace programs, sectoral responses, generalized rather than focused prevention campaigns, and antiretroviral (ARV) programs.

What Expectations/Assumptions Do Authorities in the Region Have about the Social Location of the Epidemic?

Which population sub-groups are seen by the authorities (and therefore perhaps also

TABLE 3. Social Groups in Which Epidemic Is Thought to Be Growing Rapidly

Country	IDU	FSW	Prisoners	Youth	Migrants	STDs	MSM	Blood donors
Albania					*			
Armenia	*	*	*					
Azerbaijan	*							
Belarus	*			*				
Bosnia-Herzegovina	*	*						
Czech Republic								
Georgia	*							
Kazakhstan	*							
Kosovo					*			
Kyrgyzstan	*							
Latvia	*		*					
Lithuania	*							
Moldova	*							
Poland	*							
Romania	*							
Russia	*	*	*	*		*		
Slovakia							*	*
Turkey		*		*				
Tajikistan	*	*						
Turkmenistan	NA	NA	NA	NA	NA	NA	NA	NA
Ukraine	*							
Uzbekistan	*							
Yugoslavia	*							

by the national media and general public) as the foci for the epidemic? As long as an epidemic is perceived as restricted to a number of "high-risk" groups, two things are likely to happen:

(1) Those groups may be stigmatized.
(2) The general population (including politicians, policy-makers, and other opinion-formers) may be able to deny that the epidemic affects "ordinary" people like them.

In most countries, the surveillance system follows standard epidemiological practice and focuses on the core transmitters, often assumed to be IDU. The second most commonly recorded group is blood donors and/or blood recipients; and the third group is antenatal clinic attenders and pregnant women. We can examine these data from another perspective. They are a *representation* of the situation to policymakers, politicians, and the interested public via the official reporting system. For example, Albania's epidemic is reported through tests of antenatal clinic attenders, IDU, truck drivers, military recruits, and blood donors and recipients, as is that of Azerbaijan. In contrast, Uzbekistan officially "sees" only IDU. Each view of the epidemic "shows" some groups and "excludes" others.

What else do the authorities see? Key informants were asked: "In which population sub-group(s) do you think the epidemic in your country is developing at the fastest rate?" Their responses are shown in Table 3, and demonstrate very clearly the official view in most parts of the region that this is an IDU epidemic. While this may indeed be the case, it is also possible that emphasis on this group and on other "anti-social" groups (such as prisoners and sex workers) may have the unintended consequence of diverting attention away from a growing heterosexual epidemic.

From a policy and political perspective, "the epidemic" is a matter of perception. How it is perceived is an artifact of the reporting system. The reporting system is itself a reflection of resource availability, resource allocation, and political expectations within countries. If decision-makers and opinion leaders do not "see" the epidemic, either because they do not have good data or they do not understand the available data, they will be unable to look forward and to consider its potential significance for prevention and impact mitigation purposes. (It is possible that the number of groups for which data are collected increases as the epidemic becomes, or is perceived to become, worse. This hypothesis was tested statistically and there was no linear correlation between level of HIV infection reported officially and the number of groups.) Thus, the quality of national reporting systems is naturally of great importance. However, equally significant is whether people in positions of power are sufficiently "AIDS literate" to understand why and how resources must be allocated to ensure that good information becomes available and is used to guide policy—for both prevention and impact mitigation, as appropriate.

National Surveillance Capacity

At the time of the survey, two countries, Bosnia-Herzegovina and Lithuania, did not have national systems of sero-surveillance for HIV/AIDS (Table 4). The Russian Federation, by far the largest country in the region by both population and land area, had only one site. Some of the smaller countries, notably Armenia, Latvia, and Kyrgyzstan appeared to have excellent coverage with between 120,000 and 150,000 people per site. In general, the more sites, the more fine-grained the analysis; however, more is not always better. The design of surveillance systems is also a factor. A number of countries were very poorly equipped to understand their epidemics. Furthermore, some countries, such as Ukraine, which appeared to have a reasonable number of sites (although there are over eight million people per site), did not yet have systems which enabled adequate reporting and understanding. This was due to lack of test kits, laboratory infrastructure, and the administrative resources to make good use of the available data. Some limitations of the Ukrainian system—which may be representative of other countries in the region—are discussed in Barnett and Whiteside (1997) and in Balakireva *et al.* (2001).

This is an area of policy and administration where urgent investment now could help avoid longer-term adverse impacts and make a major contribution to short- and medium-term control and prevention measures.

Surveillance information is a key to understanding the epidemic's future development. Investment in existing surveillance systems and in their capacity to build on data is urgently required. Informants were asked whether any projections had been made as to where the epidemic might go over the next decade. Projections of the number of HIV infections per year over the next ten years (until 2011) had only been attempted in six countries (Belarus, Kyrgyzstan, Moldova, Russia, Tajikistan, and Ukraine), and then only in the last two years. This means that 75% of the countries of the region had made no attempt to predict what kind of epidemic they would face in the medium term. As a matter of some urgency, national authorities would be advised to undertake such relatively low-cost exercises on a regular basis as part of an active engagement with the problem.

RESPONDING TO THE EPIDEMIC: NATIONAL INFRASTRUCTURE AND POLICY DOMAINS

How are governments responding to the epidemic? Informants in all countries surveyed, except Albania and Bosnia-Herzegovina, reported the existence of a government document on HIV/AIDS. Turkey reported having first formulated this document as early as 1992, followed by Moldova, Romania, and Slovakia in 1993. The countries reporting having first formulated this

TABLE 4. National Surveillance Systems (NSS)

Country	Existence of NSS	Number of sites	Population per site
Albania	Yes	2	1,750,000
Armenia	Yes	27	122,222
Azerbaijan	Yes	16	487,500
Belarus	Yes	6	1,716,667
Bosnia-Herzegovina	No	0	NA
Czech Republic	Yes	15	686,667
Georgia	Yes	64	78,125
Kazakhstan	Yes	21	795,238
Kosovo	No	0	NA
Kyrgyzstan	Yes	40	120,000
Latvia	Yes	16	150,000
Lithuania	No	1	3,593,000
Moldova	Yes	7	628,571
Poland	Yes	25	1,544,000
Romania	Yes	Unknown	NA
Russia	Yes	1	145,000,000
Slovakia	Yes	44	122,727
Tajikistan	Yes	24	275,000
Turkey	Yes	Unknown	NA
Turkmenistan	Yes	6	766,667
Ukraine	Yes	8	8,133,333
Uzbekistan	Yes	20	1,255,000
Yugoslavia	Yes	20	535,000

document in 2001 included Armenia, Kosovo, Russia, and Ukraine. Of those countries having such a document, all except Kosovo, Russia, and Yugoslavia reported that it included a "Statement of National policies" on HIV/AIDS. All except Ukraine, Uzbekistan, and Yugoslavia reported that the national document included strategic approaches for the health sector to respond to HIV/AIDS, and all except Azerbaijan, Kyrgyzstan, Poland, Romania, Ukraine, and Yugoslavia reported that the government document set out indicators of achievement over defined periods of time.

The effects of civil disorder and rapid political transition account for the absence of any recorded government initiative in Albania and Bosnia-Herzegovina. All other countries had developed a national policy document; some were not produced until comparatively recently. It is significant that two of the most seriously affected countries, Russia and Ukraine, had not developed their national documents until very recently indeed.

Such national documents are important frameworks for discussion and, ultimately, action. Experience elsewhere has shown that the processes whereby they are developed can be important factors in motivating government departments, the private sector, and civil society organizations to face up to the difficulties and challenges posed by the epidemic.

It is widely accepted that HIV/AIDS cannot be seen solely as a medical problem. Its implications for successful socioeconomic transition and development demand a response from across government and society. Key informants' replies provided some evidence that in many cases a multi-sectoral response, accompanied by a specification of the goals to be achieved, was being formulated. The key question for the future will be: "How effectively is this process managed, and how realistic is the assessment of progress towards both general and sectoral goals?"

The answer to this question will depend on two elements: i) political will, and ii)

TABLE 5. Budget Allocations for HIV/AIDS: Central, Regional, and Civil Society

Country	A.	B.	C.
Albania	No info	No info	No info
Armenia	Yes	No	Yes
Azerbaijan	No	No	No
Belarus	No	No	No
Bosnia-Herzegovina	No info	No info	No info
Czech Republic	No	Yes	Yes
Georgia	No	No	Yes
Kazakhstan	Yes	No	Yes
Kosovo	Yes	No	No
Kyrgyzstan	No	No	No
Latvia	No	No	No
Lithuania	No	No	No
Moldova	Yes	Yes	Yes
Poland	Yes	No	No
Romania	Unknown	No	No
Russia	Yes	Yes	Yes
Slovakia	No	No	No
Tajikistan	No	No	Yes
Turkey	No	No	No
Turkmen	No	No	Yes
Ukraine	Yes	No	No
Uzbekistan	No	No	Yes
Yugoslavia	Unknown	Unknown	Unknown

A. Are there clearly delineated HIV/AIDS related budgets for central and regional expenditure?
B. Are there clearly delineated national/regional budgets for support to HIV/AIDS-related civil society organizations?
C. Is there an established monitoring and evaluation plan for judging the effects on central and regional governmental activities in relation to HIV/AIDS?

resource allocation. It is not possible to assess the former directly. But we can arrive at some conclusions as to the latter. Table 5 shows that, in most cases, there was no clear resource allocation, either for central and regional expenditure, or for support of civil-society organizations. This disturbing finding in part answers the question of political will. Absence of resource allocation suggests political will is absent. Absence of resource allocation also means that much ground must be made up if the governments of the region are to make any headway in meeting the challenges of HIV/AIDS.

The degree of funding shortfalls was disturbing. It makes the societies more vulnerable to the impact of the epidemic than they would otherwise be. A distinction is drawn between susceptibility and vulnerability (Barnett and Whiteside, 1999; Barnett *et al.*, 2000). "Vulnerability" describes the likelihood that a social or economic entity will be adversely affected by the impact of HIV/AIDS mortality and morbidity. In the absence of funding, most countries are vulnerable to the long-term socio-economic effects of HIV/AIDS. While many countries report cross-sectoral preparation at the level of program development in relation to the epidemic, and also that ministries other than health have developed programs (Table 6), the sad reality is that lack of finance in many cases means such preparations may come to nothing.

Funding

So, what funds had been allocated? Table 7 shows that with the exception of

TABLE 6. Have Ministries Other than the Ministries of Health Developed HIV/AIDS Programs?[a]

	Education	Justice	International affairs	Economy/ finance/trade	Welfare	Labor	Culture	Youth	Sports	Information	External affairs	Defense
Belarus			*	*			*		*	*		*
Czech Republic	*	*	*	*	*							*
Kazakhstan	*						*			*		*
Kosovo								*				
Kyrgyzstan	*		*									*
Latvia	*	*										
Lithuania	*	*	*			*						
Moldova	*	*	*	*		*		*	*		*	
Romania		*										
Russia	*	*										
Slovakia	*	*	*									
Tajikistan	*	*	*	*						*		
Turkey	*											*
Turkmen	*	*	*	*	*		*				*	*
Ukraine	*	*	*	*		*				*		*
Uzbekistan	*	*	*									

[a] The following countries reported not having HIV/AIDS programs in any Ministries other than Health: Albania, Armenia, Azerbaijan, Bosnia-Herzegovina, Georgia, Poland, Yugoslavia.

Poland, Kyrgyzstan, Russia, and Ukraine, the amounts were disturbingly small. On a per capita basis, only Poland was allocating appropriate sums from its national budget. The highest amount of overseas funding, to Moldova, was very small, around $500,000 in the preceding financial year—and this was a 60% increase from the preceding year's receipts from these sources.

Vulnerability and poverty march together. Most countries in this region are poor. A few are beginning to allocate increasing amounts of funding for HIV/AIDS from central government budgets, mostly to prevention and care. Very little is being spent to mitigate the potential socio-economic impact of the epidemic. Overall, we found that Armenia's total allocation to HIV/AIDS increased by 6% between fiscal year (FY) 2000 and FY 2001; Moldova's by 20%, Latvia's by 22%, Georgia's by 10%, Poland's by 20% (from a high base), Belarus's by 4.3%, Kyrgyzstan's by a massive 114%, Lithuania's by almost 100%, and Tajikistan's by almost 12%. When we examined year-on-year increases in external funding, we found that most countries received substantial additions to funding from external sources: Armenia by 60%, Moldova by 400%, Turkmenistan by 63%, Belarus 107%, Kazakhstan almost 100%, and Tajikistan 60%.

The message here is that in the absence of external funding—multilateral, bilateral, NGO, or foundation—most of these countries do not have the resources to rise to the considerable challenges they face. And, of course, external funding is not dependable and cannot contribute to sustainable programs unless it is part of long-term assistance.

Prevention

Expenditure on HIV/AIDS is low. It is mostly targeted to prevention and care. Here, we look at how these programs are structured. For the moment, most national epidemics appear to be located among IDU, and the clear danger is that this may become a generalized, heterosexually-transmitted epidemic. In Russia and Ukraine, it is likely that this has already happened. Table 8 shows how far each country has gone in pursuing the most important steps to prevent spread from core transmitter groups into the general population using established interventions.

Most countries have programs of outreach for female sex workers (FSW), but few have such programs for male sex workers (MSW). The record on needle exchange schemes is generally good, but we have no idea of coverage and success rates. Similarly, there is an uneven record on provision of facilities for cleaning injecting equipment in prisons and in places where this is lacking, it needs strengthening. Prisons act as amplifiers of the epidemic, as people are infected in prisons through injection drug use or sex, and then transmit the disease to their sexual partners after release.

The Administrative, Policy, and Research Base for Confronting the HIV/AIDS Challenge and Mitigating the Social and Economic Consequences

The barest minimum governmental response to the epidemic is without doubt the establishment of a National AIDS Advisory Committee (NAAC) or similar body. For those countries which had established such a committee, the mean time between recording the first case and formation of the committee was 6.2 years (the shortest time period was three years and the longest was 20 years). This does not suggest that, in general, the response has been very rapid. As of 2002, six of the countries of the region had not yet established such minimal infrastructure. Five countries had only established these bodies as recently as 2001. In other words, almost 50% of the region had not developed a minimal response before 2001, despite indications from the epidemiological data that the epidemic had been developing for many years.

Where National AIDS Advisory Committees have been established, one then needs

TABLE 7. Central Government and International Funding Received by Government National AIDS Programs (US$) in Most Recent Financial Year

Country	Total population[a] (1000's)	Financial year	Amount received from Government's central budget (US$)	Amount per capita	Amount received from international sources (US$)	Amount per capita	Total received	Total amount per capita
Albania	3,145	No info	30,000	0.01	100,000	0.03	130,000	0.04
Armenia	3,788	2001	44,499	0.01	295,108	0.08	339,607	0.09
Azerbaijan	8,096	No info	No info	—	No info	—	—	—
Belarus	10,147	2000	No info	NA	794,669	0.08	—	—
Czech Republic	10,260	2001	850,000	0.08	0	0	850,000	0.08
Georgia	5,239	2001	920,000	0.18	0	0	920,000	0.18
Kazakhstan	16,095	2001	316,000	0.02	169,612	0.01	485,612	0.03
Kyrgyzstan	4,986	2001	4,132,218	0.83	No info	—	—	—
Latvia	2,406	2001	511,221	0.21	No info	—	—	—
Lithuania	3,689	2001	704,400	0.19	680,200	0.18	1,384,600	0.38
Moldova	4,285	2001	85,270	0.02	527,000	0.12	612,270	0.14
Poland	38,577	2001	13,000,000	0.34	0	0	13,000,000	0.34
Romania	22,388	No info	No info	—	No info	—	—	—
Russia	144,644	2001	5,800,000	0.04	0	0	5,800,000	0.04
Slovakia	5,430	2000	No info	—	No info	—	—	—
Tajikistan	6,135	2001	25,392	0	9,372	0.02	119,764	0.02
Turkey	67,696	2001	No separate budget for GNAP	—	9,000	0.13	9,000	—
Turkmenistan	4,835	2001	20,000	0	309,500	0.06	329,500	0.07
Ukraine	49,122	2001	1,986,283	0.04	No info	—	—	—
Uzbekistan	25,257	No info	No info	—	No info	—	—	—
Yugoslavia	10,538	2000	No info	—	No info	—	—	—

[a] Source: (UNPOP, 2001)

TABLE 8. Progress on Major Prevention Initiatives

Countries	Outreach to FSW[a]	Outreach to MSW[b]	Needle exchange program for IDU[c]	Needle exchange program operated by national government	Needle exchange program operated by local government	Needle exchange program operated by NGOs[d]	Provision in prison for cleaning of injecting equipment	National blood Transfusion service Tests all donations for HIV+?	Batch or individual testing?	Blood donation paid for or not?
Albania	Yes	No	Yes	No	No	Yes	No	Yes	Indiv	Yes
Armenia	No	No	No	—	—	—	Yes	No	—	Yes
Azerbaijan	No	No	Yes	No	No	Yes	No	No	Both	Both
Belarus	Yes	No	Yes	No	Yes	Yes	Yes	Yes	Indiv	Yes
Bosnia-Herzegovina	No	No	No	—	—	—	No	No	—	No
Czech Republic	Yes	Yes	Yes	Yes	Yes	Yes	No	Yes	Indiv	No
Georgia	Yes	Yes	Yes	No	No	Yes	Yes	No	Indiv	Yes
Kazakhstan	Yes	Yes	Yes	No	Yes	No	No	Yes	Indiv	Yes
Kosovo	No	No	No	—	—	—	No	Yes	Indiv	No
Kyrgyzstan	Yes	No	Yes	Yes	Yes	Yes	Yes	No	Indiv	Yes
Latvia	Yes	No	Yes	Yes	Yes	No	Yes	Yes	Indiv	No
Lithuania	Yes	Yes	Yes	Yes	Yes	Yes	Yes	Yes	Indiv	Yes
Moldova	No	No	Yes	Yes	Yes	Yes	Yes	Yes	Indiv	Yes
Poland	Yes	Yes	Yes	No	No	Yes	No	Yes	Indiv	No
Romania	Yes	Yes	No	—	—	—	No data	Yes	Indiv	Yes
Russia	Yes	No	Yes	No	Yes	Yes	No	Yes	Indiv	Yes
Slovakia	Yes	No	Yes	Yes	No	Yes	No	Yes	Indiv	No
Tajikistan	Yes	No	Yes	No	Yes	Yes	Yes	Yes	Indiv	No
Turkey	Yes	No	No	—	—	—	No	Yes	Batch	No
Turkmen	Yes	No	No	—	—	—	Yes	Yes	Batch	Yes
Ukraine	Yes	No	Yes	No	Yes	Yes	No	Yes	Indiv	Yes
Uzbekistan	Yes	No	Yes	Yes	Yes	Yes	No	Yes	Indiv	Yes
Yugoslavia	No	No	Yes	No	No	Yes	Yes	Yes	Indiv	No

[a] Female Sex Workers
[b] Male Sex Workers
[c] Injecting Drug Users
[d] Non-governmental Organizations

TABLE 9. National AIDS Advisory Committee (NAAC) Formation and Representation

	Is there an NAAC or similar body?	If so, what year was it established?	How many members are on the NAAC?	How many NAAC members are medically qualified?	What is the male-to-female ratio among NAAC members?	Does the NAAC include members representing PLWHA[a]?	Does the NAAC include members from faith communities?	How many members of the NAAC represent national NGOs?
Albania	No[b]	—	—	—	—	—	—	—
Armenia	No	—	—	—	—	—	—	—
Azerbaijan	No	—	—	—	—	—	—	—
Belarus	Yes	1996	17	5	14:3	No	No	0
Bosnia-Herzegovina	Yes	2002	[d]	[d]	[d]	[d]	[d]	[d]
Czech Republic	Yes	1993	22	14	15:7	Yes	Yes	5
Georgia	Yes	1996	18	4	16:2	No	No	0
Kazakhstan	Yes	1995	14	3	11:3	No	No	0
Kosovo	Yes	2001	14	12	7:7	No	No	0
Kyrgyzstan	Yes	1997	39	7	28:11	No	Yes	3
Latvia	Yes	1998	12	7	3:9	No	No	1
Lithuania	Yes	2001	10	9	8:2	No	No	0
Moldova	Yes	2001	15	5	10:5	Yes	Yes	1
Poland	Yes	1998	15	10	8:7	No	No	0
Romania	Yes	2001	29	19	15:14	Yes	No	3
Russia	No[c]	—	—	—	—	—	—	—

[a] People living with HIV/AIDS.
[b] It was reported that "some effort is going on to form such a body". However, in the year 2000, a National Interministerial committee has been established. It consists of deputy ministers from each Ministry.
[c] The UNAIDS and the Russian Ministry of Health are trying to establish such a body. "A federal commission responsible for HIV/AIDS does exist within the Ministry of Health, but it does not include participation from other stakeholders or other ministers."
[d] Not yet defined.

to ask how they are constituted, and how far they have representation from across the spectrum of stakeholders. HIV/AIDS is a disease, but confronting it, and its effects, requires engagement across the social and economic spectrum. Initial responses have usually put the burden of management of the problem onto the shoulders of the medical profession. This demands skills and knowledge they may not have, and has taken them away from their areas of expertise. Experience shows that cross-sectoral engagement must be established at the highest levels of national response. Table 9 outlines the formation and representation of NAACs in the region. The majority have a preponderance of representation from the non-medically qualified, and five have mainly medically qualified people, with Lithuania scoring highest at 10% of the total membership of its NAAC.

LOOKING TO THE FUTURE

Experience in Africa, Thailand, and Brazil shows that an HIV/AIDS epidemic is followed by medium- and long-term costs. Some of these are financial, but others are social, cultural, and what may be described as hedonic losses. Knowledge of the possibility of having to confront such burdens is uniformly poor in this region. Only in three countries, the Czech Republic, Uzbekistan, and Tajikistan, were National AIDS plans reported to contain sections dealing with the social and economic effects of the epidemic. Only in Belarus, Ukraine, Kyrgyzstan, Moldova, and Poland had any studies been made to try and explore this problem. No commercial organization anywhere in the region has considered the potential effects of HVI/AIDS on its operation. Only in Ukraine and very recently in Russia did the World Bank Country Report have a section dealing specifically with the significance and potential effects of HIV/AIDS for socio-economic development.

CONCLUSION

The region is ill-prepared to confront HIV/AIDS, despite its high human resource endowment. The challenges of "transition" and HIV/AIDS together present an enormous burden. Surveillance systems must be strengthened and prevention programs expanded; in some countries they must be adapted to take account of a looming heterosexual epidemic. Political and administrative HIV/AIDS literacy levels must be raised. In short, in many countries, the authorities must act urgently if the epidemic is not to move inexorably ahead and cause damage to society and economy—damage from which it will take many decades and many dollars to recover. As part of this engagement, the regional nature of the epidemic must be recognized.

REFERENCES

Balakireva, O., Galustian, Y., Yaremenko, O., Levchuk, N., Andruschak, L. (2001). HIV/AIDS Social and Economic Impacts in Ukraine, Kyiv, British Council and Ukrainian Institute for Social Research.

Barnett, T. and Blaikie, P.M. (1992). *AIDS in Africa: Its Present and FutureImpact*, Belhaven Press and Guilford Press, London and New York.

Barnett, T. and Whiteside, A. (1999). HIV/AIDS and Development: Case Studies and a Conceptual Framework, *European J Devel Res*. Vol. 11, No. 2, December 1999, pp. 220–234.

Barnett, T., Whiteside, A., and Decosas, J. (2000). The Jaipur Paradigm: A conceptual framework for understanding social susceptibility and vulnerability to HIV. *J South African Med Assoc*, November Vol. 90, No. 11, pp. 1098–1101.

Barnett, T. and Whiteside, A. (2002). AIDS in the 21st Century: Disease and Globalisation, London and New York, Palgrave Macmillan.

II

Molecular Epidemiology, Genetic Diversity, and Overlaps with Endemic Disease

16

Molecular Epidemiology of HIV in Asia and the Pacific

Sodsai Tovanabutra, Deborah L. Birx, and Francine E. McCutchan

US Military HIV Research Program, Rockville, Maryland, USA

INTRODUCTION

HIV-1 strains in the pandemic are genetically diverse. Nine subtypes (A, B, C, D, F, G, H, J, and K) and 15 circulating recombinant forms (CRFs) have been identified to date (Kuiken *et al.*, 2002). Figure 1 shows a phylogenetic tree of representative full-genome sequences of all of these forms, illustrating the genetic complexity of this important pathogen.

Another level of complexity is revealed by molecular epidemiological studies of the geographic distribution of the subtypes and CRF (McCutchan, 2000a; McCutchan, 2000b; McCutchan *et al.*, 2000; Peeters and Sharp, 2000). Each molecular form has a unique and distinctive distribution, prevalence, and pattern of intermixing with other forms. In addition, the majority of recombinant forms that have been identified are currently without evidence of epidemic spread; the presence of these unique recombinant forms (URFs) establishes the potential for even greater diversity in the pandemic, were circumstances to foster their expansion in new populations or geographic regions (Robertson *et al.*, 2000; McCutchan *et al.*, 2000).

Intermixing of HIV-1 strains in populations seems to have predictable consequences: the emergence of recombinant forms (Robertson *et al.*, 1995; Robertson *et al.*, 2000; McCutchan, 2000b). Many of the identified CRFs appear to have arisen soon after multiple subtypes began to circulate in the same social network; the best studied are intravenous drug user (IDU) networks, which often include producers, distributors, and users of injection drugs (Bobkov *et al.*, 1998; Yu *et al.*, 1999; Piyasirisilp *et al.*, 2000; Thomson *et al.*, 2001; Naganawa *et al.*, 2002; Tovanabutra *et al.*, 2003; Esteves *et al.*, 2003). CRF01_AE, predominant in Southeast Asia, was initially separated from subtype B in Thailand by risk group. However, soon after CRF01_AE and subtype B began to co-circulate in IDU, new recombinant forms began to arise (Tovanabutra *et al.*, 2001; Tovanabutra *et al.*, 2004), including a new CRF, called CRF15_01B (Tovanabutra *et al.*, 2003). In South Asia, the epidemic is principally subtype C, alongside subtype B in some regions. In southern China, two new BC recombinant forms, CRF07_BC and CRF08_BC (Yu *et al.*, 1999; Piyasirisilp *et al.*, 2000; McCutchan *et al.*, 2002), are now

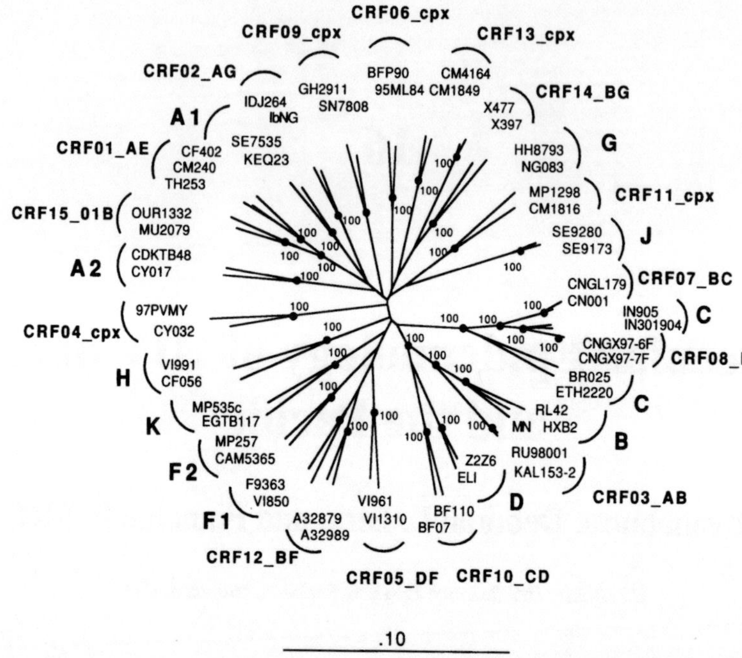

FIGURE 1. Phylogenetic Tree Showing the Global Genetic Diversity of HIV-1. The neighbor-joining tree was constructed based on near full-genome nucleotide reference sequences (HIV Sequence Compendium 2002) of the 9 subtypes (A, B, C, D, F, G, H, J, and K), 4 sub-subtypes (A1, A2, F1 and F2) and the 15 circulating recombinant forms (CRFs). Bootstrap values (over 100 replicates) are shown on clade-defining nodes. The scale bar at the bottom represents 10% genetic difference.

circulating, each predominating along a different heroin trafficking route. Subtype A, whose main focus is in east Africa, has now expanded in Eastern Europe and Central Asia (Novitsky *et al.*, 1998; Nabatov *et al.*, 2002; McCutchan *et al.*, 2003; Masharsky *et al.*, 2003). Its intersection with subtype B from Western Europe generated CRF03_AB (Liitsola *et al.*, 1998; Liitsola *et al.*, 2000).

Heterosexual networks also generate recombinant HIV, which can constitute a very substantial fraction of strains when multiple subtypes co-circulate (McCutchan *et al.*, 2000; Hoelscher *et al.*, 2001; Dowling *et al.*, 2002; Harris *et al.*, 2002; Arroyo *et al.*, 2004). Two of the six globally prevalent strains, CRF01_AE in Southeast Asia and CRF02_AG in West and Central Africa, may provide examples of extremely widespread and highly prevalent CRFs that first arose in heterosexual networks in Africa. At least half of the CRFs and most of the URFs identified to date have been found in epidemics where heterosexual transmission is the primary mode of HIV-1 spread (Kuiken *et al.*, 2002).

The complexity of the HIV-1 pandemic has been progressively unveiled through countless studies of the molecular epidemiology of HIV-1, each focussed on a particular region, population, or group. The challenge of identifying subtypes among the many recombinant forms has been met with varying success, and each entry into the database of HIV-1 sequences must be viewed through the lens of the state of knowledge at the time it was collected. Early in the epidemic, partial sequencing of HIV-1 strains, or assays that evaluated a small portion of the genome (Louwagie *et al.*, 1993; Delwart *et al.*, 1993; Gao *et al.*, 1994; Louwagie *et al.*, 1995; Gaywee *et al.*, 1996), were employed. With increasing knowledge of the diversity of subtypes and the impact of recombination, full-genome sequencing came

TABLE 1. HIV-1 Prevalence, Sequence Database, and Predominant Subtypes in Asia and the Pacific

Country/Region	HIV/AIDS cases[a]	Adult Rate (%)[a]	HIV sequences[b]	Full genome sequences	Predominant strain(s)
India	3,970,000	0.8	449	13	C
China	850,000	0.1	299	16	B, CRF01, CRF07, CRF08
Thailand	670,000	1.8	2,501	16	CRF01, B
Myanmar	400,000	n.a.	114	9	B, C, CRF01
Cambodia	170,000	2.7	32	0	CRF01
Vietnam	130,000	0.3	795	0	CRF01, B
Indonesia	120,000	0.1	37	0	CRF01, B
Philippines	94,000	<0.1	57	0	B
Pakistan	78,000	0.1	0	0	n.a.
Nepal	58,000	0.5	36	0	C
Malaysia	42,000	0.4	28	0	CRF01, B
Papua New Guinea	17,000	0.7	0	0	n.a.
Bangladesh	13,000	<0.1	35	0	C
Australia	12,000	0.1	1,616	16	B
Japan	12,000	<0.1	1,594	4	B, CRF01
Kazakhstan	6,000	0.1	0	0	n.a
Sri Lanka	4,800	<0.1	0	0	n.a.
South Korea	4,000	<0.1	919	2	B
Singapore	3,400	0.2	158	0	B, CRF01
Hong Kong	2,600	0.1	0	0	n.a.
Laos	1,400	<0.1	0	0	n.a.
New Zealand	1,200	0.1	10	0	B
Uzbekistan	740	<0.1	32	0	A
Kyrgyzstan	500	<0.1	0	0	n.a.
Tajikistan	200	<0.1	0	0	n.a.
Turkmenistan	<100	<0.1	0	0	n.a.
Taiwan	n.a.	n.a.	231	1	B, CRF01

[a] According to UNAIDS estimates at the end of 2001. Data are not available for North Korea and Hong Kong. n.a., not available.
[b] HIV sequences available in the Los Alamos database as of November, 2003 (http://hiv-web.lanl.gov).

to the forefront (Salminen *et al.*, 1995; Carr *et al.*, 1999; McCutchan *et al.*, 2000). In this review, we compile and summarize data from all stages of the HIV-1 pandemic in Asia and the Pacific, with a focus on the more recent data that may provide a more accurate picture of the composition of strains in each country and region. Where data is limited, evidence from partial sequencing or other genotyping techniques may be the only available, and is included to provide a preview where full knowledge is later to come. Finally, it must be acknowledged that the literature on HIV-1 diversity is vast, and we include here most, but not necessarily all, of the published information. The rapid evolution of knowledge in this field ensures that future reviews will complete and refine the detailed molecular picture presented here.

Statistics on the HIV-1 epidemic in Asia and the Pacific reveal extreme heterogeneity in HIV-1 prevalence. Table 1 lists HIV/AIDS cases, at the end of 2001, according to UNAIDS (UNAIDS/WHO, 2003). The countries of India, China, Thailand, Myanmar are hardest hit, followed by Cambodia, Vietnam, and Indonesia. The low number of cases reported for Central Asia may reflect less well-studied epidemics.

These data must also be considered in terms of the percent of the adult population that is HIV-1 positive (Table 1). Here Cambodia and Thailand bear the brunt of the epidemic, followed by India. Some countries with a smaller population show a relatively high rate of HIV-1 infection in adults; Malaysia, Vietnam, and Papua New Guinea are examples. By any measure, the HIV-1 epidemic is most severe in a handful of countries, with a rather low burden of cases in much of the region.

Of interest for our goal of describing the molecular forms of HIV-1 in this vast region, the database of sequences is disproportionately distributed with respect to the most severely affected countries. (Table 1). The most comprehensive database of HIV-1 sequences comes from Thailand, with 2500 entries in the Los Alamos database (http://hiv-web.lanl.gov). The relatively limited epidemics in Australia and Japan are represented by about 1600 sequences each. Severely affected India, China, Vietnam each post between 300 and 800 sequence entries. Molecular data from most other countries is extremely limited or altogether missing.

Moreover, we must consider the extent of full-genome sequence data, in light of the pervasive spread of recombinant strains in some parts of this region. Partial sequencing and other approaches have limited power to resolve pure subtypes from recombinant strains, especially URFs of unpredictable structure. At last count in December 2003, 77 full-length genomes were available, mostly from Thailand, China, India, and Australia.

An overview of the predominant HIV-1 strains by country is also provided in Table 1. CRF01_AE and subtypes B and C are the common theme, alongside CRFs derived from them. However, it can be noted that subtypes A, D, F, G, other CRFs, URFs, and HIV-2 have been detected occasionally.

From a historical perspective, the introduction of HIV-1 into Asia and the Pacific has been uneven and influenced by many different factors. The first indications of the presence of HIV-1 were in the early 1980s, mostly sporadic reports in men who have sex with men (MSM) and female sex workers (FSW). In the mid 1980s, HIV-1 began to be identified in FSW in the metropolitan areas, and IDU in Manipur State of India (Jain *et al.*, 1994). By the late 1980s, an epidemic of subtype B had exploded among IDU in Thailand and in Yunan Province, China (Shao, 1991; Ou *et al.*, 1993). Almost simultaneously, subtype E (now called CRF01_AE in acknowledgement of its recombinant structure) spread rapidly in Thailand through heterosexual transmission (Weniger *et al.*, 1994). Within epidemic centers, HIV-1 spread among high risk populations, and subsequently into the general population in the familiar pattern of FSW, clients, wives, and children. HIV-1 spread from the initial epicenters, probably in China, Thailand, and India, across borders to neighboring countries of Myanmar, Malaysia, Cambodia, Laos, and Vietnam. Travel, trafficking of women and drugs played a role in this spread. Opium cultivation in the Golden Triangle, positioned between Thailand, Myanmar, and Laos, fueled the development of recombinant HIV-1 in a mixed-subtype environment. The epidemic in India represents a major focus of subtype C, the most globally prevalent strain according to UNAIDS estimates (UNAIDS/WHO, 2003). The upsurge of IDU that followed the breakup of the Soviet Union has generated the most rapidly expanding HIV-1 epidemic in the globe, principally involving subtype A.

In contrast to these patterns of epidemic spread among neighboring countries, sometimes with identifiable avenues and linked by the circulating HIV-1 strains, much of Asia and the Pacific seems isolated from the epicenters. Strains in Australia, New Zealand, Japan, Taiwan, Korea, the Philippines, Singapore, and Indonesia are mostly subtype B, like those in North America and Western Europe.

Figure 2 shows phylogenetic relationships among HIV-1 strains from Asia and the Pacific represented by full-genome sequences. Strains from Australia, Korea, and Taiwan form a significant cluster within subtype B, suggesting linkage between these epidemics. Likewise, the CRF01_AE strains from Thailand, China, Japan, and Myanmar are significantly linked. Subtype C from India

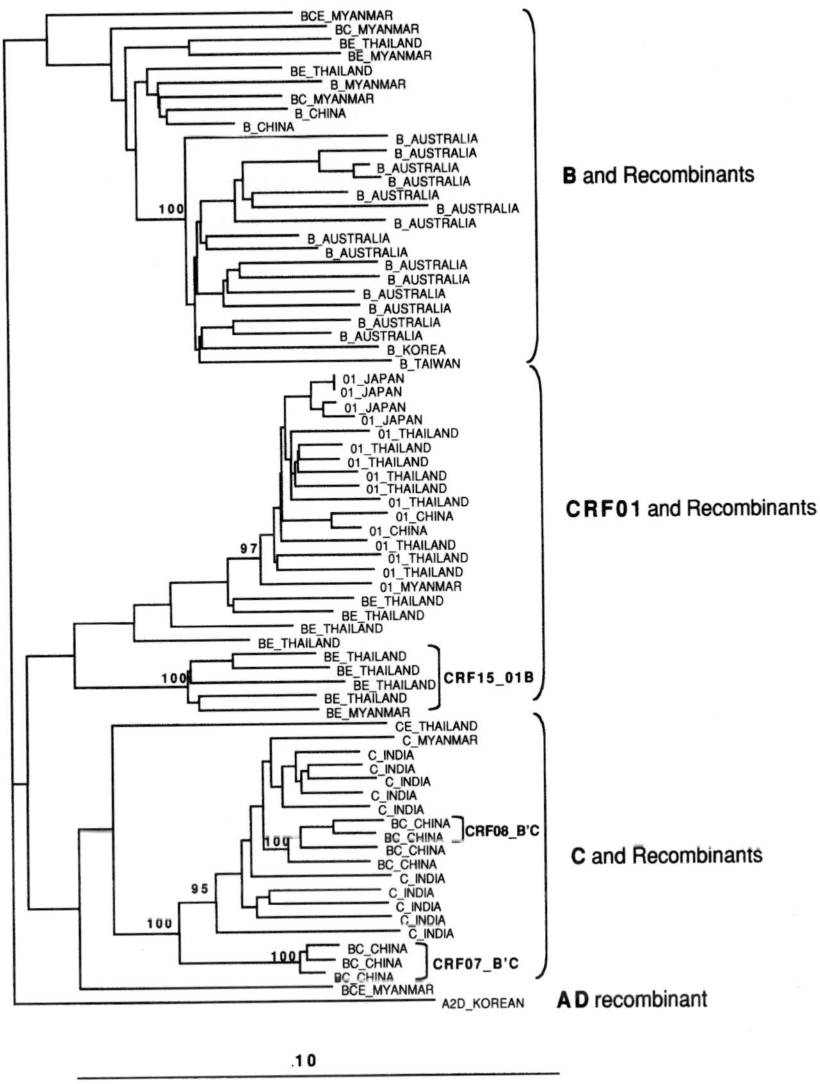

FIGURE 2. HIV-1 Genetic Diversity in Asia and the Pacific. The neighbor-joining phylogenetic tree shows the subtype distribution of all the published nearly full-genome nucleotide sequences from the region (http://hiv-web.lanl.gov). Strains are distributed into three main genetic clusters: subtype B, C and CRF01_AE. For each strain only the genotype (B: subtype B; C: subtype C; 01: CRF01_AE; BE: B/CRF01_AE recombinant; BC: B/C recombinant; BCE: B/C/CRF01_AE recombinant), and country of isolation are shown. Bootstrap values (over 100 replicates) are shown on clade-defining nodes. The tree was rooted on the Korean A2/D recombinant strain (97KR004). The scale bar at the bottom represents 10% genetic difference.

are parental strains for the two BC recombinants circulating in China, and this fact brings them into significant association in the tree. The subtype B stains from China have contributed to BC, BE, and BCE recombinants found in China, Myanmar, and Thailand. The CRF15_01B first identified in Thailand clusters with other BE recombinant strains of different structure from Thailand and Myanmar. The key subtypes have spread across borders, often recombined, and spawned new CRFs and URFs in their wake. The utility, indeed the near necessity, of full-genome sequencing is well illustrated in Figure 2, where the full web of interrelationships is starkly revealed.

In the following sections, a detailed, country-by-country review is presented for the most important centers of the HIV-1 epidemic in Asia and the Pacific, according to the molecular data available. The review is organized by region: Southeast Asia and China, South Asia, Central Asia, and Australia and the Pacific.

SOUTHEAST ASIA AND CHINA

Thailand

The HIV-1 epidemic in Thailand is the best studied in the region, due in part to early and continuous participation in the planning and execution of HIV vaccine trials in this country. The major routes of transmission are heterosexual and IDU, which both played a role in the introduction of HIV-1 into Thailand in the late 1980s. Analysis of *gag* and *env* genes of the earliest HIV-1 strains from Thailand identified subtype B in IDU and CRF01_AE, identified in Thailand before it was also detected in central Africa, in HIV acquired through sexual exposure (McCutchan *et al.*, 1992). This separation of strains by risk group (Weniger *et al.*, 1991; Ou *et al.*, 1992; McCutchan *et al.*, 1992; Ou *et al.*, 1993; Weniger *et al.*, 1994) persisted for almost a decade.

Once introduced into Thailand, the expansion of HIV-1 was rapid (Weniger *et al.*, 1994). In 1990, a survey in young military conscripts with heterosexual exposures in the north revealed a 12% HIV-1 prevalence (Nelson *et al.*, 1993; Sirisopana *et al.*, 1996), uniformly CRF01_AE according to a study of the envelope gene in incident infections (Nopkesorn *et al.*, 1998). Several studies confirmed that CRF01_AE and subtype B, with low inter-patient diversity of strains within each subtype, were circulating widely in Thailand by the early 1990s (Ou *et al.*, 1992; McCutchan *et al.*, 1992; Ou *et al.*, 1993; Bachmann *et al.*, 1994; Ichimura *et al.*, 1994; Auwanit *et al.*, 2000).

One interesting facet of the early epidemic in Thailand emerged through study of the subtype B strains. Alongside subtype B like those in North America and Europe, with their typical GPGR motif at the crown of the V3 loop, some subtype B in Thailand were divergent and had a GPGQ in V3 (Ou *et al.*, 1992; Ou *et al.*, 1993); these were termed B-prime (B') (Kalish *et al.*, 1994). It was later confirmed that envelopes from B and B' strains formed separate clusters within subtype B (Kalish *et al.*, 1994), and a full-length genome of a B' strain was found in southern China (Graf *et al.*, 1998). The interconnection of early epidemics around the Golden Triangle is reinforced by the distribution of subtype B'.

The initial classification of the heterosexually acquired HIV-1 from Thailand as subtype E, based on analysis of envelope, was re-visited when the *gag* gene of these strains was found to cluster with subtype A (Louwagie *et al.*, 1993). The first full genome sequences from Thailand and from central Africa (Gao *et al.*, 1996; Carr *et al.*, 1996), where this strain apparently arose, revealed the AE recombinant form CRF01_AE, the first in a series of circulating recombinant forms to be identified (Robertson *et al.*, 2000).

The simultaneous entry of two subtypes into Thailand set the stage for many subsequent studies comparing their distribution in different regions of the country and risk groups. The predominance of CRF01_AE in heterosexually acquired infections was documented in military cohorts (Mason *et al.*, 1998), fishermen (Entz *et al.*, 2000), female (Limpakarnjanarat *et al.*, 1999) and male sex workers (Beyrer *et al.*, 1997), and other studies of individuals at heterosexual risk (Subbarao *et al.*, 1998; Tovanabutra *et al.*, 2002). The principal strain in IDU was subtype B (Kunanusont *et al.*, 1995; Kitayaporn *et al.*, 1998; Subbarao *et al.*, 1998; Vongsheree *et al.*, 2002). Another theme repeatedly confirmed was the initially low, but slowly expanding, genetic diversity within the CRF01_AE and the subtype B components of the epidemic (Vongsheree *et al.*, 2002). Depending on the region of envelope sequenced, the mean inter-patient nucleotide sequence diversity reported within CRF01_AE and subtype B ranged from 2.3% to 3.8% in early studies (Ou *et al.*, 1992; McCutchan *et al.*, 1992), and had reached 5.7% in CRF01_AE by 1995 (Ichimura *et al.*, 1994; Subbarao *et al.*, 1998). At the amino acid level in the V3 region of CRF01_AE, the mean diversity among seroconverters was 7.8% in strains collected in 1993–1995 (Wang *et al.*, 1998) and had increased to 9.5% by 1997, compared to 4.4% among reference sequences from 1991–1992 (Auwanit *et al.*, 2000).

After the first few years, the epidemic in Thailand took a new turn. Subtype B, initially the majority strain among IDU, was joined by CRF01_AE in this risk group, CRF01_AE accounted for an increasing fraction of new infections, from 2.6% in 1988–1989 to 25.6% in 1990–1991 and 43.8% in 1992–1993 (Wasi *et al.*, 1995). In the period 1995–1998, almost 80% of new infections in IDU were CRF01_AE (Kalish *et al.*, 1995), and in the north, 90% of prevalent infections in IDU were also CRF01_AE (Tovanabutra *et al.*, 2000).

This shift in proportions and intermixing of strains produced the expected result-the appearance of recombinants between CRF01_AE and subtype B. The emergence of these strains was heralded by the detection of two individuals co-infected with CRF01_AE and subtype B in 1995 (Artenstein *et al.*, 1995b), and by a documented superinfection (serial acquisition of CRF01_AE, then B) in 2002 (Ramos *et al.*, 2002). Molecular epidemiology studies began to turn up CRF01_AE/B recombinants by 1997, not only in individuals with IDU exposures (Tovanabutra *et al.*, 2001) but, significantly, also in those with only heterosexual exposure (Viputtikul *et al.*, 2002). Recently, several subtype-discordant cases detected by screening assays turned out to be the same CRF01_AE/B recombinant form, now called CRF15_01B (Tovanabutra *et al.*, 2003). Many unique recombinants have also been identified, coming from a variety of studies in different regions of the country and risk groups. Some very recent data indicates that, currently, about one in seven new infections in Thailand may be a CRF01_AE/B recombinant strain (Tovanabutra *et al.*, 2004). Finally, one of the first HIV-1 strains collected in northern Thailand, initially characterized as CRF01_AE by partial envelope sequencing, has been shown to be one of the unique CRF01_AE/B recombinants, establishing their presence almost from the inception of the Thailand epidemic (Swanson *et al.*, 2003).

Preparation for vaccine trials in Thailand has spurred surveillance for HIV-1 subtypes in large cohorts, which provides the first substantial database of full-genome HIV-1 sequences. Among 39 incident infections from 1999–2002 among IDU in the north, 33 were CRF01_AE and 5 were CRF01_AE/B recombinants (Tovanabutra *et al.*, 2004). In Rayong and Chonburi provinces in 1999, a study of 20 incident and 7 prevalent infections showed 21 CRF01_AE, 2 subtype B, three CRF01_AE/B and one CRF01_AE/C recombinant (Watanaveeradej *et al.*, 2003; Watanaveeradej *et al.*, unpublished). The molecular picture in Thailand is changing. While CRF01_AE still predominates, it has recombined substantially with subtype B, and to some extent, subtype C, while the subtype B component of the epidemic may be decreasing.

Figure 3 shows the molecular complexity of HIV-1 strains from Thailand, based on full-genome sequences. From this phylogenetic tree it is clear that it is no longer adequate to characterize Thailand's epidemic as CRF01_AE and B. Current studies have revealed relatively few strains that are subtype B and an increasing proportion of recombinant strains; CRF01_AE/B, CRF01_AE/C, and even triple recombinants have been detected. Of interest, the CRF01_AE/B strains have most of their genome from CRF01_AE,

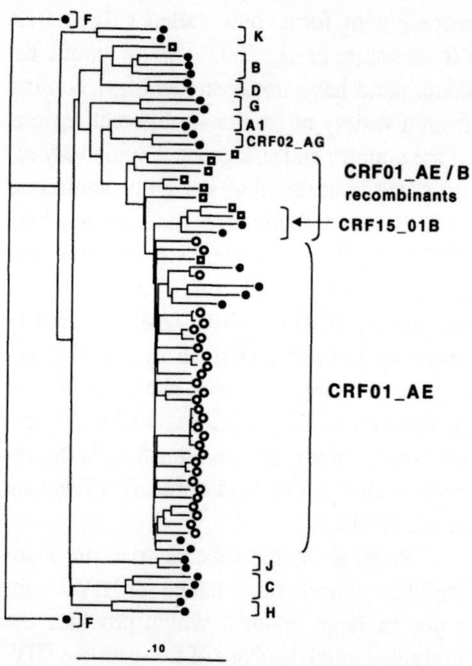

FIGURE 3. The Evolving HIV-1 Epidemic in Thailand. The neighbor-joining phylogenetic tree shows the HIV-1 subtype distribution of a set of recently sampled nearly full-genome nucleotide sequences from intravenous drug-users (IDU) from Northern Thailand. In contrast to the predominance of subtype B in IDU in the late 1980s, all of the strains are CRF01_AE (open circles) or B/CRF01_AE recombinants (squares). Among the latter, CRF15_01B (depicted by an arrow) spread into the heterosexual population. Reference strains from other subtypes are shown as black circles. Hypermutated sequences, which have artificially long branches and are not representative of within-clade diversity, are depicted by filled circles. The tree was rooted on reference subtype F strains. The scale bar at the bottom represents 10% genetic difference.

a fact reflected in their position in the tree. Only one CRF01_AE/B recombinant that is mostly subtype B has been identified to date.

This vivid picture of the dynamics of the HIV-1 epidemic in Thailand encapsulates several themes that will be reiterated again in this review. The fate of newly introduced strains can be quite disparate. Initially, the strains can maintain low diversity, but this can gradually increase over time. They can remain separated in different risk groups for a time, minimizing the opportunity for co-infection and recombination, but when intermixing occurs, recombinant strains soon arise. Many recombinants are generated, but relatively few attain epidemic spread to become CRFs. More than one variant within a subtype can be introduced (B and B', for example), but one may persist while the other wanes. New subtypes can enter, not only in their pure form, but also as recombinants with the strains already present. Finally, the proportions of strains can shift over time, often substantially. Molecular epidemiology must be ongoing, both to track changing dynamics of local epidemics and to develop a broader picture of regional epidemics and their interactions across borders.

China

Table 1 illustrates the pivotal role of the HIV-1 epidemic in China. In Asia, only India surpasses China in terms of the number of HIV/AIDS cases, but this large number of cases still represents only 0.1% of China's adult population. The number of cases could be enormous if HIV-1 were to spread freely in China. Routes of transmission are a key element to consider: it appears that China's epidemic is mostly blood-borne, with the majority of infections in IDU, followed by recipients of blood transfusions, with a minority of infections in those infected heterosexually. The social networks in which HIV-1 is spreading may initially limit the epidemic but, as seen in Thailand, whatever barriers exist between social networks can break down over time.

The first sporadic HIV cases were reported in China between 1985 and 1988. An epidemic among IDU in the southwestern province of Yunnan was documented in 1989, and in several other provinces by 1994 (Sun *et al.*, 1994). The first subtypes identified were B and B', followed by C and CRF01_AE. The B' strain recombined with subtype C to generate CRF07_BC and CRF08_BC which, alongside the initial subtypes, have become prevalent in China. Occasionally, subtypes A, D, F and G have been detected (Shao *et al.*, 1998).

The distribution of these HIV-1 strains within provinces has been studied, indicating that subtype B (mostly B') is widely distributed throughout the country, but each province presents a distinctive picture of HIV-1 strains (Shao *et al.*, 1998).

Yunnan province in the southwest harbors the full diversity of the China epidemic, but strains were apparently introduced at different times and by different routes of transmission. Drug trafficking and IDU were associated with the introduction of subtype B' in the late 1980s, subtype C in the early 1990s, and with their subsequent spread to other regions (Weniger *et al.*, 1994; Luo *et al.*, 1995; Yu *et al.*, 1998; Graf *et al.*, 1998; Shao *et al.*, 1998; Beyrer *et al.*, 2000). Both subtypes exhibited low inter-patient diversity, only 3.6% for B' and 2.6% for C by 1993 (Luo *et al.*, 1995). CRF01_AE was found among women who had been FSW in Thailand, and may have been introduced through heterosexual transmission (Cheng *et al.*, 1994). Not surprisingly, BC recombinant stains of low diversity arose in Yunnan and spread within the province. Partial sequencing of HIV from IDU showed only CRF08_BC in the eastern and southeastern prefectures of Wenshan and Honghe, respectively, while Dehong in the west, almost one third of the strains were subtype B' and the remainder were unique BC recombinants, without evidence of CRF08_BC. The dynamics of introduction, intersection and spread can quickly lead to a complex epidemiology, even in a highly circumscribed region (Yang *et al.*, 2002).

In Sichuan, another southwestern province bordering Yunnan, subtype B' and C strains of low diversity have been identified by partial envelope sequencing (Quinn, 1998). It is not clear whether these are recombinant. A large survey in northwestern Xinjiang in 1996–1997 using partial envelope sequences showed a highly homogeneous subtype C strain related to subtype C from India. Full genome sequencing of these subsequently identified CRF07_BC, related to CRF08_BC by several breakpoints but with a different structure. CRF07_BC may dominate the epidemic in Xinjiang (Piyasirisilp *et al.*, 2000; Su *et al.*, 2000; Rodenburg *et al.*, 2001; McCutchan *et al.*, 2002).

Guangxi, bordering Yunnan in the south of China, harbors the full diversity of the China epidemic like Yunnan. Again, there is heterogeneity within Guangxi province, with CRF01_AE predominant near the Vietnam border and subtype C (or recombinants containing C) near the Yunan-Guangxi border (Yu *et al.*, 1998; Yu *et al.*, 1999; Chen *et al.*, 1999). It was in Guangxi that CRF08_BC was first identified by full-genome sequencing (Piyasirisilp *et al.*, 2000), although one of the four initial strains of the CRF was found in Xinjiang (Rodenburg *et al.*, 2001).

Partial *env* or *gag* sequencing of strains from the central provinces of Hubei (Li *et al.*, 1997) and Henan (Su *et al.*, 2003) has shown subtype B'. Along the South China Sea, CRF01_AE appears to predominate, according to studies in Guangdong (Feng *et al.*, 2000) and Fujian (Yan *et al.*, 1999; Yan *et al.*, 2001) provinces. The picture changes again in Shanghai, where most blood transfusion recipients had subtype B' but CRF08_BC was found in IDU. In heterosexual and perinatal transmission cases, all of the diversity again reappeared, including a unique CRF01_AE/B recombinant (Zhong *et al.*, 2003). In eastern Shandong province, blood donors harbored B' while heterosexual infections were C, A, B, and CRF01_AE (Huang *et al.*, 2000; Liu *et al.*, 2000), and the situation in Liaoning to the north appears equally complex (Nerurkar *et al.*, 1998).

The complexity of this initial picture of HIV-1 in China suggests that in-depth and systematic molecular analysis of strains will be required to fully characterize the national epidemic. In particular, strains may circulate in risk groups that transcend provincial borders, providing a focus for interventions and a means to monitor their success. The large public health infrastructure in China provides a potential platform to achieve these goals.

Taiwan

The first indigenous AIDS case in Taiwan was reported in 1985. The largest study to date included samples from 363 HIV-1 positive individuals collected since 1990 from different risk groups, and was approached by partial sequencing of multiple genome regions. Subtype B comprised 74% of strains, and CRF01_AE accounted for 23%. Among heterosexuals, subtypes A, C, and AG recombinants were detected at low levels (Lee *et al.*, 2000a).

Likewise, a study conducted in 1993–1996, which included 288 patients attending AIDS treatment centers in different regions in Taiwan and represented half of the AIDS cases in Taiwan at the time showed a predominance of subtype B (68%) and CRF01_AE (27%). Among the 21 females in this study, CRF01_AE was found most frequently, alongside subtypes A, C, and G (Chen *et al.*, 1998).

Hong Kong

The first reported HIV/AIDS case was in 1984, and prevalence has remained low, affecting less than 0.1% of the adult population. Most of the reported cases are in men and were acquired sexually. No information is available about HIV-1 subtypes in this region.

Myanmar

An explosive HIV-1 epidemic had appeared among IDU in Myanmar by 1988, reaching more than 50% prevalence in this group (Htoon *et al.*, 1994). Early studies in the country identified B' as the predominant strain (Weniger *et al.*, 1994; Cassol *et al.*, 1996). Subsequent work has identified subtype B', C, CRF01_AE and unique recombinant forms, which differ in their distribution among risk groups and geographic regions. In the study (Kusagawa *et al.*, 1998) B' was identified as the predominant strain, accounting for 90% of infections with 10% CRF01_AE. IDU only harbored B' and CRF01_AE was predominant in FSW near the border with Thailand. In the north central city of Mandalay, from 1997–1999, CRF01-AE, B', C, and recombinant strains, including B'/CRF01_AE, B'/C, and B'/C/CRF01_AE were identified (Motomura *et al.*, 2000). A more recent study in this city showed these same patterns, and the URFs were confirmed by full genome sequencing. The emerging picture is one of extensive intermixing of stains, principally in IDU, generating many new URF in Myanmar (Takebe *et al.*, 2003).

Laos

The location of this country, bordering Thailand, Myanmar, China, Vietnam, and Cambodia, places it at the intersection of several different HIV-1 epidemics, but little data is available about the current situation. A study among commercial sex workers in the capital city of Vientiane and in Savannakhet, close to the border with Thailand, showed 1% HIV-1 prevalence (UNAIDS/WHO, 2003). It is believed that most of the transmission in the country is heterosexual. CRF01_AE was identified among pregnant women in Vientiane (Loue *et al.*, 1998).

Cambodia

Cambodia has the highest adult rate of HIV/AIDS cases in the region, according to a 2002 report by UNAIDS. The first HIV-1 infection identified was in a blood donor in Phnom Penh in 1991, and the first AIDS case was diagnosed in 1993 (Phalla *et al.*, 1998). By 1992–1995, the heterosexual risk for HIV-1 was already significant. Military personnel who had served in peacekeeping assignments in Cambodia, including six persons from the Uruguayan Army and Marine Corps and five from the French Army, acquired HIV-1 there; almost all were CRF01_AE. (Artenstein *et al.*, 1995a; Lasky *et al.*, 1997). A comprehensive study in 1996, which included more than 1000 individuals, showed a prevalence of 4.5% in women seeking reproductive health services, 12.5% in police and military groups, and 40.6% in FSW (Ryan *et al.*, 1998). The limited genetic work on HIV-1 strains in Cambodia has detected CRF01_AE almost exclusively.

Vietnam

The first HIV-1 infection was detected in Vietnam in 1990 in Ho Chi Minh City, and by 1993, AIDS cases were reported in south and south central regions (Chung *et al.*, 1998). A comprehensive study in 1992–1993 illuminated the early stages, indicating that the first explosive epidemic occurred among IDU in South Vietnam, with 7.5% infected by 1995, and the strain involved was CRF01_AE. Both FSW and IDU harbored this strain almost exclusively (Fukushima *et al.*, 1995), and in 1995, the nucleotide sequence divergence ranged from 2.5% to 4.9% by partial envelope sequencing (Nerurkar *et al.*, 1996), a finding reiterated by other studies in the region (Nerurkar *et al.*, 1997). By phylogenetic analysis, these strains found their closest counterparts in Cambodia and Thailand (Nerurkar *et al.*, 1997).

With the increase in seroprevalence among FSW in the south of Vietnam, a cross-sectional study was conducted in 1995–1996, including Ho Chi Minh City, An Giang province bordering Cambodia, and Can Tho province. The highest prevalence was in An Giang (9.5%), and among 7 strains genotypes, 6 were CRF01_AE and one was subtype B (Thuy *et al.*, 1998). By 1996–1997, HIV-1 infections were increasing in northern Vietnam (Chung *et al.*, 1998), and, like the south, CRF01_AE was found. The CRF01_AE strains in northern Vietnam were of low diversity, and by phylogenetic analysis they clustered with strains isolated from IDU in neighboring Guangxi province of China (Kato *et al.*, 1999). A signature amino acid just downstream of the V3 loop, and an I to M substitution within V3, further linked these epidemics, a finding reiterated in another study that included Lang Son and Quan Ninh provinces on the China border (Kato *et al.*, 2001).

Meanwhile, additional complexity was developing in the south. By 2001, among 25 samples collected in Ho Chi Minh City, a CRF01_AE/B recombinant was detected, and a CRF02_AG/D strain, possibly from West Africa, had been identified (Caumont *et al.*, 2001). In a study of more than 200 strains from the South in 2001–2002, in which several genome regions of each strain were partially sequenced, CRF01_AE predominated but subtype B and CRF01_AE/B recombinants were also found (Lan *et al.*, 2003).

The epidemic in Vietnam probably represents multiple introductions at different times and across different borders, but it is clear that both IDU and heterosexual exposures have played key roles in the penetration of HIV-1 into the general population in this country.

Malaysia

The historical relationship between Thailand and Malaysia, its southern neighbor, has facilitated not only trade and cultural exchanges but also trafficking of drugs and of women for the commercial sex industry and, as a consequence, HIV-1. HIV-1 had already been identified in Malaysia by 1986 (Ismail, 1998). Injection drug use seems to be the driving force, in contrast to Thailand's primarily heterosexual epidemic. Prevalence rates are highest in this group, and the majority of IDU surveyed in the northeastern state of Kelantan were crossing back and forth across the Thailand border (Singh and Crofts, 1993).

A study in 1992–1993 among IDU in Kuala Lumpur showed mostly subtype B' and some subtype C related to strains in India and like other IDU epidemics, the diversity of the B' strains was low, only 2.8% by partial *env* sequencing (Brown *et al.*, 1996). In this study the subtype C infections were in persons who reported a history of blood transfusions or organ transplantation in India.

By 1995, CRF01_AE had entered the IDU population alongside subtype B' (Tsuchie *et al.*, 1995; Kasper *et al.*, 1997), although CRF01_AE was not in the majority. This picture was confirmed by other subsequent studies, from which CRF01_AE predominated in heterosexual cases during the same period (Beyrer *et al.*, 1998; Saraswathy *et al.*, 2000).

Singapore

HIV was first detected in Singapore in 1985, but seroprevalence in the general population has remained low and was less than 1% in high risk groups in 2000. Subtype B is the predominant strain, and of note, most of this is the North American B strain, not the B' strain first identified in Thailand and southern China.

In 1998, a study of 43 HIV-1 positive individuals identified 26 subtype B, 13 CRF01_AE, 2 subtype C, and 1 subtype A. The IDU harbored B' while the heterosexually acquired HIV-1 were mostly B, consistent with two separate introductions of this subtype (Se-Thoe *et al.*, 1998). By 2002, a study of 58 infections, in which partial *env* and *gag* sequences were obtained, had been completed. The two genome regions gave concordant subtype results, indicating that recombination is still low in this population, although CRF01_AE and subtype B were present is almost equal proportions. Separation of strains by risk group may be the principal reason: B' in IDU, B in MSM, and CRF01_AE in heterosexuals (Kalish *et al.*, 2002).

SOUTH ASIA

India

The HIV epidemic in India had reached staggering proportions by 2002, with an estimated 4 million HIV/AIDS cases. First detected in 1986, HIV-1 has spread mostly through commercial sex workers, which may constitute up to 75% of cases, and in IDU, who represent 15–20%; blood transfusion risk is still high, accounting for 3–6% of the epidemic. The predominant HIV-1 strains are subtype C and B', but subtypes A, B, D, CRF01_AE, and URFs have been detected at low levels. India harbors the only major focus of HIV-2 outside West Africa.

Molecular characterization of the Indian epidemic began in the early 1990s in Mumbai, the most populous province in the country where HIV-1 prevalence had reached over 30% among FSW by 1992 (Jain *et al.*, 1994). Using serological responses to the V3 loop screening 405 non-random serum samples from this population, 76% were reactive with HIV-1, 4% with HIV-2, and 20% were dual reactive (Pfutzner *et al.*, 1992). The dual reactive samples were followed up, and genetic analysis in seven of them confirmed HIV-1 subtype C and, in five, HIV-2. Analysis of gp120 or V3 confirmed HIV-1 subtype C strains of moderate diversity (Grez *et al.*, 1994).

In Punjab, subtype C sequences of even lower diversity were found in 1995, alongside subtype B and other strains (Jameel *et al.*, 1995), and in Hyderabad, a 1994 study found principally subtype B (Baskar *et al.*, 1994). HIV-1 strains from Goa, Bihar, Haryana, West Bengal, and New Delhi states included subtypes C and B (Voevodin *et al.*, 1996), and a study in southern India in 1996 reported principally C but included subtype A (Cassol *et al.*, 1996). Similarly, among 46 sexually transmitted infection (STI) patients in Pune in 1998, 44 were subtype C, with one strain each of subtypes A and B (Gadkari *et al.*, 1998).

By 1999, the first full-genome sequences from India had been obtained, from Pune; five were subtype C and one was AC recombinant. Most of the subtype C strains from India form a significant cluster in phylogenetic analysis; the fact that this was reiterated with full-genome sequences shows that a divergent subtype C strain, rather than an undetected CRF, is responsible (Lole *et al.*, 1999).

Like other subtype C strains, those from India sometimes have unique configurations of regulatory elements in the LTR. An analysis of LTR sequences from 28 samples from Pune, Mumbai, and Vellore showed the expected third NF-kappaB binding motif, as well as six strains with insertions and deletions not previously described, one of which resembles an AP-1 binding site (Choudhury *et al.*, 2000).

A study in 1996–1997 of 322 subjects, which included IDU and their non-injecting wives, showed 72% HIV-1 seroprevalence, and the sexual transmission rate from IDU to their spouses was 45%. Using strain-specific peptide EIA, it was determined that subtype C was most common among IDU (78%) and their wives (57%), followed by subtype B' (12% and 13%, respectively) (Chakrabarti *et al.*, 2000).

Calcutta is the most populous city in the eastern part of India. In 1999, HIV clinic attendees harbored mostly subtype C, but a subtype A strain was also found. As noted before, these subtype C sequences formed a distinct lineage within subtype C. Together, these data support the concept that much of the current Indian epidemic is descended from a single introduction into the country (Shankarappa *et al.*, 2001).

More recent work at the National HIV/AIDS Reference Centre in New Delhi, Heteroduplex Mobility Analysis (HMA) of envelope gene showed that among 125 patients studied in 2002, the proportions were 78% subtype C, 9% subtype B', 2% subtype A, 2% CRF01_AE, and the remainder untypeable (Sahni *et al.*, 2002). Among FSW in Calcutta, 1998–2000, and IDU in Manipur (1996-1997), subtype C predominated, but among the IDU, subtype B' and apparent dual infections with C and B' were reported (Mandal *et al.*, 2002). Finally, a study in 2003 reported on HIV-2 in south India. Among 12 subjects with HIV-2 infection, 11 were confirmed HIV-2 by V3 region sequencing and the last was an HIV-1/HIV-2 co-infection. All were infected with HIV-2 subtype A (Kannangai *et al.*, 2003).

The unique features of HIV-1 in India can be briefly summarized. The epidemic shows a strong founder effect, with a particular subtype C strain descended from those in Africa predominating. However, a number of studies, at different stages of the epidemic and in different regions and risk groups, have revealed low levels of subtypes A, B', and CRF01_AE. The fact that one of six full-genome sequences from India was recombinant suggests undetected complexity not so far revealed by partial genome sequencing and other approaches. Finally, it must be mentioned that the number of strains genetically analyzed is very small for a country with at least 4 million HIV infections. Molecular epidemiology can contribute to a more comprehensive and accurate description as the basis for public health interventions.

Bangladesh

In densely populated Bangladesh, about 13,000 persons were living with HIV/AIDS by 2001. In 1999–2000, among IDU in central and northwest of the country, 5 subtype C and a CRF01_AE/B recombinant have been identified (Azim *et al.*, 2002). Among nine samples from 2001, one subtype A, 5 subtype C, one subtype G, and 2 unique A-containing recombinant strains were found (Ljungberg *et al.*, 2002). This study included those with a history of travel, either to India or to the Arabian Peninsula, raising the possibility that some of the detected strains may not have been acquired in Bangladesh. Nonetheless, the heterogeneity revealed by one small study is noteworthy.

Sri Lanka and Pakistan

As of 2001, these countries exhibited a low rate of HIV-1 infection; prevalences were less than 1% in FSW. No information is available about HIV-1 subtypes.

Nepal

Nepal was reported to have 58,000 HIV infections by 2001, an epidemic that includes heterosexual and IDU risk groups. A major increase in HIV-1 infection among IDU occurred in the 1990s, rising from 0% to 40% between 1995 and 1997. Partial envelope sequences in IDU indicated a homogeneous epidemic of subtype C alongside more divergent C strains, perhaps indicative of two introductions (Oelrichs *et al.*, 2000).

The extensive spread of HIV-1 in India has apparently not been reiterated throughout South Asia. A subtype C strain of low diversity, predominant in India, has apparently seeded smaller epidemics, but all of the strains present in Southeast Asia, including CRF01_AE and B', have been detected at low levels.

CENTRAL ASIA

Increasing spread of HIV-1 in Central Asia is anticipated in the wake of an upsurge of intravenous drug use and sexually transmitted diseases in the countries of Turkmenistan, Tajikistan, Kyrgyzstan, Kazakhstan, and Uzbekistan, but there is little information available about HIV seroprevalence or subtypes in most of these countries.

Turkmenistan, Tajikistan, Kyrgyzstan, and Kazakhstan

As estimated by UNAIDS at the end of 2001, the number of persons infected with HIV-1 in these countries ranged from 175 to 2522. IDU form the nucleus of these epidemics, and there is no available information about HIV-1 subtypes.

Uzbekistan

Like neighboring countries, only a few hundred HIV-1 infections are reported in Uzbekistan, mostly acquired through injecting drug use but also circulating in MSM and heterosexuals. A study of 33 strains obtained in 1999–2002 from 12 regional AIDS centers and representing all risk groups was conducted. 70% were subtype A, 27% subtype B, 3% were subtype D. Among the subtype A strains, 17 of 21 clustered closely with a subtype A strain also found in Ukranian IDU, and four of eight subtype B clustered with CRF03_AB from Russian IDU. Some of the heterosexually acquired subtype A clustered with subtype A from Africa (Kurbanov *et al.*, 2003).

The first opportunity to gain insight into the epidemiology of HIV-1 in the region has shown the interconnection of IDU networks across great distances, linking Uzbekistan with the IDU epidemics in former Soviet Republics to the west by the presence of a subtype A strain of low diversity and CRF03_AB.

AUSTRALIA AND THE PACIFIC

Japan

The HIV-1 prevalence in Japan remains low, less that 1% in high risk groups except FSW from foreign countries. The main routes of transmission have been contaminated blood products, blood transfusion, and heterosexual.

The first HIV/AIDS cases were acquired through blood products for treatment of hemophilia, imported from North America and Europe in the mid 1980s. North American subtype B was predominant at the beginning of the epidemic, but later CRF01_AE also entered through foreign travel.

In 1991, 28 HIV-1 cases acquired through contaminated blood or blood products were subtype B (Hattori *et al.*, 1991). Among 72 samples from Yokohama City collected from 1991–1997, 36 were subtype B, 35 were CRF01_AE, and one was dually infected. However, the study included 23 Thai female heterosexuals, which may have artificially expanded the CRF01_AE proportion. Among Japanese heterosexuals, subtype B was predominant until 1993, but later studies showed CRF01_AE instead (Imai *et al.*, 1997). Indeed, a study in 1998 found five of eight strains in Japanese heterosexuals were CRF01_AE (Yoshino *et al.*, 1998).

In Fukuoka in the south of Japan, far from the metropolitan area of Tokyo, most strains were subtype B by V3 loop peptide serology in 1999, a result later confirmed by partial *env* sequencing (Chijiwa *et al.*, 1999). Finally, a large study among pregnant women from 1989 to 1999 showed considerable subtype diversity, including subtypes A, B, D, G, and CRF01_AE (Hara *et al.*, 2001).

Korea

UNAIDS estimated that by 2001, there were less than 100 HIV-1 infections in North Korea (where data about HIV has remained virtually unavailable), and about 4,000 in South Korea. The first report of HIV-1 infection in South Korea was in 1985, and most reports indicate subtype B as the predominant strain. Two different subgroups have been discerned among Korean subtype B strains, and low levels of CRF01_AE, CRF02_AG, subtypes A, C, D, H and other recombinants have been reported.

Phylogenetic analysis of the *nef* gene among 46 samples collected from 1993 to 1997 in several risk groups showed 3A, 41 B, 1 D, and one unclassified strain. Most of the subtype B strains formed a sub-cluster, separate from international reference strains of this subtype (Kang *et al.*, 1998). Similarly, a study of 58 strains collected from 1986–1993, representing blood contamination and sexual exposures, showed 51 subtype B, four A, two C, and one H strain. Seven different tetrameric tips at the V3 loop were found among the subtype B strains (Kim *et al.*, 1999b). CRF01_AE was detected in Korea in a 2000 report, and phylogenetic analysis linked the strains to those from Thailand (Lee *et al.*, 2000b).

Other studies confirm the existence of a distinctive subtype B strain in Korea with a high frequency of unusual V3 loop crown motifs, while the subtype B strains not within this cluster tended to have the GPGR motif typical of North American subtype B strains (Kim *et al.*, 1999a; Oh *et al.*, 2002; Daniels *et al.*, 2003).

One of the subtype A strains identified in Korea through partial sequencing was confirmed as subtype A in *gp*120 (de Souza *et al.*, 1997) but another sequenced over the whole genome was found to be an A2/D recombinant, probably of Africa origin (Gao *et al.*, 2001).

Phylogenetic analysis of the partial *RT* genes from 29 antiretroviral naïve HIV-1 positive persons in Korea, collected from 1987 to 1992, showed 23 B, one D, one CRF02_AG, and one CRF01_AE/B recombinant and in 43 protease-inhibitor naïve patients, 41 subtype B, and one subtype A were identified. Again, the subtype B strains formed a Korean subcluster within subtype B. A study of *gp*160 revealed 32 amino acid signatures distinguishing Korean B from those in the West (Sung *et al.*, 2001; Sung *et al.*, 2003).

The Philippines

HIV-1 remains at low prevalence in the Philippines. Subtype B was first identified in the country by *gag* sequencing of samples collected between 1988 and 1992 (Louwagie *et al.*, 1993). In a study of 51 samples from Manila collected from 1987 to 1996, which included 33 persons who had lived or traveled abroad, 72% were subtype B, 16% CRF01_AE, 6% A, 4% C, and 2% D. Subtype B and C and CRF01_AE were not closely related to strains elsewhere in Asia (Paladin *et al.*, 1998).

In another study of 54 samples from 1985 to 1997 representing STI, all samples obtained prior to 1993 were subtype B, which constituted 70% of infections overall. Subsequently, CRF01_AE and subtypes F and C were detected (Santiago *et al.*, 1998). Using the approach of sequencing portions of *gag* and *env* genes, 46 samples were analyzed; the strains swere 71% subtype B, 20% CRF01_AE, subtype C, and the recombinants A/B and G/A (Espantaleon *et al.*, 2003).

Indonesia

Indonesia is among the most populous countries in the world. The low HIV-1 prevalence rate still represents a substantial number of infections, estimated at 120,000 by the end of 2001. Of note, much higher rates of infection, up to 35%, have been seen among IDU (UNAIDS/WHO, 2003). The first study of HIV-1 subtypes identified subtype B (Cassol *et al.*, 1996). In 2001, 16 samples from STI clinic attendees in West Papua subtyped in *env* and *gag* were mostly CRF01_AE of low diversity and closely related to strains from Thailand. Two subtype B were detected, including B and B' strains (Foley *et al.*, 2001).

The potential for HIV-1 to spread more widely in Indonesia's large population is apparent, and molecular epidemiology is urgently needed to better define the epidemic and provide avenues for control.

Australia

In Australia, 12,000 were infected with HIV/AIDS by 2001, with the MSM and bisexual populations most affected. Subtype B predominates in the country. By sequencing of part of the *env* gene of 17 HIV-1 seropositive individuals in Sydney, only subtype B was found in a study conducted in 1996 (Dwyer *et al.*, 1996). Among 141 samples collected between 1993 and 2002, subtype B was predominant among MSM and IDU (94% and 100%, respectively), whereas non-B subtypes were frequent in heterosexually (57%) or perinatally (22%) infected individuals. Overall, the non-B subtypes constituted 26% of strains, mostly subtype C and CRF01_AE, but also including subtypes A and G (Herring *et al.*, 2003).

This molecular picture suggests a subtype B epidemic in the country among MSM and IDU, alongside a much more diverse one in heterosexuals which still represent the minority of infections in the country.

New Zealand and Papua New Guinea

Low rates of HIV-1 infection are believed to exist in these countries, and the sparse molecular data available indicates subtype B is predominant, mostly among MSM (Dwyer *et al.*, 1996; Dwyer *et al.*, 1998). Subtype C was also identified in heterosexual females in New Zealand (Dwyer *et al.*, 1998).

CONCLUSION

In Asia and the Pacific, HIV-1 was first detected in the early 1980s. The country-by-country review provided here is a study in contrasts, with the virus infecting 4 million in India, almost 1 million in China, and more than 1 million in Southeast Asia, while in most of the region, prevalence rates remain low. Molecular epidemiology has identified subtype C, B, and CRF01_AE as the principal strains in the epicenters of the Asian epidemic. New recombinant strains have been generated and some have gained epidemic spread. Low levels of subtypes A, D, F, and G have been identified as well. With the exception of Thailand, the sequence database is not focused on the heart of the epidemic, and the paucity of full-genome sequences, especially in populations where multiple subtypes co-circulate, is evident. Virtually all of the available data comes from cross-sectional, convenience samples, often collected over a decade or more.

The spread of HIV-1 in Southeast Asia and China has been complex and uneven. Multiple introductions across borders, initial separation of strains by risk group, explosive epidemics in IDU generating strains of low diversity, and eventual intermixing leading to the generation of novel recombinant strains are often repeated themes. Overall, the dominance of CRF01_AE, subtypes B and C, and recombinants generated from them is incontrovertible. The molecular epidemiology provides a framework for intervention, and must be ongoing to capture the dynamics of this complicated regional picture.

Systematic surveillance, use of full-genome sequencing or multi-region genotyping approaches, and identification of incident strains in high risk and general population sectors are research priorities for the future.

REFERENCES

Arroyo, M.A., Hoelscher, M., Sanders-Buell, E., Herbinger, K., Samky, E., Maboko, L., Hoffmann, O., Robb, M.L., Birx, D.L., and McCutchan, F.E. (2004). HIV-1 subtypes among blood donors in the Mbeya region of southwest Tanzania. *AIDS Res Hum Retroviruses*, In press.

Artenstein, A.W., Coppola, J., Brown, A.E., Carr, J.K., Sanders-Buell, E., Galbarini, E., Mascola, J.R., VanCott, T.C., Schonbrood, P., and McCutchan, F.E. (1995a). Multiple introductions of HIV-1 subtype E into the western hemisphere. *Lancet*. 346:1197–1198.

Artenstein, A.W., VanCott, T.C., Mascola, J.R., Carr, J.K., Hegerich, P. A., Gaywee, J., Sanders-Buell, E., Robb, M.L., Dayhoff, D.E., and Thitivichianlert, S. (1995b). Dual infection with human immunodeficiency virus type 1 of distinct envelope subtypes in humans. *J Infect Dis*. 171:805–810.

Auwanit, W., Ayuthaya, P.I., Duangchanda, S., Mukai, T., Kurata, T., and Ikuta, K. (2000). Highly variable sequences in the env V3 region of HIV type 1 distributing among Thai carriers from 1995 to 1997. *AIDS Res Hum Retroviruses*. 16:283–289.

Azim, T., Bogaerts, J., Yirrell, D.L., Banerjea, A.C., Sarker, M.S., Ahmed, G., Amin, M.M., Rahman, A.S., and Hussain, A.M. (2002). Injecting drug users in Bangladesh: prevalence of syphilis, hepatitis, HIV and HIV subtypes. *AIDS*. 16:121 123.

Bachmann, M.H., Delwart, E.L., Shpaer, E.G., Lingenfelter, P., Singal, R., and Mullins, J.I. (1994). Rapid genetic characterization of HIV type 1 strains from four World Health Organization-sponsored vaccine evaluation sites using a heteroduplex mobility assay. WHO Network for HIV Isolation and Characterization. *AIDS Res Hum Retroviruses*. 10:1345–1353.

Baskar, P.V., Ray, S.C., Rao, R., Quinn, T.C., Hildreth, J.E., and Bollinger, R.C. (1994). Presence in India of HIV type 1 similar to North American strains. *AIDS Res Hum Retroviruses*. 10:1039–1041.

Beyrer, C., Artenstein, A., Kunawararak, P., VanCott, T., Mason, C., Rungreungthanakit, K., Hegerich, P., Nelson, K.E., Khamboonruang, C., and Natpratan, C. (1997). The molecular epidemiology of HIV-1 among male sex workers in northern Thailand. *J Acquir Immune Defic Syndr Hum Retrovirol*. 15:304–307.

Beyrer, C., Vancott, T.C., Peng, N.K., Artenstein, A., Duriasamy, G., Nagaratnam, M., Saw, T.L., Hegerich, P.A., Loomis-Price, L.D., Hallberg, P.L., Ettore, C.A., and Nelson, K.E. (1998). HIV type 1 subtypes in Malaysia, determined with serologic assays: 1992–1996. *AIDS Res Hum Retroviruses*. 14:1687–1691.

Beyrer, C., Razak, M.H., Lisam, K., Chen, J., Lui, W., and Yu, X.F. (2000). Overland heroin trafficking routes and HIV-1 spread in south and south-east Asia. *AIDS*. 14:75–83.

Bobkov, A., Kazennova, E., Selimova, L., Bobkova, M., Khanina, T., Ladnaya, N., Kravchenko, A., Pokrovsky, V., Cheingsong-Popov, R., and Weber, J. (1998). A sudden epidemic of HIV type 1 among injecting drug users in the former Soviet Union: identification of subtype A, subtype B, and novel gagA/envB recombinants. *AIDS Res Hum Retroviruses*. 14:669–676.

Brown, T.M., Robbins, K.E., Sinniah, M., Saraswathy, T.S., Lee, V., Hooi, L.S., Vijayamalar, B., Luo, C.C., Ou, C.Y., Rapier, J., Schochetman, G., and Kalish, M.L. (1996). HIV type 1 subtypes in Malaysia include B, C, and E. *AIDS Res Hum Retroviruses*. 12:1655–1657.

Carr, J.K., Salminen, M.O., Koch, C., Gotte, D., Artenstein, A.W., Hegerich, P.A., St Louis, D., Burke, D.S., and McCutchan, F.E. (1996). Full-length sequence and mosaic structure of a human immunodeficiency virus type 1 isolate from Thailand. *J Virol*. 70:5935–5943.

Carr, J.K., Laukkanen, T., Salminen, M.O., Albert, J., Alaeus, A., Kim, B., Sanders-Buell, E., Birx, D.L., and McCutchan, F.E. (1999). Characterization of subtype A HIV-1 from Africa by full genome sequencing. *AIDS*. 13:1819–1826.

Cassol, S., Weniger, B.G., Babu, P.G., Salminen, M.O., Zheng, X., Htoon, M.T., Delaney, A., O'Shaughnessy, M., and Ou, C.Y. (1996). Detection of HIV type 1 env subtypes A, B, C, and E in Asia using dried blood spots: a new surveillance tool for molecular epidemiology. *AIDS Res Hum Retroviruses*. 12:1435–1441.

Caumont, A., Lan, N.T., Uyen, N.T., Hung, P.V., Schvoerer, E., Urriza, M.S., Roques, P., Schrive, M.H., Lien, T.T., Lafon, M.E., Dormont, D., Barre-Sinoussi, F., and Fleury, H.J. (2001). Sequence analysis of env C2/V3, gag p17/p24, and pol protease regions of 25 HIV type 1 isolates from Ho Chi Minh City, Vietnam. *AIDS Res Hum Retroviruses*. 17:1285–1291.

Chakrabarti, S., Panda, S., Chatterjee, A., Sarkar, S., Manna, B., Singh, N.B., Naik, T.N., Detels, R., and Bhattacharya, S.K. (2000). HIV-1 subtypes in injecting drug users & their non-injecting wives in Manipur, India. *Indian J Med Res*. 111:189–194.

Chen, J., Young, N.L., Subbarao, S., Warachit, P., Saguanwongse, S., Wongsheree, S., Jayavasu, C., Luo, C.C., and Mastro, T.D. (1999). HIV type 1 subtypes in Guangxi Province, China, 1996. *AIDS Res Hum Retroviruses*. 15:81–84.

Chen, Y.M., Lee, C.M., Lin, R.Y., and Chang, H.J. (1998). Molecular epidemiology and trends of HIV-1 subtypes in Taiwan. *J Acquir Immune Defic Syndr Hum Retrovirol*. 19:393–402.

Cheng, H., Zhang, J., Capizzi, J., Young, N.L., and Mastro, T.D. (1994). HIV-1 subtype E in Yunnan, China. *Lancet*. 344:953–954.

Chijiwa, K., Ishibashi, T., Kashiwagi, S., and Mori, R. (1999). The distribution of HIV-1 subtypes in Fukuoka, Japan. *Microbiol Immunol*. 43:271–278.

Choudhury, S., Montano, M.A., Womack, C., Blackard, J.T., Maniar, J.K., Saple, D.G., Tripathy, S., Sahni, S., Shah, S., Babu, G.P., and Essex, M. (2000). Increased promoter diversity reveals a complex phylogeny of human immunodeficiency virus type 1 subtype C in India. *J Hum Virol*. 3:35–43.

Chung, A., Vu, M.Q., and Dondero, T.J. (1998). HIV epidemiologic situation in Vietnam: a review of available data. *AIDS*. 12 Suppl B:S43–S49.

Daniels, R.S., Kang, C., Patel, D., Xiang, Z., Douglas, N.W., Zheng, N. N., Cho, H.W., and Lee, J.S. (2003). An HIV type 1 subtype B founder effect in Korea: gp160 signature patterns infer circulation of CTL-escape strains at the population level. *AIDS Res Hum Retroviruses*. 19:631–641.

de Souza, M., Song, M.S., Carr, J.K., Sanders-Buell, E., Shin, Y., Artenstein, A.W., Lee, H., McCutchan, F.E., and Brown, A.E. (1997). HIV–1 subtypes A and B isolated from the Republic of Korea. *AIDS*. 11:389–391.

Delwart, E.L., Shpaer, E.G., Louwagie, J., McCutchan, F.E., Grez, M., Rubsamen-Waigmann, H., and Mullins, J.I. (1993). Genetic relationships determined by a DNA heteroduplex mobility assay: analysis of HIV-1 env genes. *Science*. 262:1257–1261.

Dowling, W.E., Kim, B., Mason, C.J., Wasunna, M., Alam, U., Elson, L., Birx, D.L., Robb, M.L., McCutchan, F.E., and Carr, J.K. (2002). Forty-one near full length HIV-1 sequences from Kenya reveal an epidemic of subtype A and A-containing recombinants. *AIDS*. 16:1809–1820.

Dwyer, D.E., Ge, Y.C., Bolton, W.V., Wang, B., Cunningham, A.L., and Saksena, N.K. (1996). Subtype B isolates of human immunodeficiency virus type 1 detected in Australia. *Ann Acad Med Singapore*. 25:188–191.

Dwyer, D.E., Herring, B.L., Ge, Y.C., Bolton, W.V., Ellis-Pegler, R.B., Thomas, M., Schroeder, B.A., Croxson, M.C., Cunningham, A.L., Mullins, J.I., and Saksena, N.K. (1998). Human immunodeficiency virus type 1 subtypes B and C detected in New Zealand. *AIDS Res Hum Retroviruses*. 14:1105–1108.

Entz, A.T., Ruffolo, V.P., Chinveschakitvanich, V., Soskolne, V., and van Griensven, G.J. (2000). HIV-1 prevalence, HIV-1 subtypes and risk factors among fishermen in the Gulf of Thailand and the Andaman Sea. *AIDS*. 14:1027–1034.

Espantaleon, A., Kageyama, S., Bernardo, M.T., Nakano, T., Leano, P.S., Alban, P., Abrenica, R., Morimatsu, S., Teraoka, H., and Agdamag, D.M. (2003). The influence of the expanding HIV genetic diversity on molecular diagnosis in the Philippines. *Int J STD AIDS*. 14:125–131.

Esteves, A., Parreira, R., Piedade, J., Venenno, T., Franco, M., Germano de Sousa, J., Patricio, L., Brum, P., Costa, A., and Canas-Ferreira, W.F. (2003). Spreading of HIV-1 subtype G and envB/gagG recombinant strains among injecting drug users in Lisbon, Portugal. *AIDS Res Hum Retroviruses*. 19:511–517.

Feng, T., Shao, Y., and Li, L. (2000). Molecular epidemiology analysis of HIV-1 subtype E strains found in Shenzhen, China. *Zhonghua Shi Yan He Lin Chuang Bing Du Xue Za Zhi*. 14:330–332.

Foley, B., Donegan, E., Silitonga, N., Wignall, F.S., Busch, M.P., and Delwart, E.L. (2001). Importation of multiple HIV type 1 strains into West Papua, Indonesia (Irian Jaya). *AIDS Res Hum Retroviruses*. 17:1655–1659.

Fukushima, Y., Takahashi, H., Hall, W.W., Nakasone, T., Nakata, S., Song, P., Dinh Duc, D., Hien, B., Nguyen, X.Q., Ngoc Trinh, T., Nishioka, K., Kitamura, K., Komuro, K., Vahlne, A., and Honda, M. (1995). Extraordinary high rate of HTLV type II seropositivity in intravenous drug abusers in south Vietnam. *AIDS Res Hum Retroviruses*. 11:637–645.

Gadkari, D.A., Moore, D., Sheppard, H.W., Kulkarni, S.S., Mehendale, S.M., and Bollinger, R.C. (1998). Transmission of genetically diverse strains of HIV-1 in Pune, India. *Indian J Med Res*. 107:1–9.

Gao, F., Yue, L., Craig, S., Thornton, C.L., Robertson, D.L., McCutchan, F.E., Bradac, J.A., Sharp, P.M., and Hahn, B.H. (1994). Genetic variation of HIV type 1 in four World Health Organization-sponsored vaccine evaluation sites: generation of functional envelope (glycoprotein 160) clones representative of sequence subtypes A, B, C, and E. WHO Network for HIV Isolation and Characterization. *AIDS Res Hum Retroviruses*. 10:1359–1368.

Gao, F., Robertson, D.L., Morrison, S.G., Hui, H., Craig, S., Decker, J., Fultz, P.N., Girard, M., Shaw, G.M., Hahn, B.H., and Sharp, P.M. (1996). The heterosexual human immunodeficiency virus type 1 epidemic in Thailand is caused by an intersubtype (A/E) recombinant of African origin. *J Virol*. 70:7013–7029.

Gao, F., Vidal, N., Li, Y., Trask, S.A., Chen, Y., Kostrikis, L.G., Ho, D.D., Kim, J., Oh, M.D., Choe, K., Salminen, M., Robertson, D.L., Shaw, G.M., Hahn, B.H., and Peeters, M. (2001). Evidence of two distinct subsubtypes within the HIV-1 subtype A radiation. *AIDS Res Hum Retroviruses*. 17:675–688.

Gaywee, J., Artenstein, A.W., VanCott, T.C., Trichavaroj, R., Sukchamnong, A., Amlee, P., de Souza, M., McCutchan, F.E., Carr, J.K., Markowitz, L.E., Michael, R., and Nittayaphan, S. (1996). Correlation of genetic and serologic approaches to HIV-1 subtyping in Thailand. *J Acquir Immune Defic Syndr Hum Retrovirol.* 13:392–396.

Graf, M., Shao, Y., Zhao, Q., Seidl, T., Kostler, J., Wolf, H., and Wagner, R. (1998). Cloning and characterization of a virtually full-length HIV type 1 genome from a subtype B'-Thai strain representing the most prevalent B-clade isolate in China. *AIDS Res Hum Retroviruses.* 14:285–288.

Grez, M., Dietrich, U., Balfe, P., von Briesen, H., Maniar, J.K., Mahambre, G., Delwart, E.L., Mullins, J.I., and Rubsamen-Waigmann, H. (1994). Genetic analysis of human immunodeficiency virus type 1 and 2 (HIV-1 and HIV-2) mixed infections in India reveals a recent spread of HIV-1 and HIV-2 from a single ancestor for each of these viruses. *J Virol.* 68:2161–2168.

Hara, T., Yoshino, N., Takayama, N., Minamitani, M., Naganawa, S., Ohkubo, H., Takizawa, M., Izumi, Y., Kantake, M., Suzuki, S., Takano, M., Kita, T., Totani, R., Nagai, Y., Honda, M., and Nakasone, T. (2001). Presence of multiple HIV type 1 subtypes among mothers and children in Japan. *AIDS Res Hum Retroviruses.* 17:569–575.

Harris, M.E., Serwadda, D., Sewankambo, N., Kim, B., Kigozi, G., Kiwanuka, N., Phillips, J.B., Wabwire, F., Meehen, M., Lutalo, T., Lane, J.R., Merling, R., Gray, R., Wawer, M., Birx, D.L., Robb, M.L., and McCutchan, F.E. (2002). Among 46 near full length HIV type 1 genome sequences from Rakai District, Uganda, subtype D and AD recombinants predominate. *AIDS Res Hum Retroviruses.* 18:1281–1290.

Hattori, T., Shiozaki, K., Eda, Y., Tokiyoshi, S., Matsushita, S., Inaba, H., Fujimaki, M., Meguro, T., Yamada, K., Honda, M., Nishikawa, K., and Takatsuki, K. (1991). Characteristics of the principal neutralizing determinant of HIV-1 prevalent in Japan. *AIDS Res Hum Retroviruses.* 7:825–830.

Herring, B.L., Ge, Y.C., Wang, B., Ratnamohan, M., Zheng, F., Cunningham, A.L., Saksena, N.K., and Dwyer, D.E. (2003). Segregation of human immunodeficiency virus type 1 subtypes by risk factor in Australia. *J Clin Microbiol.* 41:4600–4601.

Hoelscher, M., Kim, B., Maboko, L., Mhalu, F., von Sonnenburg, F., Birx, D.L., and McCutchan, F.E. (2001). High proportion of unrelated HIV-1 intersubtype recombinants in the Mbeya region of southwest Tanzania. *AIDS.* 15:1461–1470.

Htoon, M.T., Lwin, H.H., San, K.O., Zan, E., and Thwe, M. (1994). HIV/AIDS in Myanmar. *AIDS.* 8 Suppl 2:S105–S109.

Huang, T., Liu, C., Su, S., Fu, J., Liu, X., and Kang, D. (2000). Analysis on the characteristic and trend of AIDS epidemics in Shandong. *Zhonghua Liu Xing Bing Xue Za Zhi.* 21:338–340.

Ichimura, H., Kliks, S.C., Visrutaratna, S., Ou, C.Y., Kalish, M.L., and Levy, J.A. (1994). Biological, serological, and genetic characterization of HIV-1 subtype E isolates from northern Thailand. *AIDS Res Hum Retroviruses.* 10:263–269.

Imai, M., Kondo, M., Sudo, K., Saito, T., Sato, H., Takebe, Y., Noguchi, Y., Kawata, K., Ito, A., Sagara, H., and Kihara, M. (1997). Simple method for typing human immunodeficiency virus type I (B, E) by PCR and chronological change of distribution of subtype (B to E) in Japan. *Kansenshogaku Zasshi.* 71: 918–923.

Ismail, R. (1998). HIV/AIDS in Malaysia. *AIDS.* 12 Suppl B:S33–S41.

Jain, M.K., John, T.J., and Keusch, G.T. (1994). Epidemiology of HIV and AIDS in India. *AIDS.* 8 Suppl 2:S61–S75.

Jameel, S., Zafrullah, M., Ahmad, M., Kapoor, G.S., and Sehgal, S. (1995). A genetic analysis of HIV-1 from Punjab, India reveals the presence of multiple variants. *AIDS.* 9:685–690.

Kalish, M.L., Luo, C.C., Weniger, B.G., Limpakarnjanarat, K., Young, N., Ou, C.Y., and Schochetman, G. (1994). Early HIV type 1 strains in Thailand were not responsible for the current epidemic. *AIDS Res Hum Retroviruses.* 10:1573–1575.

Kalish, M.L., Baldwin, A., Raktham, S., Wasi, C., Luo, C.C., Schochetman, G., Mastro, T.D., Young, N., Vanichseni, S., Rubsamen-Waigmann, H., von Briesen, H., Mullins, J.I., Delwart, E.L., Herring, B., Esparza, J., Heyward, W.L., and Osmanov, S. (1995). The evolving molecular epidemiology of HIV-1 envelope subtypes in injecting drug users in Bangkok, Thailand: implications for HIV vaccine trials. *AIDS.* 9:851–857.

Kalish, M.L., Korber, B.T., Pillai, S., Robbins, K.E., Leo, Y.S., Saekhou, A., Verghese, I., Gerrish, P., Goh, C.L., Lupo, D., Tan, B.H., Brown, T.M., and Chan, R. (2002). The sequential introduction of HIV-1 subtype B and CRF01AE in Singapore by sexual transmission: accelerated V3 region evolution in a subpopulation of Asian CRF01 viruses. *Virology.* 304:311–329.

Kang, M.R., Cho, Y.K., Chun, J., Kim, Y.B., Lee, I., Lee, H.J., Kim, S.H., Kim, Y.K., Yoon, K., Yang, J.M., Kim, J.M., Shin, Y.O., Kang, C., Lee, J.S., Choi, K.W., Kim, D.G., Fitch, W.M., and Kim, S. (1998). Phylogenetic analysis of the nef gene reveals a distinctive monophyletic clade in Korean HIV-1 cases. *J Acquir Immune Defic Syndr Hum Retrovirol.* 17:58–68.

Kannangai, R., Shaji, R.V., Ramalingam, S., Jesudason, M.V., Abraham, O. C., George, R., Shanmugam, A.P., Schwartz, D.H., and Sridharan, G. (2003). HIV-2 subtype circulating in India (south). *J Acquir Immune Defic Syndr.* 33:219–222.

Kasper, P., Chalwatzis, N., Duraisamy, G., Ofenloch-Hahnle, B., and Faatz, E. (1997). HIV type 1 gag subtype A is predominant in Malaysian intravenous drug users. *AIDS Res Hum Retroviruses*. 13:1251–1253.

Kato, K., Shiino, T., Kusagawa, S., Sato, H., Nohtomi, K., Shibamura, K., Nguyen, T.H., Pham, K.C., Truong, X.L., Mai, H.A., Hoang, T.L., Bunyaraksyotin, G., Fukushima, Y., Honda, M., Wasi, C., Yamazaki, S., Nagai, Y., and Takebe, Y. (1999). Genetic similarity of HIV type 1 subtype E in a recent outbreak among injecting drug users in northern Vietnam to strains in Guangxi Province of southern China. *AIDS Res Hum Retroviruses*. 15:1157–1168.

Kato, K., Kusagawa, S., Motomura, K., Yang, R., Shiino, T., Nohtomi, K., Sato, H., Shibamura, K., Nguyen, T.H., Pham, K.C., Pham, H.T., Duong, C.T., Bui, D.T., Hoang, T.L., Nagai, Y., and Takebe, Y. (2001). Closely related HIV-1 CRF01_AE variant among injecting drug users in northern Vietnam: evidence of HIV spread across the Vietnam-China border. *AIDS Res Hum Retroviruses*. 17:113–123.

Kim, E.Y., Cho, Y.S., Maeng, S.H., Kang, C., Nam, J.G., and Lee, J.S. (1999a). Characterization of V3 loop sequences from HIV type 1 subtype B in South Korea: predominance of the GPGS motif. *AIDS Res Hum Retroviruses*. 15:681-686.

Kim, Y.B., Cho, Y.K., Lee, H.J., Kim, C.K., Kim, Y.K., and Yang, J.M. (1999b). Molecular phylogenetic analysis of human immunodeficiency virus type 1 strains obtained from Korean patients: env gene sequences. *AIDS Res Hum Retroviruses. 15*: 303–307.

Kitayaporn, D., Vanichseni, S., Mastro, T.D., Raktham, S., Vaniyapongs, T., Des Jarlais, D.C., Wasi, C., Young, N.L., Sujarita, S., Heyward, W.L., and Esparza, J. (1998). Infection with HIV-1 subtypes B and E in injecting drug users screened for enrollment into a prospective cohort in Bangkok, Thailand. *J Acquir Immune Defic Syndr Hum Retrovirol*. 19:289–295.

Kuiken, C.L., Foley, B., Freed, E., Hahn, B., Marx, P.A., McCutchan, F., Mellors, J.W., Wolinksy, S., and Kober, B., (eds.). (2002). *HIV Sequence Compendium 2002*. Published by Theoretical Biology and Biophysics Group, Los Alamos National Laboratory, Los Alamos, NM, LA-UR 03-3564.

Kunanusont, C., Foy, H.M., Kreiss, J.K., Rerks-Ngarm, S., Phanuphak, P., Raktham, S., Pau, C.P., and Young, N.L. (1995). HIV-1 subtypes and male-to-female transmission in Thailand. *Lancet*. 345:1078–1083.

Kurbanov, F., Kondo, M., Tanaka, Y., Zalalieva, M., Giasova, G., Shima, T., Jounai, N., Yuldasheva, N., Ruzibakiev, R., Mizokami, M., and Imai, M. (2003). Human immunodeficiency virus in Uzbekistan: epidemiological and genetic analyses. *AIDS Res Hum Retroviruses*. 19:731–738.

Kusagawa, S., Sato, H., Watanabe, S., Nohtomi, K., Kato, K., Shino, T., Thwe, M., Oo, K.Y., Lwin, S., Mra, R., Kywe, B., Yamazaki, S., and Takebe, Y. (1998). Genetic and serologic characterization of HIV type 1 prevailing in Myanmar (Burma). *AIDS Res Hum Retroviruses*. 14:1379–1385.

Lan, N.T., Recordon-Pinson, P., Hung, P.V., Uyen, N.T., Lien, T.T., Tien, H.T., Garrigue, I., Schrive, M.H., Pellegrin, I., Lafon, M.E., Aboulker, J.P., Barre-Sinousi, F., and Fleury, H.J. (2003). HIV type 1 isolates from 200 untreated individuals in Ho Chi Minh City (Vietnam): ANRS 1257 Study. Large predominance of CRF01_AE and presence of major resistance mutations to antiretroviral drugs. *AIDS Res Hum Retroviruses*. 19:925–928.

Lasky, M., Perret, J.L., Peeters, M., Bibollet-Ruche, F., Liegeois, F., Patrel, D., Molinier, S., Gras, C., and Delaporte, E. (1997). Presence of multiple non-B subtypes and divergent subtype B strains of HIV-1 in individuals infected after overseas deployment. *AIDS*. 11:43–51.

Lee, C.N., Wang, W.K., Fan, W.S., Twu, S.J., Chen, S.C., Sheng, M.C., and Chen, M.Y. (2000a). Determination of human immunodeficiency virus type 1 subtypes in Taiwan by vpu gene analysis. *J Clin Microbiol*. 38:2468–4674.

Lee, J.S., Nam, J.G., Kim, E.Y., Kang, C., Koo, B.K., and Cho, H.W. (2000b). Introduction of HIV type 1 subtype E virus into South Korea. *AIDS Res Hum Retroviruses*. 16:1083–1087.

Li, Y.W., Shao, Y.M., and Luo, X.G. (1997). Subtype and sequence analysis of the C2-V3 region of gp120 genes among HIV-1 strains in Hubei province. *Zhonghua Liu Xing Bing Xue Za Zhi*. 18:217–219.

Liitsola, K., Tashkinova, I., Laukkanen, T., Korovina, G., Smolskaja, T., Momot, O., Mashkilleyson, N., Chaplinskas, S., Brummer-Korvenkontio, H., Vanhatalo, J., Leinikki, P., and Salminen, M.O. (1998). HIV-1 genetic subtype A/B recombinant strain causing an explosive epidemic in injecting drug users in Kaliningrad. *AIDS*. 12:1907–1919.

Liitsola, K., Holm, K., Bobkov, A., Pokrovsky, V., Smolskaya, T., Leinikki, P., Osmanov, S., and Salminen, M. (2000). An AB recombinant and its parental HIV type 1 strains in the area of the former Soviet Union: low requirements for sequence identity in recombination. UNAIDS Virus Isolation Network. *AIDS Res Hum Retroviruses*. 16:1047–1053.

Limpakarnjanarat, K., Mastro, T.D., Saisorn, S., Uthaivoravit, W., Kaewkungwal, J., Korattana, S., Young, N.L., Morse, S.A., Schmid, D.S., Weniger, B.G., and Nieburg, P. (1999). HIV-1 and other sexually transmitted infections in a cohort of female sex workers in Chiang Rai, Thailand. *Sex Transm Infect*. 75:30–35.

Liu, C., Xing, H., and Su, S. (2000). Molecular epidemiological study on HIV-1 infection in Shandong

Province. *Zhonghua Shi Yan He Lin Chuang Bing Du Xue Za Zhi*. 14:231–235.

Ljungberg, K., Hassan, M.S., Islam, M.N., Siddiqui, M.A., Aziz, M.M., Wahren, B., Islam, K.B., and Leitner, T. (2002). Subtypes A, C, G, and recombinant HIV type 1 are circulating in Bangladesh. *AIDS Res Hum Retroviruses*. 18:667–670.

Lole, K.S., Bollinger, R.C., Paranjape, R.S., Gadkari, D., Kulkarni, S.S., Novak, N.G., Ingersoll, R., Sheppard, H.W., and Ray, S.C. (1999). Full-length human immunodeficiency virus type 1 genomes from subtype C-infected seroconverters in India, with evidence of intersubtype recombination. *J Virol*. 73:152–160.

Loue, S., Bounlu, K., Pholsena, V., and Mastro, T.D. (1998). HIV seroprevalence and HIV-1 subtype E among pregnant women in Vientiane, Laos. *AIDS*. 12:1403.

Louwagie, J., McCutchan, F.E., Peeters, M., Brennan, T.P., Sanders-Buell, E., Eddy, G.A., van der Groen, G., Fransen, K., Gershy-Damet, G.M., Deleys, R., and Burke, D.S. (1993). Phylogenetic analysis of gag genes from 70 international HIV-1 isolates provides evidence for multiple genotypes. *AIDS*. 7:769–780.

Louwagie, J., Janssens, W., Mascola, J., Heyndrickx, L., Hegerich, P., van der Groen, G., McCutchan, F.E., and Burke, D.S. (1995). Genetic diversity of the envelope glycoprotein from human immunodeficiency virus type 1 isolates of African origin. *J Virol*. 69:263–271.

Luo, C.C., Tian, C., Hu, D.J., Kai, M., Dondero, T., and Zheng, X. (1995). HIV-1 subtype C in China. *Lancet*. 345:1051–1052.

Mandal, D., Jana, S., Bhattacharya, S.K., and Chakrabarti, S. (2002). HIV type 1 subtypes circulating in eastern and northeastern regions of India. *AIDS Res Hum Retroviruses*. 18:1219–1227.

Masharsky, A.E., Klimov, N.A., and Kozlov, A.P. (2003). Molecular cloning and analysis of full-length genome of HIV type 1 strains prevalent in countries of the former Soviet Union. *AIDS Res Hum Retroviruses*. 19:933–939.

Mason, C.J., Kitsiripornchai, S., Markowitz, L.E., Chanbancherd, P., Supapongse, T., Jugsudee, A., Sirisopana, N., Chuenchitra, C., Torugsa, K., VanCott, T.C., Michael, R.A., and Nitayaphan, S. (1998). Nationwide surveillance of HIV-1 prevalence and subtype in young Thai men. *J Acquir Immune Defic Syndr Hum Retrovirol*. 19:165–173.

McCutchan, F.E. (2000a). HIV/AIDS. In: Thompson, R.C.A. (ed.), *Molecular Epidemiology of Infectious Diseases*. Edward Arnold Limited, London, pp. 143–167.

McCutchan, F.E. (2000b). Understanding the genetic diversity of HIV-1. *AIDS*. 14 Suppl 3:S31–S44.

McCutchan, F.E., Hegerich, P.A., Brennan, T.P., Phanuphak, P., Singharaj, P., Jugsudee, A., Berman, P.W., Gray, A.M., Fowler, A.K., and Burke, D.S. (1992). Genetic variants of HIV-1 in Thailand. *AIDS Res Hum Retroviruses*. 8:1887–1895.

McCutchan, F.E., Carr, J.K., Robb, M.L., Mascola, J., Yu, X.F., Janssens, W., Salminen, M., Albert, J., Burke, D.S., Unadis, P., and Birx, D.L. (2000). Full genome Sequencing of HIV-1 reveals new complexity in the pandemic. In *the XIII International AIDS Conference*. Durban, South Africa, 9–14 July 2000.

McCutchan, F.E., Carr, J.K., Murphy, D., Piyasirisilp, S., Gao, F., Hahn, B., Yu, X.F., Beyrer, C., and Birx, D.L. (2002). Precise mapping of recombination breakpoints suggests a common parent of two BC recombinant HIV type 1 strains circulating in China. *AIDS Res Hum Retroviruses*. 18:1135–1140.

McCutchan, F.E., Carr, J.K., Tovanabutra, S., Yu, X.F., Beyrer, C., and Birx, D.L. (2002). HIV-1 and drug trafficking: viral strains illuminate networks and provide focus for interventions. In: Effects of drug use and high-risk behavior on HIV transmission across national borders. In *the XIV International AIDS Conference*, NIDA satellite sessions, Barcelona, Spain, 7–12 July 2002.

Motomura, K., Kusagawa, S., Kato, K., Nohtomi, K., Lwin, H.H., Tun, K.M., Thwe, M., Oo, K.Y., Lwin, S., Kyaw, O., Zaw, M., Nagai, Y., and Takebe, Y. (2000). Emergence of new forms of human immunodeficiency virus type 1 intersubtype recombinants in central Myanmar. *AIDS Res Hum Retroviruses*. 16:1831–1843.

Myers, G., Korber, B., Berzofksy, J.A., Smith, R.F. and Pavlakis, G.N. (Eds.). *Human Retroviruses and AIDS 1992*: A Compilation and Analysis of Nucleic Acid and Amino Acid Sequences. Theoretical Biology and Biophysics Group, Los Alamos National Laboratory, Los Alamos, NM.

Nabatov, A.A., Kravchenko, O.N., Lyulchuk, M.G., Shcherbinskaya, A.M., and Lukashov, V.V. (2002). Simultaneous introduction of HIV type 1 subtype A and B viruses into injecting drug users in southern Ukraine at the beginning of the epidemic in the former Soviet Union. *AIDS Res Hum Retroviruses*. 18:891–895.

Naganawa, S., Sato, S., Nossik, D., Takahashi, K., Hara, T., Tochikubo, O., Kitamura, K., Honda, M., and Nakasone, T. (2002). First report of CRF03_AB recombinant HIV type 1 in injecting drug users in Ukraine. *AIDS Res Hum Retroviruses*. 18:1145–1149.

Nelson, K.E., Celentano, D.D., Suprasert, S., Wright, N., Eiumtrakul, S., Tulvatana, S., Matanasarawoot, A., Akarasewi, P., Kuntolbutra, S., Romyen, S., Sirisopana, N., and Theetranont, C. (1993). Risk factors for HIV infection among young adult men in northern Thailand. *JAMA*. 270:955–960.

Nerurkar, V.R., Nguyen, H.T., Dashwood, W.M., Hoffmann, P.R., Yin, C., Morens, D.M., Kaplan, A.H., Detels, R., and Yanagihara, R. (1996). HIV type 1 subtype E in commercial sex workers and injection drug users in southern Vietnam. *AIDS Res Hum Retroviruses*. 12:841–843.

Nerurkar, V.R., Nguyen, H.T., Woodward, C.L., Hoffmann, P.R., Dashwood, W.M., Long, H.T., Morens, D.M., Detels, R., and Yanagihara, R. (1997). Sequence and phylogenetic analyses of HIV-1 infection in Vietnam: subtype E in commercial sex workers (CSW) and injection drug users (IDU). *Cell Mol Biol* (Noisy-le-grand). 43:959–968.

Nerurkar, V.R., Wu, Z., Dashwood, W.M., Woodward, C.L., Zhang, M., Detels, R., and Yanagihara, R. (1998). Complete nef gene sequence of HIV type 1 subtype B' from professional plasma donors in the People's Republic of China. *AIDS Res Hum Retroviruses*. 14:461–464.

Nopkesorn, T., Mock, P.A., Mastro, T.D., Sangkharomya, S., Sweat, M., Limpakarnjanarat, K., Laosakkitiboran, J., Young, N.L., Morse, S.A., Schmid, S., and Weniger, B.G. (1998). HIV-1 subtype E incidence and sexually transmitted diseases in a cohort of military conscripts in northern Thailand. *J Acquir Immune Defic Syndr Hum Retrovirol*. 18:372–379.

Novitsky, V.A., Montano, M.A., and Essex, M. (1998). Molecular epidemiology of an HIV-1 subtype A subcluster among injection drug users in the Southern Ukraine. *AIDS Res Hum Retroviruses*. 14:1079–1085.

Oelrichs, R.B., Shrestha, I.L., Anderson, D.A., and Deacon, N.J. (2000). The explosive human immunodeficiency virus type 1 epidemic among injecting drug users of Kathmandu, Nepal, is caused by a subtype C virus of restricted genetic diversity. *J Virol*. 74:1149–1157.

Oh, M.D., Park, S.W., Kim, U., Kim, H.B., Choe, Y.J., Kim, E., and Choe, K. (2002). Determination of genetic subtypes of HIV type 1 isolated from Korean AIDS patients. *AIDS Res Hum Retroviruses*. 18:1229–1233.

Ou, C.Y., Takebe, Y., Luo, C.C., Kalish, M., Auwanit, W., Bandea, C., de la Torre, N., Moore, J.L., Schochetman, G., and Yamazaki, S. (1992). Wide distribution of two subtypes of HIV-1 in Thailand. *AIDS Res Hum Retroviruses*. 8:1471–1472.

Ou, C.Y., Takebe, Y., Weniger, B.G., Luo, C.C., Kalish, M.L., Auwanit, W., Yamazaki, S., Gayle, H.D., Young, N.L., and Schochetman, G. (1993). Independent introduction of two major HIV-1 genotypes into distinct high-risk populations in Thailand. *Lancet*. 341:1171–1174.

Paladin, F.J., Monzon, O.T., Tsuchie, H., Aplasca, M.R., Learn, G.H., Jr., and Kurimura, T. (1998). Genetic subtypes of HIV-1 in the Philippines. *AIDS*. 12:291–300.

Peeters, M., and Sharp, P.M. (2000). Genetic diversity of HIV-1: the moving target. *AIDS*. 14 Suppl 3:S129–S140.

Pfutzner, A., Dietrich, U., von Eichel, U., von Briesen, H., Brede, H.D., Maniar, J.K., and Rubsamen-Waigmann, H. (1992). HIV-1 and HIV-2 infections in a high-risk population in Bombay, India: Evidence for the spread of HIV-2 and presence of a divergent HIV-1 subtype. *J Acquir Immune Defic Syndr*. 5:972–977.

Phalla, T., Leng, H.B., Mills, S., Bennett, A., Wienrawee, P., Gorbach, P., and Chin, J. (1998). HIV and STD epidemiology, risk behaviors, and prevention and care response in Cambodia. *AIDS*. 12 Suppl B:S11–S18.

Piyasirisilp, S., McCutchan, F.E., Carr, J.K., Sanders-Buell, E.,Liu, W., Chen, J., Wagner, R., Wolf, H., Shao, Y., Lai, S., Beyrer, C., and Yu, X.F. (2000). A recent outbreak of human immunodeficiency virus type 1 infection in southern China was initiated by two highly homogeneous, geographically separated strains, circulating recombinant form AE and a novel BC recombinant. *J Virol*. 74:11286–11295.

Quinn, T.C. (1998). Molecular variants of HIV-1 and their impact on vaccine development. *Int J STD AIDS*. 9 Suppl 1:2.

Ramos, A., Hu, D.J., Nguyen, L., Phan, K.O., Vanichseni, S., Promadej, N., Choopanya, K., Callahan, M., Young, N.L., McNicholl, J., Mastro, T.D., Folks, T.M., and Subbarao, S. (2002). Intersubtype human immunodeficiency virus type 1 superinfection following seroconversion to primary infection in two injection drug users. *J Virol*. 76:7444–7452.

Robertson, D.L., Sharp, P.M., McCutchan, F.E., and Hahn, B.H. (1995). Recombination in HIV-1 [letter]. *Nature*. 374:124–126.

Robertson, D.L., Anderson, J.P., Bradac, J.A., Carr, J.K., Foley, B., Funkhouser, R.K., Gao, F., Hahn, B.H., Kalish, M.L., Kuiken, C., Learn, G.H., Leitner, T., McCutchan, F., Osmanov, S., Peeters, M., Pieniazek, D., Salminen, M., Sharp, P.M., Wolinsky, S., and Korber, B. (2000). HIV-1 nomenclature proposal. *Science*. 288:55–56.

Rodenburg, C.M., Li, Y., Trask, S.A., Chen, Y., Decker, J., Robertson, D.L., Kalish, M.L., Shaw, G.M., Allen, S., Hahn, B.H., and Gao, F. (2001). Near full-length clones and reference sequences for subtype C isolates of HIV type 1 from three different continents. *AIDS Res Hum Retroviruses*. 17:161–168.

Ryan, C.A., Vathiny, O.V., Gorbach, P.M., Leng, H.B., Berlioz-Arthaud, A., Whittington, W.L., and Holmes, K.K. (1998). Explosive spread of HIV-1 and sexually transmitted diseases in Cambodia. *Lancet* 351:1175.

Sahni, A.K., Prasad, V.V., and Seth, P. (2002). Genomic diversity of human immunodeficiency virus type-1 in India. *Int J STD AIDS*. 13:115–118.

Salminen, M.O., Koch, C., Sanders-Buell, E., Ehrenberg, P.K., Michael, N.L., Carr, J.K., Burke, D.S., and McCutchan, F.E. (1995). Recovery of virtually full-length HIV-1 provirus of diverse subtypes from primary virus cultures using the polymerase chain reaction. *Virology*. 213:80–86.

Santiago, M.L., Santiago, E.G., Hafalla, J.C., Manalo, M.A., Orantia, L., Cajimat, M.N., Martin, C., Cuaresma, C., Dominguez, C.E., Borromeo, M.E., De Groot, A.S., Flanigan, T.P., Carpenter, C.C., Mayer, K.H., and Ramirez, B.L. (1998). Molecular epidemiology of HIV-1 infection in the Philippines, 1985 to 1997: transmission of subtypes B and E and potential emergence of subtypes C and F. *J Acquir Immune Defic Syndr Hum Retrovirol*. 18:260–269.

Saraswathy, T.S., Ng, K.P., and Sinniah, M. (2000). Human immunodeficiency virus type 1 subtypes among Malaysian intravenous drug users. *Southeast Asian J Trop Med Public Health*. 31:283–286.

Se-Thoe, S.Y., Foley, B.T., Chan, S.Y., Lin, R.V., Oh, H.M., Ling, A.E., Chew, S.K., Snodgrass, I., and Sng, J.E. (1998). Analysis of sequence diversity in the C2-V3 regions of the external glycoproteins of HIV type 1 in Singapore. *AIDS Res Hum Retroviruses*. 14:1601–1604.

Shankarappa, R., Chatterjee, R., Learn, G.H., Neogi, D., Ding, M., Roy, P., Ghosh, A., Kingsley, L., Harrison, L., Mullins, J.I., and Gupta, P. (2001). Human immunodeficiency virus type 1 env sequences from Calcutta in eastern India: identification of features that distinguish subtype C sequences in India from other subtype C sequences. *J Virol*. *75*:10479–10487.

Shao, Y. (1991). Isolation of human immunodeficiency virus (HIV) in epidemic area of HIV infection in Yunnan Province. *Zhonghua Liu Xing Bing Xue Za Zhi*. 12:129–135.

Shao, Y., Su, L., Sun, X., Sun, H., Xing, H., Pan, P.L., Wolf, H., and Shen, J. (1998). Molecular epidemiology of HIV infection in China. In *the XII International AIDS Conference*, Geneva, Switzerland, 28 June–3 July 1998.

Singh, S., and Crofts, N. (1993). HIV infection among injecting drug users in north-east Malaysia, 1992. *AIDS Care*. 5:273–281.

Sirisopana, N., Torugsa, K., Mason, C.J., Markowitz, L.E., Jugsudee, A., Supapongse, T., Chuenchitra, C., Michael, R.A., Burke, D.S., Singharaj, P., Johnson, A.E., McNeil, J.G., McCutchan, F.E., and Carr, J.K. (1996). Correlates of HIV-1 seropositivity among young men in Thailand. *J Acquir Immune Defic Syndr Hum Retrovirol*. 11:492–498.

Su, B., Liu, L., Wang, F., Gui, X., Zhao, M., Tien, P., Zhang, L., and Chen, Z. (2003). HIV-1 subtype B' dictates the AIDS epidemic among paid blood donors in the Henan and Hubei provinces of China. *AIDS*. 17:2515–2520.

Su, L., Graf, M., Zhang, Y., von Briesen, H., Xing, H., Kostler, J., Melzl, H., Wolf, H., Shao, Y., and Wagner, R. (2000). Characterization of a virtually full-length human immunodeficiency virus type 1 genome of a prevalent intersubtype (C/B') recombinant strain in China. *J Virol*. 74:11367–11376.

Subbarao, S., Limpakarnjanarat, K., Mastro, T.D., Bhumisawasdi, J., Warachit, P., Jayavasu, C., Young, N.L., Luo, C.C., Shaffer, N., Kalish, M.L., and Schochetman, G. (1998). HIV type 1 in Thailand, 1994–1995: persistence of two subtypes with low genetic diversity. *AIDS Res Hum Retroviruses*. 14: 319–327.

Sun, X., Nan, J., and Guo, Q. (1994). AIDS and HIV infection in China. *AIDS*. 8 Suppl 2:S55–S59.

Sung, H., Foley, B.T., Bae, I.G., Chi, H.S., and Cho, Y.K. (2001). Phylogenetic analysis of reverse transcriptase in antiretroviral drug-naive Korean HIV type 1 patients. *AIDS Res Hum Retroviruses*. 17:1549–1554.

Sung, H., Foley, B.T., Ahn, S.H., Kim, Y.B., Chae, J.D., Shin, Y.O., Kang, H.I., and Cho, Y.K. (2003). Natural polymorphisms of protease in protease inhibitor-naive HIV-1 infected patients in Korea: a novel L63M in subtype B. *AIDS Res Hum Retroviruses*. *19*:525–530.

Swanson, P., Devare, S.G., and Hackett, J., Jr. (2003). Full-length sequence analysis of HIV-1 isolate CM237: a CRF01_AE/B intersubtype recombinant from Thailand. *AIDS Res Hum Retroviruses*. 19:707–712.

Takebe, Y., Motomura, K., Tatsumi, M., Lwin, H.H., Zaw, M., and Kusagawa, S. (2003). High prevalence of diverse forms of HIV-1 intersubtype recombinants in Central Myanmar: geographical hot spot of extensive recombination. *AIDS*. 17:2077–2087.

Thomson, M.M., Delgado, E., Manjon, N., Ocampo, A., Villahermosa, M.L., Marino, A., Herrero, I., Cuevas, M.T., Vazquez-de Parga, E., Perez-Alvarez, L., Medrano, L., Taboada, J.A., and Najera, R. (2001). HIV-1 genetic diversity in Galicia Spain: BG intersubtype recombinant viruses circulating among injecting drug users. *AIDS*. 15:509–516.

Thuy, N.T., Nhung, V.T., Thuc, N.V., Lien, T.X., and Khiem, H.B. (1998). HIV infection and risk factors among female sex workers in southern Vietnam. *AIDS*. 12:425–432.

Tovanabutra, S., Razak, M.H., Rungruengthanakit, K., Chanbancherd, P., de Souza, M., Jittiwutikarn, J., Suriyanon, V., Celentano, D.D., and McCutchan, F.E. (2000). HIV-1 subtype E is predominant among drug users in northern Thailand. In *the XIII International AIDS Conference*. Durban, South Africa, 9–14 July 2000.

Tovanabutra, S., Polonis, V., de Souza, M., Trichavaroj, R., Chanbancherd, P., Kim, B., Sanders-Buell, E., Nitayaphan, S., Brown, A., Robb, M.R., Birx, D.L., McCutchan, F.E., and Carr, J.K. (2001). First CRF01_AE/B recombinant of HIV-1 is found in Thailand. *AIDS*. 15:1063–1065.

Tovanabutra, S., Robison, V., Wongtrakul, J., Sennum, S., Suriyanon, V., Kingkeow, D., Kawichai, S., Tanan, P., Duerr, A., and Nelson, K.E. (2002). Male viral load and heterosexual transmission of HIV-1 subtype E in northern Thailand. *J Acquir Immune Defic Syndr*. 29:275–283.

Tovanabutra, S., Watanaveeradej, V., Viputtikul, K., de Souza, M., Razak, M.H., Suriyanon, V., Jittiwutikarn, J., Sriplienchan, S., Nitayaphan, S., Benenson, M.W., Sirisopana, N., Renzullo, P.O., Brown, A.E., Robb, M.L., Beyrer, C., Celentano, D.D., McNeil, J.G., Birx, D.L., Carr, J.K., and McCutchan, F.E. (2003). A new circulating recombinant form, CRF15_01B, reinforces the linkage between IDU and heterosexual epidemics in Thailand. *AIDS Res Hum Retroviruses*. 19:561–567.

Tovanabutra, S., Beyrer, C., Sakkhachornphop, S., Razak, M.H., Ramos, G., Vongchak, T., Rungreungthanakit, K., Saokhieo, P., Tejafong, K., Kim, B., de Souza, M., Robb, M.L., Birx, D.L., Jittiwutikarn, J., Suriyanon, V., Celentano, D.D., and McCutchan, F.E. (2004). The changing molecular epidemiology of HIV-1 among northern Thai drug users, 1999 to 2002. *AIDS Res Hum Retroviruses*. 20:465–475.

Tsuchie, H., Saraswathy, T.S., Sinniah, M., Vijayamalar, B., Maniar, J.K., Monzon, O.T., Santana, R.T., Paladin, F.J., Wasi, C., Thongcharoen, P. (1995). HIV-1 variants in South and South-East Asia. *Int J STD AIDS*. 6:117–120.

UNAIDS/WHO. *AIDS Epidemic Update: November 2003*. (http://www.unaids.org).

Viputtikul, K., de Souza, M., Trichavaroj, R., Carr, J.K., Tovanabutra, S., McCutchan, F.E., Sriplienchan, S., Buapunth, P., Chuenchitra, C., McNeil, J.G., Birx, D.L., Brown, A.E., and Nitayaphan, S. (2002). Heterosexually acquired CRF01_AE/B recombinant HIV type 1 found in Thailand. *AIDS Res Hum Retroviruses*. 18:1235–1237.

Voevodin, A., Crandall, K.A., Seth, P., and Al Mufti, S. (1996). HIV type 1 subtypes B and C from new regions of India and Indian and Ethiopian expatriates in Kuwait. *AIDS Res Hum Retroviruses*. 12:641–643.

Vongsheree, S., Phutiprawan, T., Sri-ngam, P., Thaisri, H., Puangtabtim, W., and Sawanpanyalert, P. (2002). Co-existence of HIV-1 subtypes B' and E infections among Thai injecting drug users. *Asian Pac J Allergy Immunol*. 20:29–35.

Wang, Z., Lyles, C.M., Beyrer, C., Celentano, D.D., Vlahov, D., Natpratan, C., Markham, R., Khamboonruang, C., Nelson, K., and Yu, X.F. (1998). Diversification of subtype E human immunodeficiency virus type 1 env in heterosexual seroconverters from Northern Thailand. *J Infect Dis*. 178:1507–1511.

Wasi, C., Herring, B., Raktham, S., Vanichseni, S., Mastro, T.D., Young, N.L., Rubsamen-Waigmann, H., von Briesen, H., Kalish, M.L., Luo, C.C., Pau, C.P., Baldwin, A., Mullins, J.I., Delwart, E.L., Esparza, J., Heyward, W.L., and Osmanov, S. (1995). Determination of HIV-1 subtypes in injecting drug users in Bangkok, Thailand, using peptide-binding enzyme immunoassay and heteroduplex mobility assay: evidence of increasing infection with HIV-1 subtype E. *AIDS*. 9:843–849.

Watanaveeradej, V., de Souza, M.S., Benenson, M.W., Sirisopana, N., Nitayaphan, S., Chanbancherd, P., Brown, A.E., Sanders-Buell, E., Birx, D.L., McCutchan, F.E., and Carr, J.K. (2003). Subtype C/CRF01_AE recombinant HIV-1 found in Thailand. *AIDS*. 17:2138–2140.

Watanveeradej, V., de Souza, M., Nitayaphan, S., Benenson, M.W., Sirisopana, N., Renzullo, P.O., Brown, A.E., McNeil, J.G., Birx, D.L., McCutchan, F.E., and Carr, J, K. (2003). Molecular epidemiology of HIV-1 in a vaccine candidate cohort in Thailand. Unpublished data.

Weniger, B.G., Limpakarnjanarat, K., Ungchusak, K., Thanprasertsuk, S., Choopanya, K., Vanichseni, S., Uneklabh, T., Thongcharoen, P., and Wasi, C. (1991). The epidemiology of HIV infection and AIDS in Thailand. *AIDS*. 5 Suppl 2:S71–S85.

Weniger, B.G., Takebe, Y., Ou, C.Y., and Yamazaki, S. (1994). The molecular epidemiology of HIV in Asia. *AIDS*. 8 Suppl 2:S13–S28.

Yan, Y., Zheng, Z., and Shao, Y. (1999). Analysis on the epidemic characterization and trend of AIDS in Fujian Province. *Zhonghua Liu Xing Bing Xue Za Zhi*. 20:23–26.

Yan, Y., Weng, Y., and Chen, G. (2001). Relationship between epidemiology of HIV-1 infection and HIV-1 subtypes in Fujian province. *Zhonghua Liu Xing Bing Xue Za Zhi*. 22:428–431.

Yang, R., Xia, X.,Kusagawa, S., Zhang, C., Ben, K., and Takebe, Y. (2002). On-going generation of multiple forms of HIV-1 intersubtype recombinants in the Yunnan Province of China. *AIDS*. 16:1401–1407.

Yoshino, N., Naganawa, S., Nakasone, T., mura, S., Kita, T., and Honda, M. (1998). Vertical transmission of human immunodeficiency virus type 1 in Japan, 1989–1997: presence of two subtypes B and E with subtype E predominance. National Cooperative Study Investigators on Vertical Transmission of HIV-1. *Acta Paediatr Jpn*. 40:503–509.

Yu, X. F., Chen, J., Shao, Y., Beyrer, C., and Lai, S. (1998). Two subtypes of HIV-1 among injection-drug users in southern China. *Lancet*. 351:1250.

Yu, X.F., Chen, J., Shao, Y., Beyrer, C., Liu, B., Wang, Z., Liu, W., Yang, J., Liang, S., Viscidi, R.P., Gu, J., Gurri-Glass, G., and Lai, S. (1999). Emerging HIV infections with distinct subtypes of HIV-1 infection among injection drug users from geographically separate locations in Guangxi Province, China. *J Acquir Immune Defic Syndr*. 22:180–188.

Zhong, P., Kang, L., Pan, Q., Konings, F., Burda, S., Ma, L., Xue, Y., Zheng, X., Jin, Z., and Nyambi, P. (2003). Identification and distribution of HIV type 1 genetic diversity and protease inhibitor resistance-associated mutations in Shanghai, P. R. China. *J Acquir Immune Defic Syndr*. 34: 91–101.

17

Human Genetics and HIV-1 Infection

Xu G. Yu, Marcus Altfeld, and Bruce D. Walker

Howard Hughes Medical Institute, Partners AIDS Research Center and Infectious Disease Division, Massachusetts General Hospital and Harvard Medical School, Boston, Massachusetts USA

INTRODUCTION

Even before the human genome was sequenced, there has been increasing evidence that human genetics influences infectious diseases. This review will discuss the key role of a number of genetic factors that have been shown to exert such influence, particularly in the context of HIV/AIDS.

Overview of HLA Diversity in Relation to Infectious Diseases

The Major Histocompatibility Complex (MHC) or Human Leukocyte Antigen (HLA) system is the most polymorphic of all human genetic systems, consisting of a complex 3.6 megabase genetic locus including 128 expressed genes, about 40% of which have a role in immunity (MHC Sequencing Consortium, 1999). The key role of the MHC in the adaptive immune response to pathogens makes it of critical importance for the host defense against viruses such as HIV, and may help to explain marked differences in clinical outcomes among persons suffering from the same infectious disease. Zinkernagel and Doherty's Nobel Prize-winning discovery (1974) that cellular immunity to viral infections is "restricted" by the highly variable proteins of the MHC laid a foundation for understanding general mechanisms used by the cellular immune system to recognize both foreign microorganisms and self molecules (Hill, 2001; Lipsitch *et al.*, 2003). Their observations concerning the specificity of adaptive T-lymphocyte-mediated immunity was that it explained the ability of the immune system to recognize invading microorganisms and certain forms of cancer. They also explained the ability of the immune system to react against certain kinds of self tissues in some autoimmune diseases, such as rheumatic conditions, multiple sclerosis, and diabetes.

Many studies have examined the frequency distribution of HLA alleles among ethnically diverse populations, and have determined that the frequencies of specific haplotypes can be significantly different among different human populations. A study including 1296 subjects from five major ethnic groups in the United States (African-Americans, Caucasians, Hispanics, Asians, and North American Natives) showed

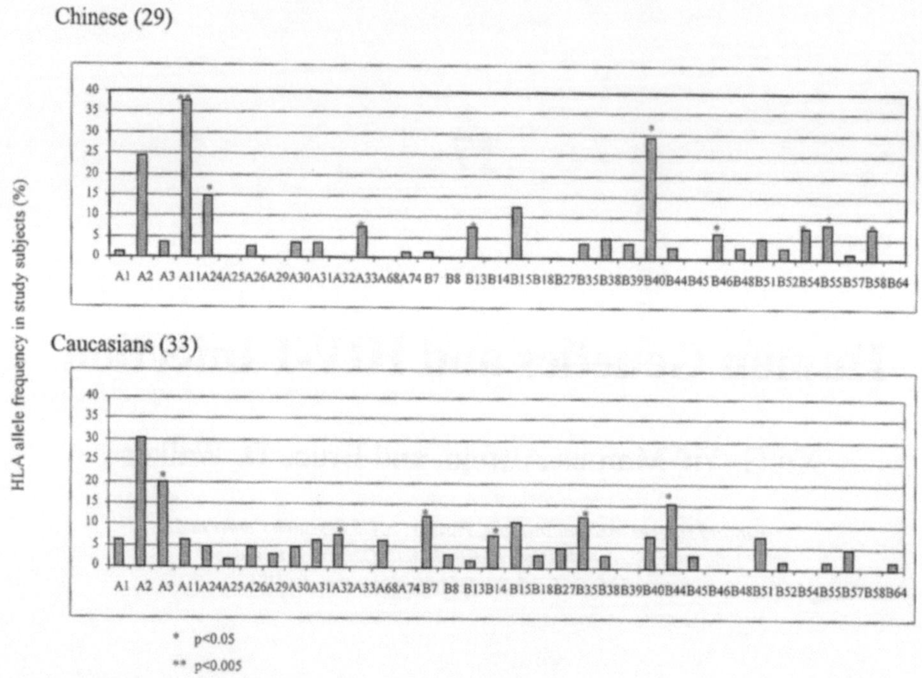

FIGURE 1. Frequency of HLA class I alleles expressed in studied Chinese and Caucasians. The HLA class I A and B alleles are represented on the χ axis, and the corresponding frequencies of each allele expressed in the studied Chinese and Caucasian population are represented on the y axis. * and ** symbolize the differences in the expression of these alleles in the two populations reaching the statistical significance.

that many HLA class I alleles are present with significantly higher frequencies in one population and completely absent in other populations (Cao *et al.*, 2001). In particular, many HLA class I alleles that appeared almost exclusively in either African Americans or Asians were not observed in Caucasians or North American Natives (Cao *et al.*, 2001).

In preliminary studies, we have begun to determine HLA types of persons of Chinese descent, and have compared these to the prevalent alleles in Caucasians. In a pilot study with 29 Chinese and 33 Caucasians (Figure 1), the predominant HLA class I alleles in the studied Chinese were HLA-A2, -A11, -A24, and -B4001, while HLA-A2, -A3, -B44, -B7, and –B35 were the predominant HLA class I alleles in Caucasians. These data indicate a marked difference in dominant HLA class I alleles in persons of diverse ethnicity. Given the central role of class I molecules in immune recognition events, these data also indicate that immune responses to pathogens such as HIV may be very different in persons of diverse ethnicities compared to populations in whom current vaccine candidates are being tested, providing rationale for more intensive studies in Chinese populations vulnerable to the expanding HIV epidemic.

Infectious diseases depend on the function of the cellular immune system and consequently on its mechanisms for specific recognition. Individual HLA alleles may be especially effective, or especially ineffective, at presenting antigens from particular infectious agents. Therefore, carrying one versus two copies of a given allele might predispose an infected individual to a more or less favorable disease outcome, since the diversity of HLA alleles influences the number of viral epitopes that can be presented to the immune system for recognition. A "population heterozygote advantage" was suggested by

TABLE 1. Some HLA Associations with Infectious Disease

Disease	HLA allele(s)[a]	Population[b]
Malaria	B53↓ DRB1*1302↓	Gambia
Tuberculosis	DR2↑	India, Russia, Indonesia
Leprosy	DR2↑	India
HIV progression	B35↑ A1-B8-DR3↑ B27↓	USA, Europe
Hepatitis B persistence	DRB1*1302↓	Gambia, Germany
Hepatitis C persistence	DR5↓	Italy, UK

Source: adapted from Hill, 1998
[a] ↑ indicates a susceptibility allele; ↓ indicates a protective allele.
[b] The population (country) in which the study was performed is shown.

Doherty and Zinkernagel (1975) soon after their discovery of MHC restriction: since each MHC allele provides an infected individual with the ability to present a particular set of antigens, individuals who are heterozygous at a particular MHC locus may mount a more diverse immune response to a given infection, resulting in a better outcome than individuals who are homozygous for either of the corresponding alleles (Lipsitch *et al.*, 2003).

A number of studies indeed suggest that HLA influences disease outcome. In the 1970s and 1980s the bacterial diseases leprosy and tuberculosis were frequently studied. It was confirmed that the HLA-DR2 is associated with susceptibility to both leprosy and tuberculosis, particularly in Asian populations (Table 1) (Bothamley *et al.*, 1989; Brahmajothi *et al.*, 1991; Khomenko *et al.*, 1990; Rani *et al.*, 1993; Singh *et al.*, 1983; Todd *et al.*, 1990; van Eden *et al.*, 1980). Another important study has demonstrated the association of HLA-B53 with resistance to severe malaria in The Gambia (Hill *et al.*, 1991). Since the 1990s, a number of studies about the association of HLA genes with various manifestations of viral infections, such as hepatitis B virus (HBV) and C virus (HCV), have been reported. HLA-DRB1*1302 was associated with clearance of HBV infection and with a decreased chance of becoming a persistent carrier, who are at high risk of chronic liver disease in The Gambia (Thursz *et al.*, 1995); while HLA-DR5 has higher allele frequency in Italian asymptomatic HCV-infected individuals or in healthy controls than those with chronic liver disease (Peano *et al.*, 1994; Zavaglia *et al.*, 1996). While most of these studies have lacked the power to detect the heterozygote advantage in infectious diseases, one recent study indicated that HLA class II homozygotes were found to be more likely to develop persistent HBV infection than were heterozygotes, supporting this hypothesis (Thursz *et al.*, 1997).

Host Genetics in HIV Infections

The AIDS pandemic has stimulated a large number of studies investigating the role of genetic host factors, including HLA and chemokine receptors or ligands in various manifestations of HIV-1 infection, disease progression, and immune defenses. Several cohort studies examining HLA associations with disease progression in HIV-1-infected individuals have suggested that heterozygosity of the HLA class I loci is associated with the delayed onset of AIDS (Carrington *et al.*, 1999b; Gao *et al.*, 2001; Hendel *et al.*, 1999; Tang *et al.*, 1999). In addition, several specific HLA alleles have been associated with different patterns of HIV-1 disease progression (Flores-Villanueva *et al.*, 2001; Hendel *et al.*, 1999; Kaslow *et al.*, 1996; Keet *et al.*, 1999). In particular, certain HLA class I alleles (HLA-B*27 and -B*5701) have been associated with low set point viremia and long-term non-progressive HIV-1 infection in multiple independent studies (Costello *et al.*, 1999; Goulder *et al.*, 1996; Goulder *et al.*, 1997a; Kaslow *et al.*, 1996; Klein *et al.*, 1998;

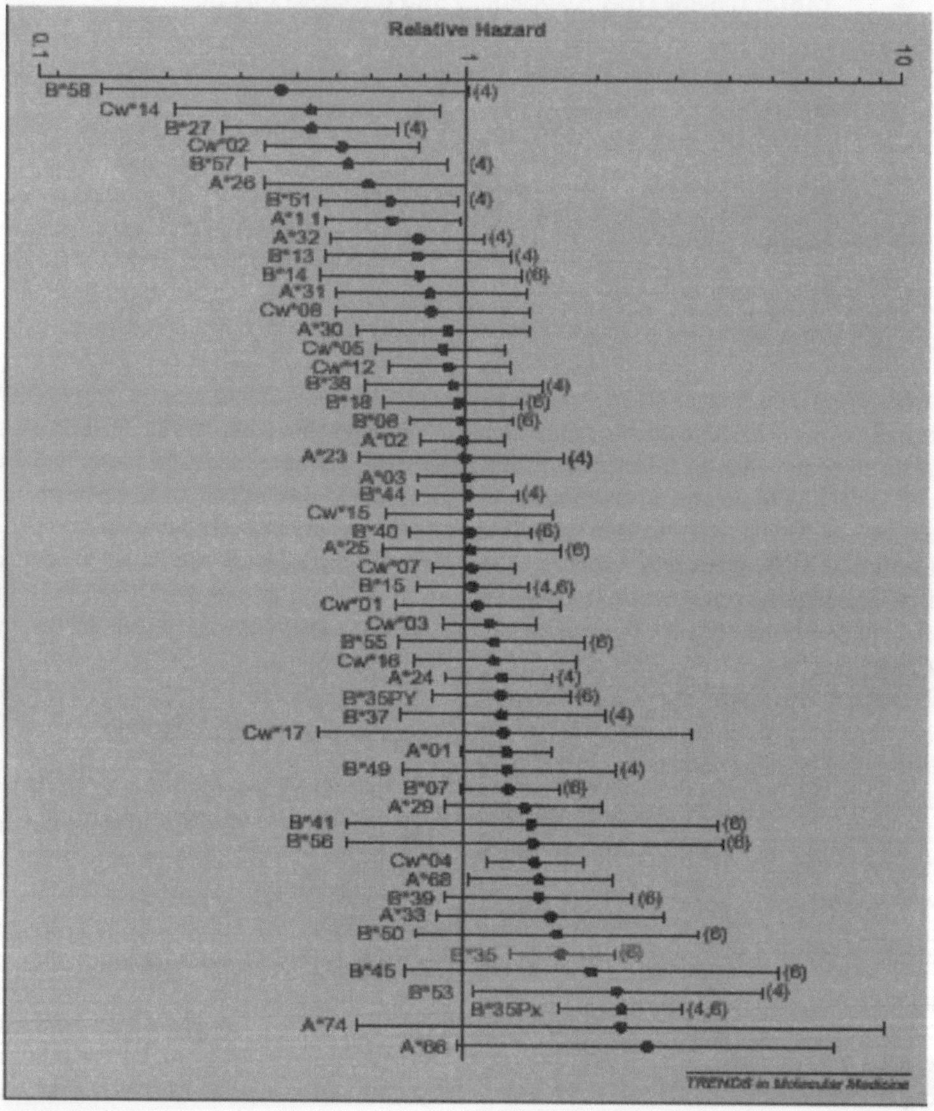

FIGURE 2. Genetic associations of HLA class I types with progression to AIDS in a group of 600 Caucasian seroconvertor patients tested by O'Brien's group. Relative hazard (RH) values were determined for each of the 54 HLA types listed. Bars represent 95% confidence intervals (CI) for each RH. Bw4/Bw6 specificities of alleles that retain them are shown in parentheses. Class I types with CI that cross the line representing a RH of 1 are not significant, whereas all others are significant at $P < 0.05$. (This figure was originally published by O'Brien et al. HLA and AIDS: a cautionary tale, Trends in Molecular Medicine, 2001: 379–381. Copyright belongs to Elsevier Inc.)

McNeil *et al.*, 1996). In contrast, HLA alleles B*35 and –Cw*04 were found to accelerate progression to AIDS (Carrington *et al.*, 1999b; Itescu *et al.*, 1992; Jeannet *et al.*, 1989; Tomiyama *et al.*, 1997). A comprehensive analysis about genetic associations of 54 HLA class I types with progression to AIDS were performed by O'Brien *et al.* (2001), in a group of 600 Caucasian HIV-1-infected individuals (Figure 2). A recent study by our group described the association of HLA-B*57 with asymptomatic acute HIV-1 infection and good control of viral replication following acute infection, suggesting a crucial impact of this allele on the course of acute infection, translating into potential favorable long-term outcome (Altfeld *et al.*, 2003). Understanding why these particular alleles are associated with different outcomes is highly relevant to understanding HIV pathogenesis and to vaccine development; yet this remains elusive.

In addition to the described impact of HLA on the speed of HIV-1 disease progression, the genetic HLA background has also been shown to influence the response of an individual to HIV-1 vaccines. Homozygosity at class I loci, although conferring an unfavorable prognosis following natural infection as discussed above, showed no disadvantage for vaccine responses (Kaslow *et al.*, 2001). However, among the individuals carrying the protected alleles like HLA-B*27 or – B*57, the proportions responding to Gag or Env after exposure to ALVAC-HIV recombinant canarypox vaccine were also significantly higher (Kaslow *et al.*, 2001). This may be due to the characteristics of these alleles in the breadth or specificity of its peptide binding repertoire (Kelleher *et al.*, 2001) or to some intrinsic ability of these alleles to present processed viral proteins (Wilson *et al.*, 2000).

In addition to HLA, polymorphisms of chemokine receptors are another important host genetic factor associated with HIV-1 pathogenesis and disease progression. The chemokine receptors CXCR4 and CCR5 were identified as co-receptors, along with CD4, for HIV-1 entry in 1996 (Alkhatib *et al.*, 1996; Choe *et al.*, 1996; Deng *et al.*, 1996; Doranz *et al.*, 1996; Dragic *et al.*, 1996; Feng *et al.*, 1996). The best example of genetic factors affecting susceptibility to HIV infection or the rate of progression to AIDS is the characterization of CCR5-delta 32 mutation, a 32 base pair deletion in the single coding exon of the gene (Dean *et al.*, 1996; Liu *et al.*, 1996; Samson *et al.*, 1996). Homozygous expression of the mutant CCR5-delta 32 allele has been shown to provide almost complete protection against HIV-1 infection by so-called R5 strains (strains using CCR5 as a coreceptor), but not X4 strains, which use the CXCR4 coreceptor for entry (Liu *et al.*, 1996). Individuals heterozygous for this mutation have been shown to experience a slower progression to AIDS (by 2–4 years on average) after HIV-1 seroconversion (Dean *et al.*, 1996; Huang *et al.*, 1996; Michael *et al.*, 1997; Zimmerman *et al.*, 1997) and protection from AIDS-related lymphoma (Dean *et al.*, 1999; Rabkin *et al.*, 1999). However, the frequency of this mutant CCR5-delta 32 allele is quite different among different populations. It was found at a high allele frequency of approximately 10% in some Northern European populations, but is rare or absent in Asia and has not been found in populations of sub-Saharan African origin (Hill, 1998; Martinson *et al.*, 1997). In the United States, the frequency of the allele is 11% in white persons but only 1.7% in individuals of African descent (Carrington *et al.*, 1999a; Hogan and Hammer, 2001). In addition, mutations in the untranslated promotor region of the CCR5 gene have been shown to impact HIV disease progression, potentially by altering CCR5 gene expression (Mummidi *et al.*, 1997). For instance, the point mutation 59029 (A to G) has been associated with a retardation of the spontaneous HIV disease process (McDermott *et al.*, 1998). Moreover, individuals with a homozygous CCR5-59356-T mutation, which is most commonly encountered in persons of African descent, have a higher risk for a perinatal HIV acquisition (Kostrikis *et al.*, 1999).

An additional genetic marker that significantly impacts spontaneous HIV disease progression is the CC-chemokine receptor 2 (CCR2) V641 mutation. This genetic alteration does not result in a differential cell surface expression of CCR2, nor does it affect the susceptibility to HIV infection; yet, in a number of epidemiological surveys, HIV-infected individuals with a heterozygous or homozygous mutation at this gene locus had a substantially slower disease progression (Hendel *et al.*, 1998; Martin *et al.*, 1998; Meyer *et al.*, 1999; Smith *et al.*, 1997). In contrast to the

CCR5Δ32 mutation, which is predominantly found in persons of Caucasoid descent, the frequency of the CCR2 V641 mutation seems to be more equally distributed over divergent ethnicities, being present in 10–25% of subjects in Caucasians and all other ethnic groups (Hogan and Hammer, 2001).

A third genetic factor that apparently influences HIV disease progression involves the stromal derived factor 1 (SDF-1). SDF-1 represents the physiologic ligand for the chemokine receptor CXCR-4, which serves as a co-receptor for viral X4 strains (Bleul *et al.*, 1996; Oberlin *et al.*, 1996). A single base mutation (SDF 1–3'a) results in an up-regulated biosynthesis of the SDF-1, which might then competitively inhibit viral binding to CXCR-4 and thus interfere with X4 viral entry into target cells (Hogan and Hammer, 2001). Individuals with a homozygous SDF 1–3'a mutation may experience a slower progression to AIDS, but seem to have an unaltered risk for the acquisition of an HIV infection (Hendel *et al.*, 1998; Martin *et al.*, 1998; Winkler *et al.*, 1998). Finally, a recent study suggested that a mutation in the CX3CR1 might also influence the dynamics of the HIV disease process: Homozygosity for the haplotype CX3CR1 I249 M280 has been shown to accelerate progression to AIDS (Faure *et al.*, 2000).

GENETICS AND IMMUNE RESPONSES TO HIV-1 INFECTION

The association between HLA type and HIV resistance implies that HLA-restricted immune responses may play a role in resistance to HIV infection, and many studies have been performed to investigate the impact of HLA-restricted cytotoxic T lymphocytes (CTL) responses on HIV infection since the first demonstration of cytotoxic T-cell immune responses to HIV in infected individuals in 1987 (Plata *et al.*, 1987; Walker *et al.*, 1987). Accumulating evidence has shown that HIV-1-specific CTL play a central role in the control of viremia after primary infection (Borrow *et al.*, 1994; Koup *et al.*, 1994) and thus in long-term AIDS-free survival from the infection (Altfeld and Rosenberg, 2000; Goulder *et al.*, 1999; McMichael *et al.*, 2000). High levels of HIV-1-specific CTL are detectable in subjects with asymptomatic chronic infection (Harrer *et al.*, 1994; Harrer *et al.*, 1996a; Harrer *et al.*, 1996b; Rinaldo *et al.*, 1995; Walker *et al.*, 1987), but generally decline with disease progression (Klein *et al.*, 1995). The critical role of virus-specific CTL responses in the control of viremia has been directly demonstrated by $CD8^+$ T cell depletion studies in SIV infection in macaques showing that $CD8^+$ T cells effectively suppress viral replication (Jin *et al.*, 1999; Schmitz *et al.*, 1999). The immune activity generated during acute infection in particular appears to be a critical determinant of the ultimate speed of progression to disease (Allen *et al.*, 2000; Barouch *et al.*, 2000; Borrow *et al.*, 1994; Borrow *et al.*, 1997; Koup *et al.*, 1994; Rosenberg *et al.*, 2000). Recent data derived from HIV-1-infected individuals who were treated during acute HIV-1 infection furthermore showed enhancement of both CTL and T helper cell responses against HIV-1 associated with at least transient viral control following supervised treatment interruptions (Rosenberg *et al.*, 2000). Therefore, the induction and maintenance of HIV-1-specific $CD8^+$ T cell responses is considered to be a key element in the development of effective HIV-1 vaccines (Allen *et al.*, 2000; Amara *et al.*, 2001; Barouch *et al.*, 2000; Barouch *et al.*, 2002; Shiver *et al.*, 2002).

There is growing evidence that there are qualitative differences in the CTL responses generated by infected individuals, and that these may influence long-term control of the infection and, ultimately, the prognosis. Studies in acute retroviral infections in animal models have suggested that $CD8^+$ T cell responses directed against immunodominant CTL epitopes may be importantly involved in the initial control of viral replication (Allen *et al.*, 2000; Barouch *et al.*, 2002). Our recent studies indicated that immunodominant viral epitopes consistently targeted during acute HIV-1 infection can be identified for certain HLA class I alleles, but that differences in the pattern of development of epitope-specific CTL responses exist among different HLA class I alleles in HIV-1 infection (Goulder *et al.*, 2001; Yu *et al.*, 2002). The strong influence of the HLA class I genotype of an individual upon the selection of HIV-1-specific immnunodominant epitopes has been observed for HLA-A2 (Goulder *et al.*, 1997b), -A3 (Yu *et al.*, 2002), -B27 (Goulder *et al.*, 1997a), -B14 (Kalams *et al.*, 1996), and many other examples in other viral infections, for example HLA-A11-restricted Epstein-Barr virus-specific responses (Levitsky *et al.*, 1996).

In addition, HLA allele frequencies at a population level may impact the clustering of HIV-1-specific T cell responses, as shown in more recent studies. While the different HIV-1 proteins are targeted at similar frequencies in Caucasians, Africans,and Chinese (Addo *et al.*, 2003; Altfeld *et al.*, 2001; Betts *et al*, 2001; Novitsky *et al.*, 2001; Novitsky *et al.*, 2002; Novitsky *et al.*, 2003; Yu, *et al.*, unpublished data), HIV-1-specific T cell responses tend to cluster in different regions of these proteins in these different ethnicities (Goulder *et al.*, 2000), as shown by the clustering of T cell responses in the whole genome for Chinese and Caucasians in Figure 1, and this differential clustering of cellular immune responses was linked to the expression of different predominant HLA class I alleles. Recent data in infected individuals of Chinese origin demonstrated that described optimal epitopes restricted by the most frequently expressed HLA class I alleles in the studied Chinese (HLA-A11, -24,and B-4001) were contained within the frequently targeted regions in infected Chinese and recognized by the corresponding virus-specific T cells. In the studies of Goulder *et al.*, the differential clustering was due to the predominance of HLA-B42- and -B81-restricted $CD8^+$ T cell responses directed against an immunodominant p24 Gag epitope in infected Africans studied, while virus-specific T cells from Caucasians targeted HLA-A2- and -A3-restricted epitopes in p17-Gag. Taken together, these data suggest that the differential clustering of virus-specific T cell responses in different ethnicities is influenced by the differences in the genetic HLA class I background in these populations.

During both acute and chronic HIV infection, the virus is under constant attack of HIV-specific $CD8^+$ T cells that can eliminate HIV-infected cells by direct MHC-class I restricted cytolysis. MHC (HLA) molecules are expressed on a variety of antigen-presenting cells and can bind viral peptides that then become visible to immune cells and can subsequently be targeted. Thus, the repertoire of HLA molecules present in an individual plays a critical role for the quality of the immune response a person is able to generate. In general, individuals with heterozygous HLA class I alleles are able to present a broader selection of viral epitopes than persons with homozygous alleles, typically resulting in a wider range of viral regions being targeted by the immune system (Bodmer, 1972). Moreover, individuals with rare HLA class I types seem to have an advantageous ability to generate effective HIV-specific immune responses, probably because the virus is less frequently exposed to immune responses generated in the context of this HLA background and therefore less able to adapt to these types of immune attack (Trachtenberg *et al.*, 2003).

At the population level, the extensive polymorphisms of the HLA gene loci ensures that HIV is targeted in every individual in a unique fashion that is determined by the HLA type class I alleles of the respective person. In other words, the heterogeneity of human HLA class I system guaranties that selected mutations in the HIV genome do not allow escape from the entire repertoire of immune responses in individuals in a given geographic location, but rather affect solely the immune responses generated in a single individual (Trachtenberg *et al.*, 2003). Recent data, however, indicate that HIV is able to specifically adapt to the repertoire of HLA class I molecules being present in a specific geographic region or ethnic constellation (Moore *et al.*, 2002). Indeed, a large analysis of viral species in Australia has recently indicated that viral mutations are frequently associated with specific HLA-class I alleles in the host (Moore *et al.*, 2002). In addition, these authors were able to show that a local or regional cluster of HLA types was linked to a geographically distinctive genetic sequence in the HIV-1 RT gene, suggesting that HLA-class I mediated immune pressure is able to shape viral gene sequences in a way that allows the virus to escape from the MHC class restricted immune pressure. A similar relationship has not yet been demonstrated in Asian countries; however, given the distinctive genetic characteristics of Asian ethnicities, it is likely that HIV-1 will similarly adapt to genetic diversity present in these communities.

GENETICS AND TREATMENT OF HIV-1 INFECTION

Ideally, one would like to be able to tailor HIV therapy based on likelihood of disease progression or based on some genetic predictor of response to a specific agent, but as yet there are insufficient data for such pharmacogenomic interventions. There are however some tantalizing associations that are being recognized that may ultimately influence clinical care. One example is hypersensitivity reactions to specific drugs. Hypersensitivity reaction is a clinical syndrome thought to be immune-mediated and described previously with many different drugs, including a number of antiretroviral agents (Balint and Gergely, 1996; Bossi *et al.*, 2000; Bourezane *et al.*, 1998; Cribb *et al.*, 1996; Demeter *et al.*, 2000; deShazo and Kemp, 1997; Goodgame *et al.*, 2000; Hamer and Morris, 1999; Herranz *et al.*, 1994; Tancrede-Bohin *et al.*, 1996; Wassef and Keiser, 1995; Weiss and Baker, 1987). About 5% (1–14%) of HIV-1-infected individuals treated with abacavir develop a hypersensitivity reaction (Mallal *et al.*, 2002), which can represent a life-threatening reaction characterized by multisystem involvement (Hetherington *et al.*, 2001a). More than 93% of abacavir hypersensitivity reactions occur within the first 6 weeks of treatment (median time to onset 11 days) (Hetherington *et al.*, 2001a). Symptoms related to the hypersensitivity reaction worsen with continued therapy and usually improve within 24 hours of abacavir discontinuation. Rechallenge with abacavir after a hypersensitivity reaction typically results in recurrence of symptoms within hours, with the potential to induce a more severe clinical syndrome with increased risk of life-threatening hypotension and death (Escaut *et al.*, 1999).

The mechanism of the hypersensitivity reaction to abacavir is not yet known. However, previous studies in the pathogenesis of several similar multisystem drug hypersensitivity reactions indicated the involvement of MHC-restricted presentation of drug or drug metabolites, with direct binding of these non-peptide antigens to MHC molecules or haptention to endogenous proteins before I cell presentation (Park *et al.*, 2001; Schnyder *et al.*, 2000; Zanni *et al.*, 1998). Several recent studies have investigated the association between genetic factors and susceptibility to hypersensitivity to abacavir. The analysis from the clinical trials involving 5332 individuals reported by Hetherington *et al.* (2001b) showed that ethnic origin might influence abacavir hypersensitivity, with about a 40% reduction in the risk associated with African descent. In a study of 200 consecutive abacavir-treated individuals in the Western Australian HIV Cohort, the presence of the HLA-B*5701, HLA-DR7, HLA-DQ3 haplotype was strongly associated with increased risk of developing the hypersensitivity reaction syndrome (Mallal *et al.*, 2002), which once again supports an important and immediately applicable clinical role for HLA typing. Therefore, administration of abacavir to patients with the HLA-B*5701, HLA-DR7,

HLA-DQ3 haplotype should be avoided. This example demonstrates that in the future, genetic factors may play a more important role in the decision-making regarding choice of antiretroviral therapy in HIV-1 infection.

CONCLUSIONS

Host genetic factors have been shown to play an important role in the control of infectious diseases. The distinct genetic background of Asian populations may have implications for HIV disease progression, the generation of HIV-1-specific cellular immune responses, the viral evolution on the population level, as well as antiretroviral treatment strategies. Moreover, the rational design of HIV-1-specific vaccines for Asian individuals may have to take the HLA diversity in these populations into account.

REFERENCES

Addo, M.M., Yu, X.G., Rathod, A., Cohen, D., Eldridge, R.L., Strick, D., Johnston, M.N., Corcoran, C., Wurcel, A.G., Fitzpatrick, C.A., Feeney, M.E., Rodriguez, W.R., Basgoz, N., Draenert, R., Stone, D.R., Brander, C., Goulder, P.J., Rosenberg, E.S., Altfeld, M. & Walker, B.D. (2003). Comprehensive Epitope Analysis of Human Immunodeficiency Virus Type 1 (HIV-1)-Specific T-Cell Responses Directed against the Entire Expressed HIV-1 Genome Demonstrate Broadly Directed Responses, but No Correlation to Viral Load. *J Virol.* 77:2081–2092.

Alkhatib, G., Combadiere, C., Broder, C.C., Feng, Y., Kennedy, P.E., Murphy, P.M. & Berger, E.A. (1996). CC CKR5: a RANTES, MIP-1alpha, MIP-1beta receptor as a fusion cofactor for macrophage-tropic HIV-1. *Science.* 272:1955–1958.

Allen, T.M., O'Connor, D.H., Jing, P., Dzuris, J.L., Mothe, B.R., Vogel, T.U., Dunphy, E., Liebl, M.E., Emerson, C., Wilson, N., Kunstman, K.J., Wang, X., Allison, D.B., Hughes, A.L., Desrosiers, R.C., Altman, J.D., Wolinsky, S.M., Sette, A. & Watkins, D.I. (2000). Tat-specific cytotoxic T lymphocytes select for SIV escape variants during resolution of primary *viraemia. Nature.* 407:386–390.

Altfeld, M. & Rosenberg, E.S. (2000). The role of CD4(+) T helper cells in the cytotoxic T lymphocyte response to HIV-1. *Curr Opin Immunol.* 12:375–380.

Altfeld, M., Addo, M.M., Eldridge, R.L., Yu, X.G., Thomas, S., Khatri, A., Strick, D., Phillips, M.N., Cohen, G.B., Islam, S.A., Kalams, S.A., Brander, C., Goulder, P.J., Rosenberg, E.S. & Walker, B.D. (2001). Vpr is preferentially targeted by CTL during HIV-1 infection. *J Immunol.* 167:2743–2752.

Altfeld, M., Addo, M.M., Rosenberg, E.S., Hecht, F.M., Lee, P.K., Vogel, M., Yu, X.G., Draenert, R., Johnston, M.N., Strick, D., Allen, T.M., Feeney, M.E., Kahn, J.O., Sekaly, R.P., Levy, J.A., Rockstroh, J.K., Goulder, P.J. & Walker, B.D. (2003). Influence of HLA-B57 on clinical presentation and viral control during acute HIV-1 infection. *AIDS.* 17:2581–2591.

Amara, R.R., Villinger, F., Altman, J.D., Lydy, S.L., O'Neil, S.P., Staprans, S.I., Montefiori, D.C., Xu, Y., Herndon, J.G., Wyatt, L.S., Candido, M.A., Kozyr, N.L., Earl, P.L., Smith, J.M., Ma, H.L., Grimm, B.D., Hulsey, M.L., Miller, J., McClure, H.M., McNicholl, J.M., Moss, B. & Robinson, H.L. (2001). Control of a mucosal challenge and prevention of AIDS by a multiprotein DNA/MVA vaccine. *Science.* 292:69–74.

Balint, G. & Gergely, P., Jr. (1996). Clinical immunotoxicity of antirheumatic drugs. *Inflamm Res.* 45 Suppl 2:S91–S95.

Barouch, D.H., Santra, S., Schmitz, J.E., Kuroda, M.J., Fu, T.M., Wagner, W., Bilska, M., Craiu, A., Zheng, X.X., Krivulka, G.R., Beaudry, K., Lifton, M.A., Nickerson, C.E., Trigona, W.L., Punt, K., Freed, D.C., Guan, L., Dubey, S., Casimiro, D., Simon, A., Davies, M.E., Chastain, M., Strom, T.B., Gelman, R.S., Montefiori, D.C. & Lewis, M.G. (2000). Control of viremia and prevention of clinical AIDS in rhesus monkeys by cytokine-augmented DNA vaccination [In Process Citation]. *Science.* 290:486–492.

Barouch, D.H., Kunstman, J., Kuroda, M.J., Schmitz, J.E., Santra, S., Peyerl, F.W., Krivulka, G.R., Beaudry, K., Lifton, M.A., Gorgone, D.A., Montefiori, D.C., Lewis, M.G., Wolinsky, S.M. & Letvin, N.L. (2002). Eventual AIDS vaccine failure in a rhesus monkey by viral escape from cytotoxic T lymphocytes. *Nature.* 415:335–339.

Betts, M.R., Ambrozak, D.R., Douek, D.C., Bonhoeffer, S., Brenchley, J.M., Casazza, J.P., Koup, R.A. & Picker, L.J. (2001). Analysis of total human immunodeficiency virus (HIV)-specific CD4(+) and CD8(+) T-cell responses: relationship to viral load in untreated HIV infection. *J Virol.* 75:11983–11991.

Bleul, C.C., Farzan, M., Choe, H., Parolin, C., Clark-Lewis, I., Sodroski, J. & Springer, T.A. (1996). The lymphocyte chemoattractant SDF-1 is a ligand for LESTR/fusin and blocks HIV-1 entry. *Nature.* 382:829–833.

Bodmer, W.F. (1972). Evolutionary significance of the HL-A system. *Nature.* 237:139–145 passim.

Borrow, P., Lewicki, H., Hahn, B.H., Shaw, G.M. & Oldstone, M.B. (1994). Virus-specific CD8+ cytotoxic T-lymphocyte activity associated with control of viremia in primary human immunodeficiency virus type 1 infection. *J Virol.* 68:6103–6110.

Borrow, P., Lewicki, H., Wei, X., Horwitz, M.S., Peffer, N., Meyers, H., Nelson, J.A., Gairin, J.E., Hahn, B.H., Oldstone, M.B. & Shaw, G.M. (1997). Antiviral pressure exerted by HIV-1-specific cytotoxic T lymphocytes (CTLs) during primary infection demonstrated by rapid selection of CTL escape virus. *Nat Med.* 3:205–211.

Bossi, P., Colin, D., Bricaire, F. & Caumes, E. (2000). Hypersensitivity syndrome associated with efavirenz therapy. *Clin Infect Dis.* 30:227–228.

Bothamley, G.H., Beck, J.S., Schreuder, G.M., D'Amaro, J., de Vries, R.R., Kardjito, T. & Ivanyi, J. (1989). Association of tuberculosis and M. tuberculosis-specific antibody levels with HLA. *J Infect Dis.* 159:549–555.

Bourezane, Y., Salard, D., Hoen, B., Vandel, S., Drobacheff, C. & Laurent, R. (1998). DRESS (drug rash with eosinophilia and systemic symptoms) syndrome associated with nevirapine therapy. *Clin Infect Dis.* 27:1321–1322.

Brahmajothi, V., Pitchappan, R.M., Kakkanaiah, V.N., Sashidhar, M., Rajaram, K., Ramu, S., Palanimurugan, K., Paramasivan, C.N. & Prabhakar, R. (1991). Association of pulmonary tuberculosis and HLA in south India. *Tubercle.* 72:123–132.

Cao, K., Hollenbach, J., Shi, X., Shi, W., Chopek, M. & Fernandez-Vina, M.A. (2001). Analysis of the frequencies of HLA-A, B, and C alleles and haplotypes in the five major ethnic groups of the United States reveals high levels of diversity in these loci and contrasting distribution patterns in these populations. *Hum Immunol.* 62:1009–1030.

Carrington, M., Dean, M., Martin, M.P. & O'Brien, S.J. (1999a). Genetics of HIV-1 infection: chemokine receptor CCR5 polymorphism and its consequences. *Hum Mol Genet.* 8:1939–1945.

Carrington, M., Nelson, G.W., Martin, M.P., Kissner, T., Vlahov, D., Goedert, J.J., Kaslow, R., Buchbinder, S., Hoots, K. & O'Brien, S.J. (1999b). HLA and HIV-1: heterozygote advantage and B*35-Cw*04 disadvantage. *Science.* 283:1748–1752.

Choe, H., Farzan, M., Sun, Y., Sullivan, N., Rollins, B., Ponath, P.D., Wu, L., Mackay, C.R., LaRosa, G., Newman, W., Gerard, N., Gerard, C. & Sodroski, J. (1996). The beta-chemokine receptors CCR3 and CCR5 facilitate infection by primary HIV-1 isolates. *Cell.* 85:1135–1148.

Costello, C., Tang, J., Rivers, C., Karita, E., Meizen-Derr, J., Allen, S. & Kaslow, R.A. (1999). HLA-B*5703 independently associated with slower HIV-1 disease progression in Rwandan women. *AIDS.* 13:1990–1991.

Cribb, A.E., Lee, B.L., Trepanier, L.A. & Spielberg, S.P. (1996). Adverse reactions to sulphonamide and sulphonamide-trimethoprim antimicrobials: clinical syndromes and pathogenesis. *Adverse Drug React Toxicol Rev.* 15:9–50.

Dean, M., Carrington, M., Winkler, C., Huttley, G.A., Smith, M.W., Allikmets, R., Goedert, J.J., Buchbinder, S.P., Vittinghoff, E., Gomperts, E., Donfield, S., Vlahov, D., Kaslow, R., Saah, A., Rinaldo, C., Detels, R. & O'Brien, S.J. (1996). Genetic restriction of HIV-1 infection and progression to AIDS by a deletion allele of the CKR5 structural gene. Hemophilia Growth and Development Study, Multicenter AIDS Cohort Study, Multicenter Hemophilia Cohort Study, San Francisco City Cohort, ALIVE Study. *Science.* 273:1856–1862.

Dean, M., Jacobson, L.P., McFarlane, G., Margolick, J.B., Jenkins, F.J., Howard, O.M., Dong, H.F., Goedert, J.J., Buchbinder, S., Gomperts, E., Vlahov, D., Oppenheim, J.J., O'Brien, S.J. & Carrington, M. (1999). Reduced risk of AIDS lymphoma in individuals heterozygous for the CCR5-delta32 mutation. *Cancer Res.* 59:3561–3564.

Demeter, L.M., Shafer, R.W., Meehan, P.M., Holden-Wiltse, J., Fischl, M.A., Freimuth, W.W., Para, M.F. & Reichman, R.C. (2000). Delavirdine susceptibilities and associated reverse transcriptase mutations in human immunodeficiency virus type 1 isolates from patients in a phase I/II trial of delavirdine monotherapy (ACTG 260). *Antimicrob Agents Chemother.* 44:794–797.

Deng, H., Liu, R., Ellmeier, W., Choe, S., Unutmaz, D., Burkhart, M., Di Marzio, P., Marmon, S., Sutton, R.E., Hill, C.M., Davis, C.B., Peiper, S. C., Schall, T.J., Littman, D.R. & Landau, N.R. (1996). Identification of a major co-receptor for primary isolates of HIV-1. *Nature.* 381:661–666.

deShazo, R.D. & Kemp, S.F. (1997). Allergic reactions to drugs and biologic agents. *JAMA* 278:1895–1906.

Doherty, P.C. & Zinkernagel, R.M. (1975). A biological role for the major histocompatibility antigens. *Lancet.* 1:1406–1409.

Doranz, B.J., Rucker, J., Yi, Y., Smyth, R.J., Samson, M., Peiper, S.C., Parmentier, M., Collman, R.G. & Doms, R.W. (1996). A dual-tropic primary HIV-1 isolate that uses fusin and the beta-chemokine receptors CKR-5, CKR-3, and CKR-2b as fusion cofactors. *Cell.* 85:1149–1158.

Dragic, T., Litwin, V., Allaway, G.P., Martin, S.R., Huang, Y., Nagashima, K.A., Cayanan, C., Maddon, P.J., Koup, R.A., Moore, J.P. & Paxton, W.A. (1996). HIV-1 entry into CD4+ cells is mediated by the chemokine receptor CC-CKR-5. *Nature.* 381:667–673.

Escaut, L., Liotier, J.Y., Albengres, E., Cheminot, N. & Vittecoq, D. (1999). Abacavir rechallenge has to be avoided in case of hypersensitivity reaction. *AIDS.* 13:1419–1420.

Faure, S., Meyer, L., Costagliola, D., Vaneensberghe, C., Genin, E., Autran, B., Delfraissy, J.F., McDermott, D.H., Murphy, P.M., Debre, P., Theodorou, I. & Combadiere, C. (2000). Rapid progression to AIDS in HIV+ individuals with a structural variant of the chemokine receptor CX3CR1. *Science.* 287:2274–2277.

Feng, Y., Broder, C.C., Kennedy, P.E. & Berger, E.A. (1996). HIV-1 entry cofactor: functional cDNA cloning of a seven-transmembrane, G protein-coupled receptor. *Science.* 272:872–877.

Flores-Villanueva, P.O., Yunis, E.J., Delgado, J.C., Vittinghoff, E., Buchbinder, S., Leung, J.Y., Uglialoro, A.M., Clavijo, O.P., Rosenberg, E.S., Kalams, S.A., Braun, J.D., Boswell, S.L., Walker, B.D. & Goldfeld, A.E. (2001). Control of HIV-1 viremia and protection from AIDS are associated with HLA-Bw4 homozygosity. *Proc Natl Acad Sci U S A.* 98:5140–5145.

Gao, X., Nelson, G.W., Karacki, P., Martin, M.P., Phair, J., Kaslow, R., Goedert, J.J., Buchbinder, S., Hoots, K., Vlahov, D., O'Brien, S.J. & Carrington, M. (2001). Effect of a single amino acid change in MHC class I molecules on the rate of progression to AIDS. *N Engl J Med.* 344:1668–1675.

Goodgame, J.C., Pottage, J.C., Jr., Jablonowski, H., Hardy, W.D., Stein, A., Fischl, M., Morrow, P., Feinberg, J., Brothers, C.H., Vafidis, I., Nacci, P., Yeo, J. & Pedneault, L. (2000). Amprenavir in combination with lamivudine and zidovudine versus lamivudine and zidovudine alone in HIV-1-infected antiretroviral-naive adults. Amprenavir PROAB3001 International Study Team. *Antivir Ther.* 5:215–225.

Goulder, P.J., Bunce, M., Krausa, P., McIntyre, K., Crowley, S., Morgan, B., Edwards, A., Giangrande, P., Phillips, R.E. & McMichael, A.J. (1996). Novel, cross-restricted, conserved, and immunodominant cytotoxic T lymphocyte epitopes in slow progressors in HIV type 1 infection. *AIDS Res Hum Retroviruses.* 12:1691–1698.

Goulder, P.J., Phillips, R.E., Colbert, R.A., McAdam, S., Ogg, G., Nowak, M.A., Giangrande, P., Luzzi, G., Morgan, B., Edwards, A., McMichael, A.J. & Rowland-Jones, S. (1997a). Late escape from an immunodominant cytotoxic T-lymphocyte response associated with progression to AIDS. *Nat Med.* 3:212–217.

Goulder, P.J., Sewell, A.K., Lalloo, D.G., Price, D.A., Whelan, J.A., Evans, J., Taylor, G.P., Luzzi, G., Giangrande, P., Phillips, R.E. & McMichael, A.J. (1997b). Patterns of immunodominance in HIV-1-specific cytotoxic T lymphocyte responses in two human histocompatibility leukocyte antigens (HLA)- identical siblings with HLA-A*0201 are influenced by epitope mutation. *J Exp Med.* 185:1423–1433.

Goulder, P.J., Rowland-Jones, S.L., McMichael, A.J. & Walker, B.D. (1999). Anti-HIV cellular immunity: recent advances towards vaccine design. *AIDS.* 13:S121–S136.

Goulder, P.J., Brander, C., Annamalai, K., Mngqundaniso, N., Govender, U., Tang, Y., He, S., Hartman, K.E., O'Callaghan, C.A., Ogg, G.S., Altfeld, M.A., Rosenberg, E.S., Cao, H., Kalams, S.A., Hammond, M., Bunce, M., Pelton, S.I., Burchett, S.A., McIntosh, K., Coovadia, H.M. & Walker, B.D. (2000). Differential narrow focusing of immunodominant human immunodeficiency virus *gag*-specific cytotoxic T-lymphocyte responses in infected African and caucasoid adults and children [In Process Citation]. *J Virol.* 74:5679–5690.

Goulder, P.J., Altfeld, M.A., Rosenberg, E.S., Nguyen, T., Tang, Y., Eldridge, R.L., Addo, M.M., He, S., Mukherjee, J.S., Phillips, M.N., Bunce, M., Kalams, S.A., Sekaly, R.P., Walker, B.D. & Brander, C. (2001). Substantial Differences in Specificity of HIV-specific Cytotoxic T Cells in Acute and Chronic HIV Infection. *J Exp Med.* 193:181–194.

Hamer, H.M. & Morris, H.H. (1999). Hypersensitivity syndrome to antiepileptic drugs: a review including new anticonvulsants. *Cleve Clin J Med.* 66:239–245.

Harrer, E., Harrer, T., Buchbinder, S., Mann, D.L., Feinberg, M., Yilma, T., Johnson, R.P. & Walker, B.D. (1994). HIV-1-specific cytotoxic T lymphocyte response in healthy, long-term nonprogressing seropositive persons. *AIDS Res Hum Retroviruses.* 10:S77–S78.

Harrer, T., Harrer, E., Kalams, S.A., Barbosa, P., Trocha, A., Johnson, R.P., Elbeik, T., Feinberg, M.B., Buchbinder, S.P. & Walker, B.D. (1996a). Cytotoxic T lymphocytes in asymptomatic long-term nonprogressing HIV-1 infection. Breadth and specificity of the response and relation to in vivo viral quasispecies in a person with prolonged infection and low viral load. *Journal of Immunology.* 156:2616–2623.

Harrer, T., Harrer, E., Kalams, S.A., Elbeik, T., Staprans, S.I., Feinberg, M.B., Cao, Y., Ho, D.D., Yilma, T., Caliendo, A.M., Johnson, R.P., Buchbinder, S.P. & Walker, B.D. (1996b). Strong cytotoxic T cell and weak neutralizing antibody responses in a subset of persons with stable nonprogressing HIV type 1 infection. *AIDS Research & Human Retroviruses.* 12:585–592.

Hendel, H., Henon, N., Lebuanec, H., Lachgar, A., Poncelet, H., Caillat-Zucman, S., Winkler, C.A., Smith,

M.W., Kenefic, L., O'Brien, S., Lu, W., Andrieu, J.M., Zagury, D., Schachter, F., Rappaport, J. & Zagury, J.F. (1998). Distinctive effects of CCR5, CCR2, and SDF1 genetic polymorphisms in AIDS progression. *J Acquir Immune Defic Syndr Hum Retrovirol.* 19:381–386.

Hendel, H., Caillat-Zucman, S., Lebuanec, H., Carrington, M., O'Brien, S., Andrieu, J.M., Schachter, F., Zagury, D., Rappaport, J., Winkler, C., Nelson, G.W. & Zagury, J.F. (1999). New class I and II HLA alleles strongly associated with opposite patterns of progression to AIDS. *J Immunol.* 162:6942–6946.

Herranz, P., Fernandez-Diaz, M.L., de Lucas, R., Gonzalez-Garcia, J. & Casado, M. (1994). Cutaneous vasculitis associated with didanosine. *Lancet.* 344:680.

Hetherington, S., McGuirk, S., Powell, G., Cutrell, A., Naderer, O., Spreen, B., Lafon, S., Pearce, G. & Steel, H. (2001a). Hypersensitivity reactions during therapy with the nucleoside reverse transcriptase inhibitor abacavir. *Clin Ther.* 23:1603–1614.

Hetherington, S., Steel, H., Lafon, S. & al, e. (2001b). Safety and tolerance of abacavir (1596, ABC) alone and in combination therapy of HIV infection. *In: Program and abstracts of the 12th International Conference on AIDS (Geneva). Stockholm: International AIDS Society [abstract 12353].*

Hill, A.V. (1998). The immunogenetics of human infectious diseases. *Annu Rev Immunol.* 16:593–617.

Hill, A. V. (2001). The genomics and genetics of human infectious disease susceptibility. *Annu Rev Genomics Hum Genet.* 2:373–400.

Hill, A.V., Allsopp, C.E., Kwiatkowski, D., Anstey, N.M., Twumasi, P., Rowe, P.A., Bennett, S., Brewster, D., McMichael, A.J. & Greenwood, B. M. (1991). Common west African HLA antigens are associated with protection from severe malaria. *Nature.* 352:595–600.

Hogan, C.M. & Hammer, S. M. (2001). Host determinants in HIV infection and disease. Part 2: genetic factors and implications for antiretroviral therapeutics. *Ann Intern Med.* 134:978–996.

Huang, Y., Paxton, W.A., Wolinsky, S.M., Neumann, A.U., Zhang, L., He, T., Kang, S., Ceradini, D., Jin, Z., Yazdanbakhsh, K., Kunstman, K., Erickson, D., Dragon, E., Landau, N.R., Phair, J., Ho, D.D. & Koup, R.A. (1996). The role of a mutant CCR5 allele in HIV-1 transmission and disease progression. *Nat Med.* 2:1240–1243.

Itescu, S., Mathur-Wagh, U., Skovron, M.L., Brancato, L.J., Marmor, M., Zeleniuch-Jacquotte, A. & Winchester, R. (1992). HLA-B35 is associated with accelerated progression to AIDS. *J Acquir Immune Defic Syndr.* 5:37–45.

Jeannet, M., Sztajzel, R., Carpentier, N., Hirschel, B. & Tiercy, J. M. (1989). HLA antigens are risk factors for development of AIDS. *J Acquir Immune Defic Syndr.* 2:28–32.

Jin, X., Bauer, D.E., Tuttleton, S.E., Lewin, S., Gettie, A., Blanchard, J., Irwin, C.E., Safrit, J.T., Mittler, J., Weinberger, L., Kostrikis, L.G., Zhang, L., Perelson, A.S. & Ho, D.D. (1999). Dramatic rise in plasma viremia after CD8(+) T cell depletion in simian immunodeficiency virus-infected macaques. *J Exp Med.* 189:991–998.

Kalams, S.A., Johnson, R.P., Dynan, M.J., Hartman, K.E., Harrer, T., Harrer, E., Trocha, A.K., Blattner, W.A., Buchbinder, S.P. & Walker, B.D. (1996). T cell receptor usage and fine specificity of human immunodeficiency virus 1-specific cytotoxic T lymphocyte clones: analysis of quasispecies recognition reveals a dominant response directed against a minor in vivo variant. *J Exp Med.* 183:1669–1679.

Kaslow, R.A., Carrington, M., Apple, R., Park, L., Munoz, A., Saah, A.J., Goedert, J.J., Winkler, C., O'Brien, S.J., Rinaldo, C., Detels, R., Blattner, W., Phair, J., Erlich, H. & Mann, D.L. (1996). Influence of combinations of human major histocompatibility complex genes on the course of HIV-1 infection [see comments]. *Nat Med.* 2:405–411.

Kaslow, R.A., Rivers, C., Tang, J., Bender, T.J., Goepfert, P.A., El Habib, R., Weinhold, K. & Mulligan, M.J. (2001). Polymorphisms in HLA class I genes associated with both favorable prognosis of human immunodeficiency virus (HIV) type 1 infection and positive cytotoxic T-lymphocyte responses to ALVAC-HIV recombinant canarypox vaccines. *J Virol.* 75:8681–8689.

Keet, I.P., Tang, J., Klein, M.R., LeBlanc, S., Enger, C., Rivers, C., Apple, R.J., Mann, D., Goedert, J.J., Miedema, F. & Kaslow, R.A. (1999). Consistent associations of HLA class I and II and transporter gene products with progression of human immunodeficiency virus type 1 infection in homosexual men. *J Infect Dis.* 180:299–309.

Kelleher, A.D., Long, C., Holmes, E.C., Allen, R.L., Wilson, J., Conlon, C., Workman, C., Shaunak, S., Olson, K., Goulder, P., Brander, C., Ogg, G., Sullivan, J.S., Dyer, W., Jones, I., McMichael, A.J., Rowland-Jones, S. & Phillips, R.E. (2001). Clustered mutations in HIV-1 *gag* are consistently required for escape from HLA-B27-restricted cytotoxic T lymphocyte responses. *J Exp Med.* 193: 375–386.

Khomenko, A.G., Litvinov, V.I., Chukanova, V.P. & Pospelov, L.E. (1990). Tuberculosis in patients with various HLA phenotypes. *Tubercle.* 71:187–192.

Klein, M.R., van Baalen, C.A., Holwerda, A.M., Kerkhof Garde, S.R., Bende, R.J., Keet, I.P., Eeftinck-Schattenkerk, J.K., Osterhaus, A.D., Schuitemaker, H. & Miedema, F. (1995). Kinetics of Gag-specific cytotoxic T lymphocyte responses during the clinical course of HIV-1 infection: a longitudinal analysis of rapid progressors and long-term asymptomatics. *J Exp Med.* 181:1365–1372.

Klein, M.R., van der Burg, S.H., Hovenkamp, E., Holwerda, A.M., Drijfhout, J.W., Melief, C.J. & Miedema, F. (1998). Characterization of HLA-B57-restricted human immunodeficiency virus type 1 Gag and RT-specific cytotoxic T lymphocyte responses. *Journal of General Virology.* 79:2191–2201.

Kostrikis, L.G., Neumann, A.U., Thomson, B., Korber, B.T., McHardy, P., Karanicolas, R., Deutsch, L., Huang, Y., Lew, J.F., McIntosh, K., Pollack, H., Borkowsky, W., Spiegel, H.M., Palumbo, P., Oleske, J., Bardeguez, A., Luzuriaga, K., Sullivan, J., Wolinsky, S.M., Koup, R.A., Ho, D.D. & Moore, J.P. (1999). A polymorphism in the regulatory region of the CC-chemokine receptor 5 gene influences perinatal transmission of human immunodeficiency virus type 1 to African-American infants. *J Virol.* 73:10264–10271.

Koup, R.A., Safrit, J.T., Cao, Y., Andrews, C.A., McLeod, G., Borkowsky, W., Farthing, C. & Ho, D.D. (1994). Temporal association of cellular immune responses with the initial control of viremia in primary human immunodeficiency virus type 1 syndrome. *Journal of Virology.* 68:4650–4655.

Levitsky, V., Zhang, Q.J., Levitskaya, J. & Masucci, M.G. (1996). The life span of major histocompatibility complex-peptide complexes influences the efficiency of presentation and immunogenicity of two class I-restricted cytotoxic T lymphocyte epitopes in the Epstein-Barr virus nuclear antigen 4. *J Exp Med.* 183:915–926.

Lipsitch, M., Bergstrom, C.T. & Antia, R. (2003). Effect of human leukocyte antigen heterozygosity on infectious disease outcome: the need for allele-specific measures. *BMC Med Genet.* 4:2.

Liu, R., Paxton, W.A., Choe, S., Ceradini, D., Martin, S.R., Horuk, R., MacDonald, M.E., Stuhlmann, H., Koup, R.A. & Landau, N.R. (1996). Homozygous defect in HIV-1 coreceptor accounts for resistance of some multiply-exposed individuals to HIV-1 infection. *Cell.* 86:367–377.

The MHC Sequencing Consortium. (1999). Complete sequence and gene map of a human major histocompatibility complex. *Nature.* 401:921–923.

Mallal, S., Nolan, D., Witt, C., Masel, G., Martin, A.M., Moore, C., Sayer, D., Castley, A., Mamotte, C., Maxwell, D., James, I. & Christiansen, F. T. (2002). Association between presence of HLA-B*5701, HLA-DR7, and HLA-DQ3 and hypersensitivity to HIV-1 reverse-transcriptase inhibitor abacavir. *Lancet.* 359:727–732.

Martin, M.P., Dean, M., Smith, M.W., Winkler, C., Gerrard, B., Michael, N.L., Lee, B., Doms, R.W., Margolick, J., Buchbinder, S., Goedert, J.J., O'Brien, T.R., Hilgartner, M.W., Vlahov, D., O'Brien, S.J. & Carrington, M. (1998). Genetic acceleration of AIDS progression by a promoter variant of CCR5. *Science.* 282:1907–1911.

Martinson, J.J., Chapman, N.H., Rees, D.C., Liu, Y.T. & Clegg, J.B. (1997). Global distribution of the CCR5 gene 32-basepair deletion. *Nat Genet.* 16:100–103.

McDermott, D.H., Zimmerman, P.A., Guignard, F., Kleeberger, C.A., Leitman, S.F. & Murphy, P.M. (1998). CCR5 promoter polymorphism and HIV-1 disease progression. Multicenter AIDS Cohort Study (MACS). *Lancet.* 352:866–870.

McMichael, A.J., Callan, M., Appay, V., Hanke, T., Ogg, G. & Rowland-Jones, S. (2000). The dynamics of the cellular immune response to HIV infection: implications for vaccination. *Philos Trans R Soc Lond B Biol Sci.* 355:1007–1011.

McNeil, A.J., Yap, P.L., Gore, S.M., Brettle, R.P., McColl, M., Wyld, R., Davidson, S., Weightman, R., Richardson, A.M. & Robertson, J.R. (1996). Association of HLA types A1-B8-DR3 and B27 with rapid and slow progression of HIV disease. *Qjm.* 89:177–185.

Meyer, L., Magierowska, M., Hubert, J.B., Theodorou, I., van Rij, R., Prins, M., de Roda Husman, A.M., Coutinho, R. & Schuitemaker, H. (1999). CC-chemokine receptor variants, SDF-1 polymorphism, and disease progression in 720 HIV-infected patients. SEROCO Cohort. Amsterdam Cohort Studies on AIDS. *AIDS.* 13:624–626.

Michael, N.L., Chang, G., Louie, L.G., Mascola, J.R., Dondero, D., Birx, D.L. & Sheppard, H.W. (1997). The role of viral phenotype and CCR-5 gene defects in HIV-1 transmission and disease progression. *Nat Med.* 3:338–340.

Moore, C.B., John, M., James, I.R., Christiansen, F.T., Witt, C.S. & Mallal, S.A. (2002). Evidence of HIV-1 adaptation to HLA-restricted immune responses at a population level. *Science.* 296:1439–1443.

Mummidi, S., Ahuja, S.S., McDaniel, B.L. & Ahuja, S.K. (1997). The human CC chemokine receptor 5 (CCR5) gene. Multiple transcripts with 5'-end heterogeneity, dual promoter usage, and evidence for polymorphisms within the regulatory regions and noncoding exons. *J Biol Chem.* 272:30662–30671.

Novitsky, V., Rybak, N., McLane, M.F., Gilbert, P., Chigwedere, P., Klein, I., Gaolekwe, S., Chang, S.Y., Peter, T., Thior, I., Ndung'u, T., Vannberg, F., Foley, B.T., Marlink, R., Lee, T.H. & Essex, M. (2001). Identification of human immunodeficiency virus type 1 subtype C Gag-, Tat-, Rev-, and Nef-specific elispot-based cytotoxic T-lymphocyte responses for AIDS vaccine design. *J Virol.* 75:9210–9228.

Novitsky, V., Cao, H., Rybak, N., Gilbert, P., McLane, M.F., Gaolekwe, S., Peter, T., Thior, I., Ndung'u, T., Marlink, R., Lee, T.H. & Essex, M. (2002).

Magnitude and frequency of cytotoxic T-lymphocyte responses: identification of immunodominant regions of human immunodeficiency virus type 1 subtype C. *J Virol.* 76:10155–10168.

Novitsky, V., Gilbert, P., Peter, T., McLane, M.F., Gaolekwe, S., Rybak, N., Thior, I., Ndung'u, T., Marlink, R., Lee, T.H. & Essex, M. (2003). Association between virus-specific T-cell responses and plasma viral load in human immunodeficiency virus type 1 subtype C infection. *J Virol.* 77:882–890.

Oberlin, E., Amara, A., Bachelerie, F., Bessia, C., Virelizier, J.L., Arenzana-Seisdedos, F., Schwartz, O., Heard, J.M., Clark-Lewis, I., Legler, D.F., Loetscher, M., Baggiolini, M. & Moser, B. (1996). The CXC chemokine SDF-1 is the ligand for LESTR/fusin and prevents infection by T-cell-line-adapted HIV-1. *Nature.* 382:833–835.

O'Brien, S.J., Gao, X. & Carrington, M. (2001). HLA and AIDS: a cautionary tale. *Trends Mol Med.* 7:379–381.

Park, B.K., Naisbitt, D.J., Gordon, S.F., Kitteringham, N.R. & Pirmohamed, M. (2001). Metabolic activation in drug allergies. *Toxicology.* 158:11–23.

Peano, G., Menardi, G., Ponzetto, A. & Fenoglio, L.M. (1994). HLA-DR5 antigen. A genetic factor influencing the outcome of hepatitis C virus infection? *Arch Intern Med.* 154:2733–2736.

Plata, F., Autran, B., Martins, L.P., Wain-Hobson, S., Raphael, M., Mayaud, C., Denis, M., Guillon, J.M. & Debre, P. (1987). AIDS virus-specific cytotoxic T lymphocytes in lung disorders. *Nature.* 328:348–351.

Rabkin, C.S., Yang, Q., Goedert, J.J., Nguyen, G., Mitsuya, H. & Sei, S. (1999). Chemokine and chemokine receptor gene variants and risk of non-Hodgkin's lymphoma in human immunodeficiency virus-1-infected individuals. *Blood.* 93:1838–1842.

Rani, R., Fernandez-Vina, M.A., Zaheer, S.A., Beena, K.R. & Stastny, P. (1993). Study of HLA class II alleles by PCR oligotyping in leprosy patients from north India. *Tissue Antigens.* 42:133–137.

Rinaldo, C., Huang, X.L., Fan, Z.F., Ding, M., Beltz, L., Logar, A., Panicali, D., Mazzara, G., Liebmann, J., Cottrill, M. & et al. (1995). High levels of anti-human immunodeficiency virus type 1 (HIV-1) memory cytotoxic T-lymphocyte activity and low viral load are associated with lack of disease in HIV-1-infected long-term nonprogressors. *J Virol.* 69:5838–5842.

Rosenberg, E.S., Altfeld, M., Poon, S.H., Phillips, M.N., Wilkes, B.M., Eldridge, R.L., Robbins, G.K., D'Aquila, R.T., Goulder, P.J. & Walker, B.D. (2000). Immune control of HIV-1 after early treatment of acute infection [In Process Citation]. *Nature.* 407:523–526.

Samson, M., Libert, F., Doranz, B.J., Rucker, J., Liesnard, C., Farber, C.M., Saragosti, S., Lapoumeroulie, C., Cognaux, J., Forceille, C., Muyldermans, G., Verhofstede, C., Burtonboy, G., Georges, M., Imai, T., Rana, S., Yi, Y., Smyth, R.J., Collman, R.G., Doms, R.W., Vassart, G. & Parmentier, M. (1996). Resistance to HIV-1 infection in caucasian individuals bearing mutant alleles of the CCR-5 chemokine receptor gene. *Nature.* 382:722–725.

Schmitz, J.E., Kuroda, M.J., Santra, S., Sasseville, V.G., Simon, M.A., Lifton, M.A., Racz, P., Tenner-Racz, K., Dalesandro, M., Scallon, B.J., Ghrayeb, J., Forman, M.A., Montefiori, D.C., Rieber, E.P., Letvin, N.L. & Reimann, K.A. (1999). Control of viremia in simian immunodeficiency virus infection by CD8+ lymphocytes. *Science.* 283:857–860.

Schnyder, B., Burkhart, C., Schnyder-Frutig, K., von Greyerz, S., Naisbitt, D.J., Pirmohamed, M., Park, B.K. & Pichler, W.J. (2000). Recognition of sulfamethoxazole and its reactive metabolites by drug-specific CD4+ T cells from allergic individuals. *J Immunol.* 164:6647–6654.

Shiver, J.W., Fu, T.M., Chen, L., Casimiro, D.R., Davies, M.E., Evans, R.K., Zhang, Z.Q., Simon, A.J., Trigona, W.L., Dubey, S.A., Huang, L., Harris, V.A., Long, R.S., Liang, X., Handt, L., Schleif, W.A., Zhu, L., Freed, D.C., Persaud, N.V., Guan, L., Punt, K.S., Tang, A., Chen, M., Wilson, K.A., Collins, K.B., Heidecker, G.J., Fernandez, V.R., Perry, H.C., Joyce, J.G., Grimm, K.M., Cook, J.C., Keller, P.M., Kresock, D.S., Mach, H., Troutman, R.D., Isopi, L.A., Williams, D.M., Xu, Z., Bohannon, K.E., Volkin, D.B., Montefiori, D.C., Miura, A., Krivulka, G.R., Lifton, M.A., Kuroda, M.J., Schmitz, J.E., Letvin, N.L., Caulfield, M.J., Bett, A.J., Youil, R., Kaslow, D.C. & Emini, E.A. (2002). Replication-incompetent adenoviral vaccine vector elicits effective anti-immunodeficiency-virus immunity. *Nature.* 415:331–335.

Singh, S.P., Mehra, N.K., Dingley, H.B., Pande, J.N. & Vaidya, M.C. (1983). Human leukocyte antigen (HLA)-linked control of susceptibility to pulmonary tuberculosis and association with HLA-DR types. *J Infect Dis.* 148:676–681.

Smith, M.W., Dean, M., Carrington, M., Winkler, C., Huttley, G.A., Lomb, D.A., Goedert, J.J., O'Brien, T.R., Jacobson, L.P., Kaslow, R., Buchbinder, S., Vittinghoff, E., Vlahov, D., Hoots, K., Hilgartner, M.W. & O'Brien, S.J. (1997). Contrasting genetic influence of CCR2 and CCR5 variants on HIV-1 infection and disease progression. Hemophilia Growth and Development Study (HGDS), Multicenter AIDS Cohort Study (MACS), Multicenter Hemophilia Cohort Study (MHCS), San Francisco City Cohort (SFCC), ALIVE Study. *Science.* 277:959–965.

Tancrede-Bohin, E., Grange, F., Bournerias, I., Roujeau, J.C. & Guillaume, J.C. (1996). Hypersensitivity syndrome associated with zalcitabine therapy. *Lancet.* 347:971.

Tang, J., Costello, C., Keet, I.P., Rivers, C., Leblanc, S., Karita, E., Allen, S. & Kaslow, R.A. (1999). HLA class I homozygosity accelerates disease progression in human immunodeficiency virus type 1 infection. *AIDS Res Hum Retroviruses.* 15:317–324.

Thursz, M.R., Kwiatkowski, D., Allsopp, C.E., Greenwood, B.M., Thomas, H.C. & Hill, A.V. (1995). Association between an MHC class II allele and clearance of hepatitis B virus in the Gambia. *N Engl J Med.* 332:1065–1069.

Thursz, M.R., Thomas, H.C., Greenwood, B.M. & Hill, A.V. (1997). Heterozygote advantage for HLA class-II type in hepatitis B virus infection. *Nat Genet.* 17:11–12.

Todd, J.R., West, B.C. & McDonald, J.C. (1990). Human leukocyte antigen and leprosy: study in northern Louisiana and review. *Rev Infect Dis.* 12:63–74.

Tomiyama, H., Miwa, K., Shiga, H., Moore, Y.I., Oka, S., Iwamoto, A., Kaneko, Y. & Takiguchi, M. (1997). Evidence of presentation of multiple HIV-1 cytotoxic T lymphocyte epitopes by HLA-B*3501 molecules that are associated with the accelerated progression of AIDS. *J Immunol.* 158: 5026–5034.

Trachtenberg, E., Korber, B., Sollars, C., Kepler, T.B., Hraber, P.T., Hayes, E., Funkhouser, R., Fugate, M., Theiler, J., Hsu, Y.S., Kunstman, K., Wu, S., Phair, J., Erlich, H. & Wolinsky, S. (2003). Advantage of rare HLA supertype in HIV disease progression. *Nat Med.* 9:928–935.

van Eden, W., de Vries, R.R., Mehra, N.K., Vaidya, M.C., D'Amaro, J. & van Rood, J.J. (1980). HLA segregation of tuberculoid leprosy: confirmation of the DR2 marker. *J Infect Dis.* 141:693–701.

Walker, B.D., Chakrabarti, S., Moss, B., Paradis, T.J., Flynn, T., Durno, A.G., Blumberg, R.S., Kaplan, J.C., Hirsch, M.S. & Schooley, R.T. (1987). HIV-specific cytotoxic T lymphocytes in seropositive individuals. *Nature.* 328:345–348.

Wassef, M. & Keiser, P. (1995). Hypersensitivity of zidovudine: report of a case of anaphylaxis and review of the literature. *Clin Infect Dis.* 20:1387–1389.

Weiss, R.B. & Baker, J.R., Jr. (1987). Hypersensitivity reactions from antineoplastic agents. *Cancer Metastasis Rev.* 6:413–432.

Wilson, J.D., Ogg, G.S., Allen, R.L., Davis, C., Shaunak, S., Downie, J., Dyer, W., Workman, C., Sullivan, S., McMichael, A.J. & Rowland-Jones, S. L. (2000). Direct visualization of HIV-1-specific cytotoxic T lymphocytes during primary infection. *AIDS.* 14:225–233.

Winkler, C., Modi, W., Smith, M.W., Nelson, G.W., Wu, X., Carrington, M., Dean, M., Honjo, T., Tashiro, K., Yabe, D., Buchbinder, S., Vittinghoff, E., Goedert, J.J., O'Brien, T.R., Jacobson, L.P., Detels, R., Donfield, S., Willoughby, A., Gomperts, E., Vlahov, D., Phair, J. & O'Brien, S.J. (1998). Genetic restriction of AIDS pathogenesis by an SDF-1 chemokine gene variant. ALIVE Study, Hemophilia Growth and Development Study (HGDS), Multicenter AIDS Cohort Study (MACS), Multicenter Hemophilia Cohort Study (MHCS), San Francisco City Cohort (SFCC). *Science.* 279:389–393.

Yu, X.G., Addo, M.M., Rosenberg, E.S., Rodriguez, W.R., Lee, P.K., Fitzpatrick, C.A., Johnston, M.N., Strick, D., Goulder, P.J., Walker, B.D. & Altfeld, M. (2002). Consistent patterns in the development and immunodominance of human immunodeficiency virus type 1 (HIV-1)-specific CD8+ T-cell responses following acute HIV-1 infection. *J Virol.* 76:8690–8701.

Zanni, M.P., von Greyerz, S., Schnyder, B., Brander, K.A., Frutig, K., Hari, Y., Valitutti, S. & Pichler, W.J. (1998). HLA-restricted, processing- and metabolism-independent pathway of drug recognition by human alpha beta T lymphocytes. *J Clin Invest.* 102:1591–1598.

Zavaglia, C., Bortolon, C., Ferrioli, G., Rho, A., Mondazzi, L., Bottelli, R., Ghessi, A., Gelosa, F., Iamoni, G. & Ideo, G. (1996). HLA typing in chronic type B, D and C hepatitis. *J Hepatol.* 24:658–665.

Zimmerman, P.A., Buckler-White, A., Alkhatib, G., Spalding, T., Kubofcik, J., Combadiere, C., Weissman, D., Cohen, O., Rubbert, A., Lam, G., Vaccarezza, M., Kennedy, P.E., Kumaraswami, V., Giorgi, J.V., Detels, R., Hunter, J., Chopek, M., Berger, E.A., Fauci, A.S., Nutman, T.B. & Murphy, P.M. (1997). Inherited resistance to HIV-1 conferred by an inactivating mutation in CC chemokine receptor 5: studies in populations with contrasting clinical phenotypes, defined racial background, and quantified risk. *Mol Med.* 3:23–36.

Zinkernagel, R.M. & Doherty, P. C. (1974). Immunological surveillance against altered self components by sensitised T lymphocytes in lymphocytic choriomeningitis. *Nature.* 251:547–548.

18

Human Immunodeficiency Virus Type 2 (HIV-2)

Biology and Pathogenesis

Phyllis J. Kanki

Department of Immunology and Infectious Diseases, Harvard School of Public Health, Harvard AIDS Institute, Boston, Massachusetts, USA

INTRODUCTION

Human immunodeficiency virus type 2 (HIV-2) is the second human immunodeficiency virus in the class of human retroviruses; it constitutes the closest known virus related to the prototype AIDS virus, HIV-1. HIV-2 is endemic in West Africa and is rare in Asia. Nevertheless, the virus demonstrates unique biologic features that inform our understanding of HIV viruses in general.

HIV-2 was first discovered based on its similarities to simian immunodeficiency virus (SIV) and cross-reactivity to HIV-1 (Barin *et al.*, 1985; Kanki *et al.*, 1985a; Kanki *et al.*, 1985b). When sera from West African female sex workers (FSW) were screened for antibodies to HIV-1 antigens, antibodies revealed extensive cross-reactivity for the virus core antigens but minimal antibody binding reactivity for the HIV-1 envelope (Barin *et al.*, 1985). Yet, when the same West African human sera were assayed on SIV antigens, they reacted strongly with the envelope proteins as well as the core antigens, suggesting infection with a virus that was more closely related to SIV than to HIV-1. Most HIV-2 isolates are essentially indistinguishable from the SIVs of such species as mangabeys and macaques, leading one to conclude that some SIVs and most HIV-2s are essentially the same virus (Essex and Kanki, 1988; Gao *et al.*, 1992a). *In vivo*, this relationship is illustrated by the ability of HIV-2s to infect and replicate in monkeys (Stahl Hennig *et al.*, 1990; Castro *et al.*, 1991). By contrast, HIV-1 does not infect in most monkey species, but does readily infect chimpanzees and gibbon apes (Alter *et al.*, 1984; Francis *et al.*, 1984; Gajdusek *et al.*, 1985; Fultz *et al.*, 1986).

HIV-2 shares many virologic and biologic features with HIV-1. Both viruses are transmitted by the same routes, they infect the same cells, and they both exhibit considerable genetic variation in the outer envelope gene. As with other retroviruses, both HIVs

TABLE 1. Biological Characteristics of HIV-2 Compared to HIV-1

Characteristic	HIV-2	HIV-1	Magnitude difference
Evolutionary Age	Older	Early 1900s	?
Geographic Distribution	West Africa Former colonial ties	Worldwide	
Age specific prevalence	Older		
Vertical Transmission	Lower		20–30 fold
Heterosexual Transmission	Lower		2–9 fold
Induction of Immunity	Robust	Variable	
Proviral Load	Similar	Similar	
Plasma Viral Load	Lower		30–40 fold
Genetic Diversity	Lower		5–10 fold
Time to AIDS	20–30 yrs	6–8 yrs	2–4 fold

Source: (Kanki *et al.*, 2002)

induce lifelong infection, with permanent integration of viral genetic material into the host cell's DNA. It was based on these initial similarities, that some believed that HIV-2 might cause a second worldwide AIDS epidemic. However, over 18 years since its discovery, research studies conducted both in the laboratory and in HIV-2-infected people have highlighted distinct biological differences between these related viruses (Essex and Kanki, 1994; Markovitz, 1993; Kanki, 1999). Some of these unique properties include a distinct global distribution of the virus with limited spread, significantly reduced perinatal and sexual transmission, slower rates of progression to AIDS and the potential protective effect of HIV-2 from subsequent HIV-1 infection (Kanki, 1999). A complete review and update of all aspects of HIV-2 infection are beyond the scope of this review, rather, we have chosen to highlight some of the biological aspects of HIV-2 which have been of most interest from a comparative perspective (Table 1). Based on our current understanding, the distinct biological differences between these related viruses suggest that viral versus host determinants may be more responsible for the unique pathogenic mechanisms employed by HIV viruses in general. It is hoped that the further characterization of such determinants will be useful for the design of effective HIV interventions.

HIV-2 VIRUS LIFE CYCLE

HIV-2s are morphologically similar to HIV-1s. They are spherical, 100–120 nm virions, and the length of the entire genome of HIV-2 is about 9 kilobases which is similar to the length of HIV-1. The open reading frames of HIV-2 are also similar to those of HIV-1 (Figure 1). For different HIV-1, HIV-2, and SIVs, the genes may be in different reading frames, but the level of conservation within each gene is still high. The *gag* and *pol* messages are unspliced, the *env* singly spliced, and the major regulatory genes doubly spliced and made from multiple messages. The regulatory gene sequences appear to vary more among HIV-2s when compared with HIV-1s (Zagury *et al.*, 1988; Tristem *et al.*, 1989; Kirchhoff *et al.*, 1990). HIV-1 has one gene, vpu, which is not found in HIV-2 (Matsuda *et al.*, 1988; Strebel *et al.*, 1989; Cohen *et al.*, 1988). However, the function of the HIV-1 vpu, namely the ability to increase viral particle release, may be provided by the HIV-2 envelope (Bour and Strebel, 1996). HIV-2 has one gene, vpx, which is not found in HIV-1 (Franchini *et al.*, 1989; Yu *et al.*, 1988; Henderson *et al.*, 1988; Kappes *et al.*, 1988).

The replication cycle of HIV-2 includes: *a*) adsorption to CD4 and the relevant coreceptor with subsequent fusion with the cell surface; *b*) penetration and uncoating;

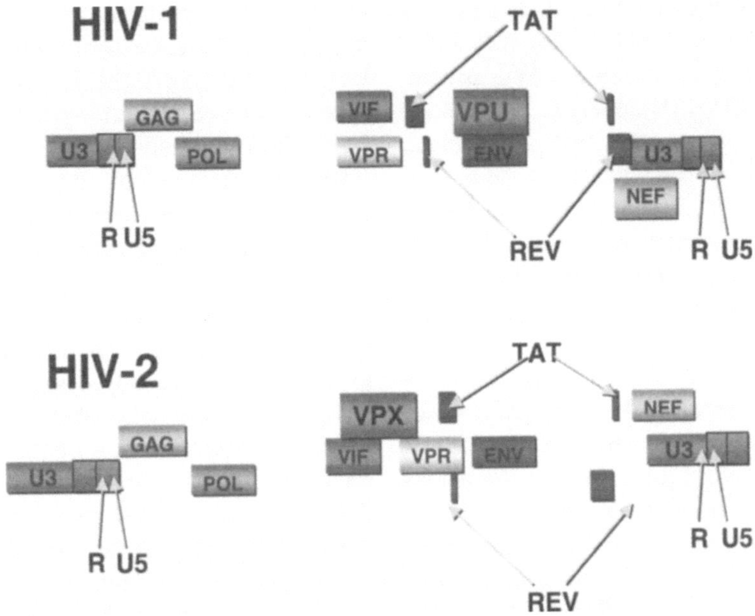

FIGURE 1. Genomic structure of HIV-1 and HIV-2 (Kanki *et al.*, 2002)

c) reverse transcription; *d*) transport of viral DNA to nucleus; *e*) chromosomal integration; *f*) transcription of viral mRNA and splicing; *g*) translation of regulatory and structural proteins; *h*) transport of structural proteins to the cytoplasmic membrane and virus assembly; and *i*) budding, maturation, and release.

Receptors and Co-receptors

HIV-2 infects the same range of cells as HIV-1 CD4 positive helper lymphocytes, monocytes, macrophages, and microglia cells in the central nervous system. Although HIV-2 infects through the same CD4 receptor, it apparently does so with a 10 to100-fold greater affinity than HIV-1 (Moore, 1990; Morikawa *et al.*, 1992; Bahraoui *et al.*, 1992). Although the HIV-2 envelope protein appears to be slightly less glycosylated than HIV-1, this does not appear to account for their differences in binding efficiency (Bahraoui *et al.*, 1992). It is believed that infection by HIV-2 is inhibited more efficiently by soluble CD4 than is HIV-1 (Looney *et al.*, 1990).

Several members of the chemokine receptor family have been shown to function in association with CD4 to permit HIV-1 entry and infection in various types of cells (Feng *et al.*, 1996; Clapham *et al.*, 1992; Looney *et al.*, 1990). Like HIV-1, certain HIV-2s have been shown to utilize Fusin/CXCR4, as both a co-receptor (in the presence of CD4) and as an alternative receptor, in the absence of CD4 (Feng *et al.*, 1996; Endres *et al.*, 1996). HIV-2 viruses appear to be more promiscuous in their utilization of various co-receptors, compared with HIV-1, including CXCR4, CCR1-5, and the co-receptors designated BONZO/STRL33 and BOB/GPR15 (Bron *et al.*, 1997; Endres *et al.*, 1996; Feng *et al.*, 1996). Most CCR5-requiring isolates are non-syncytium inducing, whereas isolates utilizing multiple co-receptors were syncytium inducing. However, the efficiency with which the co-receptors are utilized by HIV-2 appears to vary greatly between various isolates (Heredia *et al.*, 1997).

In vitro studies of HIV-2 isolates by a number of laboratories have described differences in the cytopathicity of HIV-2 as compared with HIV-1 (Evans *et al.*, 1988a; Kong *et al.*, 1988; Albert *et al.*, 1990; Albert *et al.*, 1996). In some cases related to the clinical stage of the HIV-2 -infected individual, HIV-2 isolates demonstrate decreased cell killing, less syncytial cell formation, reduced virus replication, and differences in interaction with CD4 (Albert *et al.*, 1996).

The V3 loop of rapid/high HIV-2 isolates differs significantly from slow/low isolates in that the V3 sequence is more heterogeneous and has a higher net charge. Mutations at amino acid positions 313 and 314, to positively charged amino acids, has also been significantly associated with the rapid/high phenotype, similar to that of HIV-1 (Albert *et al.*, 1996). These amino acid changes in the V3 loop of HIV-2 also appear to determine the co-receptor usage for CXCR4 and CCR5. The distinct co-receptor usage of two reference HIV-2 molecular clones, GH-1 and ROD, allowed the identification of the region of gp120 which is important for co-receptor specificity. By constructing a series of chimeric viruses between GH-1 and ROD, the C-terminal half of the V3 loop region of gp120 was found to determine the differential co-receptor usage between GH-1 and ROD. Notably, the shift in the co-receptor usage from CCR5 to CXCR4 was associated with an increase in the net positive charge in the V3 region (Isaka *et al.*, 1999).

HIV-2 Polymerase Gene

The HIV pol gene encodes three proteins: protease, reverse transcriptase(which also has RNase H activity), and endonuclease/integrase. The HIV-2 protease, as expressed in yeast, was also shown to be efficient at hydrolyzing HIV-1 peptide junctions (Pichuantes *et al.*, 1990). This suggests that the substrate specificities of both viral proteins are analogous. The reverse transcriptase/RNase H molecule of HIV-2 is similar in size to the HIV-1 reverse transcriptase and is serologically cross-reactive with human antibodies (Allan *et al.*, 1987). The HIV-2 polymerase appears to be equally error-prone to that of HIV-1 (Bakhanashvili and Hizi, 1992). The fidelity of mis-insertion and mis-pair extension throughout DNA synthesis exhibited by mutants of the reverse transcriptase of HIV-2 resistant to nucleoside analogs has been studied. The Val74 mutant of HIV-1 reverse transcriptase (RT) has previously been shown to display a substantially enhanced fidelity, whereas the comparable mutant of HIV-2 RT has fidelity similar to that of the wild-type RT. Depending on the assay employed and the DNA sequences extended, most other mutants of HIV-2 RT displayed moderate affects on the enzyme, leading to mild increases in fidelity of DNA synthesis. This implies a more complex and less distinctive correlation between drug-resistance, mis-insertion, and mis-pair extension in HIV-2 RT in contrast to HIV-1 RT, and it provides evidence for potential biochemical differences between these two related RTs (Taube *et al.*, 1997).

As for other retroviral reverse transcriptases, the DNA polymerase is associated with the amino terminus of the molecule and RNase H is associated with the carboxy terminus (Hizi *et al.*, 1991a). However, the specific RNase H activity of HIV-2 appears to be about ten-fold lower than the comparable activity of the HIV-1 enzyme (Hizi *et al.*, 1991b).

HIV-2: Structural Genes—*gag* and *env*

The *gag* gene products are essentially the same for HIV-1 and HIV-2 (Voss *et al.*, 1992) and are highly conserved. A 55-kD precursor is myristoylated and cleaved by the viral protease to form p17 (MA), p24 (CA), p2, p7 (NC), p1, and p6. The matrix protein (MA) p17 is at the amino terminus, and in its cleaved form it surrounds the nucleocapsid. The capsid (CA) p24 is slightly larger for HIV-2 or SIV and is sometimes described as p26/27 (Barin *et al.*, 1985; Henderson *et al.*,

1990). It provides the structure for the core that contains the genome and the polymerase and integrase enzymes (Haseltine, 1992). Researchers have identified (NC) p7–8 as a nucleic acid-binding protein (Gorelick *et al.*, 1990), and both zinc finger motifs are involved with the specificity of packaging the genomic viral RNA into the virions (Komatsu *et al.*, 1996).

The envelope glycoprotein precursor is slightly smaller for HIV-2, as are the external glycoprotein and the transmembrane protein. Although usually described using the terminology for HIV-1 (gp160, gp120, gp41, respectively), the HIV-2 glycoproteins are sometimes designated with lower sizes (e.g., gp140–145, gp105–110, gp32–40). Analysis of the primary amino acid sequence for N-linked glycosylation sites shows the HIV-2 and SIV gp120s have significantly fewer conserved sites. This could presumably account for the lower molecular weight of the HIV-2 gp120, as carbohydrates make up 50% or more of the HIV-1 gp120 (Lee *et al.*, 1992a; Lee *et al.*, 1992b; Leonard *et al.*, 1990).

HIV-2 envelope sequences vary to approximately the same degree as HIV-1 sequences (Guyader *et al.*, 1987; Zagury *et al.*, 1988; Franchini *et al.*, 1989; Kuhnel *et al.*, 1989; Hasegawa *et al.*, 1989; Kumar *et al.*, 1990; Klemm *et al.*, 1988; Boeri *et al.*, 1992; Sankalé *et al.*, 1996). Although the V3 regions correspond in both virus types, HIV-2s do not have the conserved GPGR amino acid sequence at the tip of the V3 loop (Franchini *et al.*, 1989; Boeri *et al.*, 1992). External glycosylation sites appear to be conserved between HIV-1 and HIV-2 as are the sites for CD4 binding (Kirchhoff *et al.*, 1990; Franchini *et al.*, 1987), precursor processing (Steffy *et al.*, 1992), fusion (Steffy *et al.*, 1992), principal neutralizing domain at V3 (Boeri *et al.*, 1992; Robert-Guroff *et al.*, 1992; Bjorling *et al.*, 1991), cytolytic T cell activity (Nixon *et al.*, 1990; Cao *et al.*, 1997), and perhaps antibody-dependent cell cytotoxicity (Bjorling *et al.*, 1991; Norley *et al.*, 1990; Ljunggren *et al.*, 1988). Much of the envelope glycoprotein of HIV-1 appears to generate binding antibodies. Antibodies from people infected with HIV-2, demonstrate binding activity concentrated in the middle of gp120, including the V3 loop (Huang *et al.*, 1991; Mannervik *et al.*, 1992), as well as the amino terminus of the transmembrane protein (Huang *et al.*, 1991; Norrby *et al.*, 1991). Another region, the carboxy terminus of gp120, may be slightly less immunogenic, but it appears to be the most cross-reactive between HIV-1 and HIV-2 (Norrby *et al.*, 1991).

The most type-specific region of HIV-2 gp120, the V3 loop region, is also the principal neutralizing domain, as it is for HIV-1 (Boeri *et al.*, 1992; Robert-Guroff *et al.*, 1992; Bjorling *et al.*, 1991). Two distinct antigenic sites in the V3 of HIV-2 have been identified that appear to correspond to the principal neutralizing determinant (PND) of HIV-1; the conserved Phe-His-Ser-Gln and Trp-Cys-Arg motifs (positions 315–318 and 329–331) possibly interact to form a discontinuous antigenic site based on computer simulation modeling (Bjorling *et al.*, 1999). However, other neutralizing regions of lower activity have been described, including a linear epitope in V2 and one conformational epitope outside V1, V2, and V3 (Bjorling *et al.*, 1991; McKnight *et al.*, 1996). Some investigators have described cross-neutralization between HIV-1 and HIV-2 with human antibodies (Weiss *et al.*, 1988; Bottiger *et al.*, 1989). Although weakly bidirectional, they appear stronger for serum from HIV-2-infected people for cross-neutralization of HIV-1 (Weiss *et al.*, 1988; Bottiger *et al.*, 1989).

Although the fusion domains for syncytia induction have been mapped to the hydrophobic amino terminus of the transmembrane protein, loss of syncytia-inducing ability does not appear to have much of an effect on the infectivity of HIV-2 (Steffy *et al.*, 1992). Both HIV-1 and HIV-2 have a long cytoplasmic domain on the transmembrane protein. This often becomes truncated, at least when culturing the virus in T cell lines. Even small truncations of this sort appear to enhance fusion activity (Mulligan *et al.*, 1992; Kong *et al.*, 1988). Whether this has any importance *in vivo* is still unclear.

GENETIC PEDIGREE OF HIV-2

It has been estimated that the HIV-1 and HIV-2/SIV groups of viruses might have diverged from each other as recently as 50–60 years ago (Smith *et al.*, 1988; Myers *et al.*, 1992). The SIVs of mangabeys and macaques are the closest relatives of HIV-2s (Essex and Kanki, 1988; Gao *et al.*, 1992b; Marx *et al.*, 1991). As a group, the SIVs apparently vary more between different species and subspecies of monkeys than different HIVs vary from each other (Essex and Kanki, 1988; Marx *et al.*, 1991; Emau *et al.*, 1991; Allan *et al.*, 1990). As HIV-2s appear to be largely limited to West Africa, it is not surprising that they are most closely related to SIVs originating from monkeys in that region (Essex and Kanki, 1988; Gao *et al.*, 1992b; Marx *et al.*, 1991). The only exception may be the macaque SIV, which is also closely related to both HIV-2 and mangabey SIV (*Cercoebus atys*). As SIVs have never been observed in wild Asian monkeys such as macaques, it appears likely that infection of this species occurred accidentally in captivity from African monkeys or human tissues originating from West Africa (Essex and Kanki, 1988). The entire genome of HIV-2 is about 40–45% related to HIV-1 at the nucleotide sequence level (Franchini *et al.*, 1987).

The antigenic relatedness of both SIV and HIV-2 to the prototype HIV-1 virus prompted both the discovery and further classification of these related viruses (Barin *et al.*, 1985; Kanki *et al.*, 1987a; Biberfeld *et al.*, 1987). As with HIV-1, nucleoside sequence data indicate significant genetic variability amongst HIV-2 strains (Franchini *et al.*, 1987; Boeri *et al.*, 1992). As more sequence data have become available from various HIV-2 and SIV strains, it has also become apparent that no branching order of divergence can be specified, and that these virus types may, in fact, share a common ancestor (Kirchhoff *et al.*, 1990; Gao *et al.*, 1992b).

In comparison to HIV-1, the genetic diversity of HIV-2 is less extensive and only two subtypes (A and B) have been well characterized. Other studies have reported the existence of four additional subtypes (C, D, E, and F), but different attempts to isolate viruses or obtain additional samples to sequence from these identified subtypes have been unsuccessful (Gao *et al.*, 1994). An unusual HIV-2 isolate, Abt96, from an asymptomatic blood donor from Ivory Coast has been sequenced, and phylogenetic data suggests a novel HIV-2 subtype, preliminarily designated as subtype G (Yamaguchi *et al.*, 2000).

Thus far, HIV-2 subtype A is the most characterized subtype and appears to be the major variant circulating in West Africa (Sankalé *et al.*, 1995; Sarr *et al.*, 2000; Norrgren *et al.*, 1997; Peeters *et al.*, 1998; Xiang *et al.*, 1997). At present, the Ghanaian isolates, subtype B (Dietrich *et al.*, 1989; Kawamura *et al.*, 1992) are believed to be most distant from the prototype HIV-2/mangabey/macaque virus (Essex and Kanki, 1988). A recent study from Ivory Coast suggests a predominance of HIV-2 subtype B in this country (Pieniazek *et al.*, 1999). Like the situation with HIV-1 subtypes, the potential impact of subtype differences on the epidemiology, pathogenicity, and transmission of HIV-2 is not yet well appreciated.

HIV-2 DIAGNOSIS

Studies of HIV-2 epidemiology and natural history are heavily dependent on accurate HIV-2 viral diagnosis. The same procedures for serologic testing, virus culture, and genetic diagnosis that were developed for HIV-1 (such as polymerase chain reaction [PCR]) have been modified for HIV-2 diagnosis and have improved over the years. The close relationship of HIV-2 to HIV-1 on a genetic and antigenic level has necessitated the development and implementation of type-specific diagnostic assays. Because most of the tests were developed for HIV-1 using HIV-1 antigens, the degree of cross-reactivity and specificity for HIV-2 is variable. Most of the first generation tests used whole virus antigens in which core antigens, such as p24 and pol p66/p51, are well represented. These antigens are more strongly cross-reactive than envelope antigens, especially gp120 (Barin *et al.*, 1985; Kanki, 1987; Bottiger *et al.*, 1990; Holzer *et al.*, 1990).

Blood bank screening for HIV-2 was instituted in the United States in 1990, following the lead of many European nations. As a result, the vast majority of commercial HIV enzyme-linked immunosorbent assays (ELISA) utilize a combined antigen source that incorporates HIV-2-specific antigens. Confirmation of HIV-2 serostatus requires an HIV-2-specific immunoblot assay, or specific peptide assays. Immunoblots demonstrating a profile of major structural gene product recognition are typically used to confirm HIV-1 and HIV-2 diagnosis using standard criteria. HIV-2-specific diagnosis by immunoblot requires antibody reactivity to *env* ± *gag* ± *pol* antigens. In the absence of reactivity to *gag* or *pol* antigens, the presence of reactivity to two envelope antigens is required (gp120 and gp32) (WHO, 1990).

Various investigations have focused on identifying type-specific antigens to allow confirmatory tests that will distinguish between HIV-1 and HIV-2. Most have been made as synthetic peptides (Baillou *et al.*, 1991b; Baillou *et al.*, 1991a; Ayres *et al.*, 1990; Broliden *et al.*, 1991), but some were larger, bacterially expressed peptides (Gueye-Ndiaye *et al.*, 1993; Zuber *et al.*, 1990) that vary in sensitivity and specificity. As most were selected for specificity, sensitivity could be compromised. Thus, although appropriate for type-specific confirmation, they may not be as useful as larger HIV-2-specific antigens for initial screening.

For HIV investigators working in Africa where HIV-1 and HIV-2 infections are prevalent, it has been critical to identify cost-efficient alternative antibody testing strategies for screening, confirmation, and discrimination of HIV-1 and HIV-2 infections. These strategies have included rapid simple tests (RST) as well as ELISA. In a study of 1110 consecutive sera from Bissau, Guinea Bissau, 198 (17.8%) were found HIV-seropositive: 52 (4.7%) HIV-1, 120 (10.8%) HIV-2, and 26 (2.3%) HIV-1/HIV-2 dually reactive. Western blot was used as a gold standard for confirming the reactivity of the specimens. The sensitivities of all assays were 100%. The specificities of the screening assays at initial and repeated testing was 98.0% and 99.7%, respectively. The specificities for Enzygnost and for Capillus were 99.8 and 99.9%, respectively. The various combinations of two or three assays showed specificities of 99.2–100%. Serodiagnostic strategies for HIV can be based on RST alone, and differentiation between HIV-1 and HIV-2 can be achieved as part of these strategies. However, the considerable variability in the capacity of individual assays to discriminate between HIV-1 and HIV-2 needs to be considered in design and interpretation of such data (Andersson *et al.*, 1997).

When human serum samples have been tested in places such as Ivory Coast, Senegal, and Burkina Faso, a disproportionately large fraction of the samples often test as "dual positive" because they appear reactive on both HIV-1 and HIV-2 confirmatory tests (Kanki, 1987; Denis *et al.*, 1987; Zuber *et al.*, 1990; Kanki *et al.*, 1999). These sites have significant rates of both HIV-1 and HIV-2, and distinction of viruses and designation of dual reactivity remains a diagnostic challenge for the typical HIV laboratory. The HIV dual antibody profile is characterized by antibodies with strong reactivity to the *env* antigens of both HIV-1 and HIV-2 by immunoblot and/or radioimmunoprecipitation analysis (RIPA) (Barin *et al.*, 1985; Kanki *et al.*, 1986; Holzer *et al.*, 1990;

Tedder *et al.*, 1988; Kanki *et al.*, 1988; Gueye-Ndiaye *et al.*, 1993). Several possible biologic explanations for this phenomenon can be entertained, including extensive cross reactivity by either of the HIV's, dual infection, or infection with a recombinant virus.

Isolation of both HIV-1 and HIV-2 has been reported from selected HIV-dual cases and PCR evidence of both viruses has ranged from 30–80% in serologically-defined dual reactives reported from similar populations (Evans *et al.*, 1988b; Peeters *et al.*, 1992; Rayfield *et al.*, 1988). It is unclear whether the low and variable rate of concordance between serology and PCR is due to extensive HIV-1 cross reactivity, misclassification of samples based on serodiagnosis, or insensitivity of the PCR assays. Improvement of PCR assays with southern blot detection or nested primer sets has maximized the sensitivity and specificity for HIV-2 provirus detection (Dieng-Sarr, 1998; Dieng-Sarr *et al.*, 1999). The further development of such assays will be critical to studies that seek to characterize HIV-2 biology and its interaction with HIV-1 *in vivo*. Largely due to the need for further studies, it has been difficult to predict from the published literature what the interactions of these two distinct HIV type viruses would be in human populations. In the absence of HIV-2 infection alone, it seems clear that reports of dual infection in certain parts of Africa and the rest of the world, were more likely misinterpreted laboratory data than a true biological entity.

EPIDEMIOLOGY AND GLOBAL DISTRIBUTION

The isolation of a second retrovirus, HIV-2, led to fears that a second AIDS pandemic would occur, and would be similar in scope and magnitude to that caused by HIV-1. However, the peculiar biologic properties of HIV-2, namely the lower transmissibility of this virus through both sexual and vertical routes, contributed to a more regionalized endemic distribution of the virus. Studies conducted shortly after the discovery of HIV-2 found significant rates of HIV-2 in a number of West African countries, frequently with low to absent rates of HIV-1 (Kanki, 1987; Harrison *et al.*, 1991). In the late 1980s, in countries such as Guinea Bissau, The Gambia, Cape Verde and Senegal, the prevalence of HIV-2 infection exceeded that of infection with HIV-1. But in most instances, HIV-1 infection has now increased and exceeded rates of HIV-2 infection (Kanki, 1987; Naucler *et al.*, 1990; Denis *et al.*, 1987; Pepin *et al.*, 1991b). Rates of HIV-2 infection are highest in sexually active populations such as FSW, sexually transmitted disease patients, prisoners, and people hospitalized with infectious diseases (Kanki, 1987; Romieu *et al.*, 1990; Naucler *et al.*, 1989; Denis *et al.*, 1987; Kanki and DeCock, 1994). These risk groups usually have seroprevalence rates that are five-to ten-fold higher than the general population, which is often represented by blood donors and pregnant women.

In 1985, the discovery of HIV-2 in West Africa prompted numerous serologic studies to determine the geographic distribution of the virus. Since that time, significant HIV-2 infection has been well documented in most West African countries which, surprisingly, is a distinctly different worldwide distribution than HIV-1 (Kanki, 1999). Largely due to relatively low prevalence rates in most places outside of West Africa, it has been difficult to compare the prevalence rates in different countries due to differences in study design and diagnostic methodologies. Often times serosurveys were conducted with methods that failed to distinguish HIV-1 from HIV-2. Thus erroneously reported type-specific prevalence rates, or difficulties with diagnosis and distinction of HIV-dual infections resulted from the lack of HIV-specificity in the serologic or nucleic-acid based assays.

In most countries of West Africa such as Burkina Faso, Ghana, Ivory Coast, Nigeria, and Mali, infection with HIV-1 is more prevalent than infection with HIV-2 and ranges from a 32- to 24-fold rate ratio (HIV-1 versus HIV-2) (Kanki *et al.*, 1990; Kanki and DeCock, 1994; Ankrah *et al.*, 1994; Olaleye *et al.*, 1993; Maiga *et al.*, 1993; Kanki, 1999). For example, in a study from Bamako, Mali, HIV-2 infection was found in 3.9% of 176 FSW, in contrast to the 20.45% HIV-1 infection in the same group. Comparison of HIV-1 and HIV-2 seroprevalence data from our study with previous data from Mali shows a significant rise in HIV-1 prevalence and a significant decrease in HIV-2 prevalence and confirms similar trends observed in neighboring countries (Peeters *et al.*, 1998).

The existence of significant rates of HIV-1 and HIV-2 in many of these countries raised the question of what outcome would result from the interaction of these viruses at the population level. Anderson and May (1996) analyzed the available biological and epidemiological data on the pathogenicity, transmissibility, and antigenic similarity of HIV-1 and HIV-2, and used simple mathematical models to study the competition between the two viral types. The mathematical model of the concomitant transmission of the two viruses transmitted within the same sexually active population, suggested a positive association between pathogenicity and reproductive success, suggesting that HIV-1 would competitively displace HIV-2 in the longer term. This finding is supported by studies that measure and compare the rates of sexual and perinatal transmission of the two viruses, as well as the temporal falling trends of HIV-2 prevalence through the region (Kanki *et al.*, 1994; Andreasson *et al.*, 1993; Ngagne *et al.*, 1995; Adjorlolo-Johnson *et al.*, 1994). The current data suggests that in order to establish endemic infection HIV-2 has been present in certain populations for a long time and its spread outside of these endemic areas is limited by a low transmission potential. It therefore seems unlikely that this virus will cause a global pandemic similar to that of HIV-1.

A second epidemiologic pattern of HIV-2 infection has been suggested from reports of HIV-2 in Portugal, Mozambique, Angola, southwestern India, and Brazil, all areas with former ties to Portugal (Smallman-Raynor and Cliff, 1991; Santos-Ferreira *et al.*, 1990; Victorino *et al.*, 1992; Rubsamen-Waigmann *et al.*, 1991). This pattern appears to have low but stable rates of HIV-2 in the population; (Kanki and DeCock, 1994; Santos-Ferreira *et al.*, 1990; Victorino *et al.*, 1992). These countries once shared political ties and have economic relationships that still exist today. HIV-2 has also been detected in the large cities of southwestern India (Rubsamen-Waigmann *et al.*, 1991), perhaps because of exchange with the former Portuguese colonies of Africa. Goa, a former Portuguese colony, situated south of Bombay on the western coast, has reported 4.9% HIV-2 and 9.8% HIV-1 infection in sexually transmitted infection (STI) patients (Rubsamen-Waigmann *et al.*, 1994). Significant HIV-2 infection has not been reported in other parts of Asia to date.

Geographically, the distribution of HIV-2 seems to be totally independent from the distribution of HIV-1 (Kanki, 1987; Smallman-Raynor and Cliff, 1991; Kanki and DeCock, 1994; Kanki, 1999). Countries in central or eastern Africa appear to be relatively free of HIV-2, as are most regions of Europe and North America. In these very low risk regions, almost all of the HIV-2 infections observed are either in West African immigrants or in individuals who had contact with West Africans.

France was one of the first countries to institute HIV-2 testing in blood donors, and as a result of testing several HIV-2 cases were identified (Courouce *et al.*, 1989). Of 75 HIV-2-infected persons studied in Paris, 58 were of African origin, 12 European, and 5 Caribbean (Matheron *et al.*, 1993). To a lesser degree, other European countries have reported sporadic cases of HIV-2 infection in large serosurveys, and these cases usually have a link to West Africa (Kanki *et al.*, 1990; De Cock and Brun-Vezinet, 1989; Smallman-Raynor and Cliff, 1991). The first cases of HIV-2 infection in Spain were identified in 1988 in 3

African immigrants living in Barcelona. By 1999, 92 cases had been reported (Machuca *et al.*, 1999). In 22 subjects, HIV-2 subtyping was performed on proviral DNA. 16 subjects were found to be infected with subtype A, and of those, 8 were Spanish-born and 8 were African immigrants. The remaining subjects were infected with HIV-2 subtype B, and of those two were Spanish-born and 4 originated from Equatorial Guinea (Machuca *et al.*, 1999).

TRANSMISSION OF HIV-2

Although HIV-2 is transmitted by sex and blood, as is HIV-1, the rate of infection in West Africa appears more stable than that of HIV-1. In Senegal, during an eight-year period of follow-up, there was a 26-fold increase in HIV-1, whereas the rate of increase in HIV-2 infection remained relatively constant (Kanki *et al.*, 1994; Donnelly *et al.*, 1993). This implies that HIV-2 may have been in the human population in Africa at least as long as HIV-1, and in West Africa HIV-2 has apparently been present considerably longer. The relative lack of significant HIV-2 prevalence in Europe, North America, and Asia as compared to the expansion of HIV-1 in the same continents also supports the general observation that HIV-2 is spread less efficiently than HIV-1 (Smallman-Raynor and Cliff, 1991; Kanki, 1987; Kanki *et al.*, 1994; Hendry *et al.*, 1991; Kvinesdal *et al.*, 1992; Georgoulias *et al.*, 1990; Costigliola *et al.*, 1992; Estebanez *et al.*, 1992; Downing and Biryahwaho, 1990; O'Brien *et al.*, 1992; Anderson and May, 1996).

Case reports of HIV-2 transmitted by blood and blood products have been published, however widespread HIV testing in blood bank settings has limited the risk of this mode of transmission (Parkman, 1990; Dufoort *et al.*, 1988). The most common modes of HIV transmission in HIV-2 endemic areas are perinatal and heterosexual transmission. Since most West African countries have been afflicted with both HIV-1 and HIV-2 infections, direct comparison of transmission rates between the two viruses has been possible. In Senegalese FSW followed over an 11-year period, the annual incidence of HIV-1 dramatically increased, with a 1.18-fold increased risk per year and a 13-fold increase in risk over the entire study period. The incidence of HIV-2 remained stable, despite higher HIV-2 prevalence (Kanki *et al.*; 1994, Kanki, 1997). In this high risk group the heterosexual transmission of HIV-2 was significantly slower than that of HIV-1, which strongly suggests differences in the infectivity potential of these two related immunodeficiency viruses (Kanki *et al.*, 1994; Kanki, 1997). Using mathematical modeling techniques, the efficiency of heterosexual transmission of HIV-2 has been estimated to range from five to nine times less than that of HIV-1 per sexual act with an infected partner (Donnelly *et al.*, 1993). This has been recently corroborated using newer methods with fewer assumptions (Gilbert *et al.*, 2002).

The sexual transmission of HIV-2, like HIV-1, appears to be enhanced by the presence of other sexually transmitted diseases such as chancroid or syphilis (Pepin *et al.*, 1992). Enhanced risk for infection with HIV-2 was also associated with an increase in years of sexual activity and non-Senegalese nationality. Additionally, HIV-2-infected women tend to be older than HIV-1-infected women (Kanki *et al.*, 1992). Similarly, in a cross-sectional discordant couple study of HIV-2 transmission, older women were more likely to have a seropositive spouse than younger women (Aaby *et al.*, 1996).

Maternal or neonatal transmission of HIV-2 also occurs (Morgan *et al.*, 1990), but it appears to be less efficient than that of HIV-1 (Gayle *et al.*, 1992; Del Mistro *et al.*, 1992; Poulsen *et al.*, 1992). Prospective studies of HIV-2 perinatal transmission have been conducted in Guinea Bissau, Ivory Coast, France, and Senegal, all demonstrating extremely low rates of perinatal transmission of HIV-2 (0–3.7% transmission) in contrast to that of

HIV-1 (15–45% transmission) (Andreasson *et al.*, 1993; Adjorlolo-Johnson *et al.*, 1994; Ngagne *et al.*, 1995; Abbott *et al.*, 1994). In studies that measured perinatal transmission of both viruses, the rate of HIV-1 transmission was 10 to20-fold higher than that of HIV-2.

In a Gambian study of HIV-2 and HIV-1 perinatal transmission, the antenatal geometric mean plasma viral load of 94 HIV-1-infected women was 15,100 copies per ml (95% CI 10,400-19,000) which was much higher than that of 60 randomly selected HIV-2-infected women, which was 410 copies per ml (95% CI 150–910) ($P < 0.001$). The estimated transmission rate of HIV-1 was 24.4% (95% CI 14.6–33.9) and that of HIV-2 was 4% (95% CI 1.9–7.4). Five of 17 HIV-1-positive, and three of eight HIV-2-positive babies were infected after 2 months of age, presumably by breast milk. Birth in the rainy season (odds ratio (OR) 2.9; 95% CI 1.2–7.2), a low postnatal CD4 cell percentage (OR for a 10% drop 2.4; 95% CI 1.1–5.1), and a high maternal plasma viral load (OR for a ten-fold increase 2.9; 95% CI 1.1–7.8) were risk factors for transmission that applied equally to both viruses. Low maternal HIV-2 RNA levels, which on average was 37-fold less than in HIV-1 infection, were thought to explain the low rates of mother-child transmission in HIV-2 infection (O'Donovan *et al.*, 2000).

PATHOGENESIS OF HIV-2

During the late 1980s and early 1990s, natural history studies of HIV-1 infection conducted in the developed world provided important data on the pathogenesis of HIV-1 infection *in vivo*. Although numerous cross sectional studies of HIV-2 infection were conducted in the late 1980s, they were intrinsically limited in their ability to describe the natural history of HIV-2 infection, which required prospective studies (Romieu *et al.*, 1990). Studies concerning the natural history of chronic infections such as HIV are difficult to achieve particularly with minimal loss to follow-up. Not surprisingly, such studies have been rare in developing countries, where viruses such as HIV-2 can be studied. Very few studies have evaluated deterioration of the immune system and/or alternatives in the virus load over time in HIV-2-infected people.

In cross-sectional studies, T4 lymphocyte counts and T4:T8 ratios appear reduced in HIV-2-infected healthy carriers, but less dramatically than in HIV-1-infected carriers (Marlink *et al.*, 1994; Lisse *et al.*, 1990; Kestens *et al.*, 1992; Pepin *et al.*, 1991b). Alterations in T-cell subsets evaluated prospectively have shown similar results, where immunosuppression in HIV-2-infected people was significantly slower than HIV-1 and could not be demonstrated in all followed subjects (Lisse *et al.*, 1996; Traore *et al.*, 1996). Skin test anergy to various antigens is also less pronounced in HIV-2 infection (Marlink *et al.*, 1994; Pepin *et al.*, 1991a).

The degree of immune activation and apoptosis in lymphocytes were compared in healthy West African patients infected with HIV-1 or -2. The lower decline of CD4 T cells in HIV-2 compared with HIV-1-infected donors was associated with lower levels of immune activation, evaluated by HLA-DR expression on lymphocytes and sera concentrations of IgG and beta2 microglobulin (Kestens *et al.*, 1992; Pepin *et al.*, 1991b; Victorino *et al.*, 1992). *Ex vivo* apoptosis was found in both infections in all lymphocyte subsets, including CD4 and CD8 T cells, as well as B cells, but was lower in HIV-2 than in HIV-1 infection (Michel *et al.*, 2000). These observations support the hypothesis that long-term activation of the immune system, weaker in HIV-2 infection, significantly contributes to T cell deletion and disease evolution (Michel *et al.*, 2000). The HIV-2 envelope has also been shown to have an inhibitory affect on T cell proliferation and the up-regulation of CD40L and OX40, which are co stimulatory molecules important in the activation and differentiation of the T cell response; this effect was accompanied by a reduced level of apoptosis (Cavaleiro *et al.*, 2000).

HIV-2 REPLICATION AND GENETIC DIVERSITY

It is now well established that new genotypes of HIV-1 evolve over time in the same individual after infection. The earliest isolates generally grow in macrophages as well as lymphocytes. They do not cause syncytia in established T cell lines and are associated with a "slow-low" phase where the load of virus in blood and blood cells is very low. As disease develops, HIV-1s that have changes in the envelope V3 loop evolve. These viruses are often associated with higher virus loads in blood and syncytia induction in T cell lines, and they are called "rapid-high" viruses (Asjo *et al.*, 1986; Fenyo *et al.*, 1989). The ability of HIV-2s to induce syncytia may be lower than for HIV-1s (Mulligan *et al.*, 1990). HIV-2 is more difficult to isolate from asymptomatic people than is HIV-1; but when it is isolated, it appears to show the "slow-low" pattern (Albert *et al.*, 1990; Schulz *et al.*, 1990). Similarly, the "rapid-high" isolates were more likely to be from HIV-2-infected people with disease. The determinants of cell tropism and replication capacity for HIV-2 have not yet been mapped. However, a correlation between the number of charged residues in the V3 loop, the nature of the residues at positions 18 and 19 of the V3 loop, and the phenotype of HIV-2 isolates have been described (Albert *et al.*, 1996; Sankalé *et al.*, 1996).

As with HIV-1, the polymerase activity of HIV-2 is error-prone, and as a result, extensive variation occurs between isolates (Bakhanashvili and Hizi, 1992). This is primarily exhibited in the envelope gene against which much of the selective pressure of the immune system is exerted. This results in differences in *env* of as much as 1% per year for evolutionary selection (Myers and Pavlakis, 1992; Boeri *et al.*, 1992). Limited studies on the inter-patient variability of HIV-2 have shown that the range of variability in the envelope V3 sequence is similar to the inter-patient variability of HIV-1 (Boeri *et al.*, 1992; Sankalé *et al.*, 1995). Tissue-specific quasi species have been identified in HIV-1 infection *in vivo*, and this has also been demonstrated in the analysis of blood and brain viral sequences from an HIV-2-infected individual (Sankalé *et al.*, 1996; Sankalé *et al.*, 1998). Evaluation of intra-patient variation in the V3 envelope region of HIV-2 in asymptomatic and symptomatic individuals followed over time has shown a lower variation when compared to HIV-1 (Sankalé *et al.*, 1995). This lower intra-patient variation appears to be a distinct feature of HIV-2 infection that may result from decreased viral burden and also contribute to lower rates of transmission and disease development.

In evaluation of paired blood and cervical lavage samples, the rate of viral shedding was 36.4% for HIV-1 and 16% for HIV-2, after repeat PCRs (Sankalé *et al.*, 1998). In most cases, phylogenetic analysis showed that the viral sequences from blood and genital secretions were intermingled, and subclusters did not segregate according to sample site. In rare cases, however, tissue-specific sequences were observed, suggesting a complex relationship between quasi species in the two sites where preferential transmission of HIV variants may be due to multiple factors.

Evidence for a lower viral burden in HIV-2-infected individuals has been reported from both virus isolation and PCR studies (Simon *et al.*, 1993; Berry *et al.*, 1994; Dieng-Sarr *et al.*, 1999; Popper *et al.*, 1999; Dieng-Sarr *et al.*, 1998; Berry *et al.*, 1998). The isolation rate of HIV-2 from peripheral blood mononuclear cells or plasma of asymptomatic HIV-2-infected individuals was lower than the isolation rate for HIV-1 (Simon *et al.*, 1993). At lower CD4+ lymphocyte counts, virus isolation was equally efficient in both infections. Studies in the Gambia and Senegal suggest that proviral HIV-2 copies increase with the development of the disease and the drop of CD4+ lymphocytes (Berry *et al.*, 1994; Dieng-Sarr *et al.*, 1999).

In our studies that compared the HIV-2 proviral loads in HIV-2 singly and dually infected individuals, we found that the median proviral loads differed significantly, with those in the HIV-2 group ranging from 63.2 to 669.8 copies/10^5 CD4+ cells, demonstrating an inverse correlation with the CD4+ lymphocyte count. The HIV dually infected persons showed less variation in viral load, ranging from 9.9 to 43.3 copies/10^5 CD4+ cells. In contrast, among the HIV dually infected persons, low HIV-2 proviral load was correlated with low CD4+ lymphocyte counts. The HIV-2 proviral loads in HIV dually infected persons were significantly lower than those in HIV-2 monotypically infected individuals ($P < .0001$), despite comparable CD4+ lymphocyte counts. These results suggest that different HIV-2 proviral dynamics prevail in HIV dual infection (Dieng-Sarr *et al.*, 1999).

HIV-2 is less pathogenic than HIV-1, but the mechanisms underlying this difference have not been defined. We developed an internally controlled quantitative reverse transcriptase-polymerase chain reaction to measure HIV-2 viral load and determined levels of plasma virus in a cohort of registered FSW in Dakar, Senegal (Popper *et al.*, 1999). The assay has a lower limit of detection of 100 copies/ml and is linear over 4 logs. HIV-2 viral RNA was detectable in 56% of all samples tested; the median load was 141 copies/ml. Levels of viral RNA in the plasma were inversely related to CD4+ cell counts. HIV-2 and HIV-1 viral loads were compared among the seroincident women in the cohort; the median viral load was 30-fold lower in the HIV-2-infected women ($P<0.001$, Wilcoxon rank sum test), irrespective of the length of time infected. This suggests that plasma viremia is linked to the differences in the pathogenicity of the 2 viruses (Popper *et al.*, 1999).

Using an LTR-based RT-PCR assay, Berry *et al.* (1998) reported a cross-sectional study of HIV infected patients stratified according to percent CD4 T-lymphocytes (CD4%). HIV-2-infected individuals had lower plasma RNA levels than HIV-1-infected persons at lower CD4% levels, while at higher CD4% levels the plasma RNA levels were similar. Likewise, in studies of HIV-2 patients in Portugal, plasma viremia could be detected in only ten of 30 subjects (33%), a rate much lower than that seen in HIV-1 infection. Virus was isolated from 16 of 30 patients (53.3%). A significant correlation was found between CD4+ counts, clinical status, rate of virus isolation, and plasma viral load (Soriano *et al.*, 1998). In a study of known seroconverters, HIV-2-infected individuals demonstrated a viral setpoint ~28-fold lower than HIV-1-infected individuals in the same study (Andersson *et al.*, 2000).

Levels of virus in the plasma are closely related to the pathogenicity of HIV-1, and infection with HIV-2 leads to significantly lower plasma viral load. To further identify the source of this difference, we measured both viral RNA and proviral DNA in matched samples from 34 HIV-2-infected individuals. The median level of HIV-2 RNA for the group was 189 copies/ml. Levels of HIV-2 RNA were below the limit of detection in nearly half the women which was consistent with what we had previously reported in this population (Popper *et al.*, 2000). Levels of HIV-2 proviral DNA were similar to that of HIV-1 but failed to correlate with levels of viral RNA. Thus, it appears that significant differences occur upon expression, release, and/or maintenance of virions in the bloodstream. It is possible that shifts in splicing patterns could be responsible for the differences in virion production, but further studies would be required to verify such an explanation for the current data. Comparative studies of both viral and host factors that may affect expression will be useful for understanding the differences between HIV-1 and HIV-2 pathogenesis.

HIV-2 CLINICAL OUTCOME

Early surveys included various case reports with AIDS in HIV-2-infected people (Romieu *et al.*, 1990; Clavel *et al.*, 1986; Saimot *et al.*, 1987). The disease characteristics, including tuberculosis, chronic diarrhea,

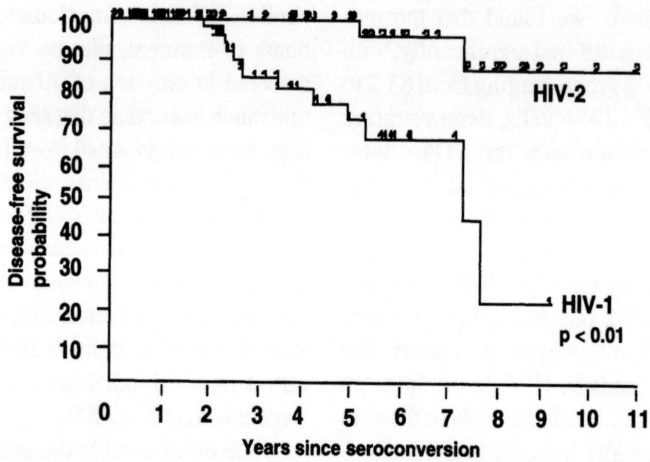

FIGURE 2. Kaplan-Meier AIDS-free survival probability comparing incident HIV-1 and HIV-2 infected individuals. Wilcoxon-Gehan, p value <0.01. (Kanki *et al.*, 2002)

and *Candida* infections, seemed similar to diseases seen in HIV-1-associated AIDS (Romieu *et al.*, 1990; De Cock *et al.*, 1990; Le Guenno *et al.*, 1991). Central nervous system involvement was also occasionally seen in HIV-2-infected people (Schneider *et al.*, 1990; Dwyer *et al.*, 1992). However, classical African AIDS-associated diseases, such as tuberculosis, often had only a weak epidemiological association with HIV-2, even in HIV-2 endemic areas (Marlink *et al.*, 1988; Marlink *et al.*, 1994; Kanki, 1999).

Our prospective studies conducted in a registered FSW cohort in Dakar, Senegal has provided the unique opportunity to measure the infection and progression rates of both HIV-1 and HIV-2 infections (Marlink *et al.*, 1988; Marlink *et al.*, 1994; Traore *et al.*, 1996). Importantly, these prospective studies have compared disease progression in individuals with a known time of infection, and the cohort has been observed for over 15 years, representing one of the longest HIV natural history studies in the field. The Kaplan-Meier analysis of HIV-2 incident infected individuals indicates that 85% (95%CI = 50 – 96%) remain AIDS-free after 8 years of HIV-2 infection (Figure 2) (Kanki *et al.*, 1999). These differences in survival probabilities between HIV-2 and HIV-1 were also seen for CDC IV disease and CD4+ lymphocyte counts below 400 cells/mm^3 and CD4+ lymphocyte counts below 200 cells/mm^3.

In our prospective study of HIV-2-infected individuals, we have also identified individuals that fit a definition of long-term, non-progression, and can therefore determine a rate of this phenotype in the study population (Marlink *et al.*, 1994; Traore *et al.*, 1996). Employing a definition of long-term non-progression as $\geq$8 years infection in the absence of AIDS or related symptoms and stable CD4+ lymphocytes >500 cells/mm^3, we have found 39 of 41 (95%) of the women studied would be classified as long-term non-progressors. This dramatic difference in pathogenicity provides a unique opportunity to identify viral and host immune mechanisms involved in a closely related and relevant virus system that is predicted to have a significantly slower course of progression (Figure 2).

Since slower disease course appears to be common in HIV-2 infection, we reasoned that certain subsets of the population would possess host characteristics that might be predisposed to a more rapid disease course. We conducted a case-control study investigating possible associations between HLA and the risk of disease progression in HIV-2 (Diouf *et al.*, 2002). The HLA class I status was molecularly typed in 62 FSW from the Dakar, Senegal cohort; lack of antibodies to the HIV-2 antigen p26 was used as the surrogate marker for risk of disease progression (Popper *et al.*, 1998). Statistical analysis showed that HLA B35 was associated with a lack of p26 antibodies ($p < 0.05$) and a higher risk of disease progression. The same association was found for the class I haplotypes B35-Cw4 and A23-Cw7 ($p < 0.05$), similar to the association with HIV-1 (Carrington *et al.*, 1999). Our data shows that certain HLA molecules are associated with risk of disease progression in HIV-2, and that some of the alleles and haplotypes involved in susceptibility to disease are similar for both HIV-1 and HIV-2.

HIV-2 IMMUNITY

The attenuated phenotype of HIV-2 infection in vivo has sparked considerable interest in understanding the immunopathogenesis of this particular HIV infection. Although certain viral determinants appear to be central to the lower replicative capacity *in vivo*, the virus appears uniquely immunogenic, inducing significant immunity which may be central to the explanation of the weaker, more attenuated phenotype of HIV-2 compared with HIV-1. As with HIV-1, the antibody response to most viral structural proteins occurs shortly after infection and is thought to persist. In HIV-2 infection, over 90% of seropositives evaluated in Senegal demonstrated strong antibodies to *gag*, *pol* and *env*-encoded antigens (Kanki *et al.*, 1987b; Essex *et al.*, 1988). As already noted, the cross-reactive response to analogous HIV-1 antigens is significant in highly conserved gene products such as *gag* and *pol* and less with envelope antigens.

Previously, circulating p24 antigen of HIV-1 has been useful as a marker of virus replication *in vivo*, although in recent times, this has been partially replaced with more direct measurements of virion particles using PCR technology. Analogous studies with HIV-2 have not been described, perhaps because antibodies to p26 are found in the majority of HIV-2-infected sera, and therefore it has been assumed that complexing by free circulating p26 is less frequent. In our studies, we have found that the lack of antibodies to p26 is a fixed phenotype, not resultant from complexing of free p26, and predictive of a more rapid disease course (Popper *et al.*, 1998; Diouf *et al.*, 2002).

HIV-2 neutralizing antibodies have been described (Robert-Guroff *et al.*, 1992; Bjorling *et al.*, 1993; Bjorling *et al.*, 1994; Weiss *et al.*, 1988; Bottiger *et al.*, 1989), and in studies with fresh isolates, the broadness of the HIV-2 neutralizing response has been unusual and distinct from the neutralizing antibody response to HIV-1 (Fenyo and Putkonen, 1996). Virus neutralization studies have shown that a proportion of HIV-2 sera are also capable of cross-neutralizing HIV-1 isolates in addition to HIV-2 isolates .(Weiss *et al.*, 1988; Bottiger *et al.*, 1990). The degree to which HIV-1 positive sera can cross-neutralize HIV-2 isolates remains controversial. It is still not known whether some of the conserved domains of *env* will be capable of eliciting a cross-protective response to both viruses.

Studies of HIV-2 humoral immunity have now been extended to evaluate the highly related mucosal immune response (Belec *et al.*, 1996). Evaluation of HIV-2 antibody responses in cervicovaginal secretions have shown that only a third of infected women generate IgA responses to HIV-2 envelope antigens in this compartment, suggesting lower levels of viral replication compared to HIV-1. Of interest, the cross-reactivity by IgG and IgA to heterologous envelope antigens was more frequent with HIV-2 infection (Belec *et al.*, 1996). Cervicovaginal cross-reactivity was more pronounced for HIV-2-specific antibodies to HIV-1 epitopes than for the converse. Such features could be relevant to a differential heterosexual transmission of one type of HIV in an individual infected by the other type, in accordance with epidemiologic studies showing that HIV-2 infection protects from HIV-1 infection, and that

HIV-1 infection does not appear to protect significantly from HIV-2 infection.

Knowledge of immune mechanisms responsible for the cross-protection between highly divergent viruses such as HIV-1 and HIV-2 may contribute to an understanding of whether virus variability may be overcome in the design of vaccine candidates which are broadly protective across the HIV subtypes. In early CTL studies of HIV-2, responses against HIV-2 *gag*, *pol* and *nef* proteins were described; when HLA-B53 was restricted, HIV-2 *gag*-specific CTLs did not recognize target cells expressing HIV-1 *gag* proteins, suggesting the absence of a cross-protective cellular response (Gotch *et al.*, 1993). More recently, Bertoletti and colleagues (1998) also working in the Gambia, have shown that the majority of HIV-2-infected individuals with different HLA molecules possess a dominant cytotoxic T-cell response which is able to recognize HIV-1 *gag* protein. Furthermore, HLA-B5801-positive subjects have shown broad cross-recognition of HIV-1 subtypes since they mounted a T-cell response that tolerated extensive amino acid substitutions within HLA-B5801-restricted HIV-1 and HIV-2 epitopes. These results suggest that HLA-B5801-positive HIV-2-infected individuals have an enhanced ability to react with HIV-1 that could play a role in cross-protection (Bertoletti *et al.*, 1998).

We have applied the sensitive ELISPOT technique to further quantify the HIV-2-specific CTL response in HIV-2-infected individuals (Dieng-Sarr *et al.*, 2000b). To assess the antigen delivery system using the modified non-toxic form of the anthrax toxin, we fused the HIV-2 *gag* (P-26) to the terminal domain of the Lethal Factor (LFn; 255 aa). The LFn-HIV-2 recombinant proteins were expressed and used as antigens to stimulate CTL in a ELISPOT assay in comparison to the classic delivery system using recombinant vaccinia virus (rVV) expressing HIV-2 *gag*. We found that 87.5% of individuals in our study showed a specific *gag* CTL response. Our results have shown that priming cells with the LFn-P-26 creates better sensitivity and resolution when subjects have a low frequency of CTL precursors. Interestingly, we found that the group with strong cellular immune response had no detectable HIV-2 plasma load.

PROTECTIVE IMMUNITY—IMPLICATIONS FOR VACCINE

Global statistics of the HIV epidemic continue to underscore the urgency for an effective HIV vaccine. The developing world, particularly regions of Africa, continue to bear a significant portion of the global HIV burden, and they are unlikely to benefit from recent advances in therapeutic regimes in the foreseeable future. Important to vaccine design is the understanding of pathogenic mechanisms of HIV infection and the potential immunologic responses or correlates necessary for HIV containment. The identification of such correlates has been hampered by relatively rare instances of natural immunity that have withstood the challenge of viral exposure. In the early 1800s, Jenner's identification of the protected milkmaids provided the characterization of cowpox, later utilized for vaccination against the antigenically related smallpox for its ultimate eradication.

Demonstrated differences in the infectivity and disease potential of HIV-2 compared to HIV-1 support the notion that the mechanism for such protection might be analogous to the attenuated virus vaccine model. In our studies of the FSW cohort in Dakar, Senegal we tested the hypothesis that the attenuated phenotype of HIV-2 infection might protect from subsequent HIV-1 infection (Travers *et al.*, 1995). HIV-1 infection in previous HIV negatives along with superinfection of HIV-2infected subjects was documented over the study period with both serology and PCR assays. A Poisson regression model was used to estimate the independent effect of demographic, behavioral, and biologic variables on the risk of HIV-1 infection. Despite higher incidence of other sexually transmitted diseases,

HIV-2-infected women had a lower incidence of HIV-1 than seronegatives, with an incidence rate ratio (IRR) of 0.32 ($p = 0.008$). This analysis led to the conclusion that HIV-2 infection conferred a significant reduction in the subsequent risk of HIV-1 infection. Continued analysis of the Dakar cohort has extended the initial observation period of the first published report to over 13 years and in that time HIV-2 protection rates range from 52–74% depending on the method of analysis (Travers *et al.*, 1995; Travers and Eisen, 1998; Kanki, 1999).

The generalizability these findings has been questioned by studies from other West African sites. In Ivory Coast, Guinea Bissau, and the Gambia, studies originally designed as cross-sectional surveys were analyzed for short periods of longitudinal observation (Wiktor *et al.*, 1999; Aaby *et al.*, 1997; Ariyoshi *et al.*, 1997), as a result of their design they failed to possess sufficient statistical power, capable only of detecting an extremely high protected fraction (>99%) of HIV-1 infection due to HIV-2 infection (Travers and Eisen, 1998). In addition, a mixture of serologic methods were employed by these studies, failing to meet the PCR-based, gold standard for diagnosis of dual infection which is critical to the objective evaluation of HIV-2 protection *in vivo* (Wiktor *et al.*, 1999; Aaby *et al.*, 1997; Ariyoshi *et al.*, 1997). In a longitudinal study conducted in police officers in Guinea Bissau, Norrgren *et al.* (1999) failed to report a statistically significant result; however, only a portion of the samples were diagnosed by PCR technology. Unbiased, powerful studies, using sensitive and specific classification methods, will effectively address the generalizability of the observation of HIV-2's protective efficacy against subsequent HIV-1 infection. Despite these findings, the observation of the Dakar cohort continues to document a protective effect. The long person-time of observation with few losses to follow-up and rigorous PCR testing has supported these important findings in people (Kanki *et al.*, 1999).

Studies from other research groups including our own have described in vitro interactions of HIV-1 and HIV-2 that support our *in vivo* observations, these range from virus–virus interactions to potential immune-mediated mechanisms for HIV-2 protection. Arya and Gallo (1996) have reported that HIV-2 inhibits the replication of HIV-1 at the molecular level. This inhibition was selective, dose-dependent, and nonreciprocal. Though the exact mechanism remains to be defined, the inhibition appeared to be mainly due to an intracellular molecular event, because it could not be explained solely on the basis of cell surface receptor mediated interference. The results support the notion that the inhibition likely occurred at the level of viral RNA, possibly involving competition between viral RNAs for some transcriptional factor essential for virus replication (Arya and Gallo, 1996; Rappaport *et al.*, 1995).

We also suspected that viral determinants might play a role in HIV-2 protection, whereby one might hypothesize that HIV-2 would differentially protect from certain HIV-1 subtypes better than others. To investigate the HIV-1 subtypes involved in dual HIV-1 and HIV-2 infections, we sequenced the *env* region from 29 dually infected FSW from Senegal (Dieng-Sarr *et al.*, 2000a; Dieng-Sarr *et al.*, 2000b). The majority of women, 23 of 29, (79.3%) were infected by HIV-1 subtype A; within the HIV-1 subtype A sequences, 14 of 23 (60.8%) clustered with the West African associated A/G recombinant form (IbNG), and 9 of 23 (39.2%) formed a separate cluster distinct from the A/G IbNG. In contrast, in HIV-1 singly infected individuals, non-IbNG subtype A was found in only 13 of 98 (13.3%). Therefore, the lack of protection and/or interaction with HIV-2 was associated with a distinct HIV-1 A genotype. These results suggest differences in the biological properties of HIV-1 genotypes and their *in vivo* interaction with HIV-2 (Dieng-Sarr *et al.*, 2000b).

Beta-chemokines have now been identified as potent soluble suppressors of macrophage-tropic HIV infection *in vitro*. Studies of multiply exposed, uninfected individuals have implicated the role of elevated β-chemokines in HIV resistance, in many cases, independent of genetic mutations in the chemokine receptor (Paxton *et al.*, 1996; Cocchi *et al.*, 1995; Zagury *et al.*, 1998). Macaque studies have also suggested a role for β-chemokines in vaccine-induced protective immunity using a variety of vaccine candidates and live virus challenge (Lehner *et al.*, 1996). We used an HIV-1 *in vitro* challenge system to determine if PBMCs from HIV-2-infected individuals showed altered susceptibility to HIV-1 infection (Kokkotou *et al.*, 2000). Peripheral blood mononuclear cells were stimulated and infected with either R5 or X4 HIV-1 viruses. Fourteen of 28 (50%) HIV-2 PBMCs demonstrated over 90% inhibition of R5/HIV-1 infection compared to 0 of 19 HIV negative controls (Fisher exact test, p value = 0.0002). In contrast, HIV-2 positive and HIV negative control cells were equally susceptible to HIV-1/X4 infection. RANTES, MIP1α, MIP1β, the natural ligands of the CCR5 receptor, were measured in culture supernatant by ELISA, and supernatant levels of MIP-1β ($r = -0.56$, $p = 0.03$) and MIP-1α ($r = -0.69$, $p = 0.004$) were inversely correlated with HIV-1 replication. Using polyclonal antibodies to RANTES, MIP1α, and MIP1β, resistance was neutralized. A significant proportion of HIV-2-infected PBMCs demonstrate HIV-1 resistance *in vitro*; this resistance was β-chemokine dependent (Kokkotou *et al.*, 2000). Further studies are needed to characterize this potent anti-viral activity, and to determine its potential contribution to in vivo protection.

HIV-2 infection might dramatically influence β-chemokine production by enhancing it in magnitude and duration, thus enabling HIV-2-infected individuals to cope favorably with subsequent exposure to HIV-1. This is supported by the studies demonstrating that binding of the HIV-2 envelope to the alpha chain of CD8 stimulates dramatic levels of β-chemokine production in comparison to HIV-1 gp120 activity (Neoh *et al.*, 1997). This suggests a novel viral suppressive mechanism, one that may be adapted for immunoprophylaxis. Antiretroviral vaccine strategies that incorporate β-chemokine induction or other receptor-blocking functions raise some encouraging possibilities for vaccine design and development.

HIV-2-infected baboons (Papio cynocephalus) provide a valuable animal model for the study of HIV pathogenesis, since many features of disease progression resemble HIV-1 infection of humans. In some HIV-2-infected baboons that are clinically healthy, a CD8+ cell antiviral response that was partly mediated by a soluble factor, appeared to control viral replication in vitro. A soluble factor was found to be active against the chemokine-resistant, syncytium-inducing HIV-1 isolates and was relatively heat stable. Therefore, the soluble suppressing activity of CD8+ cells in HIV-2-infected baboons may be analogous to the CD8+ cell antiviral factor described in human HIV-infected asymptomatic people (Locher *et al.*, 1997).

HIV-2 is primarily in West Africa, where it infects an estimated 1–2 million people. It is spread less efficiently than HIV-1, making projections for future infections much lower than for HIV-1. For these reasons, development of an HIV-2 vaccine has not been a high research priority. However, HIV-2 infects monkeys whereas HIV-1 does not, and the SIV vaccine model uses viruses that are closer to HIV-2 than HIV-1. The development and testing of an HIV-2 vaccine might therefore be simpler than the development of an HIV-1 vaccine. A few reports about HIV-2 have described experimental studies with limited vaccine protection (Putkonen *et al.*, 1990; Putkonen *et al.*, 1991), but immune correlates of protection have not been identified (Andersson *et al.*, 1996; Biberfeld *et al.*, 1996; Myagkikh *et al.*, 1996). Nonetheless, the data from human studies suggesting that HIV-2 may afford protection from HIV-1 indicates that a candidate vaccine based on HIV-2 might provide necessary cross-immunity for HIV-1 protection and is worthy of further consideration.

HIV-2 THERAPY

Drugs that have efficacy against HIV-1 are generally assumed to be effective against HIV-2. However, with a few exceptions of *in vitro* analysis (De Clercq *et al.*, 1992), most HIV-1 drugs have not been tested for activity against HIV-2. A case can therefore be made that HIV-2 infection in monkeys also provides a valuable *in vivo* model for drug testing that is not readily available for HIV-1 (Bottiger *et al.*, 1992). Anti-retroviral therapy has been infrequently reported in HIV-2 infection. A recent report of two HIV-2 AIDS cases undergoing zidovudine-treatment in The Netherlands demonstrated mutations in the RT genes similar to those associated with zidovudine resistance in HIV-1 (Schutten *et al.*, 2000).

Unlike HIV-1, there is limited clinical experience with antiretroviral therapy in HIV-2 infection. This is at least partially due to the African distribution of the virus and the paucity of AIDS-related cases in developed country settings. Further, treatment decisions have been difficult in the absence of a commercially available HIV-2 plasma viral load assay. We have had limited experience in the therapy of HIV-2 patients in the US, where it appears that standard HAART (highly active antiretroviral therapy) can readily reduce viral load levels below detection (Ayanian *et al.*, 1989; Clark *et al.*, 1998).

The reverse transcriptase (RT) and protease genes from 12 HIV-2-infected individuals who had been exposed to antiretroviral drugs were examined for the presence of mutations that could be involved in drug resistance. Four individuals carried virus genotypes with amino acid substitutions potentially associated with resistance to nucleoside analogues: two at codon 70 (K–>R) and two at codon 184 (M–>V); the latter two patients harbored a codon Q151M mutation which has been associated with multi-drug resistance in HIV-1. Substitutions associated with resistance to protease inhibitors at codon 46 were observed in all individuals. Moreover, minor resistance mutations, as well as new ones, were often seen in the protease gene. Thus, amino acid changes in the HIV-2 RT and protease genes, which could be associated with drug resistance seems to occur at positions identical to those for HIV-1 (Rodes *et al.*, 2000).

Smith and colleagues (2001) have reported on the clinical management of seven HIV-2-infected patients on antiretroviral therapy followed in the U.K. HIV-2 viremia was detectable only at CD4 counts $<300 \times 106$/ml. Two patients with high load ($>50{,}000$ copies/ml) failed to respond to therapy, although these patients were given suboptimal therapy. One of these patients had a viral load $>50{,}000$ copies/ml and a CD4 count of 66. His initial regimen was dual therapy followed by sequential single drug switches. Drug resistance data on this patient's virus demonstrated 20-fold higher $IC_{50}$to 3TC (after six months of therapy) and ten-fold higher IC_{50} for SQV after nine months of therapy. In four patients, ARV therapy led to a fall in viral load and a rise in CD4 cell count, although all had initial viral load levels of $<50{,}000$ copies/ml. From the few published studies, including our own, we are not able to adequately assess the clinical utility of the NNRTI (Non-Nucleoside Reverse Transcriptase Inhibitors) class of antivirals as a treatment option for HIV-2, although *in vitro* data suggests that this class of drugs may be less efficacious with HIV-2 than HIV-1. Similar to our observations, it appears that HIV-2 differs from HIV-1 in the risk of disease progression at any given CD4 cell count and may therefore have different implications for the timing and management of ARV therapy (Mullins *et al.*, in press).

SUMMARY

HIV-2 was first described in West Africa in 1985. Since that time there has been considerable progress made in understanding the virology and epidemiology of HIV-2. The data suggests differences between HIV-2 and HIV-1 in geographic distribution, distinct epidemic trends, perinatal transmission rates, and incubation periods to the development of AIDS. The virologic determinants and mechanisms for these apparent biological differences are still unknown. However, an understanding of how HIV-2 differs from HIV-1 is essential for interpretations of comparative virologic studies. We are hopeful that such comparative studies will yield important information on the pathogenic mechanisms employed by HIV viruses, and will lead the way to the development of effective interventions for the prevention of AIDS. This is best exemplified in the studies that indicate that this close relative of HIV-1 infection, via its attenuated phenotype, may confer significant protection from subsequent HIV-1 infection. This further suggests that understanding HIV-2 immunity and cross-immunity may be useful for HIV vaccine design and development. Finally, our appreciation of the biologic diversity found in closely related HIV viruses may better help us to anticipate the future consequences of HIV infections at the host and population level.

Acknowledgements. This work results from the Inter-University Convention for the Research of AIDS and other Viral Induced Diseases (Dakar and Harvard) and the continual support from the Senegalese Ministry of Health. The research was supported in part by DAMD 17-95-C-5005, NO1-A1-35173 and 5D43 TW00004.

REFERENCES

Aaby, P., Ariyoshi, K., Buckner, M., Jensen, H., Berry, N., Wilkins, A., Richard, D., Larsen, O., Dias, F., Melbye, M., and Whittle, H. (1996). Age of wife as a major determinant of male-to-female transmission of HIV-2 infection: a community study from rural West Africa. *AIDS* 10(13): 1585–1590.

Aaby, P., Poulsen, A.G., Larsen, O., Christiansen, C.B., Jensen, H., Melbye, M., Naucler, A., and Dias, F. (1997). Does HIV-2 protect against HIV-1 infection? [letter] [see comments]. Comment in: AIDS 1998 Jan 22;12(2):224-5. *AIDS* 11(7): 939–940.

Abbott, R.C., Ndour-Sarr, A., Diouf, A., Ndoye, T., Ba, D., Tall, N., Mbaye, N., Kébé, F., Diadhiou, F., Essex, M., Marlink, R., Mboup, S., and Kanki, P. (1994). Risk Determinants for HIV Infection and Adverse Obstertrical Outcomes in Pregnant Women in Dakar, Senegal. *JAIDS* 7: 711–717.

Adjorlolo-Johnson, G., De Cock, K.M., Ekpini, E., Vetter, K.M., Sibailly, T., Brattegaard, K., Yavo, D., Doorly, R., Whitaker, J.P., Kestens, L., and Projet RETRO-CI. (1994). Prospective comparison of mother-to-child transmission of HIV-1 and HIV-2 in Abidjan, Ivory Coast [see comments] [published erratum appears in JAMA 1994 Nov 16;272(19):1482]. Comment in: JAMA 1994 Aug 10;272(6):487–8. *Jama* 272(6): 462–466.

Albert, J., Naucler, A., Bottiger, B., Broliden, P., Albino, P., Ouattara, S., Bjorkegren, C., Valentin, A., Biberfeld, G., and Fenyo, E. (1990). Replicative capacity of HIV-2, like HIV-1, correlates with severity of immunodeficiency. *AIDS* 4(4): 291–295.

Albert, J., Stalhandske, P., Marquina, S., Karis, J., Fouchier, R.A., Norrby, E., and Chiodi, F. (1996). Biological phenotype of HIV type 2 isolates correlates with V3 genotype. *AIDS Res Hum Retroviruses* 12(9): 821–828.

Allan, J.S., Coligan, J.E., Lee, T.H., Barin, F., Kanki, P., Mboup, S., McLane, M.F., Groopman, J.E., and Essex, M. (1987). Immunogenic Nature of a *pol* Gene Product of HTLV-III/LAV. *Blood* 69: 331–333.

Allan, J.S., Kanda, P., Kennedy, R.C., Cobb, E.K., Anthony, M., and Eichberg, J.W. (1990). Isolation and characterization of simian immunodeficiency viruses from two subspecies of African green monkeys. *AIDS Res Hum Retroviruses* 6: 275–285.

Alter, H.J., Eichberg, J.W., Masur, H., Saxinger, W.C., Gallo, R.C., Lane, H.C., and Fauci, A.S. (1984). Transmission of HTLV-III from human plasma to chimpanzees: an animal model for AIDS. *Science* 226: 549–552.

Anderson, R.M., and May, R.M. (1996). The population biology of the interaction between HIV-1 and HIV-2: coexistence or competitive exclusion? *AIDS* 10(14): 1663–1673.

Andersson, S., da Silva, Z., Norrgren, H., Dias, F., and Biberfeld, G. (1997). Field evaluation of alternative testing strategies for diagnosis and differentiation of HIV-1 and HIV-2 infections in an HIV-1 and HIV-2-prevalent area. *AIDS* 11(15): 1815–1822.

Andersson, S., Makitalo, B., Thorstensson, R., Franchini, G., Tartaglia, J., Limbach, K., Paoletti, E., Putkonen, P., and Biberfeld, G. (1996). Immunogenicity and protective efficacy of a human immunodeficiency virus type 2 recombinant canarypox

(ALVAC) vaccine candidate in cynomolgus monkeys. *J Infect Dis* 174(5): 977–985.

Andersson, S., Norrgren, H., da Silva, Z., Biague, A., Bamba, S., Kwok, S., Christopherson, C., Biberfeld, G., and Albert, J. (2000). Plasma viral load in HIV-1 and HIV-2 singly and dually infected individuals in Guinea Bissau, West Africa: significantly lower plasma virus set point in HIV-2 infection than in HIV-1 infection. *Arch Intern Med* 160: 3286–3293.

Andreasson, P., Dias, F., Naucler, A., Anderson, S., and Biberfeld, G. (1993). A prospective study of vertical transmission of HIV-2 in Bissau, Guinea-Bissau. *AIDS* 7: 989.

Ankrah, T., Roberts, M., Antwi, P., Atubrah, M.P., Bawuah, P.P., Kotoh, S., Acheampong, J.W., Wood, J.G., Boateng, K.A., and Mingle, J.A. (1994). The African AIDS case definition and HIV serology in medical in-patients at Komfo Anokye Teaching Hospital, Kumasi, Ghana. *West Afr J Med* 13: 98.

Ariyoshi, K., van der Loeff, M., Sabally, S., Cham, F., Corrah, T., and Whittle, H. (1997). Does HIV-2 infection provide cross-protection against HIV-1 infection? (letter). *AIDS* 11:1053–1054.

Arya, S.K., and Gallo, R.C. (1996). Human immunodeficiency virus (HIV) type 2-mediated inhibition of HIV type 1: a new approach to gene therapy of HIV-infection. *Proc Natl Acad Sci USA* 93(9): 4486–4491.

Asjo, B., Albert, J., Karlsson, A., Morfeldt-Manson, L., Biberfeld, G., Lidman, K., and Fenyo, E.M. (1986). Replicative capacity of human immunodeficiency virus from patients with varying severity of HIV infection. *Lancet* ii: 660–662.

Ayanian, J.Z., Maguire, J.H., Marlink, R., Essex, M., and Kanki, P. (1989). HIV-2 Infection in the United States. *N Engl J Med* 320: 1422–1423.

Ayres, L., Avillez, F., Garcia Benito, A., Deinhardt, F., Gurtler, L., Denis, F., Leonard, G., Ranger, S., Grob, P., and Joller Jemelka, H. (1990). Multicenter evaluation of a new recombinant enzyme immunoassay for the combined detection of antibody to HIV-1 and HIV-2. *AIDS* 4: 131–138.

Bahraoui, E., Benjouad, A., Guetard, D., Kolbe, H., Gluckman, J.C., and Montagnier, L. (1992). Study of the interaction of HIV-1 and HIV-2 envelope glycoproteins with the CD4 receptor and role of N-glycans. *AIDS Res Hum Retroviruses* 8(5): 565–573.

Baillou, A., Janvier, B., Leonard, G., Denis, F., Goudeau, A. and Barin, F. (1991a). Fine serotyping of human immunodeficiency virus serotype 1 (HIV-1) and HIV-2 infections by using synthetic oligopeptides representing an immunodominant domain of HIV-1 and HIV-2/simian immunodeficiency virus. *J Clin Microbiol* 29(7): 1387–1391.

Baillou, A., Janvier, B., Mayer, R., Kanki, P., Mboup, S., Denis, F., Goudeau, A., Essex, M. and Barin, F. (1991b). Site-Directed Serology Using Synthetic Oligopeptides Representing the C-terminus of the External Glycoproteins of HIV-1, HIV-2, or SIV_{mac} May Distinguish Subtypes Among Primate Lentiviruses. *AIDS Res Hum Retroviruses* 7: 767–772.

Bakhanashvili, M. and Hizi, A. (1992). Fidelity of the RNA-dependent DNA synthesis exhibited by the reverse transcriptases of human immunodeficiency virus types 1 and 2 and of murine leukemia virus: mispair extension frequencies. *Biochemistry* 31(39): 9393–9398.

Barin, F., Mboup, S., Denis, F., Kanki, P., Allan, J.S., Lee, T.H. and Essex, M. (1985). Serological Evidence for Virus Related to Simian T-Lymphotropic Retrovirus III in Residents of West Africa. *Lancet* ii: 1387–1390.

Belec, L., Tevi-Benissan, C., Dupre, T., Mohamed, A.S., Prazuck, T., Gilquin, J., Kanga, J.M. and Pillot, J. (1996). Comparison of cervicovaginal humoral immunity in clinically asymptomatic (CDC A1 and A2 category) patients with HIV-1 and HIV-2 infection. *J Clin Immunol* 16(1): 12–20.

Berry, N., Ariyoshi, K., Jobe, O., Ngum, P., Corrah, T., Wilkins, A., Ngum, P., Corrah, T., Wilkins, A., Whittle, H. and Tedder, R. (1994). HIV Type 2 Proviral Load measured by Quantitative Polymerase Chain Reaction correlates with CD4+ Lymphopenia in HIV Type 2-Infected Individuals. *AIDS Res Hum Retroviruses* 10: 1031–1037.

Berry, N., Ariyoshi, K., Jaffar, S., Sabally, S., Corrah, T., Tedder, R. and Whittle, H. (1998). Low peripheral blood viral HIV-2 RNA in individuals with high CD4 percentage differentiates HIV-2 from HIV-1 infection. *J Hum Virol* 1(7): 457–468.

Bertoletti, A., Cham, F., McAdam, S., Rostron, T., Rowland-Jones, S., Sabally, S., Carrah, T., Ariyoshi, K., and Whittle, H. (1998). Cytotoxic T cells from human Immunodeficiency virus type 2 infected patients frequently cross-react with different human immunodeficiency virus type 1 clades. *J Virol* 72(3): 2439–2448.

Biberfeld, G., Brown, F., Esparza, J., Essex, M., Gallo, R., Montagnier, L., Najera, R., Risser, R., and Schild, G. (1987). Meeting Report, WHO working group on characterization of HIV-related, retroviruses: Criteria for characterization and proposal for a nomenclature system. *AIDS* 1: 189–190.

Biberfeld, G., Thorstensson, R., and Putkonen, P. (1996). Protection against human immunodeficiency virus type 2 and simian immunodeficiency virus in macaques vaccinated against human immunodeficiency virus type 2. *AIDS Res Hum Retroviruses* 12(5): 443–446.

Bjorling, E., Broliden, K., Bernardi, D., Utter, G., Thorstensson, R., Chiodi, F., and Norrby, E. (1991). Hyperimmune antisera against synthetic peptides representing the glycoprotein of human immunodeficiency virus type 2 can mediate neutralization and antibody-dependent cytotoxic activity. *Proc Natl Acad Sci USA* 88: 6082–6086.

Bjorling, E., Chiodi, F., Utter, G. and Norrby, E. (1994). Two neutralizing domains in the V3 region of the envelope glycoprotein gp125 of HIV-2 type 2. *J Immunol* 152: 1952–1959.

Bjorling, E., Scarlatti, G., von Gegerfelt, A., Albert, J., Biberfeld, G., Chiodi, F., Norrby, E. and Fenyo, E.M. (1993). Autologous neutralizing antibodies prevail in HIV-2 but not in HIV-1 infection. *Virology* 193(1): 528–530.

Bjorling, E., von Garrelts, E., Morner, A., Ehnlund, M. and Persson, M.A. (1999). Human neutralizing human immunodeficiency virus type 2-specific Fab molecules generated by phage display. *J Gen Virol* 80(Pt 8): 1987–1993.

Boeri, E., Giri, A., Lillo, F., Ferrari, G., Varnier, O., Ferro, A., Sabbatani, S., Saxinger, W.C. and Franchini, G. (1992). In vivo genetic variability of the human immunodeficiency virus type 2 V3 region. *J Virol* 66: 4546–4550.

Bottiger, B., Karlsson, A., Andreasson, P.A., Naucler, A., Costa, C.M. and Biberfeld, G. (1989). Cross-neutralizing antibodies against HIV-1 (HTLV-IIIB and HTLV-IIIRF) and HIV-2 (SBL-6669 and a new isolate SBL-K135). *AIDS Res Hum Retroviruses* 5: 525–533.

Bottiger, B., Karlsson, A., Andreasson, P.A., Naucler, A., Costa, C.M., Norrby, E. and Biberfeld, G. (1990). Envelope cross-reactivity between human immunodeficiency virus types 1 and 2 detected by different serological methods: correlation between cross-neutralization and reactivity against the main neutralizing site. *J Virol* 64: 3492–3499.

Bottiger, D., Putkonen, P. and Oberg, B. (1992). Prevention of HIV-2 and SIV infections in cynomolgus macaques by prophylactic treatment with 3'-fluorothymidine. *AIDS Res Hum Retroviruses* 8(7): 1235–1238.

Bour, S. and Strebel, K. (1996). The human immunodeficiency virus (HIV) type 2 envelope protein is a functional complement to HIV type 1 Vpu that enhances particle release of heterologous retroviruses. *J Virol* 70(12): 8285–8300.

Broliden, P.A., Ruden, U., Ouattara, A.S., de The, G., Solver, E., Trojnar, J. and Wahren, B. (1991). Specific synthetic peptides for detection of and discrimination between HIV-1 and HIV-2 infection. *JAIDS* 4(10): 952–958.

Bron, R., Klasse, P.J., Wilkinson, D., Clapham, P.R., Pelchenmatthews, A., Power, C., Wells, T.N.C., Kim, J., Peiper, S.C., Hoxie, J.A. and Marsh, M. (1997). Promiscuous Use Of Cc and Cxc Chemokine Receptors In Cell-to-Cell Fusion Mediated By a Human Immunodeficiency Virus Type 2 Envelope Protein. *J Virol* 71(11): 8405–8415.

Cao, H., Kanki, P., Sankale, J.-L., Dieng-Sarr, A., Mazzara, G.P., Kalams, S.A., Korber, B., MBoup, S. and Walker, B.D. (1997). Cytotoxic T-lymphocyte cross-reactivity among different human immunodeficiency virus type 1 clades: implication for vaccine development. *J. Virol.* 71(11): 8615–8623.

Carrington, M., Nelson, G.W., Martin, M.P., Kissner, T., Vlahov, D., Gowdert, J., Kaslow, R., Buchbinder, S., Hoots, K., and O'Brien, S. (1999). HLA and HIV-1: heterozygote advantage and B*35-Cw*04 disadvantage. *Science* 283: 1748–1752.

Castro, B.A., Nepomuceno, M., Lerche, N.W., Eichberg, J.W., and Levy, J.A. (1991). Persistent infection of baboons and rhesus monkeys with different strains of HIV-2. *Virology* 184(1): 219–226.

Cavaleiro, R., Sousa, A., Loureiro, A., and Victorino, R. (2000). Marked immunosuppressive effects of the HIV-2 envelope protein in spite of the lower HIV-2 pathogenicity. *AIDS* 14: 2679–2686.

Chang, Y., and Jeang, K.T. (1992). The basic RNA-binding domain of HIV-2 Tat contributes to preferential trans-activation of a TAR2-containing LTR. *Nucleic Acids Res* 20: 5465–5472.

Clapham, P., McKnight, A. and Weiss, R.A. (1992). Human immunodeficiency virus type 2 infection and fusion of CD4-negative human cell lines: induction and enhancement by soluble CD4. *J Virol* 66: 3531–3537.

Clark, N.M., Dieng Sarr, A., Sankale, J.L., Kanki, P.J., Kazanjian, P., Winfield, R., and Markovitz, D.M. (1998). Immunologic and virologic response of HIV-2 infection to antiretroviral therapy [letter]. *AIDS* 12(18): 2506–2507.

Clavel, F., Guetard, D., Brun-Vezinet, F., Chamaret, S., Rey, M.A., Santos-Ferreira, M.O., Laurent, A.G., Dauguet, C., Katlama, C., and Rouzioux, C. (1986). Isolation of a new human retrovirus from West African patients with AIDS. *Science* 233: 343–346.

Cocchi, F., DeVico, A.L., Garzino-Demo, A., Arya, S.K., Gallo, R.C., and Lusso, P. (1995). Identification of RANTES, MIP-1 alpha, and MIP-1 beta as the major HIV-suppressive factors produced by CD8+ T cells. *Science* 270(5243): 1811–1815.

Cohen, E.A., Terwilliger, E.F., Sodroski, J.G., and Haseltine, W.A. (1988). Identification of a protein encoded by the vpu gene of HIV-1. *Nature* 334: 532–534.

Costigliola, P., Ricchi, E., Manfredi, R., Tumietto, F., Barelli, A., Borri, A., De Rosa, V., and Chiodo, F. (1992). No evidence of HIV-2 infection amongst HIV-1 Ab positive people in the largest cities of north-eastern Italy. *Eur J Epidemiology* 8(1): 140–141.

Courouce, A.M., Barin, F., Baudelot, J., Chamaret, S., Gueguen, M., Janot, C., Lemaire, J.M., Maniez, M., Mesnier, F., and Mouillot, L. (1989). HIV-2 infection among blood donors and other subjects in France. *Transfusion* 29: 368.

De Clercq, E., Yamamoto, N., Pauwels, R., Baba, M., Schols, D., Nakashima, H., Balzarini, J., Debyser, Z., Murrer, B.A., and Schwartz, D. (1992). Potent and selective inhibition of human immunodeficiency virus (HIV)-1 and HIV-2 replication by a class of bicyclams interacting with a viral uncoating event. *Proc Natl Acad Sci USA* 89(12): 5286–5290.

De Cock, K., and Brun-Vezinet, F. (1989). Epidemiology of HIV-2 Infection. *AIDS* 3(supl 1): S89–S95.

De Cock, K., Odehouri, K., Colebunders, R., Adjorlolo, G., Lafontaine, M., Porter, A., Gnaore, E., Diaby, L., Moreau, J., and Heyward, W. (1990). A comparison of HIV-1 and HIV-2 infections in hospitalized patients in Abidjan, Cote d'Ivoire. *AIDS* 4: 443.

Del Mistro, A., Chotard, J., Hall, A.J., Whittle, H., De Rossi, A., and Chieco-Bianchi, L. (1992). HIV-1 and HIV-2 seroprevalence rates in mother-child pairs living in The Gambia (west Africa). *J Acquir Immune Defic Syndr* 5(1): 19–24.

Denis, F., Barin, F., Gershy-Damet, G., Rey, J.L., Lhuillier, M., Mournier, M., Leonard, G., Sangaré, A., Goudeau, A., Mboup, S., Kanki, P., and Essex, M. (1987). Prevalence of Human T-Lymphotropic Retroviruses Type III (HIV) and Type IV in Ivory Coast. *Lancet* i: 408–411.

Dieng-Sarr, A.H.D., Thior, I., Kokkotou, E., Sankale, J.L., Marlink, R., Coll-Seck, E.M., Essex, M., Siby, T., NDoye, I., Mboup, S., and Kanki, P. (1998). HIV-1 and HIV-2 dual infection: lack of HIV-2 provirus correlates with low CD4+ lymphocyte counts. *AIDS* 12(2): 131–137.

Dieng-Sarr, A., Popper, S., Thior, I., Hamel, D.J., Sankalé, J.-L., Siby, T., Marlink, R., Essex, M., MBoup, S. and Kanki, P. (1999). Relationship between HIV-2 proviral load and CD4+ lymphocytes differs in HIV monotypic and dual infection. *J Hum Virol* 2(1): 45–51.

Dieng-Sarr, A., Sankalé, J.-L., Hamel, D.J., Guèye-NDiaye, A., Essex, M., MBoup, S. and Kanki, P.J. (2000a). Genetic Analysis of HIV Type 2 in Monotypic and Dual HIV Infections. *AIDS Res Hum Retroviruses* 16(3): 297–300.

Dieng-Sarr, A., Sankalé, J.-L., Hamel, D.J., Travers, K., Guèye-NDiaye, A., Essex, M., MBoup, S., and Kanki, P.J. (2000b). Interaction with Human Immunodeficiency Virus (HIV) Type 2 Predicts HIV Type 1 Genotype. *Virology* 268: 402–410.

Dietrich, U., Adamski, M., Kreutz, R., Seipp, A., Kuhnel, H., and Rubsamen Waigmann, H. (1989). A highly divergent HIV-2-related isolate. *Nature* 342: 948–950.

Diouf, K., Dieng-Sarr, A., Popper, S., Eisen, G., and Kanki, P.J. (2002). Associations between MHC Class I and Susceptibility to HIV-2 Disease Progression. *J Hum Virol* 5: 1–7.

Donnelly, C., Leisenring, W., Kanki, P., Awerbuch, T., and Sandberg, S. (1993). Comparison of transmission rates of HIV-1 and HIV-2 in a cohort of prostitutes in Senegal. *Bull Math Bio* 55(4): 731–743.

Downing, R.G., and Biryahwaho, B. (1990). No evidence for HIV-2 infection in Uganda. *Lancet* 336(8729): 1514–1515.

Dufoort, G., Courouce, A., Ancelle-Park, R., and Beltry, O. (1988). No Clinical Signs 14 years after HIV-2 transmission via Blood Transfusion. *Lancet* 2: 510.

Dwyer, D., Matheron, S., Bakchine, S., Bechet, J., Montagnier , L., and Vazeux, R. (1992). Detection of human immunodeficiency virus type 2 in brain tissue. *J Infect Dis* 166: 888.

Emau, P., McClure, H.M., Isahakia, M., Else, J.G., and Fultz, P.N. (1991). Isolation from African Sykes' monkeys (Cercopithecus mitis) of a lentivirus related to human and simian immunodeficiency viruses. *J Virol* 65(4): 2135–2140.

Endres, M.J., Clapham, P.R., Marsh, M., Ahuja, M., Turner, J.D., McKnight, A., Thomas, J.F., Stoebenau-Haggarty, B., Choe, S., Vance, P.J., Wells, T.N., Power, C.A., Sutterwala, S.S., Doms, R.W., Landau, N.R., and Hoxie, J.A. (1996). CD4-independent infection by HIV-2 is mediated by fusin/CXCR4. *Cell* 87(4): 745–756.

Essex, M., and Kanki, P. (1988). The Origins of the AIDS Virus. *Sci Am* 259: 64–71.

Essex, M., and Kanki, P. (1994). Human Immunodeficiency Virus Type 2 (HIV-2). *Textbook of AIDS Medicine*. S. Broder, T. Merigan and D. Bologencsi. Baltimore, Williams & Wilkins: 873–886.

Essex, M., Kanki, P., Barin, F., Chou, M.J., and Lee, T.H. (1988). Immunogenicity of HIV-1 and HIV-2 Antigens and Relationship to Disease Development. *2e Colloque des ≪Cent Gardes≫: Retroviruses of Human A.I.D.S. and Related Animal Diseases*. M. Girard and L. Vallette. Paris, Marnes-la-Coquette: 219–220.

Estebanez, P., Sarasqueta, C., Rua-Figueroa, M., Fitch, K., Eugenia, P.V., Varela, J.M., Contreras, G., Casado, C., Perez, L., and Najera, R. (1992). Absence of HIV-2 in Spanish groups at risk for HIV-1 infection. *AIDS Res Hum Retroviruses* 8(4): 423–424.

Evans, L., Moreau, J., Odehouri, K., Legg, H., Barboza, A., Cheng-Mayer, C., and Levy, J.A. (1988a). Characterization of a Noncytopathic HIV-2 Strain with Unusual Effects on CD4 Expression. *Science* 240: 1522–1525.

Evans, L., Moreau, J., Odehouri, K., Seto, D., Thomson-Honnebier, G., Legg, H., Barboza, A.,

Cheng-Mayer, C., and Levy, J. (1988b). Simultaneous isolation of HIV-1 and HIV-2 from an AIDS patient.*Lancet* ii: 1389–1391.

Feng, Y., Broder, C.C., Kennedy, P.E. and Berger, E.A. (1996). HIV-1 entry cofactor: functional cDNA cloning of a seven-transmembrane, G protein-coupled receptor. *Science* 272(5263): 872–877.

Fenyo, E., Albert, J. and Asjo, B. (1989). Replicative capacity, cytopathic effect and cell tropism of HIV. *AIDS* 3(suppl 1): S5–S12.

Fenyo, E.M. and Putkonen, P. (1996). Broad cross-neutralizing activity in serum is associated with slow progression and low risk of transmission in primate lentivirus infections. *Immunol Lett* 51(1–2): 95–99.

Franchini, G., Collalti, E., Arya, S.K., Fenyö, E.M., Biberfeld, G., Zagury, J.F., Kanki, P., Wong-Staal, F. and Gallo, R.C. (1987). Genetic Analysis of a New Subgroup of Human and Simian T-Lymphotropic Retroviruses: HTLV-IV, LAV-2, SBL6669, and STLV-III_{AGM}. *AIDS Res Hum Retroviruses* 3: 11–17.

Franchini, G., Fargnoli, K.A., Giombini, F., Jagodzinski, L., De Rossi, A., Bosch, M., Biberfeld, G., Fenyo, E.M., Albert, J. and Gallo, R.C. (1989). Molecular and biological characterization of a replication competent human immunodeficiency type 2 (HIV-2) proviral clone. *Proc Natl Acad Sci USA.* 86: 2433–2437.

Francis, D.P., Feorino, P.M., Broderson, J.R., McClure, H.M., Getchell, J.P., McGrath, C.R., Swenson, B., McDougal, J.S., Palmer, E.L., Harrison, A.K., Barre-Sinoussi, F., Chermann, J.-C., Montagnier, L., Curran, J.W., Cabradilla, C.D. and Kalyanaraman, V.S. (1984). Infection of chimpanzees with lymphadenopathy-associated virus. *Lancet* ii: 1276–1277.

Fu, G.K. and Markovitz, D.M. (1996). Purification of the pets factor. A nuclear protein that binds to the inducible TG-rich element of the human immunodeficiency virus type 2 enhancer. *J Biol Chem* 271(32): 19599–19605.

Fultz, P.N., McClure, H.M., Swenson, R.B., McGrath, C.R., Brodie, A., Getchell, J.P., Jensen, F.C., Anderson, D.C., Broderson, J.R. and Francis, D.P. (1986). Persistent infection of chimpanzees with human T-lymphotropic virus type III/lymphadenopathy-associated virus: a potential model for acquired immunodeficiency syndrome. *J Virol* 58(1): 116–124.

Gajdusek, D.C., Amyx, H.L., Gibbs, C.J.J., Asher, D.M., Rodgers-Johnson, P., Epstein, L.G., Sarin, P.S., Gallo, R.C., Maluish, A., Arthur, L.O., Montagnier, L. and Mildvan, D. (1985). Infection of chimpanzees by human T-lymphotropic retroviruses in brain and other tissues from AIDS patients. *Lancet* i: 55–56.

Gao, F., Yue, L., Robertson, D.L., Hill, S.C., Hui, H., Biggar, R.J., Neequaye, A.E., Whelan, T.M., Ho, D.D., and Shaw, G.M. (1994). Genetic diversity of human immunodeficiency virus type 2: evidence for distinct sequence subtypes with differences in virus biology. *J Virol* 68: 7433–7447.

Gao, F., Yue, L., White, A., Pappas, P.G., Barchue, J., Hanson, A.P., Greene, B.M., Sharp, P.M., Shaw, G.M. and Hahn, B.H. (1992). Human infection by genetically diverse SIVSM-related HIV-2 in West Africa. *Nature* 358: 495–499.

Gayle, H., Gnaore, E., Adjorlolo, G., Ekpini, E., Coulibaly, R., Porter, A., Braun, M., Zabban, M., Andou, J. and Timite, A. (1992). HIV-1 and HIV-2 infection in children in Abidjan, Cote D'Ivoire. *JAIDS* 5: 513.

Georgoulias, V., Agelakis, A., Fountouli, P., Darivianakis, K., Bibakis, K., Nikoloudis, E., Ammar, A., Bertoli, A.M. and Malliarakis-Pinetidou, E. (1990). Seroprevalence of HIV-2 infection in Greece (Crete). *JAIDS* 3(12): 1188–1192.

Gilbert, P., McKeague, I., Eisen, G., Mulllins, C., Guéye-Ndiaye, A., Mboup, S. and Kanki, P. (2002). Comparison of HIV-1 and HIV-2 infectivity from a prospective cohort study in Senegal. *Stat Med* in press.

Gorelick, R.J., Nigida, S.M., Jr., Bess, J.W., Jr., Arthur, L.O., Henderson, L.E. and Rein, A. (1990). Noninfectious human immunodeficiency virus type 1 mutants deficient in genomic RNA. *J Virol* 64(7): 3207–3211.

Gotch, F., McAdam, S.N., Allsopp, C.E., Gallimore, A., Elvin, J., Kieny, M.P., Hill, A.V., McMichael, A.J. and Whittle, H.C. (1993). Cytotoxic T cells in HIV2 seropositive Gambians. Identification of a virus-specific MHC-restricted peptide epitope. *J Immunol* 151(6): 3361–3369.

Gueye-Ndiaye, A., Clark, R., Samuel, K., NDour-Sarr, A.N., Ouangre, A., Sangare, L., Mboup, S., Marlink, R., Papas, R., Child, R., Coll-Seck, A., Essex, M. and Kanki, P. (1993). Cost-Effective Diagnosis of HIV-1 and HIV-2 By Recombinant-Expressed env Peptide (566/966) Dot Blot Analysis. *AIDS* 7: 481–495.

Guyader, M., Emerman, M., Sonigo, P., Clavel, F., Montagnier, L. and Alizon, M. (1987). Genome organization and transactivation of the human immunodeficiency virus type 2. *Nature* 326: 662–669.

Harrison, L.H., José da Silva, A.P., Gayle, H.D., Albino, P., George, R., Lee-Thomas, S., Rayfield, M.A., Castillo, F.D. and Heyward, W.L. (1991). Risk factors for HIV-2 infection in Guinea-Bissau. *JAIDS* 4(11): 1155–1160.

Hasegawa, A., Tsujimoto, H., Maki, N., Ishikawa, K., Miura, T., Fukasawa, M., Miki, K. and Hayami, M. (1989). Genomic divergence of HIV-2 from Ghana. *AIDS Res Hum Retroviruses* 5(6): 593–604.

Haseltine, W.A. (1992). The molecular biology of HIV-1. *AIDS, etiology, diagnosis, treatment and prevention*. V.T. DeVita, Jr., S. Hellman, S.A. Rosenberg, J. Curran, M. Essex and A.S. Fauci. Philadelphia, J.B. Lippincott Co.: 39–59.

Henderson, L., Sowder, R., Copeland, T., Benveniste, R. and Oroszlan, S. (1988). Isolation and characterization of a novel protein (X-ORF product) from SIV and HIV-2. *Science* 241: 199–201.

Henderson, L., Sowder, R., Copeland, T., Oroszlan, S. and Benveniste, R. (1990). Gag precursors of HIV and SIV are cleaved into six proteins found in the mature virions. *J Med Primatol* 19: 411–419.

Hendry, R., Parks, D., Campos Mello, D., Quinnan, G. and Balao Castro, B. (1991). Lack of evidence for HIV-2 infection among at-risk individuals in Brazil. *JAIDS* 4: 623.

Heredia, A., Vallejo, A., Soriano, V., Epstein, J.S. and Hewlett, I.K. (1997). Chemokine receptors and HIV-2 [letter]. *AIDS* 11(9): 1198–1199.

Hizi, A., Tal, R. and Hughes, S.H. (1991a). Mutational analysis of the DNA polymerase and ribonuclease H activities of human immunodeficiency virus types 2 reverse transcriptase expressed in Escherichia coli. *Virology* 180(1): 339–346.

Hizi, A., Tal, R., Shaharabany, M. and Loya, S. (1991b). Catalytic properties of the reverse transcriptase of human immunodeficiency viruses type 1 and type 2. *J Biol Chem* 266(10): 6230–6239.

Holzer, T., Allen, R., Heynen, C., Kennedy, M., Knigge, M., Paul, D. and Dawson, G. (1990). Discrimination of HIV-2 infection from HIV-1 infection by western blot and radioimmuno-precipitation analysis. *AIDS Res Hum Retroviruses* 6: 515–524.

Huang, M., Essex, M. and Lee, T.H. (1991). Localization of immunogenic domains in the human immunodeficiency virus type 2 envelope. *J Virol* 65: 5073–5079.

Isaka, Y., Sato, A., Miki, S., Kawauchi, S., Sakaida, H., Hori, T., Uchiyama, T., Adachi, A., Hayami, M., Fujiwara, T. and Yoshie, O. (1999). Small amino acid changes in the V3 loop of human immunodeficiency virus type 2 determines the coreceptor usage for CXCR4 and CCR5. *Virology* 264(1): 237–243.

Kanki, P. (1987). West African Human Retroviruses Related to STLV-III. *AIDS* 1: 141–145.

Kanki, P. (1996). Epidemiology and Natural History of HIV-2. *AIDS: Etiology, Diagnosis, Treatment and Prevention*. V. DeVita, S. Hellman and S. Rosenberg. Philadelphia, J. B. Lippincott Co.: 97–108.

Kanki, P. J. (1999). Human Immunodeficiency Virus Type 2, (HIV-2). *AIDS Reviews* 1 (20): 101–108.

Kanki, P. (1997). Epidemiology and Natural History of HIV-2. *In AIDS: Etiology, Diagnosis, Treatment and Prevention*. V. J. DeVita, S. Hellman and S. Rosenberg. Philadelphia, PA, J.B. Lippincott Co 127–135.

Kanki, P. and DeCock, K.M. (1994). Epidemiology and Natural History of HIV-2. *AIDS* 8(suppl.): S1–S9.

Kanki, P., McLane, M.F., King, N.W.J., Letvin, N.L., Hunt, R.D., Sehgal, P., Daniel, M.D., Desrosiers, R.C. and Essex, M. (1985a). Serologic Identification and Characterization of a Macaque T-Lymphotropic Retrovirus Closely Related to HTLV-III. *Science* 228: 1199–1201.

Kanki, P.J., Kurth, R., Becker, W., Dreesman, G., McLane, M.F. and Essex, M. (1985b). Antibodies to simian T-lymphotropic retrovirus type III in African green monkeys and recognition of STLV-III viral proteins by AIDS and related sera. *Lancet* 1(8441): 1330–1332.

Kanki, P.J., Barin, F., M'Boup, S., Allan, J.S., Romet-Lemonne, J.L., Marlink, R., McLane, M.F., Lee, T.H., Arbeille, B., Denis, F. and Essex, M. (1986). New human T-lymphotropic retrovirus related to simian T-lymphotropic virus type III (STLV-IIIAGM). *Science* 232(4747): 238–243.

Kanki, P., Barin, F., Mboup, S. and Essex, M. (1987a). Relationship of Simian T-Lymphotropic Virus Type III to Human Retroviruses in Africa. *Antibiot Chemother* 38: 21–27.

Kanki, P., Essex, M. and Barin, F. (1987b). Antigenic Relationships Between HTLV-3/LAV, STLV-3, and HTLV-4. *Vaccines 87: Modern Approaches to New Vaccines*. R.M. Chanock, R.A. Lerner, F. Brown and H. Ginsberg. Cold Spring Harbor, Cold Spring Harbor Laboratory: 185–187.

Kanki, P., Mboup, S., Barin, F., Denis, F., Marlink, R., Romet-Lemonne, J.L. and Essex, M. (1988). The Biology of HIV-1 and HIV-2 in Africa. *AIDS and Associated Cancers in Africa*. G. Giraldo, E. Beth-Giraldo, N. Klumeck, M.D.R. Gharbi, S.K. Kyalwazi and G. de Thé. Basel, S. Karger: 230–236.

Kanki, P., Marlink, R., Siby, T., Essex, M. and Mboup, S. (1990). Biology of HIV-2 Infection in West Africa. *Gene Regulation and AIDS*. T.S. Papas. Houston, Portfolio Publishing Company of Texas: 255–271.

Kanki, P., Mboup, S., Marlink, R., Travers, K., Hsieh, C.C., Gueye, A., Boye, C., Sankale, J.L., Donnelly, C., Leisenring, W., Siby, T., Thior, I., Dia, M., Gueye, E.H., N'Doye, I. and Essex, M. (1992). Prevalence and Risk Determinants of Human Immunodeficiency Virus Type 2 (HIV-2) and Human Immunodeficiency Virus Type 1 (HIV-1) in West African Female Prostitutes. *Am J Epidemiol* 136: 895–907.

Kanki, P., Travers, K., Hernandez-Avila, M., Marlink, R., Mboup, S., Gueye-Ndiaye, A., Siby, T., Thior, I., Sankalé, J.L., Ndoye, I., Hsieh, C.C. and Essex, M. (1994). Slower Heterosexual Spread of HIV-2 Compared with HIV-1. *Lancet* 343: 943–946.

Kanki, P.J., Hamel, D.J., Sankalé, J.-L., Hsieh, C.-C., Thior, I., Barin, F., Woodcock, S.A., Guèye-NDiaye, A., Zhang, E., Montano, M., NDoye, I., Essex, M.E.

and Mboup, S. (1999). Human Immunodeficiency Virus Type 1 Subtypes Differ in Disease Progression. *J Infect Dis* 179: 68–73.

Kanki, P.J., Sankale, J-L., Mboup, S. (2002). Biology of Human Immunodeficiency Virus Type 2 (HIV-2). In: Essex, M. Mboup, S., Kanki, P.J., Marlink, R. and Tlou, S. (Eds.) *AIDS in Africa*, Second Edition. Kluwer Academic/Plenum Publishers, New York.

Kappes, J., Morrow, C., Lee, S., Jameson, B., Kent, S., Hood, L., Shaw, G.M. and Hahn, B.H. (1988). Identification of a novel retroviral gene unique to human immunodeficiency virus type 2 and simian immunodeficiency virus SIVMAC. *J Virol* 62: 3501–3505.

Kawamura, M., Katahira, J., Fukasawa, M., Sakuragi, J., Ishikawa, K., Nakai, M., Mingle, J.A., Osei-Kwasi, M., Netty, V.B. and Akari, H. (1992). Isolation and characterization of a highly divergent HIV-2[GH-2]: generation of an infectious molecular clone and functional analysis of its rev-responsive element in response to primate retrovirus transactivators (Rev and Rex). *Virology* 188(2): 850–853.

Kestens, L., Brattegard, K., Adjorlolo, G., Ekpini, E., Sibailly, T., Diallo, K., Gigase, P., Gayle, H. and De Cock, K.M. (1992). Immunological comparison of HIV-1, HIV-2 and dually-reactive women delivering in Abidjan, Cote d'Ivoire. *AIDS* 6: 803–807.

Kirchhoff, F., Jentsch, K.D., Bachmann, B., Stuke, A., Laloux, C., Luke, W., Stahl Hennig, C., Schneider, J., Nieselt, K. and Eigen, M. (1990). A novel proviral clone of HIV-2: biological and phylogenetic relationship to other primate immunodeficiency viruses. *Virology.* 177: 305–311.

Klemm, E., Schneweis, K.E., Horn, R., Tackmann, W., Schulze, G. and Schneider, J. (1988). HIV-II infection with initial neurological manifestation. *J Neurol* 235: 304–307.

Kokkotou, E.G., Sankalé, J.-L., Mani, I., MBoup, S., Guèye-Ndiaye, A., Schwartz, D., Essex, M. and Kanki, P.J. (2000). In vitro correlates of HIV-2 mediated HIV-1 protection. *Proc Natl Acad Sci USA* 97(12): 6797–6802.

Komatsu, H., Tsukahara, T. and Tozawa, H. (1996). Viral RNA binding properties of human immunodeficiency virus type-2 (HIV-2) nucleocapsid protein-derived synthetic peptides. *Biochem Mol Biol Int* 38(6): 1143–1154.

Kong, L., Lee, S., Kappes, J., Parkin, J.S., Decker, D., Hoxie, J.A., Hahn, B.H. and Shaw, G.M. (1988). West African HIV-2-related human retrovirus with attenuated cytopathicity. *Science* 240: 1525–1529.

Kuhnel, H., von Briesen, H., Dietrich, U., Adamski, M., Mix, D., Biesert, L., Kreutz, R., Immelmann, A., Henco, K. and Meichsner, C. (1989). Molecular cloning of two west African human immunodeficiency virus type 2 isolates that replicate well in macrophages: a Gambian isolate, from a patient with neurologic acquired immunodeficiency syndrome, and a highly divergent Ghanian isolate. *Proc Natl Acad Sci USA* 86: 2383–2387.

Kumar, P., Hui, H.X., Kappes, J.C., Haggarty, B.S., Hoxie, J.A., Arya, S.K., Shaw, G.M. and Hahn, B.H. (1990). Molecular characterization of an attenuated human immunodeficiency virus type 2 isolate. *J Virol* 64: 890–901.

Kvinesdal, B.B., Worm, A.M., Lindhardt, B.O., Jensen, B.L., Nielsen, C.M. and Poulsen, A.G. (1992). HIV-2 infection in Denmark. *Scandinavian J Infect Dis* 24(4): 419–421.

Le Guenno, B.M., Barabe, P., Griffet, P.A., Guiraud, M., Morcillo, R.J., Peghini, M.E., Jean, P.A., M Baye, P.S., Diallo, A. and Sarthou, J.-L. (1991). HIV-2 and HIV-1 AIDS Cases in Senegal: Clinical patterns and immunological perturbations. *JAIDS* 4(4): 421–427.

Lee, W.R., Syu, W.J., Du, B., Matsuda, M., Tan, S., Wolf, A., Essex, M. and Lee, T.H. (1992a). Nonrandom distribution of gp120 N-linked glycosylation sites important for infectivity of human immunodeficiency virus type 1. *Proc Natl Acad Sci USA* 89(6): 2213–2217.

Lee, W.R., Yu, X.F., Syu, W.J., Essex, M. and Lee, T.H. (1992b). Mutational analysis of conserved N-linked glycosylation sites of human immunodeficiency virus type 1 gp41. *J Virol* 66(3): 1799–1803.

Lehner, T., Wang, Y., Cranage, M., Bergmeier, L.A., Mitchell, E., Tao, L., Hall, G., Dennis, M., Cook, N., Brookes, R., Klavinskis, L., Jones, I., Doyle, C. and Ward, R. (1996). Protective mucosal immunity elicited by targeted iliac lymph node immunization with a subunit SIV envelope and core vaccine in macaques. *Nat Med* 2(7): 767–775.

Leonard, C.K., Spellman, M.W., Riddle, L., Harris, R.J., Thomas, J.N. and Gregory, T.J. (1990). Assignment of intrachain disulfide bonds and characterization of potential glycosylation sites of the type 1 recombinant human immunodeficiency virus envelope glycoprotein (gp120) expressed in Chinese hamster ovary cells. *J Biol Chem* 265(18): 10373–10382.

Lisse, I.M., Poulsen, A.-G., Aaby, P., Normark, M., Kvinesdal, B., Dias, F., Molbak, K. and Knudsen, K. (1990). Immunodeficiency in HIV-2 infection: a community study from Guinea-Bissau. *AIDS* 4: 1263–1266.

Lisse, I.M., Poulsen, A.G., Aaby, P., Knudsen, K. and Dias, F. (1996). Serial CD4 and CD8 T-lymphocyte counts and associated mortality in an HIV-2-infected population in Guinea-Bissau. *JAIDS* 13(4): 355–362.

Ljunggren, K., Chiodi, F., Biberfeld, G., Norrby, E., Jondal, M. and Fenyo, E.M. (1988). Lack of cross-reaction in antibody-dependent cellular cytotoxicity between human immunodeficiency virus (HIV) and

HIV-related West African strains. *J Immunol* 140(2): 602–605.

Locher, C.P., Blackbourn, D.J., Barnett, S.W., Murthy, K.K., Cobb, E.K., Rouse, S., Greco, G., Reyesteran, G., Brasky, K.M., Carey, K.D. and Levy, J.A. (1997). Superinfection With Human Immunodeficiency Virus Type 2 Can Reactivate Virus Production In Baboons But Is Contained By a Cd8 T Cell Antiviral Response. *J Infect Dis* 176(4): 948–959.

Looney, D.J., Hayashi, S., Nicklas, M., Redfield, R.R., Broder, S., Wong Staal, F. and Mitsuya, H. (1990). Differences in the interaction of HIV-1 and HIV-2 with CD4. *JAIDS* 3: 649–657.

Machuca, A., Soriano, V., Guti rrez, M., Holguin, A., Aguilera, A., Caballero, E. and Cilla, G. (1999). Human immunodeficiency virus type 2 infection in Spain. The HIV-2 Spanish Study Group. *Intervirology* 42(1): 37–42.

Maiga, Y., Sissoko, Z. and Maiga, M. (1993). *Etude de la seroprevalence de l'Infection a VIH dans les 7 regions economiques du Mali.* VIIIth International Conference on AIDS in Africa/VIIIth African Conference on Sexually Transmitted Diseases, Marrakech.

Mannervik, M., Putkonen, P., Ruden, U., Kent, K.A., Norrby, E., Wahren, B. and Broliden, P.A. (1992). Identification of B-cell antigenic sites on HIV-2 gp125. *J AIDS* 5(2): 177–187.

Markovitz, D.M. (1993). Infection with the human immunodeficiency virus type 2. [Review] [131 refs]. *Ann Intern Med* 118(3): 211–218.

Marlink, R.G., Ricard, D., M'Boup, S., Kanki, P.J., Romet-Lemonne, J.-L., N'Doye, I., Diop, K., Simpson, M.A., Greco, F., Chou, M.J., DeGruttola, V., Hsieh, C.-C., Boye, C., Barin, F., Denis, F., McLane, M.F. and Essex, M. (1988). Clinical, hematologic, and immunologic cross-sectional evaluation of individuals exposed to human immunodeficiency virus type 2 (HIV-2). *AIDS Res Hum Retroviruses* 4: 137–148.

Marlink, R., Kanki, P., Thior, I., Travers, K., Eisen, G., Siby, T., Traore, I., C.C., H., MC., D., Gueye, E.H., Hellinger, J., Gueye, -. N.A., Sankalé, J.L., Ndoye, I., Mboup, S. and Essex, M. (1994). Reduced Rate of Disease Development with HIV-2 Compared to HIV-1. *Science* 265: 1587–1590.

Marx, P., Li, Y., Lerche, N., Sutjipto, S., Gettie, A., Yee, J.A., Brotman, B.H., Prince, A., Hanson, A., Webster, R.G., and Desrosiers, R. (1991). Isolation of a simian immunodeficiency virus related to human immunodeficiency virus type 2 from a west African pet sooty mangebey. *J Virol* 65: 4480–4485.

Matheron, S., Simon, F., Sassi, G. and *et al.* (1993). *Infection HIV-2 chez l'adulte; etude de cohorte; Paris:1986–1993.* VIIIth International Conference on AIDS in Africa and VIIIth African Conference on Sexually Transmitted Diseases, Marrakech.

Matsuda, Z., Chou, M.J., Matsuda, M., Huang, J.H., Chen, Y.M., Redfield, R., Mayer, K., Essex, M. and Lee, T.H. (1988). Human immunodeficiency virus type 1 has an additional coding sequence in the central region of the genome. *Proc Natl Acad Sci USA* 85: 6968–6972.

McKnight, A., Shotton, C., Cordell, J., Jones, I., Simmons, G. and Clapham, P.R. (1996). Location, exposure, and conservation of neutralizing and non-neutralizing epitopes on human immunodeficiency virus type 2 SU glycoprotein. *J Virol* 70(7): 4598–4606.

Michel, P., Balde, A.T., Roussilhon, C., Aribot, G., Sarthou, J.L. and Gougeon, M.L. (2000). Reduced immune activation and T cell apoptosis in human immunodeficiency virus type 2 compared with type 1: correlation of T cell apoptosis with beta2 microglobulin concentration and disease evolution. *J Infect Dis* 181(1): 64–75.

Moore, J.P. (1990). Simple methods for monitoring HIV-1 and HIV-2 gp120 binding to soluble CD4 by enzyme-linked immunosorbent assay: HIV-2 has a 25-fold lower affinity than HIV-1 for soluble CD4. *AIDS* 4: 297–305.

Morgan, G., Wilkins, H.A., Pepin, J., Jobe, O., Brewster, D. and Whittle, H. (1990). AIDS following mother-to-child transmission of HIV-2. *AIDS* 4(9): 879–882.

Morikawa, Y., Moore, J.P., Fenouillet, E. and Jones, I.M. (1992). Complementation of human immunodeficiency virus glycoprotein mutations in trans. *J Gen Virol* 73(Pt 8): 1907–1913.

Mulligan, M.J., Kumar, P., Hui, H.X., Owens, R.J., Ritter, G.D., Jr., Hahn, B.H. and Compans, R.W. (1990). The env protein of an infectious noncytopathic HIV-2 is deficient in syncytium formation. *AIDS Res Hum Retroviruses* 6: 707–720.

Mulligan, M.J., Ritter, G.D., Chaikin, M.A., Yamshchikov, G.V., Kumar, P., Hahn, B.H., Sweet, R.W. and Compans, R.W. (1992). Human immunodeficiency virus type 2 envelope glycoprotein: differential CD4 interactions of soluble gp120 versus the assembled envelope complex. *Virology* 187: 233–241.

Mullins, C.M., Eisen, G., Popper, S., Dieng Sarr, A., Sankale, J.L., Berger, J., Brodie, S., Chang, H., Collison, A., Cooley, T., Dailey, R., Rice, P., Skolnik, P., Sullivan, M. and Kanki, P.J. HAART Therapy and viral response in Human Immunodeficiency Virus Type 2 Infection. *Clin Infect Dis.* (in press).

Myagkikh, M., Alipanah, S., Markham, P.D., Tartaglia, J., Paoletti, E., Gallo, R.C., Franchini, G. and Robert-Guroff, M. (1996). Multiple immunizations with attenuated poxvirus HIV type 2 recombinants and subunit boosts required for protection of rhesus macaques. *AIDS Res Hum Retroviruses* 12(11): 985–992.

Myers, G., MacInnes, K. and Korber, B. (1992). The emergence of simian/human immunodeficiency viruses. *AIDS Res Hum Retroviruses* 8(3): 373–386.

Myers, G. and Pavlakis, G.N. (1992). Evolutionary potential of complex retroviruses. *The retroviridae*. J. A. Levy. Plenum Press, New York, pp. 1–37.

Nabel, G. and Baltimore, D. (1987). An inducible transcription factor activates expression of human immunodeficiency virus in T cells. *Nature* 326: 711–713.

Naucler, A., Albino, P., Da Silva, A.P., Andreasson, P., Andersson, S. and Biberfeld, G. (1990). HIV-2 infection in hospitalized patients in Bissau, Guinea-Bissau. *AIDS* 5: 301–304.

Naucler, A., Andreasson, P.A., Costa, C.M., Thorstensson, R. and Biberfeld, G. (1989). HIV-2-associated AIDS and HIV-2 seroprevalence in Bissau, Guinea-Bissau. *JAIDS* 2: 88–93.

Neoh, L.P., Akimoto, H., Kaneko, H., Hishikawa, T., Hashimoto, H., Hirose, S., Kaneko, Y., Yamamoto, N. and Sekigawa, I. (1997). The production of beta-chemokines induced by HIV-2 envelope glycoprotein [letter]. *Aids* 11(8): 1062–1063.

Ngagne, M., Diouf, A., Kebe, F. and *et al.* (1995). *Histoire Naturelle de la transmission verticale VIH1 et VIH 2 a Dakar*. IXth International Conference on AIDS and Associated Cancers in Africa, Kampala, Uganda.

Nixon, D.F., Huet, S., Rothbard, J., Kieny, M.P., Delchambre, M., Thiriart, C., Rizza, C.R., Gotch, F.M. and McMichael, A.J. (1990). An HIV-1 and HIV-2 cross-reactive cytotoxic T-cell epitope. *AIDS* 4(9): 841–845.

Norley, S.G., Mikschy, U., Werner, A., Staszewski, S., Helm, E.B. and Kurth, R. (1990). Demonstration of cross-reactive antibodies able to elicit lysis of both HIV-1- and HIV-2-infected cells. *J Immunol* 145: 1700–1705.

Norrby, E., Putkonen, P., Bottiger, B., Utter, G. and Biberfeld, G. (1991). Comparison of linear antigenic sites in the envelope proteins of human immunodeficiency virus (HIV) type 2 and type 1. *AIDS Res Hum Retroviruses* 7(3): 279–285.

Norrgren, H., Marquina, S., Leitner, T., Aaby, P., Melbye, M., Poulsen, A.G., Larsen, O., Dias, F., Escanilla, D., Andersson, S., Albert, J. and Naucler, A. (1997). HIV-2 genetic variation and DNA load in asymptomatic carriers and AIDS cases in Guinea-Bissau. *JAIDS: J Acquir Immune Defic Syndr* 16(1): 31–38.

Norrgren, H., Andersson, S., Biague, A.J., da Silva, Z.J., Dias, F., Naucler, A. and Biberfeld, G. (1999). Trends and interaction o fhIV-1 and HIV-2 in Guinea-Bissau, West Africa: No protection of HIV-2 against HIV-1 infection. *AIDS* 13: 701–707.

O'Brien, T.R., George, J.R., Epstein, J.S., Holmberg, S.D. and Schochetman, G. (1992). Testing for antibodies to human immunodeficiency virus type 2 in the United States. *MMWR—Morb Mortal Wkly Rep* 41(RR-12): 1–9.

O'Donovan, D., Ariyoshi, K., Milligan, P., Ota, M., Yamuah, L., Sarge-Njie, R. and Whittle, H. (2000). Maternal plasma viral RNA levels determine marked differences in mother-to-child transmission rates of HIV-1 and HIV-2 in The Gambia. MRC/Gambia Government/University College London Medical School Working Group on Mother–Child Transmission of HIV. *AIDS* 14(4): 441–448.

Olaleye, O., Bernstein, L., Ekweozor, C., Sheng, Z., Omilabu, S.A., Li , X.Y., Sullivan-Halley, J. and Rasheed, S. (1993). Prevalence of human immunodeficiency virus types 1 and 2 infections in Nigeria. *J Infect Dis* 167: 710.

Parkman, P.D. (1990). *Recommendations for the prevention of human immunodeficiency virus (HIV) transmission by blood and blood products*, Food and Drug Administration, Center for Biologics Evaluation and Research, Bethesda, MD.

Paxton, W.A., Martin, S.R., Tse, D., O'Brien, T.R., Skurnick, J., VanDevanter, N.L., Padian, N., Braun, J.F., Kotler, D.P., Wolinsky, S.M. and Koup, R.A. (1996). Relative resistance to HIV-1 infection of CD4 lymphocytes from persons who remain uninfected despite multiple high-risk sexual exposure. *Nat Med* 2(4): 412–417.

Peeters, M., Gershy-Damet, G.M., Fransen, K., Koffi, K., Coulibaly, M., Delaporte, E., Piot, P. and van der Groen, G. (1992). Virological and polymerase chain reaction studies of HIV-1/HIV-2 dual infection in Cote d'Ivoire. *Lancet* 340(8815): 339–340.

Peeters, M., Koumare, B., Mulanga, C., Brengues, C., Mounirou, B., Bougoudogo, F., Ravel, S., Bibollet-Ruche, F. and Delaporte, E. (1998). Genetic subtypes of HIV type 1 and HIV type 2 strains in commercial sex workers from Bamako, Mali. *AIDS Res Hum Retroviruses* 14(1): 51–58.

Pepin, J., Dunn, D., Gaye, I., Alonso, P., Egboga, A., Tedder, R., Piot, P., Berry, N., Schellenberg, D. and Whittle, H. (1991a). HIV-2 infection among prostitutes working in The Gambia: association with serological evidence of genital ulcer diseases and generalized lymphadenopathy. *AIDS* 5: 69.

Pepin, J., Morgan, G., Dunn, D., Gevao, S., Mendy, M., Gaye, I., Scollen, N., Tedder, R. and Whittle, H. (1991b). HIV-2-induced immunosuppression among asymptomatic West African prostitutes: evidence that HIV-2 is pathogenic, but less so than HIV-1. *AIDS* 5: 1165–1172.

Pepin, J., Quigley, M., Todd, J., Gaye, I., Janneh, M., Van Dyck, E., Piot, P. and Whittle, H. (1992). Association between HIV-2 infection and genital ulcer diseases among male sexually transmitted disease patients in The Gambia. *AIDS* 6(5): 489–493.

Pichuantes, S., Babe, L.M., Barr, P.J., DeCamp, D.L. and Craik, C.S. (1990). Recombinant HIV2 protease processes HIV1 Pr53gag and analogous junction peptides in vitro. *J Biol Chem* 265: 13890–13898.

Pieniazek, D., Ellenberger, D., Janini, L., Ramos, A., Nkengasong, J. and al., e. (1999). Predominance of Human Immunodeficiency Virus Type 2 Subtype B in Abidjan, Ivory Coast. *AIDS Res Hum Retroviruses* 15(603–608).

Popper, S., Sankalé, J.L., Thior, I., Siby, T., MBoup, S., Essex, M. and Kanki, P. (1998). Vpx reactivity as a predictor of disease progression in HIV-2 infection. *AIDS Res Hum Retroviruses* 14(13): 1157–1162.

Popper, S.J., Dieng-Sarr, A., Travers, K.U., Guèye-NDiaye, A., MBoup, S., Essex, M. and Kanki, P.J. (1999). Lower HIV-2 viral load reflects the difference in pathogenicity of HIV-1 and HIV-2. *J Infect Dis* 180: 1116–1121.

Popper, S.J., Dieng-Sarr, A., Guèye-NDiaye, A., MBoup, S., Essex, M. and Kanki, P.J. (2000). Low Plasma HIV-2 viral load is independent of proviral load: low virus production in vivo. *J Virol* 74(3): 1554–1557.

Poulsen, A.G., Kvinesdal, B.B., Aaby, P., Lisse, I.M., Gottschau, A., K., M., Dias, F. and Lauritzen, E. (1992). Lack of evidence of vertical transmission of human immunodeficiency virus type 2 in a sample of the general population in Bissau. *JAIDS* 5: 25–30.

Putkonen, P., Thorstensson, R., Albert, J., Hild, K., Norrby, E., Biberfeld, P. and Biberfeld, G. (1990). Infection of cynomolgus monkeys with HIV-2 protects against pathogenic consequences of a subsequent simian immunodeficiency virus infection. *AIDS* 4(8): 783–789.

Putkonen, P., Thorstensson, R., Walther, L., Albert, J., Akerblom, L., Granquist, O., Wadell, G., Norrby, E. and Biberfeld, G. (1991). Vaccine protection against HIV-2 infection in cynomolgus monkeys. *AIDS Res Hum Retroviruses* 7(3): 271–277.

Rappaport, J., Arya, S.K., Richardson, M.W., Baier-Bitterlich, G. and Klotman, P. E. (1995). Inhibition of HIV-1 expression by HIV-2. *J Mol Med* 73(12): 583–589.

Rayfield, M., De Cock, K., Heyward, W., Goldstein, L., Krebs, J., Kwok, S., Lee, S., McCormick, J., Moreau, J.M. and Odehouri, K. (1988). Mixed human immunodeficiency virus (HIV) infection in an individual: demonstration of both HIV type 1 and type 2 proviral sequences by using polymerase chain reaction. *J Infect Dis* 158: 1170–1176.

Robert-Guroff, M., Aldrich, K., Muldoon, R., Stern, T.L., Bansal, G.P., Matthews, T.J., Markham, P.D., Gallo, R.C. and Franchini, G. (1992). Cross-neutralization of human immunodeficiency virus type 1 and 2 and simian immunodeficiency virus isolates. *J Virol* 66(6): 3602–3608.

Rodes, B., Holguin, A., Soriano, V., Dourana, M., Mansinho, K., Antunes, F. and Gonzalez-Lahoz, J. (2000). Emergence of drug resistance mutations in human immunodeficiency virus type 2-infected subjects undergoing antiretroviral therapy. *J Clin Microbiol* 38(4): 1370–1374.

Romieu, I., Marlink, R., Kanki, P., M'Boup, S. and Essex, M. (1990). HIV-2 link to AIDS in West Africa. *JAIDS* 3: 220–230.

Rubsamen-Waigmann, H., Briesen, H., Maniar, J., Rao, P., Scholz, C. and Pfutzner, A. (1991). Spread of HIV-2 in India. *Lancet* 337: 550–551.

Rubsamen-Waigmann, H., Maniar, J., Gerte, S., Brede, H.D., Dietrich, U., Mahambre, G. and Pfutzner, A. (1994). High proportion of HIV-2 and HIV-1/2 double-reactive sera in two Indian states, Maharashtra and Goa: first appearance of an HIV-2 epidemic along with an HIV-1 epidemic outside of Africa. *Zentralbl Bakteriol.* 280: 398–402.

Saimot, A.G., Coulaud, J.P., Mechali, D., Matheron, S., M.C., D., Rey, M.A., Brun-Vezinet, F. and Leibowitch, J. (1987). HIV-2/LAV-2 in Portuguese man with AIDS (Paris, 1978) who had served in Angola in 1968–74. *Lancet* i: 688.

Sankalé, J.L., Sallier de la Tour, R., Renjifo, B., Siby, T., Mboup, S., Marlink, R., Essex, M. and Kanki, P. (1995). Intra-patient Variability of the Human Immunodeficiency Virus Type-2 (HIV-2) Envelope V3 Loop. *AIDS Res Hum Retroviruses* 11(5): 617–623.

Sankalé, J.L., De La Tour, R.S., Marlink, R.G., Scheib, R., Mboup, S., Essex, M.E. and Kanki, P.J. (1996). Distinct quasi-species in the blood and the brain of an HIV-2-infected individual. *Virology* 226(2): 418–423.

Sankalé, J.L., MBoup, S., Marlink, R., Essex, M. and Kanki, P. (1998). HIV-2 and HIV-1 Quasispecies in cervical secretions and blood. *AIDS Res Hum Retroviruses* 14(16): 1473–1481.

Santos-Ferreira, M., Cohen, T., Lourenco, M., Matos Almedia, M., Camaret, S. and Montagnier, L. (1990). A study of seroprevalence of HIV-1 and HIV-2 in six provinces of People's Republic of Angola: Clues to the spread of HIV infection. *J AIDS* 3: 780.

Sarr, A.D., Sankale, J.L., Gueye-Ndiaye, A., Essex, M., Mboup, S. and Kanki, P.J. (2000). Genetic analysis of HIV type 2 in monotypic and dual HIV infections. *AIDS Res Hum Retroviruses* 16(3): 295–298.

Schneider, J., Luke, W., Kirchhoff, F., Jung, R., Jurkiewicz, E., Stahl-Hennig, C., Nick, S., Klemm, E., Jentsch, K.D. and Hunsmann, G. (1990). Isolation and characterization of HIV-2 obtained from a patient with predominantly neurological defects. *AIDS* 4: 455.

Schulz, T., Whitby, D., Hoad, J., Corrah, T., Whittle, H. and Weiss, R.A. (1990). Biological and molecular variability of human immunodeficiency virus type 2 isolates from The Gambia. *J Virol.* 64: 5177–5182.

Schutten, M., van der Ende, M.E. and Osterhaus, A.D. (2000). Antiretroviral therapy in patients with dual infection with human immunodeficiency virus types 1 and 2 [letter]. *N Engl J Med* 342(23): 1758–1760.

Simon, F., Matheron, S., Tamalet, C., Loussert, A.I., Bartczak, S., Pepin, J., Dhiver, C., Gamba, E., Elbim, C. and Gastaut, J.A. (1993). Cellular and Plasma Viral Load in Patients Infected with HIV-2. *AIDS* 7: 1411–1417.

Smallman-Raynor, M. and Cliff, A. (1991). The Spread of Human Immunodeficiency Virus Type 2 into Europe: A Geographical Analysis. *Int J Epidemiol.* 20: 480.

Smith, N.A., Shaw, T., Berry, N., Vella, C., Okorafor, L., Taylor, D., Ainsworth, J., Choudhury, A., Daniels, R.S., El-Gadi, S., Fakoyoa, A., Moyle, G., Oxford, J.S., Tedder, R., O'Shea, S., de Ruiter, A. and Breuer, J. (2001). Antiretroviral Therapy for HIV-2 Infected Patients. *J Infect* 42: 126–133.

Smith, T.F., Srinivasan, A., Schochetman, G., Marcus, M. and Myers, G. (1988). The phylogenetic history of immunodeficiency viruses. *Nature* 333: 573–575.

Soriano, V., Gomes, P., Holguin, A., Mansinho, K., Lourenco, N. H., Garcia-Lerma, G., Heneine, W. and Antunes, F. (1998). HIV-2 in Portugal: circulating subtypes, virus isolation, plasma viral load, and clinical spectrum (the HIV-2 Iberian Project). *Int Conf AIDS* 12: 269 (abstract no. 21154).

Stahl Hennig, C., Herchenroder, O., Nick, S., Evers, M., Stille Siegener, M., Jentsch, K.D., Kirchhoff, F., Tolle, T., Gatesman, T.J. and Luke, W. (1990). Experimental infection of macaques with HIV-2ben, a novel HIV-2 isolate. *AIDS* 4: 611–617.

Steffy, K., Kraus, G., Looney, D. and Wong-Staal, F. (1992). Role of the fusogenic peptide sequence in syncytium induction and infectivity of human immunodeficiency virus type 2. *J Virol.* 66: 4532–4535.

Strebel, K., Klimkait, T., Maldarelli, F. and Martin, M.A. (1989). Molecular and biochemical analyses of human immunodeficiency virus type 1 vpu protein. *J Virol* 63: 3784–3791.

Taube, R., Avidan, O. and Hizi, A. (1997). The fidelity of misinsertion and mispair extension throughout DNA synthesis exhibited by mutants of the reverse transcriptase of human immunodeficiency virus type 2 resistant to nucleoside analogs. *Eur J Biochem* 250(1): 106–114.

Tedder, R., O'Connor, T., Hughs, A., N'Hjie, H., Corrah, T. and Whittle, H. (1988). Envelope cross-reactivity in western blot for HIV-1 and HIV-2 may not indicate dual infection. *Lancet* ii: 927–930.

Tong-Starksen, S., Welsh, T. and Peterlin, M. (1990). Differences in transcriptional enhancers of HIV-1 and HIV-2 response to T-cell activation signals. *J Immunol* 145: 4348–4354.

Traore, I., Marlink, R., Thior, I., Siby, T., Ndoye, I., Mboup, S., Essex, M., and Kanki, P. (1996). *HIV-2 as a model for long term non-progression.* XI International Conference on AIDS, Vancouver, Canada.

Travers, K. and Eisen, G., Marlink, R., Kanki, P., MBoup, S. (1998). Protection from HIV-1 infection by HIV-2. *AIDS* 12: 224–225.

Travers, K., MBoup, S., Marlink, R., Gueye-NDiaye, A., Siby, T., Thior, I., Traore, I., Dieng-Sarr, A., J.L., S., Mullins, C., NDoye, I., Hsieh, C.C., Essex, M. and Kanki, P. (1995). Natural Protection Against HIV-1 Infection Provided by HIV-2. *Science* 268: 1612–1615.

Tristem, M., Mansinho, K., Champalimaud, J.L., Ayres, L. and Karpas, A. (1989). Six new isolates of human immunodeficiency virus type 2 (HIV-2) and the molecular characterization of one (HIV-2CAM2). *J Gen Virol* 70: 479–484.

Victorino, R., Guerreiro, D., Pinto, L., Covas, M.J., Lourenco, M.H., Ferreira, M.O. and Teles, L.C. (1992). Clinical, immunological and epidemiological assessment of women with indeterminate western blots for HIV antibodies. *Int Conf AIDS* 8(3): 160 (abstract no. PuC 8046).

Voss, G., Kirchhoff, F., Nick, S., Moosmayer, D., Gelderblom, H. and Hunsmann, G. (1992). Morphogenesis of recombinant HIV-2 gag core particles. *Virus Res* 24(2): 197–210.

Weiss, R.A., Clapham, P.R., Weber, J.N., Whitby, D., Tedder, R.S., O'Connor, T., Chamaret, S. and Montagnier, L. (1988). HIV-2 antisera cross-neutralize HIV-1. *AIDS* 2: 95–100.

Wiktor, S.Z., Nkengasong, J.N., Ekpini, E.R., Adjorlolo-Johnson, G.T., Ghys, P.D., Brattegaard, K., Tossou, O., Dondero, T.J., De Cock, K.M. and Greenberg, A.E. (1999). Lack of protection against HIV-1 infection among women with HIV-2 infection. *AIDS* 13(6): 695–699.

World Health Organization (1990). AIDS: Recommendations for interpretation of HIV-2 western blot results. *Who Weekly Epidemiol Rec* 65: 74–75.

Xiang, Z., Ariyoshi, K., Wilkins, A., Dias, F., Whittle, H. and Breuer, J. (1997). HIV type 2 pathogenicity is not related to subtype in rural Guinea Bissau. *AIDS Res Hum Retroviruses* 13(6): 501–505.

Yamaguchi, J., Devare, S. and Brennan, C. (2000). Identification of a new HIV-2 subtype based on phylogenetic analysis of full-length genomic sequence. *AIDS Res Hum Retroviruses* 16(9): 925–930.

Yu, X.F., Ito, S., Essex, M. and Lee, T.H. (1988). A naturally immunogenic virion-associated protein specific for HIV-2 and SIV. *Nature* 335: 262–265.

Zagury D, L.A., Chams V., Fall L., Bernard J., Zagury J.-F., Bizzini B, Gringeri A (1998). C-C chemokines, pivotal in protection against HIV type 1 infection. *Proc. Natl. Acad. Sci. USA* 95: 3857–3861.

Zagury, J.F., Franchini, G., Reitz, M., Collalti, E., Starcich, B., Hall, L., Fargnoli, K., Jagodzinski, L., Guo, H.G. and Laure, F. (1988). Genetic variability between isolates of human immunodeficiency virus (HIV) type 2 is comparable to the variability among HIV type 1. *Proc Natl Acad Sci USA* 85: 5941–5945.

Zuber, M., Samuel, K.P., Lautenberger, J.A., Kanki, P.J. and Papas, T.S. (1990). Bacterially produced HIV-2 env polypeptides specific for distinguishing HIV-2 from HIV-1 infections. *AIDS Res Hum Retroviruses* 6: 525–534.

19

Tuberculosis Control, HIV/TB, and India

Sriram P. Tripathy[1] and Srikanth P. Tripathy[2]

[1]*Indian Council of Medical Research (ICMR), Pune, India*
[2]*National AIDS Research Institute, Bhosari, Pune, India*

INTRODUCTION

Tuberculosis as a Killer Disease in India

Tuberculosis (TB) is known to have existed in India for at least two thousand years and was the leading cause of death from communicable as well as non-communicable diseases. The ancient treatises such as *Charaka* described the disease under the names *"rajayakshma"* (king of diseases) and *"Kshyaya"* (wasting) and regarded the disease as difficult to cure. Because of the high mortality associated with the disease, TB control and research has always received high priority in India's national agenda, politically, managerially, and in the health system. A major part of the activities of the Indian Council of Medical Research, the research wing under the Government of India, was directed towards TB research during the last fifty years.

Commitment to TB Control

The advent of modern, specific antituberculosis drugs in the second half of the 20th century provided a stimulus to Indian authorities to conduct research leading to the formulation of appropriate control strategies for reducing TB morbidity, mortality, and the risk of transmission to others. Despite the meager resources of the country, elimination of TB was accorded a high priority under the 20-point Program in the Development Plan of India, with appropriate budgetary allocations and backed by strong political will at the level of the President and the Prime Minister of India.

Research Goals in TB

The major concern in TB management in the early 1950's was the large disparity between the millions of cases of active TB and the miniscule number (23,000) of TB beds available in the entire country. This disparity made it impossible for most patients to receive treatment in the sanatorium, then believed to be the most effective way to treat cases of TB. The Tuberculosis Research center, established in Chennai in 1956 under the Indian Council of Medical Research, conducted a carefully designed controlled clinical trial which provided irrefutable evidence that TB patients treated in their homes with a regimen of PAS (Para-aminosalicylic Acid) plus isoniazid daily for 12 months responded to treatment as effectively as those treated in the sanatorium with the same regimen (Tuberculosis Research Centre, 1959). Furthermore, these patients did not transmit TB to their family contacts in greater frequency than those patients treated in the sanatorium. This finding revolutionized the management of TB in control programs in India and other countries; domiciliary treatment became accepted as the best way to manage TB. The Tuberculosis Research Centre conducted a series of controlled clinical trials for formulating effective and affordable treatment regimens with a low frequency of adverse reactions to drugs and a capacity for administration of drugs on a mass scale. Notable among the achievements of the Centre were: (a) demonstration that monotherapy with isoniazid was associated with failure and emergence of isoniazid resistance and that multi-drug treatment was essential in TB; (b) demonstration of concealed drug-irregularity associated with self-administered regimens; (c) the formulation of effective regimens administered twice weekly without reducing their efficacy (Tuberculosis Research Centre, 1964); (d) the need for administering drugs under supervision, to overcome drug-irregularity and patient non-compliance; and (e) shortening the duration of chemotherapy to 6 months, ensuring better patient adherence than 12 month regimens. These findings have provided the scientific bases for modern management of TB. The entire world has benefited from the research contributions of the Tuberculosis Research Centre. Combinations of findings culled from different trials helped India to establish the current Revised National Tuberculosis Control Program (RNTCP) where fully potent anti-TB drugs are administered to patients under direct observation (DOTS) on an intermittent basis—three times weekly—for a duration of six or eight months.

Support from Global Scientific Community

Several international agencies and scientists provided financial and technical support and actively contributed to the successful execution of the trials conducted by the Tuberculosis Research Centre and its sister institution, National Tuberculosis Institute, Bangalore. The latter institution guided the Government in the formulation, establishment, and management of the National Tuberculosis Program (NTP), with its components of passive case-finding, treatment with 12-month regimens self-administered at home, and a large dependence on BCG immunization program to prevent TB. More recently, the NTP has been progressively replaced by the current RNTCP in a planned and phased manner. Under the RNTCP, the emphasis is on curing TB patients and reducing TB death rates by employing highly effective short-course regimens of six or eight months under direct observation—DOTS (Directly Observed Treatment, Short-course) and monitoring the outcome of treatment (Khatri and Frieden, 2002a). Several scientists and international agencies including the British Medical Research Council, World Health Organization (WHO), the United Nations Development Program, and the United States Public Health Service collaborated with India in TB research activities and control.

TB DISEASE BURDEN IN INDIA

India has over 12 million cases of TB accounting for over one-third of prevalent cases globally. Each year about 2 million new cases occur. Of these, less than half are detected under the program and are placed under treatment. The RNTCP started in 1993 as a pilot trial and has been expanding in a phased manner to provide coverage to larger populations (Khatri and Frieden, 2002b). With proper implementation of the RNTCP, it is expected that the reproductive rate of the disease will be reduced to less than 1, with each case of TB producing less than one secondary case, and thus meeting the essential epidemiological pre-requisite for reduction of the TB burden in successive years. However, the emergence of the HIV/AIDS epidemic in India is posing a grave threat to the timeframe of achieving TB control in India, especially in certain areas with high prevalence of HIV.

Incidence of Infection

India has a high incidence of annual risk of infection (ARI), with about 2% of the population getting infected with tubercle bacilli annually in the past. The ARI was about 1.8% per year during the past 3 decades, and has recently been estimated at 1.5% (WHO, 2003a).

Prevalence of Infection

Over one-third of India's population of about one billion are infected with the tubercle bacillus, and can be identified through assessment of reaction to an intradermal test dose of tuberculin (usually 1 TU RT 23 in India). The prevalence of infection increases with age, with reactivity rates as high as 80% of males or 70% of females in the age group of over 50 years (Tuberculosis Prevention Trial, 1980). The average positivity rate for all age groups is 40%. The large group of latent TB infection, at risk of developing active TB, forms the reservoir of TB. Most clinical cases of TB in India arise from among those with latent infection, due to reactivation of dormant bacilli which survive in equilibrium with the host for several decades. Such reactivation, however, is spread out over several years, with only about 10% of the infected pool developing active TB over a lifetime. Malnutrition, adverse conditions of stress, and lowered immunity are some of the risk factors associated with reactivation. Since the remaining 90% of the infected do not develop TB, it has not been clear whether the bacilli failed to survive in them or were alive but held in check by an efficient immune system. That the latter is true has been proven by the recent experience in HIV/TB dually infected persons, as virtually all persons with latent TB infection have been found to develop active TB as a part of the manifestation of AIDS. The incidence of TB in people living with HIV/AIDS (PLWHA) more or less corresponds to the prevalence of TB infection in the adult population in India.

TABLE 1. Estimates of TB Burden in India—2001

New cases of TB	All forms[a]	Smear positive
Number of cases (in thousands)	1820	815
Incidence rate (per 100,000)	178	79
Prevalence rate (per 100,000)	444	199

Source: WHO Global TB Control Report, 2003

[a] All forms include pulmonary, smear negative, pulmonary smear positive, smear negative extrapulmonary tuberculosis: includes sputum smear positive pulmonary tuberculosis.

Incidence of Disease

WHO estimates of the TB burden in India in 2001 are provided in Table 1 (WHO, 2003b). About 1.8 million cases of TB of all forms occur annually, of which about 815,000 are smear-positive. About 454,000 persons die of TB each year, including 24,000 who die of HIV-related TB.

Although only 10% of adult HIV/AIDS deaths are due to TB, TB is a major clinical manifestation of AIDS in Indian subjects, considering the high levels of TB infection in adults. Infection rates of over 50% in adults over 20, and 70–80% in persons aged 50 years or more have been documented (Tuberculosis Prevention Trial, 1980).

Prevalence of TB

The only national survey to measure TB disease prevalence was conducted during 1955–58 (Indian Council of Medical Research, 1958). Several regional surveys have been conducted since then, but their methods were not uniform. Even so, surveys have not shown much change in the disease burden over the past several decades. Longitudinal disease prevalence surveys (1962–2001) in Thiruvallur district in Tamil Nadu showed an annual decline of 1.8% in the prevalence of culture positive TB over the last three decades and a decline of 2.1% in the prevalence of smear-positive TB cases (Tuberculosis Research Centre, 2001).

WHO estimates of TB burden published in the global TB report of 2003 indicate a prevalence of all forms of TB and smear-positive TB as 444/100,000 and 199/100,000 population respectively (Table 1). Considering a decline of ARI to 1.5% (nationally), the estimates for 2002 have since been revised, indicating a lower prevalence of 379 and 170, respectively.

Primary Drug Resistance

Information on the prevalence of primary drug resistance in different parts of India has been unclear. Recent surveys on primary drug resistance indicate an alarmingly high prevalence of isoniazid-resistance, ranging from 10% to 23% in different parts of India. However, prevalence of primary multi-drug resistance is under 3%, and may pose no major threat to the overall success of the treatment regimens under the TB Control Program (WHO/IUATLD Global Project on Anti-Tuberculosis Drug Resistance Surveillance, 2000).

HIV BURDEN IN INDIA

Prevalence of HIV

Since the first report on indigenously infected HIV-positive cases in India in 1986 from Chennai in Tamil Nadu, the numbers of reported HIV infections have been steadily rising, with the current estimates of the HIV-positive population being about 4.6 million. The distribution of HIV infections, unlike TB, is not uniform in different parts of the country. While cases of HIV/AIDS have been reported in all States in the country, six states—Maharastra, Karnataka, Andhra Pradesh, Tamil Nadu, Manipur, and Nagaland—have had the highest burden, with prevalence of over 1% in the general population as assessed by sentinel surveillance in antenatal mothers. Recent data from Mizoram, Goa, and Dadra/Nagar Haveli indicate that HIV prevalence in 2003 has crossed the level of 1%. About 95% of the HIV/AIDS cases in India are in adults (National AIDS Control Organization [NACO], 2003a), and in the adult population the prevalence of TB infection is high (over 50%) (Tuberculosis Prevention Trial, 1980). Consequently, over two million HIV-infected persons are also infected with TB ("dual infection").

Impact of HIV on TB in India

Incidence of TB

In most persons infected with TB the bacilli remain dormant and produce no disease; only about 10% have a lifetime risk of developing TB. It has now been established that the risk is considerably increased in immuno-suppression due to HIV infection, with accelerated rates of reactivation of TB occurring at the rate of 10% annually among those dually infected persons. The two million HIV-positive Indians dually infected with HIV/TB are therefore likely to contribute about 200,000 new cases of TB in addition to the 815,000 new smear positive cases occurring each year without HIV, i.e., about a 25% increase in the TB burden. Further, due to the uneven distribution of HIV, the increase will be mostly in the six Indian states with high HIV burden.

HIV Seropositivity in TB Patients

As a consequence of the additional load of TB cases attributable to HIV, the proportion of HIV positives among the TB patients

TABLE 2. Trends in HIV Sero-positivity in TB patients in Pune, India[a]

Author	Period of study	No. of TB patients	% HIV-positive
Paranjape *et al.* (1997)	1991	344	3.2
	1992	187	5.9
	1993	395	5.0
	1994	1046	10.0
	1995	1189	15.5
National AIDS Research	1996	800	18.6
Institute, Pune	1997	400	21.5
	1998	400	29.5
(1996–97, 1998, 1999, 2000, 2001)	1999	1965	26.4
	2000	400	28.7
	2001	1588	30.4

[a] Data collected on HIV seroprevalence in TB patients presenting to chest clinics at Sassoon Hospital, Pune, in successive years. All forms of tuberculosis were included– pulmonary and extrapulmonary.

will be higher than in the general population in the six states with high HIV burden. High rates of HIV seropositivity in TB patients attending chest clinics have been reported from Mumbai, Tamil Nadu, Rajasthan, and other parts of India (Narain *et al.*, 2002).

The patterns of HIV in TB patients have been studied systematically in Pune in Maharashtra state.

The National AIDS Research Institute, in collaboration with the Sassoon General Hospital in Pune has investigated the HIV seropositivity rates among the TB patients attending the chest clinic at the Sassoon General Hospital in Pune over the period 1991–2001 (Paranjape *et al.*, 1997; National AIDS Research Institute, 1996–97, 1998, 1999, 2000, 2001). There has been a steady increase from 3.2% in 1991 to 31% in 2001 (Table 2). There is some indication that the increase has reached a plateau, possibly due to a concerted AIDS Control Programme in Pune and the rest of Maharastra state.

TB among Patients with AIDS

The high incidence of TB in HIV-positive persons is largely due to reactivation of latent TB in dually infected persons, but also includes a proportion of cases occurring due to exogenous TB infection in PLWHA, with infection progressing to primary TB in a high proportion of new infections due to the immuno-suppressed state of the host. PLWHA may have a greater risk of exposure to TB through the health care facilities handling HIV/AIDS and HIV/TB cases.

TB is a major clinical feature in AIDS patients in India, occurring in over half the patients (Table 3). In many of them, TB is the first clinical manifestation of immunosuppression.

Impact of HIV on TB Control

In parts of India with high HIV/TB burden, TB control activities could be adversely affected due to over diagnosis of sputum smear-negative pulmonary TB, low treatment success rates, high mortality rates during treatment, high default rates due to adverse drug reactivity, high relapse rates, and increased emergence of drug resistance (Central TB Division, 2002).

TB CONTROL PROGRAM IN INDIA

The TB control program is based on a system of passive case finding of TB among patients presenting to health care facilities with symptoms suggestive of pulmonary TB, such as cough of two weeks or longer

TABLE 3. Tuberculosis incidence in HIV/AIDS cases in India[a]

Author	Place	Period	No. of patients	% with TB
Arora, Kumar (1999)	Pondicherry	1991–97	190	65%
Kumarasamy *et al.* (1995)	Chennai	1987–93	100	61%
Kumarasamy *et al.* (2000)	Chennai	1999	156	58%
Agarwal, A. (1998)	Manipur	1993–95	31	45%
Bhagyawati Devi *et al.* (2003)	Manipur	2002–03	100	55%

[a] Data collected from adult PLWHA with clinical manifestation of AIDS in areas of high HIV prevalence. In most of them, TB was due to reactivation; in some, TB may have occurred due to uncontrolled progression of new infection to primary tuberculosis.

duration, fever, weight loss, and haemoptysis. Sputum smear examination by microscopy is the sheet anchor of TB control in India. Patients are identified as having bacteriologically-confirmed pulmonary TB if their sputum smear shows acid-fast bacilli. Such patients form the bulk of the patients treated under the program; in addition, clinically ill sputum-negative pulmonary TB and extrapulmonary TB patients are also managed under the Program. Patients are managed under a RNTCP wherein all are provided with free diagnosis and free treatment by the program (Khatri and Frieden, 2002a).

DOTS under RNTCP in India

The NTP was established across the country with implementation of a District Tuberculosis Program, using a District Tuberculosis Centre as the unit, and providing domiciliary treatment to patients diagnosed with active TB. The program was rated as scientifically sound and was adopted not only by India but also by other countries. Symptomatic patients attending health care facilities were provided free sputum smear microscopy, and those diagnosed as smear-positive were offered a 12-month regimen of drugs for self-administration at home. The program made no significant reduction in prevalence and incidence over three decades, since under the program conditions the regimens provided a cure in only 30–50% cases, largely because of inadequate compliance by patients. Also, only about one-third of the prevalent cases were diagnosed and treated under the program conditions. However, the program is a dynamic one and constantly is being reviewed and revised. In 1993, the program underwent major policy changes, with the implementation of the RNTCP and its increased resources, improved laboratory based diagnosis, use of effective standardized rifamycin-containing regimens of short duration of six or eight months, direct observation of treatment, and rigid reporting procedures. The RNTCP uses the sub-district as the basic unit for TB control and is being expanded in a systematically planned and phased manner ensuring that each new site is fully ready and prepared to implement all the components of the DOTS strategy recommended by the WHO and adopted by India. Components include political commitment to the program, establishment of good microscopy centers, high quality microscopy of sputum smears, administration of all the scheduled doses of drugs under direct supervision, uninterrupted supply of high quality anti-TB drugs, establishment of proper recording systems, and monitoring treatment outcomes. Currently, over 70% of India is covered by DOTS and by the end of 2004, the entire country will be covered by DOTS (Khatri and Frieden, 2002b; Central TB Division, 2003).

Treatment under RNTCP

Patients diagnosed as having active TB are offered treatment based on their classification as pulmonary or extrapulmonary, sputum smear-positive or sputum smear-

TABLE 4. Treatment Outcomes of RNTCP, India, Second Quarter, 2002

Patients	Cured	Completed treatment	Died	Remained Smear-positive	Defaulted	Transferred Out
New Cases						
Smear-positive	85.6%	0.8%	4.3%	2.8%	6.3%	0.4%
Smear-negative	—	87.5%	3.6%	1.0%	7.6%	0.3%
EPT[a]	—	91.9%	2.1%	0.2%	5.4%	0.2%
Retreatment Cases						
Relapsed Smear-positive	72.9%	2.4%	6.9%	5.3%	11.9%	0.5%
Failure Smear- positive	57.1%	3.0%	8.3%	14.1%	16.6%	0.7%
Default Smear-positive	67.7%	3.6%	6.9%	4.8%	16.3%	0.6%
Other Smear-positive	69%	73.7%	5.3%	1.0%	12.1%	0.4%

[a] EPT = Extrapulmonary TB
Source: RNTCP – Treatment outcomes of RNTCP India 4th Quarter 1993 – 2nd quarter 2002.

negative, history of previous treatment–new or re-treatment, and clinical severity of their disease. Patients are categorized into three treatment groups.

The first category includes new pulmonary sputum-positive, seriously ill sputum-negative pulmonary, and seriously ill extra pulmonary cases. These patients receive a six month regimen, consisting of an initial phase of isoniazid, rifampicin, pyrazinamide, and ethambutol administered thrice weekly for two months, following a continuation phase of isoniazid and rifamycin thrice weekly for four months (2 $H_3R_3Z_3E_3$/4 H_3R_3).

(R = rifampicin, H = isoniazid, Z = pyrazinamide, E = ethambutol, S = Streptomycin; the prefix indicates the duration of chemotherapy in months; the subscript indicates the number of doses per week).

The second treatment category includes re-treatment cases of all forms. Patients in this category are offered an eight-month regimen of 2 $S_3H_3R_3Z_3E_3$/1 $H_3R_3Z_3E_3$/5 $H_3R_3E_3$.

The third treatment category includes sputum smear-negative pulmonary cases, and extrapulmonary cases who are not seriously ill. These patients receive the regimen 2 $H_3R_3Z_3$/4 R_3H_3—i.e., same as Category I regimen excluding ethambutol during the first two months.

In each category, every dose of drug in the initial intensive phase is taken under direct observation by a health care professional or by an authorized drug provider; in the continuation phase, at least the first of the three doses of each weekly schedule is taken under direct observation.

Treatment Outcomes

The successful outcome of treatment is recorded as the proportion of smear-positive cases who become smear-negative and are classified as "cured," and the proportion of smear-negative cases who complete their course of treatment.

With the adoption of DOTS strategy and effective implementation of DOTS, the currently operative RNTCP has been successful in achieving the targeted cure rates of 85% in new smear-positive cases (RNTCP Report, 2003) (Table 4).

Although the cure rates for different types of re-treatment cases, are lower (57%–73%), these results are considerably better than what had been achieved before the introduction of DOTS in India. As the new cases form the bulk of those under treatment, the overall success rate for all patients is encouragingly high. The findings are highly encouraging and suggest attainment of the TB elimination goal in the future. However, the onset of HIV/AIDS epidemic and its spread to different parts of India may seriously undermine the success of the DOTS strategy and delay the achievement of the goal.

MANAGEMENT OF HIV/TB

Challenges

The state of immuno-suppression in HIV seropositive subjects leads to uncontrolled multiplication of tubercle bacilli resulting in the accumulation of large numbers of viable tubercle bacilli, a situation similar to lepromatous leprosy. Disseminated TB is common, with many patients presenting with extra pulmonary TB with or without pulmonary TB. This poses diagnostic and management challenges, especially since many HIV/TB cases with pulmonary TB may present with smear-negative disease and uncharacteristic radiological features of TB.

The very large number of bacilli attained in the pathologic organs may favor the emergence of drug-resistance during treatment; however, since the bacilli are multiplying rapidly, they respond very well to multidrug therapy with rifampicin and isoniazid-containing regimens. With four potent drugs employed in the RNTCP regimen, the chances of emergence of drug resistance are small. The drug regimens are likely to be as effective in the treatment of HIV/TB patients as in TB patients without HIV with no additional risk of emergence of drug-resistance. Since relapses that occur after the scheduled six or eight months of chemotherapy may occur with greater frequency, extension of the duration of treatment may be desirable. Further, many HIV/TB patients, while responding to TB chemotherapy, suffer from concurrent opportunistic infections with other microbes such as *P. carinii, S. aureus, Legionella, Listeria* and others, and die from non-TB causes. Since many of these deaths can be prevented by concurrent chemoprophylaxis with antibiotics such as cotrimoxazole, identification of HIV/TB patients among TB patients would provide scope for better management of dually infected patients and prolong their life. Strategies for controlling HIV/TB should therefore include identification of HIV-positive individuals and screening these PLWHA for TB.

Diagnosis of Active TB in Presence of HIV Infection

The absence of cavities in most cases, a high frequency of smear-negative pulmonary TB, the greater frequency of extra pulmonary TB and atypical radiologic presentations pose difficulties in diagnosis of TB in HIV-positive people. In early stages of HIV infection with mild immuno-suppression, the presentation of TB may be classical, with smear positivity, cavitation, and upper lobe infiltration. In the severely immuno-compromised subjects, the radiological appearances are generally atypical. While pulmonary TB is the most common form of TB in PLWHA, extrapulmonary TB is seen frequently and indeed, in many cases, occurs even in the absence of pulmonary TB. In addition to sputum smear examination, dually infected persons would require diagnostic aids such as radiological examination, microscopy, culture, and histopathological examination of pleural fluid and other biopsy specimens. In many cases, diagnoses would be presumptive.

All patients presenting with cough of more than two weeks duration should have their sputum (three specimens) examined for acid-fast bacilli, and if found positive, should be treated with anti-TB drugs. If negative, they should receive a course of broad-spectrum antibiotics, and if symptoms persist, can have radiological examination of the chest.

TB Chemotherapy for HIV/TB

All anti-TB drugs are as effective in HIV-positive subjects as in those without HIV, and can be used in the treatment of HIV/TB (National AIDS Control Organization and Central TB Division, 2002). The high frequency of serious adverse reactions associated with thiacetazone precludes its use in HIV/TB subjects. The drug is no longer used in the National TB Control Program in India and its use in the six high prevalent states of India has been specifically banned. The use of ketoconazole for treatment of fungal infections in HIV/TB patients should be avoided since the drug causes reduction in the blood levels of rifampicin.

The anti-TB drug regimens used in the RNTCP are to be used for dually infected patients, using the same categorization principles. Smear-negative cases, if seriously ill, will be classified as Category I patients and treated accordingly. Clinicians, at their discretion, may continue the treatment for a longer duration, extending the continuation of treatment for four months to six to seven months (National AIDS Control Organization and Central TB Division, 2002). In addition to the standard anti-TB regimens, HIV/TB patients need to be provided with appropriate care for management of HIV infection, including counseling, advice for prevention of transmission to others, diagnosis and management of other opportunistic infections, and advice on antiretroviral therapy (ART) if required.

Treatment with Antiretroviral Therapy in TB Patients

There is considerable debate regarding the stage of HIV infection when ART is to be initiated. Initiation of ART is recommended only if there is evidence of serious immunosuppression, e.g., in patients with CD_4^+ lymphocyte counts below 200/ mm^3, since the long-term use of most antiretroviral drugs is associated with adverse reactions, duration of ART is lifelong, emergence of resistance to ART drugs is frequent, and because they may not be necessary in the presence of moderate immunity (World Health Organization Regional Office for South-East Asia, 2002).

ART in the Indian Program

Until recently, antiretroviral drugs were not provided to PLWHA under the National Program. The high cost of these drugs and the need for lifelong treatment precluded their use under the National Program. Recent negotiations between the Clinton Foundation and Indian Pharmaceutical concerns have resulted in a drastic reduction in the cost of ART to 38 US cents per day for a three-drug combination for export to other countries. Similar negotiations with the Government of India have offered the prospect of further reducing drug costs. Encouraged by these developments, the Government of India announced on the eve of the World AIDS Day in December 2003 that AIDS patients in India will receive ART, free of cost, beginning April 1st 2004. Since TB is the most common manifestation of AIDS in India, most HIV/TB patients will be eligible for ART in addition to anti-TB therapy.

Co-Administration of Rifampicin with ART

The ART drugs fall into three major classes—protease inhibitors (PI), nucleoside reverse transcriptase inhibitors (NRTI) and non-nucleoside reverse transcriptase inhibitors (NNRTI) (NACO, 2003b; NACO, 2003c). Some ART drugs in the PI and NNRTI categories may reduce the serum concentration of rifamycins, and rifampicin in turn, may substantially decrease blood levels of the ART drugs. The drug rifabutin is a less potent inhibitor of cytochrome P450 than rifampicin and may be used to replace rifampicin in dually infected patients receiving both anti-TB treatment and ART, but this drug is not available in India. In such patients, rifampicin can be substituted by streptomycin. In HIV/TB patients who are already on anti-TB treatment (ATT) and are yet to receive ART, WHO recommends that initiation of ART may be delayed till the course of ATT is completed. If however, there is high risk of HIV disease progression (e.g. CD4 count less than 200/mm^3), ART and ATT can be given concurrently (World Health Organization Regional Office for South East Asia, 2002).

TB Case Finding in PLWHA

The TB control program in India is based on passive case finding among symptomatic patients presenting to health care facilities. Active case finding is limited to examination of close family members of TB patients and offering treatment to those with active TB. Chemoprophylaxis (with isoniazid or any other anti-TB drug or drug combinations) is not recommended for asymptomatic TB-infected persons (detected through tuberculin testing), as most of them are unlikely to develop active TB and hence would not benefit from chemoprophylaxis. Active case finding for TB will, however, be cost effective in the case of PLWHA, since each year as many as 10% of the tuberculin positives among them will develop active TB, most of which can be prevented by chemoprophylaxis with isoniazid. There is, therefore, a case for active case finding in PLWHA; as soon as people are identified as HIV-positive, they may be screened for active TB in HIV care facilities. Patients with active TB may be referred to TB care facilities for treatment and those who do not have active TB may be offered chemoprophylaxis with isoniazid and cotrimoxazole. Routine tuberculin testing of subjects and limiting isoniazid prophylaxis to tuberculin reactors may not be practical; giving isoniazid prophylaxis to all subjects without tuberculin testing will provide protection to tuberculin reactors against endogenous reactivation and exogenous TB infection, and to tuberculin non-reactors against exogenous infection. Further, tuberculin reaction as a means of detecting latent TB infection is not reliable in HIV-positive persons, and is often associated with false negative reactions (Centers for Disease Control, 1991).

Benefits from HIV Screening in TB Patients

In parts of India where HIV prevalence is low, routine screening of TB patients for HIV is not necessary. In high HIV-prevalence areas, however, there are substantial benefits in identification of HIV infection among TB patients. Dually infected patients undergoing treatment for TB respond well and become smear-negative, and yet many patients die during the first year due to TB unrelated causes (Harries *et al.*, 2001). Undoubtedly, some of these deaths could be prevented by diagnosis and management of other opportunistic infections which are the most frequent causes of death in HIV/TB patients cured of TB. Proper counseling of all TB patients can motivate such patients to agree to screening for HIV. The scope for management of opportunistic infections and the availability of ART when needed may motivate most TB patients to agree to screening. Currently, TB in most PLWHA is identified during the late stages of HIV infection. Screening of TB patients for HIV would result in earlier identification of PLWHA, greater chances of reduction in HIV transmission, better quality of life, and longer survival through better management of HIV.

Need for Confidentiality

Despite the considerable amount of health education and awareness campaigns in the AIDS control program and the legal protection available to PLWHA, HIV-related discrimination in employment opportunities and in the workplace, and marginalization of HIV-positive people in the community are frequently observed in the Indian setting. Any HIV screening program for TB patients must ensure maintenance of strict confidentiality of HIV status on a "need to know" basis, and restrict the HIV status information to relevant health care personnel and select family members. The patient should be assured that in addition to the TB condition, his/her HIV-related non-TB clinical episodes will be promptly attended to, either by TB care personnel or by referral to appropriate health care facilities, and that s/he would qualify for ART under the program when needed.

Chemoprophylaxis with Cotrimoxazole

Some programs in African countries have accepted the recommendation of WHO/UNDP for routine administration of cotrimoxazole to patients on ATT with the object of preventing some opportunistic infections and thereby improving the quality of life and increasing their life span. India has not yet made any decision in this regard. The Tuberculosis Research Centre in Madras is currently investigating the role of cotrimoxazole prophylaxis for HIV/TB in an ongoing study. More such studies are needed for obtaining evidence on this subject. Cotrimoxazole is inexpensive, well tolerated, and effective against many common organisms such as *P. carinii, S. aureus, Legionella, Listeria*, and other agents causing opportunistic infections in PLWHA (Bartlett and Gallant, 2003). Routine administration of cotrimoxazole may therefore be expected to benefit PLWHA, including dually infected patients.

STRATEGIES IN THE MANAGEMENT OF HIV/TB IN INDIA

Policy Formulation

African countries which had not yet established national TB programs and HIV/AIDS programs found it easy to establish a joint TB and HIV/AIDS program efficiently, with integration of activities in the two disease areas. India already had a well-established national TB program for decades and an equally strong national AIDS control program, both functioning independently and having different lines of control. Integrating the two programs would have been counterproductive. Instead, a policy decision was made to strengthen each of the two programs, permitting them to retain their independence and authority and devise appropriate collaborative mechanisms so that responsibilities were apportioned to the two programs to undertake activities according to their expertise and strengths. Both programs operate under the authority of the Ministry of Health and Family Welfare. Coordination between the two programs is therefore possible. Modalities of collaboration have been agreed to at high-level meetings for policy formulation and the evolution of a joint HIV/TB action program.

Collaboration between NACO and RNTCP

Realizing the urgency of the need for HIV/TB collaboration, the Government of India has taken appropriate steps to ensure coordination between the TB and HIV control programs, with an initial focus on the six Indian states with high prevalence of HIV. Workshops have been held, HIV/TB training modules have been prepared, and training programs have been formulated. Modes of establishing referral linkages between Voluntary Counseling and Testing Centres (VCTC) and RNTCP sputum microscopy centres have been established. The VCTC have proved an important source for detection of active TB, with 5–15% of PLWHA attending VCTC found to have active pulmonary TB. Future plans include further strengthening of the collaboration between the two programs at the State, district, and sub district levels in the six States, and expansion of the collaboration to the rest of the country in a phased manner.

SUMMARY

India has a large TB burden, with over 12 million cases of active TB requiring treatment. The current program—Revised National Tuberculosis Control Program—is poised to tackle the TB epidemic effectively through coverage of the entire country with the DOTS strategy within a year. The program is run efficiently, and cure rates have exceeded the targeted figure of 85% in many parts of the country. Over the past few decades, there has been a reduction in the ARI, prevalence, incidence, and mortality of TB; and the magnitudes of reduction are expected to increase substantially through universal application of DOTS.

The HIV epidemic in India is threatening to impede the progress and achievements of DOTS in several parts of India. Six states in the country—Maharashtra, Tamil Nadu, Karnataka, Andhra Pradesh, Manipur, and Nagaland–have a high HIV burden, with a prevalence of over 1% in the general population. While the entire country is taking steps to strengthen activities in TB control, HIV/AIDS control, and HIV/TB control, the six states with high HIV burden are tackling the HIV/TB menace on a priority basis with close collaboration between the TB and the HIV/AIDS control programs. With DOTS coverage of the entire country and availability of ART drugs to all HIV/AIDS patients, including HIV/TB patients in 2004, morbidity and mortality due to TB and HIV/TB are likely to be substantially reduced. TB transmission in the community is likely to be reduced, thus brightening the prospect of achieving elimination of TB as a major public health problem in India in the coming years.

REFERENCES

Bartlett, J.G., and Gallant, J.E. (2003). *Medical Management of HIV Infection.* Johns Hopkins University Press, Baltimore, MD, p. 317.

Centers for Disease Control. (1991). Purified Protein Derivative (PPD) tuberculin anergy and HIV infection: Guidelines for anergy testing and management of anergic persons at risk of tuberculosis. *MMWR* 41:27–32.

Central TB Division, Directorate General of Health Services. (2002). Revised National Tuberculosis Control Program. Training manual for medical officers on HIV/AIDS, Ministry of Health and Family Welfare, New Delhi, pp. 5–36.

Central TB Division, Directorate General of Health Services. (2003). TB India 2003 – RNTCP status report. Central TB Division, Directorate General of Health Services, Ministry of Health and Family Welfare, New Delhi, pp. 1–64.

Harries, A.D., Hargreaves, N.J., Gausi, F., Fwanjana, J.H., and Salonipani, F.M. (2001). High early death rates in tuberculosis patients in Malawi. *Intl J Tuberc Lung Dis* 5:1000–1005.

Indian Council of Medical Research. Tuberculosis in India—A sample survey 1955–58. Special Report Series No.34, ICMR, New Delhi, pp. 1–121.

Khatri, G.R., and Frieden, T.R. (2000b). Rapid DOTS expansion in India. *Bull. World Health Org.* 80:457–463.

Khatri, G.R., and Frieden, T.R. (2002a). Controlling tuberculosis in India. *N Engl J Med* 347:1420–1425.

Narain, J.P., Tripathy, S., and Pontali, E. (2002). Tuberculosis and HIV infection. In: Narain, J.P. (ed.), *Tuberculosis Epidemiology and Control.* World Health Organization, Regional Office for South East Asia, pp. 83–104.

National AIDS Control Organization. (2003a). HIV/AIDS Indian Scenario. HIV/AIDS Surveillance in India (as reported to NACO as of September 30, 2003).

National AIDS Control Organization. (2003b). National guidelines for clinical management of HIV/AIDS. Ministry of Health and Family Welfare, New Delhi, pp. 1–113.

National AIDS Control Organization. (2003c). Guidelines on rational use of antiretroviral drugs. Ministry of Health and Family Welfare, Government of India, New Delhi, pp. 5–23.

National AIDS Control Organization and Central TB Division, Ministry of Health and Family Welfare, Nirman Bhavan, New Delhi. (2002). Treatment guidelines for TB in HIV infected, pp. 1–12.

National AIDS Research Institute, Pune, Indian Council of Medical Research, Pune, India (1996–97) Annual Report, p. 4–5.

National AIDS Research Institute, Pune, Indian Council of Medical Research, Pune, India. (1998). Annual Report, p. 2–3.

National AIDS Research Institute, Pune, Indian Council of Medical Research, Pune, India. (1999). Annual Report, p. 14.

National AIDS Research Institute, Pune, Indian Council of Medical Research, Pune, India. (2000). Annual Report, p. 4.

National AIDS Research Institute, Pune, Indian Council of Medical Research, Pune, India. (2001). Annual Report, pp. 2–4.

Paranjape, R.S., Tripathy, S.P., Menon, P.A., Mehendale, S.M., Khatawkar, P., Joshi, D.R., Patil, U., Gadkari, D.A., and Rodrigues, J.J. (1997). Increasing trend of HIV seroprevalence among pulmonary tuberculosis patients in Pune, India. *Indian J. Med. Res.* 42:117–20.

RNTCP. (2002). Treatment outcomes of RNTCP India 4th Quarter 1993—2nd Quarter 2002.

Tuberculosis Chemotherapy Centre. (1959). A concurrent comparison of home and sanatorium treatment of pulmonary tuberculosis in South India. *Bull. World Health Org.* 21:51–144.

Tuberculosis Chemotherapy Centre. (1964). A concurrent comparison of intermittent (twice-weekly) isoniazid plus streptomycin and daily izoniazid plus

PAS in the domiciliary treatment of pulmonary tuberculosis. *Bull World Health Org*. 31:247–271.

Tuberculosis Prevention Trial, Madras. (1980). Trial of BCG vaccines in South India for tuberculosis prevention. *Indian J. Med. Res.* 72(suppl): 1–74.

Tuberculosis Research Centre (2001). Trends in the prevalence and incidence of tuberculosis in South India. *Int J Tuberc Lung Dis* 5:142–157.

World Health Organization (WHO) Regional Office for South-East Asia, New Delhi. (2002). The use of antiretroviral therapy: A simplified approach for resource constrained countries, pp. 53–54.

World Health Organization (WHO). (2003a). Provisional estimates of Annual Risk of Tuberculosis Infection. Presented to Joint Monitoring Mission, RNTCP India, New Delhi (September 16–25, 2003).

World Health Organization (WHO). (2003b). Global TB Control Report, 2003. (January 28, 2004); http://www.who.int//tbestimates.

WHO / IUATLD Global Project on Anti-Tuberculosis Drug Resistance Surveillance. (2000). Anti-Tuberculosis Drug Resistance in the World, Report No.2. Prevalence and trends. WHO/CDS/TB/2000.278.

20

Infectious Diseases and the Development of Health Systems in Thailand

Visanu Thamlikitkul[1], Viroj Tangcharoensathien[2], and Natth Bhamarapravati[3]

[1]*Siriraj Hostpital, Mahidol University, Bangkok, Thailand*
[2]*Ministry of Public Health, Nonthaburi, Thailand*
[3]*Mahidol University Salaya, Nakhonpathom, Thailand*

HISTORY AND CURRENT STATUS OF INFECTIOUS DISEASES IN THAILAND

Infectious diseases have been a major public health problem in Thailand for the past several centuries. Most infectious diseases in earlier days were food and water-borne diseases, vector-borne diseases, and infectious diseases related to poor sanitation (Wright and Breakspears, 1903; Beek, 2001). Some infectious diseases have now been eradicated, for example smallpox. The last case of smallpox in Thailand was documented in 1962. Some diseases have been brought under control by vaccines, such as diphtheria, pertussis, tetanus, poliomyelitis, and measles. However many infectious diseases continue to be public health problems such as acute respiratory tract infections, acute diarrhea, tuberculosis, dengue hemorrhagic fever, malaria, endemic infectious diseases such as melioidosis, and parasitic infestation e.g., opisthorchiasis. Like other countries, Thailand is faced with emerging infectious diseases, especially HIV/AIDS, and re-emerging diseases such as leptospirosis. Several emerging infectious diseases originating in neighboring countries such as severe acute respiratory syndrome (SARS), avian flu, and Nipah virus infections are also a threat to Thai people. Moreover, infectious diseases due to drug resistant microorganisms e.g., drug resistant *Streptococcus pneumoniae*, methicillin-resistant *Staphylococcus aureus*, and multi-drug resistant gram-negative bacilli have also been increasing.

There are 47 infectious diseases documented in the current Thai Communicable Diseases Act. These include cholera, plaque, smallpox, yellow fever, meningococcal infections, diphtheria, pertussis, tetanus, poliomyelitis, measles, rubella, mumps, chicken pox, influenza, encephalitis, dengue fever, rabies, hepatitis, hemorrhagic conjunctivitis, food poisoning, dysentery, amoebiasis, typhoid fever, paratyphoid fever, typhus fever due to *Rickettsia prowazekii*, scrub typhus, murine typhus, tuberculosis, leprosy, malaria, anthrax, trichinosis, yaws, leptospirosis, syphilis, gonorrhea, non-specific urethritis, chancroid, granuloma inguinalae, lymphogranuloma venereum, relapsing fever, acute diarrhea, chronic tropical ulcer, filariasis, HIV/AIDS, acute flaccid paralysis and SARS. Five diseases are classified as dangerous diseases, namely cholera, plaque, smallpox, yellow fever, and SARS. Any cases of the following diseases must be reported to the local health authority: cholera, plaque, smallpox, yellow fever, diphtheria, tetanus neonatorum, poliomyelitis, encephalitis, rabies, typhus fever due to *Rickettsia prowazekii*, anthrax, trichinosis, meningococcal infections, yaws, acute flaccid paralysis, and SARS.

According to the official documents of the Ministry of Public Health (MoPH) on the Burden of Disease and Injuries in Thailand in 1999, infectious diseases comprised 21% of the total of 9.6 million Disability Adjusted Life Years (2 million DALYs) (MoPH, Thailand, 2002; MoPH, Thailand, 2003a). HIV/AIDS accounted for a majority of the infectious disease burden, with 1.3 million DALYs, or 72% of the total infectious disease burden. The other major infectious diseases that contributed to the DALYs in Thailand were acute respiratory tract infections in children, and tuberculosis. Although HIV/AIDS has been the major infectious disease problem in Thailand over the past decade, it will be addressed elsewhere. This chapter will focus primarily on epidemiology and the current status of infectious diseases other than HIV/AIDS in Thailand over the past several decades, during which time a disease surveillance system has been well established. Some major infectious diseases under surveillance will be described. Morbidity and mortality data for most of the infectious diseases described in this chapter come from the annual epidemiological surveillance report prepared by the Bureau of Epidemiology, Department of Disease Control, MoPH from 1977 to 2002. It should be mentioned that the morbidity and mortality data collected by the MoPH is likely to be an under-estimate, and this data should therefore be considered as a minimum estimate of what is probably the actual reality.

Acute Gastroenteritis

Acute gastroenteritis includes acute diarrhea, food poisoning, dysentery and severe diarrhea. Cholera was the major leading cause of morbidity and mortality in Thailand in the 1900s. An epidemic of cholera in 1890 resulted in moving the Thai capital from Uthong to Krungsri Ayudaya. The morbidity rate of acute gastroenteritis per 100,000 population has been increasing, from 264 in 1977 to 1800 in 1991, to 2000 in 2002 as shown in Figure 1. However the case fatality rate has been decreasing, from 0.5% in 1977–1978 to 0.1% or less since 1982. The decrease in the case fatality rate was primarily due to improvements in sanitation and personal hygiene, and oral rehydration therapy.

Acute gastroenteritis is still a common cause of morbidity and mortality in children under age five. The common micro-organisms causing acute gastroenteritis documented by stool or rectal swab cultures in 1998 and in 1999 collected from 23 hospitals located in all regions of Thailand revealed that 18%–38% were *Salmonella* (more than 90% were non-typhoidal *Salmonella*), 21%–36% were *Vibrio parahemolyticus*, 8–12% were *Escherichia coli*, 9%–22% were *Shigella* (most of them were *Shigella sonnei* and *Shigella flexneri*), 2%–5% were *Aeromonas* 2%–3% were *Plesiomonas* and 3%–5% were *Vibrio cholerae* (Ministry of Public Health (MoPH), Thailand, 1998; MoPH, Thailand, multiple years). There were nine major outbreaks of cholera during 1900 to 1980, which infected more than 80,000 patients and caused more than 30,000 deaths. The case fatality rate decreased from 72% in 1918 to 3% in 1980. The first six major outbreaks were caused by the *Vibrio cholerae* serogroup O1 biotype classical whereas the *Vibrio cholerae* serogroup O1 biotype El-Tor serotype Ogawa and Inaba was the cause of the cholera since 1963. El Tor cholera usually causes less severe diarrhea

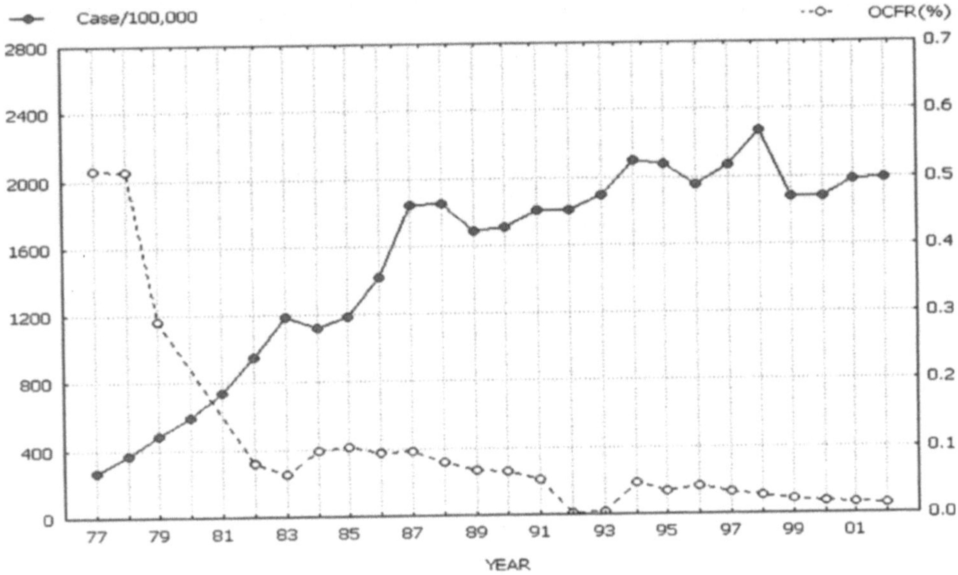

FIGURE 1. Morbidity and case fatality rate (CFR) for acute gastroenteritis (Ministry of Public Health, Thailand, 1997–2002)

with a much lower case fatality rate than classical cholera. *Vibrio cholerae* serotype Ogawa was a predominant serotype during 1993–1994 epidemic, whereas serotype Inaba has been the most common serotype ever since.

The cholera epidemics during 1992 and 1994 were caused by *Vibrio cholerae* non-O1 (O139) and since that time this strain of *Vibrio cholerae* has been found only rarely. Diarrheagenic *E.coli* strains isolated from patients with acute diarrhea in 1998 were enteropathogenic *E.coli* (86%), enteroaggregative *E.coli* (11%), enterotoxigenic *E.coli* (2%) and enteroinvasive *E.coli* (1%). Less than 50% of *Shigella* isolated from stools was sensitive to ampicillin, tetracycline and co-trimoxazole whereas 40% to 75% of non-typhoidal *Salmonella* was sensitive to ampicillin and co-trimoxazole. Nearly all strains of non-typhoidal *Salmonella* and *Shigella* were sensitive to fluoroquinolones and third generation cephalosporins (MoPH, Thailand, 1998; MoPH, Thailand, 1999; Isenbarger *et al.*, 2002). Susceptibility of *Aeromonas* to ampicillin, co-trimoxazole and norfloxacin were 10%, 70%, and 85% respectively. The *Vibrio cholerae* serotype Ogawa was susceptible to tetracycline and co-trimoxazole prior to 1996. Since 1996, more than 70% of *Vibrio cholerae* serotype Ogawa have been resistant to co-trimoxazole. Resistance to tetracycline was up to 50% in 2000 and then declined to 10% in 2002. Most strains of the *Vibrio cholerae* serotype Inaba were still sensitive to tetracycline and co-trimoxazole. *Vibrio cholerae* O139 was usually resistant to co-trimoxazole but still sensitive to tetracycline. Almost all strains of *Vibrio cholerae* were sensitive to fluoroquinolones. Antibiotic susceptibility profiles of *Vibrio cholerae*, non-typhoidal *Salmonella Shigella Aeromonas* against ampicillin, tetracycline and co-trimoxazole may vary according to geographical areas and species of the organism. *Vibrio parahemolyticus* is almost always sensitive to tetracycline, co-trimoxazole, and fluoroquinolones.

Studies of acute gastroenteritis in children have elucidated many trends and characteristics of the disease. *Campylobacter jejuni* was isolated in 27% of children presenting with dysentery at Children's Hospital in Bangkok during 1998–2000. *Campylobacter*

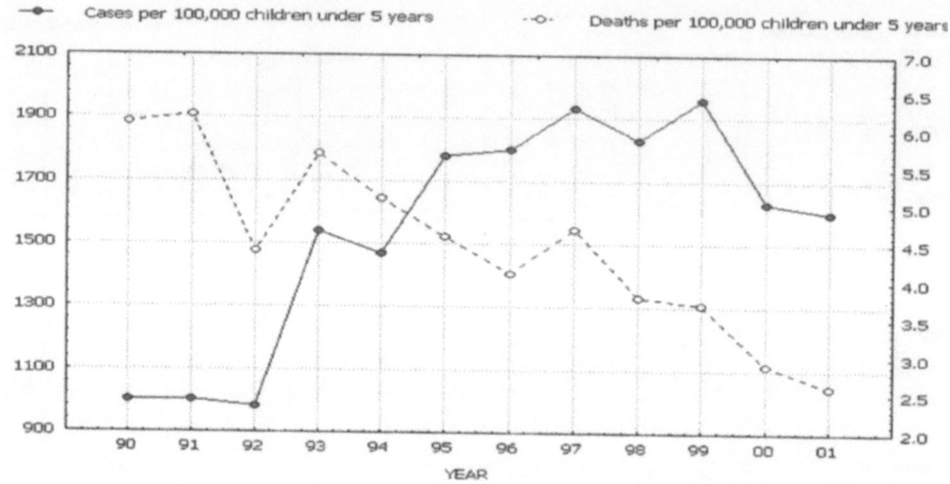

FIGURE 2. Morbidity and mortality rate for acute respiratory tract infections in children under 5 years (Ministry of Public Health, Thailand, 1997–2002)

jejuni was also a causative agent in a small outbreak of acute diarrhea in US troops deployed to Thailand in 1994 and it was the most common pathogen of acute dysentery in children (Bodhidatta *et al.*, 2002; Murphy *et al.*, 1996). Most of the *Campylobacter* isolates were resistant to ciprofloxacin but some were resistant to macrolides. Rotavirus accounted for 6%–7% of acute diarrhea in children attended Children's Hospital in Bangkok in 2000 & 2001, and it was the third most common cause next to *Aeromonas* (13%) and *Salmonella* (10.5%) (Children's Hospital, 2000 and 2001). Rotavirus was found in 27% to 34% of cases of acute diarrhea in young children and G1 was the most prevalent serotype followed by G2, G4 and G3, respectively (Maneekarn and Ushijima, 2000). Toxins produced by *S.aureus*, *E.coli*, *Bacillus cereus*, *Clostridium perfringens* in addition to enteric bacteria, cause food poisoning.

Acute Respiratory Tract Infections (ARI) in Children under Age Five

Acute respiratory infections are the most common illnesses in childhood, comprising approximately 50% of all illnesses in children under age five and 30% in children ages five through twelve. The incidence of pneumonia in children under age five was 1%–1.9% during 1990 and 2001 as shown in Figure 2. The death rate per 100,000 children under age five due to pneumonia during the same period decreased from six deaths in 1990 to 2.6 deaths in 2001 as shown in Figure 2. This data indicated that the morbidity of pneumonia in children under age five has not changed while mortality has decreased. The causative agents of ARI in Thai children are bacteria and viruses (MoPH, Thailand, 1981; Sunakorn *et al.*, 1990; Suwanjutha *et al.*, 1990; Suwanjutha *et al.*, 2002; Siritantikorn *et al.*, 2002; Vathanophas *et al.*, 1990). Otitis media and sinusitis are caused by *Streptococcus pneumoniae* and *Haemophilus influenzae*, whereas *Streptococcus pyogenes* is found in patients with pharyngitis and tonsillitis. Pneumonia and empyema may be caused by *Staphylococcus aureus*, *Streptococcus pneumoniae*, and *Haemophilus influenzae*. Nasopharyngeal swabs obtained from children under age five with upper respiratory infections (URI) and pneumonia during 1993 and 1994 revealed that *S. pneumoniae* was recovered in 37% of URI patients and 31% of pneumonia patients, and *H. influenzae* was recovered in 40% of URI patients and 37% of pneumonia patients (Bamrungtrakul *et al.*, 1994). Thirty-seven percent of *S. pneumoniae* isolates were resistant to penicillin (MIC ≥ 0.1 μg/ml) and 26% to co-trimoxazole. Twenty-one percent of *H. influenzae* isolates were resistant to ampicillin and 24% to co-trimoxazole. Most penicillin resistant *S. pneumoniae* belonged to the Spanish pandemic clone 23F and Spanish-French international clone 9V (Dejsirilert *et al.*, 1999). The prevalence of penicillin resistant *S. pneumoniae* in Thailand has been increasing to 56% in 1997 and 61% in 2000. The overuse of antibiotics is a major contributing factor to this high prevalence of antibiotic resistant *S. pneumoniae*. Between 30% and 60% of children with upper respiratory infections that were usually caused by viruses have been treated with antibiotics. *Chlamydia trachomatis* is also a causative agent of lower respiratory infections in children (MoPH, Thailand, 1998). The common cold, bronchitis, bronchiolitis and pneumonia are caused by viruses, especially the respiratory syncytial virus (RSV), influenza, parainfluenza, and adenovirus (MoPH, Thailand, 1981; Sunakorn *et al.*, 1990; Suwanjutha *et al.*, 1990; Suwanjutha *et al.*, 2002; Siritantikorn *et al.*, 2002; Vathanophas *et al.*, 1990).

Tuberculosis (TB)

Prevention and control of tuberculosis in Thailand was officially endorsed by Prince Mahidol in 1920. Tuberculosis was the second most common cause of death in Thais after malaria at the end of the World War II. The anti-TB society and hospitals for TB were established later. TB centers were founded in various parts of the country. The three national surveys of tuberculosis done in 1962, 1977, and 1991 revealed that the morbidity rate diagnosed by chest x-ray was 2.1%, 1.4%, and 1.01%, and the infectious case rate was 0.5%, 0.31%, and 0.24% respectively (Sriyabhaya *et al.*, 1993). The infection rate of children 0–14 years of age was found to be 15.2% in 1977; 8.9% in 1983; and 5.18% in 1987, making the annual risk of infection 4.9%, 2.3%, and 2.0% respectively (Sriyabhaya *et al.*, 1993). These observations showed a significant reduction in the TB burden in Thailand. However the annual morbidity rate of tuberculosis since 1992 has increased from 20,000 cases (35 per 100,000 population) to more than 30,000 cases (50 per 100,000 population) in 1999 and thereafter, as shown in Figure 3. Based on prevalence and incidence rates, it is estimated that 80,000 to 100,000 people are infected with tuberculosis every year.

The primary reasons for this reemergence of tuberculosis in Thailand are HIV infections, and the influx of migrants and illegal workers from neighboring countries. A strong association between HIV infection and a rapid increase in TB cases has been observed (Siriarayapon *et al.*, 2002). The TB registry data from a hospital in northern Thailand showed that the annual number of TB cases nearly doubled between 1990 and 1994 and the prevalence of HIV-seropositive TB patients rose from 1.5% of all TB patients in 1990 to 45.5% in 1994 (Yanai *et al.*, 1996). The prevalence of HIV infections in new cases of TB at the Chest Hospital in central Thailand was 22% during 1995 and 1996 (Punnotok *et al.*, 2000). The clinical manifestations of TB in HIV infected patients on initial presentation included a low-grade fever, cough, weight loss, lymphadenopathy with pancytopenia, and lung infiltrates (Putong *et al.*, 2002). The prevalence of primary drug resistance to TB during 1996 and 1998 at a hospital in northern Thailand was 13.2% to isoniazid, 10.8% to rifampicin, 15.6% to streptomycin, 5.8% to ethambutol; and multidrug resistance (MDR), i.e., resistance to at least both isoniazid and rifampicin, was observed in 6.3% of cases (Yoshiyama *et al.*, 2001). HIV infection was found to be a risk factor for infection with resistant *M. tuberculosis* (Yoshiyama *et al.*, 2001). A study conducted in 1995–1996 demonstrated that HIV-positive patients with first-episode TB were more likely to have resistant *Mycobacterium tuberculosis* strains when compared to TB patients without HIV infection (Punnotok

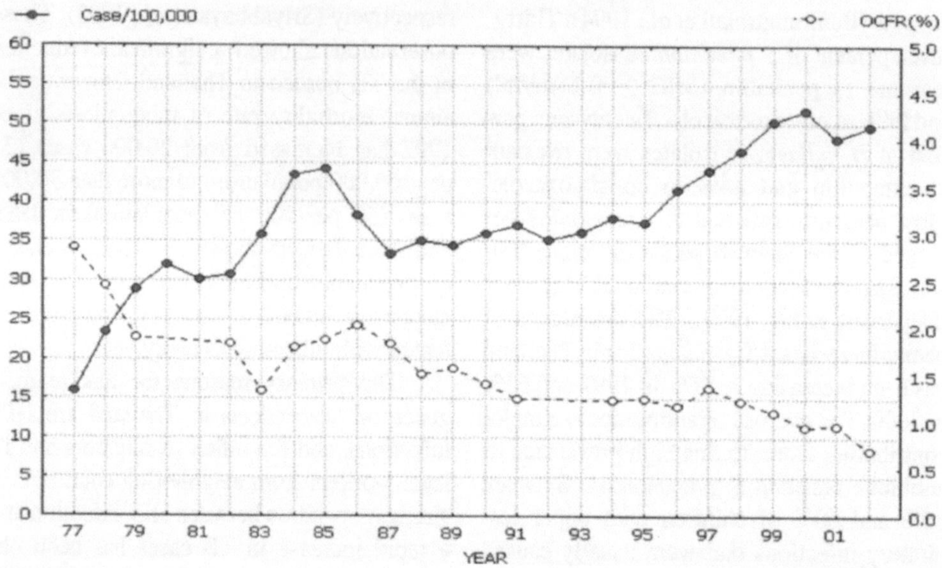

FIGURE 3. Morbidity and case fatality rate (CFR) for tuberculosis (Ministry of Public Health, Thailand, 1997–2002)

et al., 2000). The prevalence of drug resistance in patients with HIV infection as compared to patients without HIV infection was10.9% vs 3.5% for isoniazid, 9.4% vs 2.9% for rifampicin, and 5.2% vs 0.4% for at least isoniazid and rifampicin (multidrug-resistant TB). A study on drug resistant *M. tuberculosis* in a university hospital in northeastern Thailand between 1995 and 2000 revealed the prevalence of 8.2% resistance to rifampicin, 4.2% to isoniazid, 4.3% to ethambutol, 3.7% to streptomycin, 3% to kanamycin, 2.3% to ofloxacin, and 2.4% to at least isonazid and rifampicin (Reechaipichitkul, 2002). The factors associated with drug resistant tuberculosis were HIV infection and having a history of prior treatment. A high prevalence of MDR TB, 19.5%, was reported in 154 consecutive tuberculosis prisoners in central Thailand in 2000 (Pleumpanupat *et al.*, 2003).

Treatment of drug resistant TB in HIV infected patients was costly and the outcome was unsatisfactory (Yanai *et al.*, 1996; Putong *et al.*, 2002; Reechaipichitkul, 2002; Kamolratanakul *et al.*, 2002). Although TB chemoprophylaxis had been found to be beneficial in HIV infected patients with a previous exposure to *M. tuberculosis*, this preventive measure has a limited use in Thailand due to a low predictive value in detecting *M. tuberculosis* infection in HIV-infected persons by tuberculin skin test and a high prevalence of primary drug resistance (Yanai *et al.*, 1997). Tuberculosis is not only a threat to patients with HIV infection but also to the general public who come in contact with the patients, especially health care workers (Yanai *et al.*, 2003).

Rabies

The first report of a victim of human rabies in Thailand was a Thai princess who was bitten by a rabid dog in 1912. She did not receive any post-exposure treatment since rabies vaccine and rabies anti-serum were not available in Thailand at that time. She developed rabies and died three months after being bitten by the dog. Her death resulted in the establishment of the Queen Sauvabha Memorial Institute. Since that time, a diagnostic laboratory for rabies and rabies vaccine

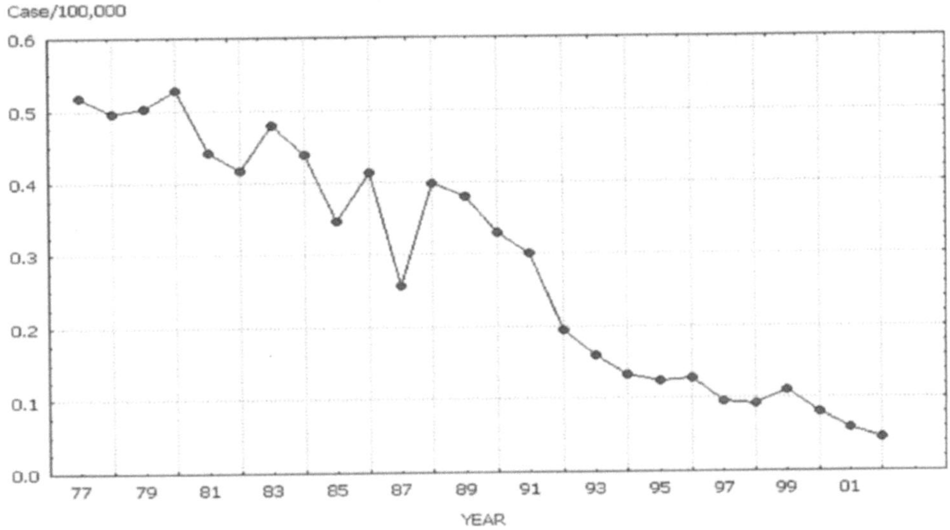

FIGURE 4. Morbidity rate for rabies (Ministry of Public Health, Thailand, 1997–2002)

production has been established in this institute. Since 1967, there have been 250 to 300 cases of human rabies per year, a rate of 0.6–0.7 per 100,000 population (MoPH, multiple years). During 1977 to 1991, approximately 200 cases of human rabies per year, a rate of 0.5 per 100,000 population, were identified. Since 1992 the number of human rabies has been decreasing, from 113 cases (0.2 per 100,000 population) in 1992 to 28 cases (0.05 per 100,000 population) in 2002 as shown in Figure 4.

Rabies in humans is more common in males than females and is more common in children aged 10 years old and under. Human rabies has been reported in all regions of Thailand, year round, with a slight increase from November to March. The continuous decrease in human rabies cases is primarily due to post-exposure treatment with vaccination and immuno-prophylaxis. Rabies post-exposure vaccinations were given to 35,000; 70,000; 130,000; 160,000; 200,000 and more than 300,000 dog bite patients in 1967, 1981, 1993, 1994, 1999 and 2001, respectively (Panichabhongse, 2001). This observation implies that the number of dog bite victims has been increasing and rabid dogs are still prevalent. Rabies vaccinations have been given to dogs since 1956. The rate of rabies in dogs has decreased yearly since 1993, from 52 per 100,000 dog population in 1993 to 21 in 1999 (Panichabhongse, 2001).

Submission of 4000 dog brains for rabies virus detection revealed a positive rate of 33% in 1997; the rate has decreased to 29% in 2001 (Kingnate *et al.*, 1997). Dogs are the main reservoir species for rabies and are responsible for 96% of human deaths. Cats are responsible for 3%–4% of human deaths and other animals and wildlife for 1%. Dogs without an owner were 2.2 times more likely to have rabies than dogs with an owner.

Acute Pyrexia of Unknown Origin (PUO)

Fifty to eighty thousand cases of patients with acute pyrexia of unknown origin were reported during 1977 and 1979 (MoPH, multiple years). The number increased from 100,000 to 200,000 cases between 1980 and 1984, and to over 200,000 cases per year since 1985. The annual rate has been about 400 per 1000,000 population since 1984, as shown in Figure 5. However, the case fatality rate was less than 0.1%, as also shown in Figure 5.

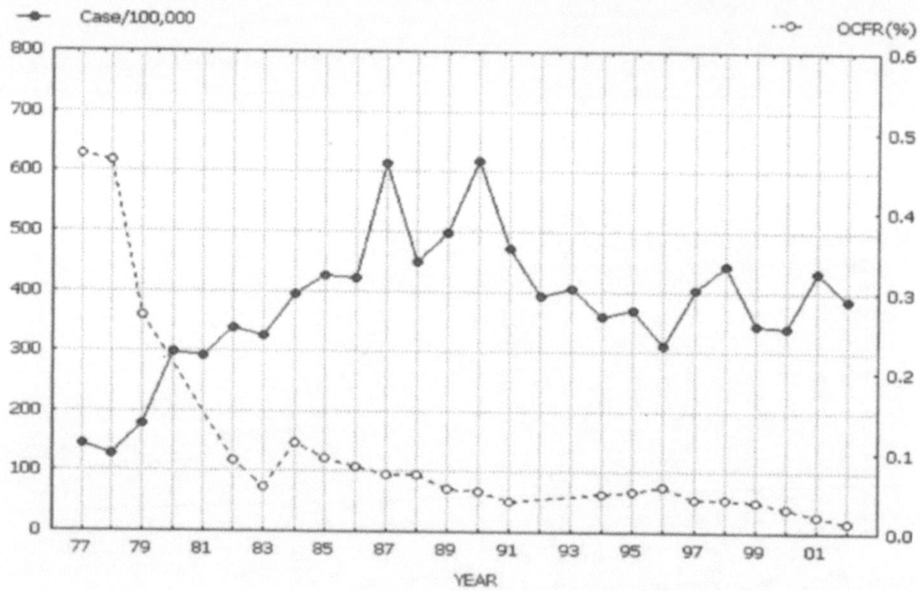

FIGURE 5. Morbidity and case fatality rate (CFR) for acute pyrexia of unknown origin (Ministry of Public Health, Thailand, 1997–2002)

Several attempts have been made to determine the cause of fever in these patients. A study of 294 acute PUO cases during 1966–1968 revealed arbovirus infections in 16.3%–18.7%, scrub typhus in 9.7%–14.2%, leptospirosis in 2.2%–5.8%, murine typhus in 0.7%–1.2%, and brucellosis in 0.6%. A study of 1218 patients with acute PUO during 1991–1992 revealed that the cause was known in 38.7% of cases. The causes of acute PUO were scrub typhus 7.5%, influenza 6%, dengue 5.7%, murine typhus 5.3%, bacteremia 3%, enteric fever 1.9%, chikungunya 1.1%, leptospirosis 1.1%, melioidosis 0.9%, Japanese Encephalitis virus infection 0.6%, and unknown in 61.3% of cases (Leelarasamee, 2000).

A recent study during 2001–2002 revealed that 31.1% of PUO cases were associated with leptospirosis, 20.7% were associated with rickettsioses which included scrub typhus, murine typhus and the spotted fever group, 2.4% were bacterial infections, 3.9% were associated with miscellaneous causes, and 41.9% were unknown (Yupin Suputtamongkol, personal communication, June 2003). Several other studies have also shown that leptospirosis, rickettsioses including the spotted fever group and arbovirus infections were causes of acute PUO (Silpapojakul *et al.*, 1993; Sirisanthana *et al.*, 1994; Silpapojakul *et al.*, 1991; Watt and Jongsakul, 2003; Endy *et al.*, 2002). Q fever was recently found to be the cause of fever in nine patients with acute PUO (Suputtamongkol *et al.*, 2003). Acute PUO continues to be a common public health problem and further research on its epidemiology and causes are still needed.

Dengue Hemorrhagic Fever (DHF)

The first case of DHF in Thailand was reported at Siriraj Hospital in 1951. There was an epidemic of DHF in Bangkok and Thonburi in 1958. This epidemic affected 2418 patients with 240 deaths. Since 1958, there have been epidemics of DHF every other year or every several years, and the number of cases have increased as more areas of the country experience epidemics. DHF has become an endemic disease in Thailand with periodic epidemic outbreaks. The endemic mode of DHF

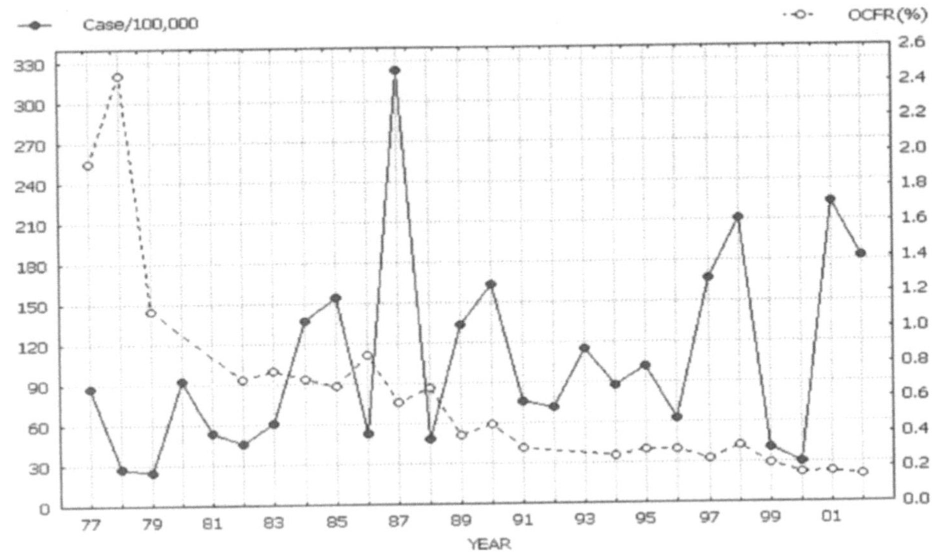

FIGURE 6. Morbidity and case fatality rate (CFR) for dengue hemorrhagic fever (Ministry of Public Health, Thailand, 1997–2002)

corresponds to the cyclic seasonal pattern, with incidence reaching its peak during the hot and rainy seasons (May–October). The epidemic mode is a non-cyclic pattern and corresponds to important non-seasonal rises in the incidence of DHF. Major epidemics over the past several decades occurred in 1977, 1980, 1984, 1985, 1987, 1989, 1990, 1993, 1995,1997, 1998, 2001, and 2002, as shown in Figure 6. During 1958 and 1963, the number of cases per year was 1,000 to 4,000. Since 1964, the number of cases for each epidemic has been over 10,000 cases. The 1987 epidemic was the worst, with 152,840 cases and 785 deaths (Ungchusak and Kunasol, 1987).

A retrospective study of spatial and temporal variations of DHF incidence in Thailand during1983 and 1995 revealed that 52.4% of DHF cases occurred during epidemic months (Barbazan *et al.*, 2002). From 1983 to 1990, three major epidemics lasting 10–12 months occurred at 10- to 15-month intervals and affected almost the entire country simultaneously (50–70 provinces). From 1991 to 1995, epidemics did not affect as many provinces simultaneously (less than 30), and were less differentiated than during the inter-epidemic periods. In many provinces a 2- to 4-month interruption was observed during the dry and cold seasons, the incidence decreasing to the "normal" level, followed by a short re-emergence (lasting 2–3 months) of the epidemic pattern.

Most of the DHF cases have been in children under 15 years old. DHF is characterized by fever, bleeding diathesis with thrombocytopenia, and a tendency to develop hypovolemia due to vasculopathy. Primary dengue infection is usually less severe than a secondary infection. Preexistent dengue immunity is a risk factor for developing dengue hemorrhagic fever. The risk of developing dengue shock syndrome (DSS) is greatest following an anamnestic dengue infection, particularly if the most recent infection was with the dengue 2 virus. Only 1% to 3% of patients with dengue fever develop DSS. Most of the infected patients are mildly symptomatic and the early symptom complex of acute dengue virus infection is protean and difficult to distinguish from other causes of febrile childhood illnesses (Endy *et al.*, 2002).

Unusual manifestations of DHF, especially cerebral and hepatic manifestations were not infrequently observed (Nimmannitya *et al.*, 1987; Pancharoen and Thisyakorn, 2001). Classical HLA class I alleles were associated with the clinical outcome of exposure to dengue virus in previously exposed and immunologically primed individuals (Stephens *et al.*, 2002). An increased dengue disease severity was correlated with a high viremia titer, secondary dengue virus infection, and DEN-2 virus type (Vaughn *et al.*, 2000). DHF was caused by Dengue virus type 1, 2, 3, 4. DEN-3 was the most frequent serotype in primary dengue, DEN-2 in secondary and in dengue hemorrhagic fever (Nisalak *et al.*, 2003). The predominant dengue serotype varied by year: DEN-1 from 1990–92, DEN-2 from 1973–86 and 1988–89; DEN-3 in 1987 and 1995–99; and DEN-4 from 1993–94. Only DEN-3 was associated with severe outbreak years. The case fatality rate of DHF has decreased from 10% to 3% during the 1960s, to 2% in the 1970s, to 0.7% in the 1980s, and to 0.3% or less since1991 as shown in Figure 6.

Prevention and control of DHF depends on control of the female Ades mosquito vector and vaccine. Currently the only effective way to avoid dengue infection in areas where the disease is endemic or epidemic is to avoid being bitten by infected *Ades egypti* mosquitoes through the use of personal insect repellent and other insect barriers. There is no dengue vaccine currently available for widespread public health use. Thai researchers have developed a dengue tetravalent live-attenuated vaccine (Sabchareon *et al.*, 2002). A study of the safety and immunogenicity of two doses of vaccine in flavivirus-seronegative Thai adults showed that the first dose was the more reactogenic and 58% of the recipients seroconverted against 3 or more serotypes; 35% seroconverted against all four. After the second dose, seroconversion was 76% and 71%, respectively. All subjects seroconverted to serotype 3 after one dose. Serotype 4 elicited the lowest primary response but the highest increase in seroconversion after the second dose (Sabchareon *et al.*, 2002).

Further research and development on a safe and efficacious dengue vaccine is urgently needed. DHF continues to be a heavy health burden in terms of high morbidity and huge socioeconomic impact (Kantachuvessiri, 2002). The goals of the Thai National Dengue Prevention and Control Plan (NDPCP) for DHF are to reduce the morbidity rate of dengue infection to 50 or less per 100,000 population, and the case fatality rate to 0.2% or less; and to reduce the mosquito breeding places measured by the Breteau index to below 50 and the container index to below 10. Interventions aimed at achieving the aforementioned goals have been employed. In addition to DHF, a disease caused by the chikungunya virus, which has similar clinical manifestations and transmission, was observed to be prevalent in Thailand (Thaikruea *et al.*, 1997).

Malaria

Malaria was first documented in Thailand in 1660 and it remains a significant infectious disease leading to morbidity and mortality in Thailand. In 1947, there were 52,000 deaths due to malaria, with a death rate of 297 per 100,000 population; the number of malaria cases was 3.8 million in 1949 (Bumrasnaradul, 1967). The morbidity rate was higher than 200 cases per 100,000 population during 1980 and 1990 and decreased to less than 100 since 2000 as shown in Figure 7. However, the morbidity rate in 1998 and 1999 increased to more than 100 per 100,000 population due to imported cases along the international borders and a reduction in vector control during the economic crisis in Thailand (Chareonviriyaphap *et al.*, 2000; Wiwanitkit, 2002).

Malaria occurs more frequently in the summer and rainy seasons (March to September). Males are more affected, and the disease affects all age groups, though it is found more frequently in those aged 15 to 44. All four human malaria parasites cause diseases in Thailand. *Plasmodium falciparum* and *Plasmodium vivax* account for more than 95% of

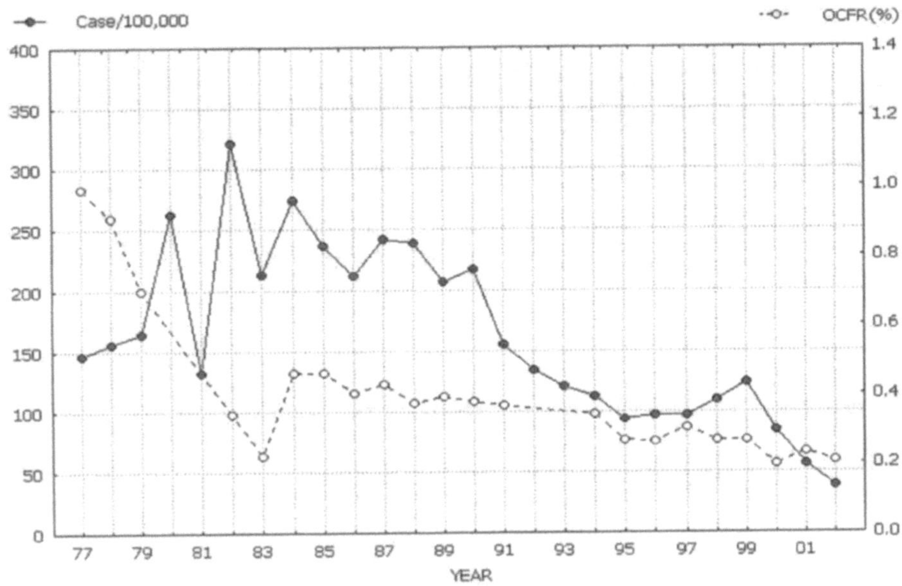

FIGURE 7. Morbidity and case fatality rate (CFR) for malaria (Ministry of Public Health, Thailand, 1997–2002)

the cases whereas *Plasmodium malariae* and *Plasmodium ovale* are very rare. During 1978 and 1985, *P falciparum* accounted for 60%–80% of cases, but after 1985 until 2002 *P falciparum* was responsible for 40%–60% of infections.

Drug resistant malaria has posed one of the most difficult problems in malaria control over the past decades (Wongsrichanalai *et al.*, 2002). Chloroquine resistant *Plasmodium falciparum* was first reported in Thailand in 1961 and chloroquine is no longer effective for falciparum malaria. Resistance to sulfadoxine-pyrimethamine was first noted on the Thai-Cambodian border and more than 90% of *P. falciparum* were resistant after this drug replaced chloroquine for a decade (Wongsrichanalai *et al.*, 2002). Mefloquine had been effective for therapy of falciparum malaria until the late 1980s when resistance was first observed near the Thai-Cambodian border. Mefloquine alone is no longer effective on the Thai-Myanmar and Thai-Cambodian borders, although it is still moderately useful in some endemic areas in and around Thailand. The role of mefloquine nowadays is to be used in combination with artemisinin derivatives. Resistances to quinine and artemisinin derivatives are considered uncommon and both drugs are still very effective if they are used in combination with another anti-malarial. *P. falciparum* resistant to more than two operational antimalarial compounds of different chemical classes (multi-drug resistance) is common at the Thai-Myanmar and Thai-Cambodia borders.

The factors that have contributed to widespread drug resistance in Thailand include wide availability of drugs, poor compliance, inappropriate therapy and self-treatment. Multidrug-resistant *P. falciparum* is being controlled within the framework of a general malaria containment program i.e., rapid case detection and treatment, and vector control in areas where transmission occurs. The currently effective regimen for therapy of falciparum malaria in Thailand, especially in the area with multi-drug resistance, is artesunate plus mefloquine or quinine plus tetracycline for uncomplicated falciparum malaria and intravenous quinine

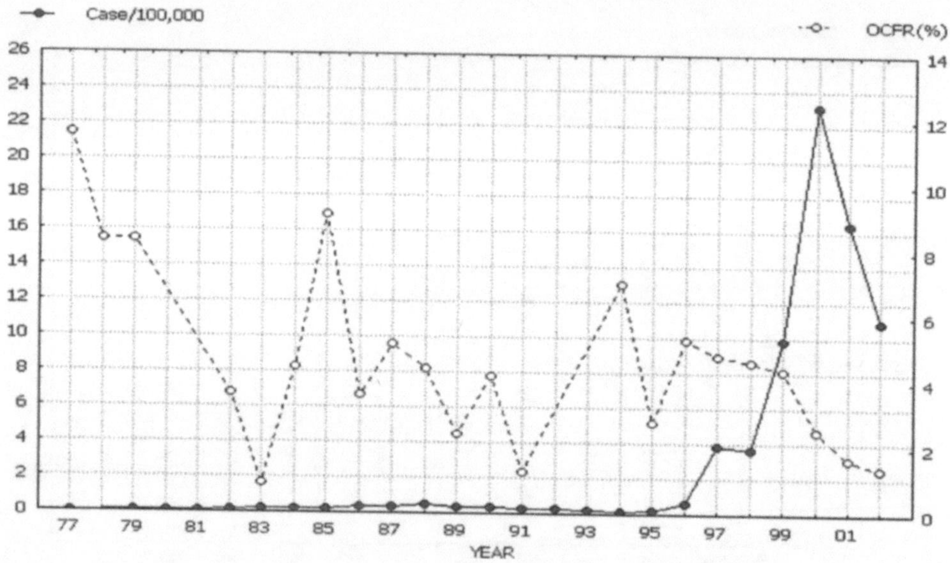

FIGURE 8. Morbidity and case fatality rate (CFR) for leptospirosis (Ministry of Public Health, Thailand, 1997–2002)

or artemisinin derivatives in cases of severe malaria. The cloroquine-primaquine regimen is still effective for therapy of vivax malaria (Congpuong *et al.*, 2002).

The mortality rate of malaria in 1930 was greater than 400 cases per 100,000 population. The mortality rate per 100,000 population has been steadily decreasing to nearly 300 cases in 1947, 14 in 1975, 8 in 1980, 2.3 in 1990 and 1.3 in 1997. The case fatality rate has been decreasing from 1% in 1977 to 0.2% in 2002 as shown in Figure 7. Fatality is usually due to cerebral malaria and severe and complicated malaria. The reduction of morbidity and case fatality in malaria is partly due to programs using chemical insecticide to spray inside houses, promotion of bed-nets often impregnated with permethrin, establishment of a surveillance and control system through more than 500 malaria clinics and more than 15,000 malaria village volunteers, and the availability of more powerful antimalarials such as artemisinin derivatives. Biological control and environmental management to control malaria vectors have also been attempted. Vector control remains to be an important strategy in the fight against malaria in Thailand.

Leptospirosis

Leptospirosis was first reported in Thailand in four patients who developed the disease during the flood in Bangkok in 1942; two patients died (Yunibandu, 1943). Prior to 1996, there were fewer than 200 cases of leptospirosis per year, and more cases were usually observed after flooding. The number of leptospirosis patients has increased to 14,285 (23 cases per 100,000 population) in 2000, as shown in Figure 8. This is clearly a reemerging disease. Geographic variability in the distribution of cases has been noted, i.e., more than 80% of cases were localized to the northeastern region. The demographic profiles of leptospirosis cases during epidemics remain unchanged. The disease is usually diagnosed during August to November. A high-risk group was found to be male farmers aged 15 to 45 years old. Risk factors for acquiring leptospirosis are walking through water, applying fertilizer in wet fields for more

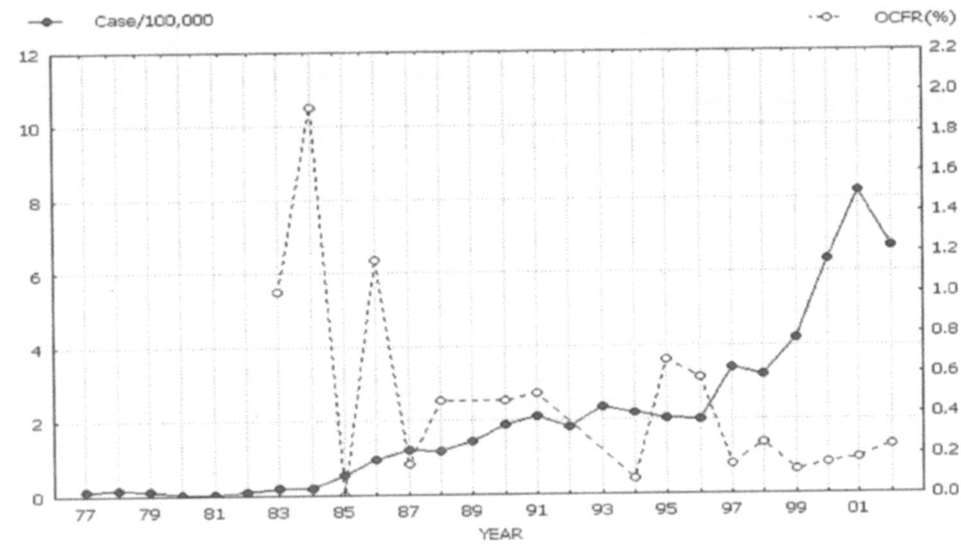

FIGURE 9. Morbidity and case fatality rate (CFR) for scrub typhus (Ministry of Public Health, Thailand, 1997–2002)

than 6 hours a day, plowing in wet fields for more than 6 hours a day, pulling out rice plant sprouts in wet fields for more than 6 hours a day, and traveling on potholed roads within 2 weeks (Tangkanakul *et al.*, 2000; Tangkanakul *et al.*, 2001).

Current clinical manifestations are not significantly different from cases recognized prior to 1996. Yet, pulmonary complications seem to be more frequent and pulmonary hemorrhage is the leading cause of death. Microagglutination test of serum samples from patients revealed that the common serovars were *bratislava, sejroe* and *pyrogenes* which were different from *icterohaemorrhagia* and *bataviae* which were reported serovars in the past (Tangkanakul, 2002). However the most common serogroup of the leptospires isolated from patients' blood was *autumnalis* (Y. Suputtamongkol, personal communication, June 2003). The case fatality rate varied from 1% to 20%. The case fatality rate during epidemics has been 1% to 10% as shown in Figure 8. Penicillin G and doxycycline are still the first line antibiotics used for therapy. Ceftriaxone has been demonstrated to be efficacious as well (Panaphut *et al.*, 2003). Marked differences in rodent population density and number of infected animals between epidemic and non-epidemic sub-districts have been found. Serological studies in rodents trapped in urban and rural areas in Thailand revealed that *pyrogenes, sejroe* and *bataviae* were *predominant* serovars (Wangroongsarb *et al.*, 2002; Kositanont *et al.*, 2003). The leptospires isolated from 14% of the rodents during 1999 and 2000 were mostly *bataviae* and *pyrogenes serovars* (Phulsuksombati *et al.*, 2001). Leptospires were also isolated from cows and buffaloes from the rice-fields. Research and development on rapid diagnostics and prevention and control of leptospirosis are being actively carried out in Thailand.

Scrub Typhus

Scrub typhus is the most common rickettsial infection in Thailand. It was first reported in Thailand in 1952 (Thainua, 1952). Prior to 1984, less than 100 cases were reported annually. The number of patients with scrub typhus has been increasing steadily since 1985 as shown in Figure 9. This was due to an increased awareness and an improvement in laboratory diagnosis. It is likely that many cases of scrub typhus prior to 1984 were reported as acute pyrexia of unknown origin. It should be emphasized that scrub typhus is a common cause of acute pyrexia of unknown origin, as mentioned earlier. Cases were reported from all regions but more cases have been observed in the northeastern region, especially from the areas close to Cambodia and in the central region; this geographic distribution is similar to that of leptospirosis. The disease usually peaks during the rainy season of June and October. Most of the cases are among male farmers. Clinical features of scrub typhus are protean, and eschar (scab) is found in 0–55% of the patients (Sirisanthana and Poneprasert, 1989; Supparatpinyo *et al.*, 1990; Silpapojakul *et al.*, 1991).

Some patients with unrecognized scrub typhus may develop complications such as pneumonia, encephalitis, and meningitis. Doxycycline has been the antibiotic of choice for treating scrub typhus with a rapid clinical response. However *Orientia tsutsugamushi* is probably resistant to doxycycline; this has been observed in patients living in the northern part of Thailand (Watt *et al.*, 1996). Macrolides such as azithromycin could be an alternative to doxycycline for treating scrub typhus (Watt *et al.*, 1999). The case fatality rate over the past 6 years has usually been less than 0.5%, as shown in Figure 9.

DEVELOPMENT OF HEALTH SYSTEMS IN THAILAND

The Socioeconomic and Health Context

Thailand, classified by the World Bank as a lower-middle income country, had a remarkable economic achievement during the 1980s to the mid 1990s. Gross Domestic Product (GDP) per capita increased from 861 USD in 1986 to a peak of 3060 USD in 1996. The 1997 financial crisis in Thailand triggered the Asian economic crisis. In 1999, the GDP per capita was 6132 US$PPP (purchasing power parity). Income distribution and poverty alleviation were among major government policies. Poverty reduction (in terms of the number of poor households) has been quite successful, but there has not been much achievement in improving income distribution. The discrepancy gap of income between the richest 10% to poorest 10% was 11.6. Data from the United Nations Development Program's Human Development Report shows that the gap between the richest 20% to poorest 20% was 7.6, with a slowly improving GINI index of 41.4. In 2000 and 2001, per capita GDP dropped to the level of 1992 (1846 USD). GDP growth in 1997 and 1998 was minus 1.7% and minus 10.8%. The economic recession had major negative consequences for all sectors of Thai society, including the health sector (Tangcharoensathien *et al.*, 2000).

Since 2002, there have been promising signs of economic recovery. GDP growth in 2002 was 3.5% and was expected to increase to more than 5% in 2003. The economic crisis had a major impact on the social sector but a lesser impact on the health sector despite government fiscal constraints (Tangcharoensathien *et al.*, 2000).

Thailand has achieved a medium human development level, as measured by Human Development Index (HDI), of 0.757 in 1999. According to the UNDP's Human Development Report, there was a steady increasing trend of the HDI over the past two decades, rising from 0.603 in 1975 to 0.749 in 1995. Thailand achieved the rank of 74 in the global league table of HDI for 2001, with an index of 0.768. Life expectancy at birth in 2001 was 68.9 years, the adult literacy rate was 95.7, the combined primary, secondary, and tertiary gross enrollment ratio was 72, and GDP per capita US$PPP was 6400 (United Nations Development Program, 2003).

Health achievement over the past two decades has also been also remarkable. A consistent reduction in total fertility rate (TFR) has been observed. The average TFR for 1995–2000 was 1.9, with a contraceptive prevalence rate of 72% (Population Reference Bureau, 2000). A health status profile indicated an infant mortality rate of 26/100,000, an under five child mortality rate of 30/100,000, and the maternal mortality rate in 1980–99 was 44/100,000. The measles immunization rate for children aged one was as high as 94% and was sustained at this level for more than 10 years, while the percentage of births attended by skilled health staff in 1995–99 was 95% (United Nations Development Program, 2003).

In terms of health care resources, there were an average of 24 physicians per 100,000 population for 1990–99. In 1998, the total health expenditure indicated that public sources comprised 1.9% of GDP, while private sources comprised 4.1% of GDP (notably household out of pocket). Per capita health expenditure was 349 US$PPP. In 1999, the number of People Living with HIV/AIDS aged 15–49 was 2.15%, along with 305,000 women and 13,900 children 0–14. The adult infection rate declined to 1.8% in 2001 (United Nations Development Program, 2003).

Healthcare Delivery System

Thailand has a pluralistic healthcare delivery system. Though the public sector, notably the Ministry of Public Health (MoPH), played a very key role in healthcare provision, the private sector, notably for-profit providers, also played an increasing role especially in the urban cities. Private hospital sector growth has been significant due to increased demand for private care among the middle classes, especially during the economic boom.

Since the five-year National Socio-Economic Development Plan of 1981–86, successive governments have placed a high importance on the development of the healthcare system, especially in the rural areas at district and sub-district level. A policy framework was laid out to achieve full coverage of district hospitals in all districts throughout the country in three successive five-year plans. The policy was implemented through adequate and sustained provision of financial and human resources. Since the early 1980s, the government has invested enormously in construction of 10 to 90 bed district hospitals in all districts. Subsequent policy also focused on full coverage of sub-district health centers to adequately provide care to local populations of about 5000 Thais. By the 7th National Socio-Economic Development Plan (1991–1996), healthcare infrastructure accomplished a very high geographical coverage (Ministry of Public Health, 2001). By 2001, there were 92 hospitals in 75 provinces outside Bangkok (25 regional and 67 general hospitals), 720 district hospitals in 795 districts (91% coverage), and 9738 health centers in 7255 sub-districts (100% coverage). These infrastructures served as important hubs for the provision of integrated healthcare services including prevention, promotion, and curative services throughout the country. Subsequently, these hubs also enabled social mobilization towards good health.

The public sector played a major role in healthcare provision. In 2000, 67% of total hospitals were owned by MoPH, 26% by the private sector, and 7% by other ministries. Some 64% of total hospital beds were owned by MoPH, 22% by private sector, and 14% by other ministries especially teaching hospitals. Private hospital bed share increased from 13% in 1991 to 22% in 2000 due to increasing demand for private medical care. Demand for private medical care was income elastic, and affected by the economic bust in 1998. Private healthcare market shrank significantly after the crisis, and a shift of utilization from private to public hospitals was observed (Putthasri *et al.*, 2003).

It should be noted that local elected governments (especially municipalities) were comparatively weak in terms of healthcare service provision, leaving the MoPH to play a significant role. A Devolution Act was promulgated recently to increasingly transfer healthcare service responsibility to local elected governments, but local governments' readiness and capacity to handle healthcare services remains in question.

Private hospitals have expanded their services in more affluent areas, such as provincial cities and metropolitan areas. A symbiotic relationship between public and private hospitals has been observed. Public doctors are allowed to have private practices during off-hours either in their own private clinics or in private hospitals.

Since 1972, the government has enforced a three-year mandatory rural service among new medical, nursing, pharmacist, and dental graduates. Young graduates are posted in district hospitals all over the country. Positive incentives are included, such as a hardship allowance, and non-private practice incentives. Financial fines are levied against violators. This has significantly improved access to quality medical services by the vast majority of Thailand's rural population.

District health systems, typically comprised of district hospitals and 8–10 sub-district health centers, contributed to the remarkable achievements of the Thailand National Family Planning policy in the last 25 years, as evidenced by the low TFR and a very high contraceptive prevalence rate. Nurses, midwives and doctors were trained to provide temporary and permanent methods of contraception through static clinics and mobile campaigns. District health systems also contributed to the achievement of high immunization coverage, significant reduction of vaccine preventable diseases, and mortality among children under age five. District health systems also serve as a major hub for disease surveillance, integrated control of diseases, and primary health care implementation.

District health systems have played a significant role in HIV/AIDS control and prevention, voluntary counseling and testing, primary prevention, safe sex campaigns, and treatment of opportunistic infections. It took only one year to scale up the Vertical Transmission Prevention Program of HIV throughout the country in 2001. Success factors were high antenatal care coverage, geographically accessible health centers, medical teams who provide counseling services, distribution of AZT, and breast milk substitution. This reflected the system's resilience to successfully accommodate new programs in a short period. In 2003, district and provincial hospitals were major hubs for the provision of universal antiretroviral treatment.

Healthcare services were organized in three levels to promote rational use of resources and to foster effective referral systems. At the primary level, health centers provide primary care, and focus on prevention and promotion services, no hospitalization services are available. At the second level, district hospitals, staffed by several general practitioners, pharmacists, dentists, and a cadre of professional nurses provide secondary care including ambulatory, basic surgery, and hospitalization services. At the third level, provincial general hospitals staffed with specialists provide more sophisticated tertiary and sub-specialty medical services. MoPH regional hospitals and teaching hospitals mostly provide super-specialty care through referral systems.

Human Resources for Health

The government finances the education of most categories of health professionals including physicians, dentists, pharmacists, nurses and other paramedics, through general tax revenue. Student's tuition fees are low and do not reflect the true cost of education. Private nursing colleges play a very minor role in producing nurses. One difficulty is a national policy that fails to understand the demand for manpower in the private sector. In addition, there is neither a clear national policy toward private sector growth nor a strong regulatory capacity to steer and maximize the contributions of the private sector. As a result, there has been an internal brain drain of well-trained public Thai healthcare professionals toward the private sector, especially during the economic and private hospital boom periods. The heavy workload and relatively low pay scale and incentives in the public sector, contrasted with lower workload and higher

TABLE 1. Top Twenty Conditions that Contribute to DALY in Thailand

Rank	Male DALY	DALY	%	Female DALY	DALY	%
1	HIV/AIDS	960,087	17%	HIV/AIDS	372,947	9%
2	Traffic accidents	510,907	9%	Stroke	280,673	7%
3	Stroke	267,567	5%	Diabetes	267,158	7%
4	Liver cancer	248,083	4%	Depression	145,336	4%
5	Diabetes	168,372	3%	Liver cancer	118,384	3%
6	Ischemic heart disease	164,094	3%	Osteoarthritis	117,994	3%
7	COPD (emphysema)	156,861	3%	Traffic accidents	114,963	3%
8	Homicide and violence	156,371	3%	Anemia	112,990	3%
9	Suicide	147,988	3%	Ischemic heart diseases	109,592	3%
10	Drug dependence	137,703	2%	Cataracts	96,091	2%
11	Alcohol dependence	130,654	2%	COPD	93,387	2%
12	Cirrhosis	117,527	2%	Deafness	87,612	2%
13	Lung cancer	106,120	2%	Lower respiratory tract infections	84,819	2%
14	Drowning	98,464	2%	Low birth weight	83,879	2%
15	Depression	95,530	2%	Dementia	70,191	2%
16	Osteoarthritis	93,749	2%	Anxiety disorders	66,992	2%
17	Tuberculosis	93,695	2%	Schizophrenia	60,800	2%
18	Deafness	93,497	2%	Tuberculosis	60,643	2%
19	Low birth weight	91,934	2%	Birth trauma and asphyxia	57,488	1%
20	Anemia	87,610	2%	Nephritis and nephrosis	55,258	1%
	Total top 20	3,926,813	70%		2,457,197	62%
	Total national	5,600,000	100%		3,980,000	100%

Source: Ministry of Public Health, Thailand, 2003b

pay in the private sector are primarily responsible for this internal drain. So far there has been no effective mechanism to prevent and mitigate this brain-drain problem. Policy solutions focus on a systematic analysis of part-time and full-time manpower arrangements between the two sectors. However, this solution faced very rigid bureaucratic rules and regulations.

Burden of Diseases

For the past 25 years, the development of Thailand's healthcare system focused on physical service expansions. There was an urgent need to look at how healthcare could better cope with the changing epidemiological profiles and burden of diseases. Rapid epidemiological transitions have occurred in Thailand, as the burden of disease shifts from communicable to non-communicable and lifestyle-related diseases. HIV/AIDS, Tuberculosis, Dengue hemorrhagic fever, and Leptospirosis comprise an unfinished agenda of infectious diseases, while maternal and child health and nutritional problems have been significantly addressed.

A recent study on burden of disease (BOD) in 1999 estimated a total number of 5.6 million Disabled Adjusted Life Year (DALY) losses among men, and 4 million DALY losses among women (Ministry of Public Health, Thailand 2002). The top ten leading causes account for 52% and 44% of total national burden among men and women (Table 1).

In 1999, the three leading causes of DALY among men were HIV/AIDS, traffic injuries, and stroke. Among women, HIV/AIDS, stroke, and diabetes were three leading causes of DALY. Many of these causes are preventable by primary reduction of risks, notably through safe sex, effective traffic injury prevention, and tobacco consumption controls.

Three major risks contributing to Thailand's BOD were unsafe sex, alcohol, and tobacco among men, unsafe sex, high blood pressure, and overweight including obesity among women (Ministry of Public Health, 2003a). Alcohol was the second contributing risk factor for BOD among men. It can lead to domestic violence, major economic and life loss, and disability due to alcohol related injuries. Recent campaigns against drunk driving were not particularly successful and tougher law enforcement was required. Despite a decreasing trend in tobacco consumption due to successful public campaigns and tough law enforcement, the high prevalence of tobacco consumption in the past decades indicates that tobacco was the third and fourth major contributing factor for BOD in Thailand.

In summary, increasing Thailand's healthcare system capacity to effectively cope with chronic diseases such as diabetes, hypertension, and cardiovascular diseases is a major millennium challenge. In addition, enabling the system to provide primary prevention and risk reduction through social mobilization and behavior modification programs are further challenges, requiring a new mix of skills, attitudes and conceptual thinking among Thai healthcare workers and policymakers.

Financing Healthcare, Insurance Coverage, and Recent Reform toward Universal Coverage

Early in Thailand's healthcare history, user charges to patients were introduced and culturally accepted by patients. In the past, user charges were made on a voluntary basis through donation boxes or contribution in kind; subsequently charges became more formalized as bills. Revenue generated through user charges is kept at facility level to improve services. Non-budget revenue played a significant role in financing healthcare facilities. The government's policy on charging patients has been accompanied by an exemption policy for the poor. Exemption started first in 1975, at the discretion of healthcare workers, as there were no government regulations. In 1981, exemption was implemented through a formal mechanism of means-testing for the issuance of a free care card for low-income households; an annual earmarked budget for free care to the poor was allocated to public health facilities. One article in the Thai Constitution stipulated clearly the government's responsibility to ensure the poor access to free care when needed.

Past governments employed a "piecemeal targeting approach" to increasing coverage for specific target population groups, starting first with a tax-financed Social Welfare Scheme for the poor (Tangcharoensathien *et al.*, 2003). This is a means-testing scheme for low-income households. In 1992, the Scheme expanded to cover all elderly Thais over age 60, acknowledging the population's lack of cash income to access healthcare. Children under age 12 were another targeted population for expansion in 1994. Though local leaders participated in the means-testing exercises and recommended eligible households to the district authorities, due to nepotism at the very local level, the scheme neither adequately covered the real poor nor effectively excluded the non-poor from enjoying the Scheme (Tangcharoensathien *et al.*, 2003).

Introduced in 1983, the Voluntary Health Card Scheme covers borderline populations who were not eligible for the social welfare scheme due to their income. This scheme has not performed well in term of coverage expansion and financing viability due to its structure. The voluntary nature of the scheme results in "adverse selection", whereby the sick participate and the healthy opt out the scheme. This results in financial non-viability in spite of more than 50% government subsidies. Stagnated coverage expansion has been observed.

Introduced in 1990, the Social Security Scheme (SSS) covers private sector employees. This is a tripartite (by the employee, the employer and the government) contributory scheme legislated in 1990. It gradually expanded coverage from private enterprises having more than twenty workers to ten, to five, and finally to one employee by April 2002. Unfortunately, beneficiaries are only the workers; to date no serious efforts have been made by the social security administration to expand its healthcare coverage to workers' spouses and dependents, despite huge surpluses of the social security fund. The strengths of the scheme were the application of a capitation contract model. It could very well contain healthcare costs, with simple and low administrative costs. Decent quality of care was provided to the social security workers though "cost-quality trade off" was one of the major weaknesses of the capitation system.

The employer liability Workmen Compensation Scheme, the predecessor of the Social Security Scheme, was designed to cover the work-related illnesses, injuries, disabilities, and death compensation to private sector employees. Employer contributions were formulated to account for the risk of each industry/business, plus an experience rate. Experience rate was meant to be a financial incentive (and vice versa disincentive) to encourage employers to introduce safety measures, but it was unsuccessful (Chunharas *et al.*, 1999).

A tax financed Civil Servant Medical Benefit Scheme (CSMBS) generously covers current public employees, retired officials, and their three generation dependents, including spouses, parents, and three children under age 20. This was a non-contributory welfare scheme. Inefficiency and poor financing value was observed in CSMBS, as it applied a "fee for service" retrospective reimbursement model.

During the past ten years of government efforts on coverage expansion, human resources were strengthened, experience was gained in insurance management, and lessons were learned about the strengths and weaknesses of different provider payment methods, notably fee for service and capitation models. Despite efforts made during the past 20 years, prior to October 2001, almost 30% of the population was not covered by any healthcare policy (Tangcharoesnathien *et al.*, 2001). By October 2001, three major public schemes were covering the entire 62.5 million population, the UC, the CSMBS, and SSS. Figure 10 depicts the relationship among the three parties concerned—the insurance or purchaser agencies, the beneficiaries and patients, and the public-private health care providers. Flow of funds and services among these three stakeholders clearly illustrates their relationship (Tangcharoensathien *et al.*, 2002).

The design of the benefits package and magnitude of the budget subsidy endorsed the "convergence principle" of closing down the existing gap of inequity among the three public insurance schemes (CSMBS, SSS and UC). Table 2 shows the trend of healthcare financing during 1995–2000 (WHO, 2002). WHO referred to National Health Account studies in 1994, 1996 and 1998 (Tangcharoensathien *et al.*, 1999; Pongpanich *et al.*, 2000), and reports on Thailand Health Profile (Ministry of Public Health, 2001). Total Health expenditure ranged 3.4% to 3.7% of GDP in 1995 to 2000. Government expenditure on health as percent of total health expenditure increased from 48.9% to 57.4% in this period, as private expenditure on health declined.

When its targeting policies were exhausted, Thailand boldly adopted a policy of universal healthcare coverage. With strong political will by the major party-led coalition government, Thailand adopted universal healthcare coverage (UC) in October 2001. The UC incorporated the Social Welfare Scheme, the Voluntary Health Card Scheme, and the uninsured into a single form of coverage, to be financed by general tax revenue. It applied a low cost capitation contract model for ambulatory care, whereby beneficiaries were required to be registered with a provider, typically with a district health system (OECD, 1994). It also applied a global budget and case-mix (diagnostic related group) for inpatient services. A nominal payment (30 Baht, approximately 70 US cents) per ambulatory visit or admission at point of service was

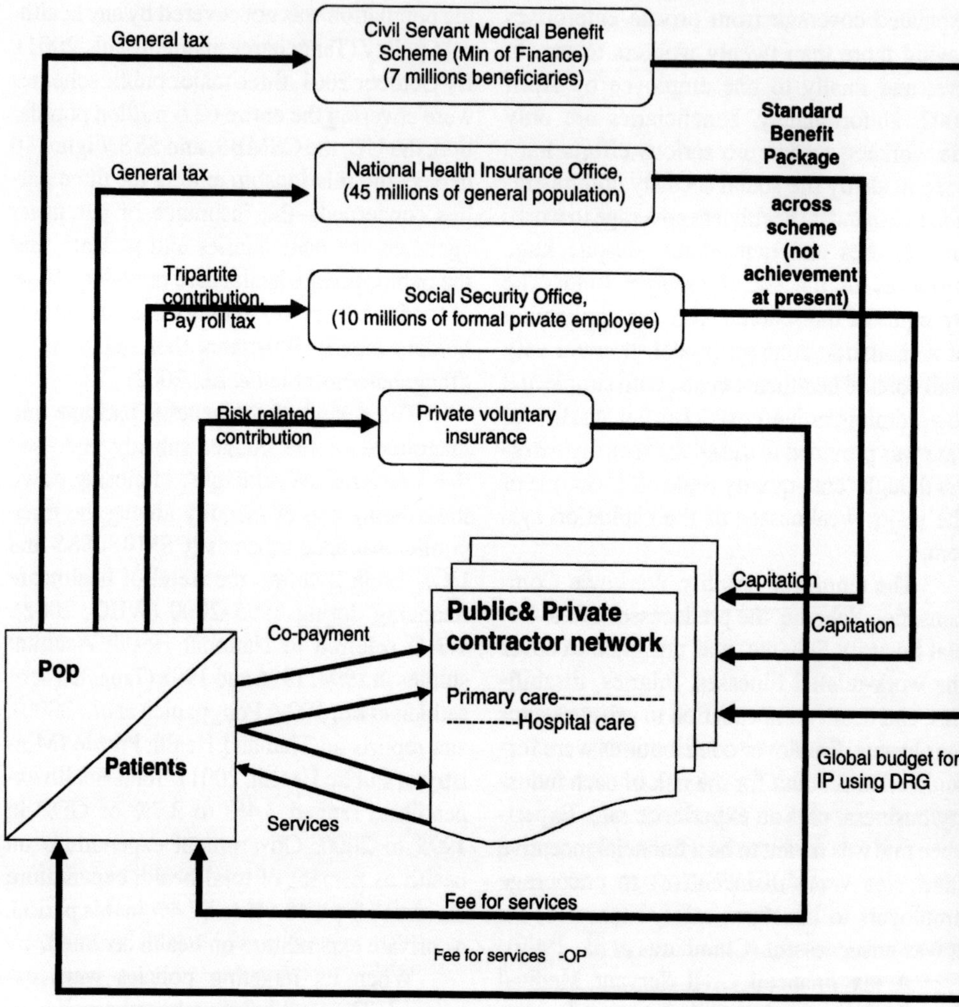

FIGURE 10. Model of health insurance system in Thailand, 2002 (Tangcharoensathien *et al.*, 2002)

introduced, and again, the poor were exempted from this nominal fee.

Future Challenges

UC might significantly change the profile of Thailand's healthcare financing from the dominant role of household out-of-pocket payment towards tax funded public health insurance. Policy makers expect to see a diminishing proportion of households facing catastrophic illnesses. However, researchers need to monitor the beneficiaries of public spending, whether they are rich or poor, through Benefit Incidence Analysis. Several national databases and household interview surveys are conducted by the National Statistical Office to provide evidence for policy monitoring and modification.

The low cost capitation contract model applied by both the Social Health Insurance plan in 1990 and more recently by the UC Scheme provided an enabling environment towards a more efficient healthcare system with rational use of resources. However, the possibility exists of a "cost quality tradeoff" of providing inadequate and poor services, under-prescription, and postponement

TABLE 2. National Expenditure on Health in Thailand, 1995–2000, Current Year Price

Expenditure ratios & per capita levels	1995	1996	1997	1998	1999	2000
Total Expenditure on Health (THE) % GDP	3.4	3.6	3.7	3.9	3.7	3.7
Government Expenditure on Health (GGHE) % THE	48.9	51.1	57.2	61.4	58.3	57.4
Private Expenditure on Health (PvtHE) % THE	51.1	48.9	42.8	38.6	41.7	42.6
GGHE % General Government Expenditure (GGE)	8.1	9.6	10.9	13.3	11.4	11.4
Social Security Expenditure on Health (SSHE) % GGHE	26.5	27.9	30.2	25.8	26.3	26.4
External Resources funded Expenditure on Health (ExtFHE) % GGHE	0.2	0.6	0.5	0.7	0.9	0.9
Private Prepaid Plans Expenditure on Health (PvtPPHE) % PvtHE	7.6	7.8	8.6	9.7	9.7	9.6
Net Out-Of-Pocket Spending on health (OOPS) % THE	44.7	42.6	36.9	32.7	35.3	36.2
THE per capita at Exchange rate (US$)	97	110	93	71	73	71
GGHE per capita at Exchange-rate (US$)	47	56	53	44	43	41
THE per capita at International Dollar rate ($)	210	237	242	228	229	240
GGHE per capita at International Dollar rate ($)	103	121	138	140	133	138

Source: Vasavid *et al.*, 2003

of elective surgeries. This threat warrants prompt policy attention toward quality monitoring, accreditation of healthcare institutions, and audit. However, the geographical monopoly whereby consumers had no choice but their local District Health System, challenges attempts for tougher measures on quality. This requires a strong grievance mechanism and monitoring of performance among contractors.

Health systems need to address priority health problems indicated by BOD measurements. Social mobilization and empowerment of individuals and communities are the most crucial tools to increase societal momentum towards a healthy life style, physical fitness, and mental well-being. Additional government strategies include legislation and law enforcement to provide a favorable, healthy, and safe environment for all Thai citizens.

LESSONS LEARNED FROM AIDS

Thailand's knowledge of HIV/AIDS has increased significantly over the course of the epidemic. The following are some of the most important lessons that can be instructive to other countries as they cope with emerging HIV/AIDS issues.

It is important to accelerate surveillance of different phases of the disease as much as possible. In Thailand, the first government approach was one of denial of the possible consequences, and took about five years. Part of this time was spent performing seroepidemiology on a handful of cases in men having sex with men (MSM). A few small-scale studies showed low levels of prevalence among male sex workers. Later studies found high incidences in female sex workers in the Northern province. Ideally, primary phases of surveillance should be shortened through improvements of the surveillance systems.

A cohesive understanding of the extent to which HIV/AIDS can cause social, economical, ethical, legal, and international issues as well as medical and health problems, must be developed.

Top-level policymaking is also a highly desirable objective. One mechanism may be a national AIDS policy commission. Top politicians may lead this commission; in some countries, the prime minister may head this committee. Alternately, a Minister of Public Health or Minister without portfolio may be asked to lead the commission. It is very important to put such a commission in place as early as possible.

The composition of a National AIDS policy commission will have to be diverse, and include representatives of non-governmental organizations (NGO), and others with a depth of knowledge about HIV/AIDS.

A National AIDS Commission should be able to bear some influence on the provincial level policymakers and staff. A provincial commission that is responsive to the national commission and able to implement policies is essential.

An important responsibility of a national HIV/AIDS policy commission is the allocation of the budget. The budget should be formulated as a % of GDP or % of the annual national budget.

It is necessary to realize that shifts in policy are possible at any time, depending on national and international politics, and other factors.

Major HIV/AIDS policy shifts can occur when there is a major shift in the healthcare structure of the country. For example, this has happened with the universal coverage policy in Thailand. There is currently controversy about whether AIDS patients will be covered in this scheme or not (WHO, 2002).

Increasing condom usage among sex workers has been successful, but programs propagating widespread use of condoms in the general population may not be as successful. As the epidemic changes and affects different sectors of Thai society, flexible policies and models of prevention are increasingly important.

Antiretroviral therapy for HIV/AIDS will occupy more of the AIDS budget as time goes on. The same may be true for the use of drugs to prevent mother to child transmission.

Acknowledgements. The authors would like to thank Dr. Kumnuan Ungchusak and Dr. Waraluk Tangkanakul for valuable advice, Ms. Patcharin Tubviroj for secretarial assistance.

REFERENCES

Bamrungtrakul, T., Sunakorn, P., Sareebutara, W., Vejabhuti, A., Lochindarat, S., Teeraratkul, A., Kittikhun, P., Pinyosmosorn, R., Wasanawat, S., Darnswang, S.A., Chupuppakarn, S., Kusum, M., and Dejsirilert, S. (1994). Surveillance of antimicrobial resistance of *Streptococcus pneumoniae* and *Haemophilus influenzae* in Thailand. *J Med Assoc Thai.* 77:572–579.

Barbazan, P., Yoksan, S., and Gonzalez, J.P. (2002). Dengue hemorrhagic fever epidemiology in Thailand: Description and forecasting of epidemics. *Microbes and Infection* 4(7): 699–705.

Beek, S.V. (2001). *Fears and Concerns in Bangkok Then and Now.* AB Publications, Nonthaburi, Thailand. pp. 85–93.

Bodhidatta, L., Vithayasai, N., Eimpokalarp, B., Pitarangsi, C., Serichantalergs, and Isenbarger, D.W. (2002). Bacterial enteric pathogens in children with acute dysentery in Thailand: Increasing importance of quinolone-resistant Campylobacter. *Southeast Asian J Trop Med Public Health* 33(4): 752–757.

Bumrasnaradul, P. (1967). In memory of Ministry of Public Health's 25th Anniversary. Mitrnara Printing, Bangkok, pp. 672–676.

Chareonviriyaphap, T., Bangs, M.J., and Ratanatham, S. (2000). Status of malaria in Thailand. *Southeast Asian J Trop Med Public Health* 31(2): 225–237.

Children's Hospital, Bangkok. (2000). Annual Report. Bangkok.

Children's Hospital, Bangkok. (2001). Annual Report. Bangkok.

Chunharas, S., Charoenparij, S., Donaldson, D., Kraushaar, D., Pinjaroen, S., Srivanichakorn, S., Suriyawongpaisal, P., Pannorunothai, S., Tangcharoensathien, V., and Valyasevi, A. (1999). Thailand: Health Management and Financing Study Project ADB no. 2997—The final integrated report. February 23, 1999. Health Systems Research Institute and MSH, Bangkok.

Congpuong, K., Na-Bangchang, K., Thimasarn, K., Tasanor, U., and Wernsdorfer, W.H. (2002). Sensitivity of *Plasmodium vivax* to chloroquine in Sa Kaeo Province, Thailand. *Acta Trop.* 83(2): 117–121.

Dejsirilert, S., Overweg, K., Sluijter, M., Saengsuk, L., Gratten, M., Ezaki, T., and Hermans, P.W. (1999). Nasopharyngeal carriage of penicillin-resistant *Streptococcus pneumoniae* among children with acute respiratory tract infections in Thailand: A molecular epidemiological survey. *Journal of Clinical Microbiology* 37(6): 1832–1838.

Endy, T.P., Chunsuttiwat, S., Nisalak, A., Libraty, D.H., Green, S., Rothman, A.L., Vaughn, D.W., and Ennis, F.A. (2002). Epidemiology of inapparent and symptomatic acute dengue virus infection: A prospective study of primary school children in Kamphaeng Phet, Thailand. *Am J Epidemiol.* 156(1): 40–51.

Isenbarger, D.W., Hoge, C.W., Srijan, A., Pitarangsi, C., Vithayasai, N., Bodhidatta, L., Hickey, K.W., and Cam, P.D. (2002). Comparative antibiotic resistance of diarrheal pathogens from Vietnam and Thailand, 1996–1999. *Emerg Infect Dis.* 8(2): 175–180.

Kamolratanakul, P., Hiransuthikul, N., Singhadong, N., Kasetjaroen, Y., Akksilp, S., and Lertmaharit, S. (2002). Cost analysis of different types of tuberculosis patients at tuberculosis centers in Thailand. *Southeast Asian J Trop Med Public Health* 33(2): 321–330.

Kantachuvessiri, A. (2002). Dengue hemorrhagic fever in Thai society. *Southeast Asian J Trop Med Public Health* 33(1): 56–62.

Kingnate, D., Sagarasaeranee, P., and Choomkasien, P. (1997). Thailand Rabies control (human side). In: Third International Symposium on Rabies Control in Asia, Wuhan, China. Elsevier, Paris, pp. 194–196.

Kositanont, U., Naigowit, P., Imvithaya, A., Singchai, C., and Puthavathana, P. (2003). Prevalence of antibodies to Leptospira serovars in rodents and shrews trapped in low and high endemic areas in Thailand. *J Med Assoc Thai.* 86(2): 136–142.

Kusum, M. (1999). National Antimicrobial Resistance Surveillance, Thailand. Ministry of Public Health, Department of Medical Sciences, Thailand.

Leelarasamee, A. (2000). Acute febrile illness of unknown origin: A prevalence study in Thailand. In: Aswapokee, N., Leelasupasri, S., Likitnukul, S., (eds.), *Infectious Diseases beyond 2000.* Holistic Publishings Co., Bangkok, pp. 59–78.

Maneekarn, N., and Ushijima, H. (2000). Epidemiology of rotavirus infection in Thailand. *Pediat Int.* 42(4): 415–421.

Ministry of Public Health, Thailand. (1977–2002). Annual Epidemiological Surveillance Reports. Bureau of Epidemiology, Department of Disease Control. (multiple years).

Ministry of Public Health, Thailand. (1981). Division of Communicable Diseases Control, Proceedings of National Workshop on Acute Respiratory Infections in Children. Sahaprachapanich Printing, Bangkok.

Ministry of Public Health, Thailand. (1998). Drug Resistance Surveillance. Department of Medical Sciences.

Ministry of Public Health, Thailand. (2001). Health Policy and Planning Bureau. Thailand Health Profile. Nonthaburi, Thailand.

Ministry of Public Health, Thailand. (2002). Burden of Disease and Injuries in Thailand, Priority Setting for Policy. The Thai Working Group on Burden of Disease and Injuries, Bureau of Health Policy and Planning. (November 2002).

Ministry of Public Health, Thailand. (2003a). Attributable risk for burden of disease in Thailand, A preliminary report. The Thai Working Group on Burden of Disease and Injuries, Bureau of Health Policy and Planning, Thailand.

Ministry of Public Health, Thailand. (2003b). The Burden of Diseases in Thailand. Thai Working Group on Burden of Disease and Injuries, Bureau of Health Policy and Planning, Nonthaburi.

Murphy, G.S. Jr., Echeverria, P., Jackson, L.R., Arness, M.K., LeBron, C., and Pitarangsi, C. (1996). Ciprofloxacin- and azithromycin-resistant Campylobacter causing traveler's diarrhea in U.S. troops deployed to Thailand in 1994. *Clin Infect Dis.* 22(5): 868–869.

Nimmannitya, S., Thisyakorn, U., and Hemsrichart. V. (1987). Dengue haemorrhagic fever with unusual manifestations. *Southeast Asian J Trop Med Public Health* 18(3): 398–406.

Nisalak, A., Endy, T.P., Nimmannitya, S., Kalayanarooj, S., Thisayakorn, U., Scott, R.M., Burke, D.S., Hoke, C.H., Innis, B.L., and Vaughn, D.W. (2003). Serotype-specific dengue virus circulation and dengue disease in Bangkok, Thailand. *Am J Trop Med Hyg.* 68(2): 191–202.

Organization of Economic Cooperation and Development. (1994). The Reform of Seven OECD countries. OECD Publishing, Paris.

Panaphut, T,. Domrongkitchaiporn, S., Vibhagool, A., Thinkamrop, B., and Susaengrat, W. (2003). Ceftriaxone compared with sodium penicillin g for treatment of severe leptospirosis. *Clin Infect Dis.* 36(12): 1507–1513.

Pancharoen, C., and Thisyakorn, U. (2001). Neurological manifestations in dengue patients. *Southeast Asian J Trop Med Public Health* 32(2): 341–345.

Panichabhongse, P. (2001). The Epidemiology of Rabies in Thailand. A thesis presented in partial fulfilment of the requirement for the degree of Master of Veterinary Studies, Massey University, Palmerston North, New Zealand. (unpublished paper).

Phulsuksombati, D., Sangjun, N., Khoprasert, Y., Kingnate, D., and Tangkanakul, W. (2001). Leptospires in rodent, northeastern region 1999–2000. *Health Sci.* 10(3): 516–525.

Pleumpanupat, W., Jittimanee, S., Akarasewi, P., Rienthong, S., Jittimanee, S., Chiewlian, Y., Phunpruk, S., Malainual, C., Ngamtrairai, N., and Adedipe, A. (2003). Resistance to anti-tuberculosis drugs among smear-positive cases in Thai prisons 2 years after the implementation of the DOTS strategy. *Int J Tuberc Lung Dis.* 7(5): 472–477.

Pongpanich, S., Tantigate, N., Srithamrongsawat, S., Vasavid, C., and Vimolkij, D. (2000). National Health Accounts for 1998 and 1999. A Research

Report. Health Systems Research Institute, Bangkok.

Population Reference Bureau. (2000). The 2000 World Population Data Sheet of the Population Bureau. PBR, Washington DC.

Punnotok, J., Shaffer, N., Naiwatanakul, T., Pumprueg, U., Subhannachart, P., Ittiravivongs, A., Chuchotthaworn, C., Ponglertnapagorn, P., Chantharojwong, N., Young, N.L., Limpakarnjanarat, K., and Mastro, T.D. (2000). Human immunodeficiency virus-related tuberculosis and primary drug resistance in Bangkok, Thailand. *Int J Tuberc Lung Dis.* 4(6): 537–543.

Putong, N.M., Pitisuttithum, P., Supanaranond, W., Phonrat, B., Tansuphasawadikul, S., Silachamroon, U., Yuda, H.C., Bussaratid, V., and Aswapokee, N. (2002). *Mycobacterium tuberculosis* infection among HIV/AIDS patients in Thailand: clinical manifestations and outcomes. *Southeast Asian J Trop Med Public Health* 33(2): 346–351.

Putthasri, W., Saithanu, S., and Tangcharoensathien, V. (2003). Private Industry in Thailand after the economic crisis (1996–2001): Role and coping mechanisms. International Health Policy Program, Nonthaburi, Thailand.

Reechaipichitkul, W. (2002). Multidrug-resistant tuberculosis at Srinagarind Hospital, Khon Kaen, Thailand. *Southeast Asian J Trop Med Public Health* 33(3): 570–574.

Sabchareon, A., Lang, J., Chanthavanich, P., Yoksan, S., Forrat, R., Attanath, P., Sirivichayakul, C., Pengsaa, K., Pojjaroen-Anant, C., Chokejindachai, W., Jagsudee, A., Saluzzo, J.F., and Bhamarapravati, N. (2002). Safety and immunogenicity of tetravalent live-attenuated dengue vaccines in Thai adult volunteers: Role of serotype concentration, ratio, and multiple doses. *Am J Trop Med Hyg.* 66(3): 264–272.

Silpapojakul, K., Chupuppakarn, S., Yuthasompob, S., Varachit, B., Chaipak, D., Borkerd, T., and Silpapojakul, K. (1991). Scrub and murine typhus in children with obscure fever in the tropics. *Ped Infect Dis J.* 10(3): 200–203.

Silpapojakul, K., Chayakul, P., Krisanapan, S., and Silpapojakul, K. (1993). Murine typhus in Thailand: Clinical features, diagnosis and treatment. *Quarterly Journal of Medicine* 86(1): 43–47.

Siriarayapon, P., Yanai, H., Glynn, J.R., Yanpaisarn, S., and Uthaivoravit, W. (2002). The evolving epidemiology of HIV infection and tuberculosis in northern Thailand. *J Acquir Imm Defic Syndr.* 31(1): 80–89.

Sirisanthana, T., Pinyopornpanit, V., Sirisanthana, V., Strickman, D., Kelly, D.J., and Dasch, G.A. (1994). First cases of spotted fever group rickettsiosis in Thailand. *Am J Trop Med Hyg.* 50(6): 682–686.

Sirisanthana, V., and Poneprasert, B. (1989). Scrub typhus in the children at Chiang Mai University Hospital. *J Infect Antimicrob Agents* 6: 22–27.

Siritantikorn, S., Puthavathana, P., Suwanjutha, S., Chantarojanasiri, T., Sunakorn, P., Ratanadilok Na Phuket, T., Nawanopparatsakul, S., Teeyapaiboonsilpa, P., Taveepvoradej, S., Pengmesri, J., and Pongpate, S. (2002). Acute viral lower respiratory infections in children in a rural community in Thailand. *J Med Assoc Thai.* 85(Suppl 4): S1167–S1175.

Sriyabhaya, N., Payanandana, V., Bamrungtrakul, T., and Konjanart, S. (1993). Status of tuberculosis control in Thailand. *Southeast Asian J Trop Med & Public Health* 24(3): 410–419.

Stephens, H.A., Klaythong, R., Sirikong, M., Vaughn, D.W., Green, S., Kalayanarooj, S., Endy, T.P., Libraty, D.H., Nisalak, A., Innis, B.L., Rothman, A.L., Ennis, F.A., and Chandanayingyong, D. (2002). HLA-A and -B allele associations with secondary dengue virus infections correlate with disease severity and the infecting viral serotype in ethnic Thais. *Tissue Antigens* 60(4): 309–318.

Sunakorn, P., Chunchit, L., Niltawat, S., Wangweerawong, M., and Jacobs, R.F. (1990). Epidemiology of acute respiratory infections in young children from Thailand. *Ped Infect Dis J.* 9(12): 873–877.

Supparatpinyo, K., Horsin, P., and Hirunsri, P. (1990). Scrub typhus at Maharaj Nakorn Chiang Mai Hospital : A study of 60 cases. *Internal Medicine* 6: 6–10.

Suputtamongkol, Y., Rolain, J.M., Losuwanaruk, K., Niwatayakul ,K., Suthinont, C., Chierakul, W., Pimda, K., and Raoult, D. (2003). Q fever in Thailand. *Emerg Infect Dis.* 9(9): 1186–1188.

Suwanjutha, S., Chantarojanasiri, T., Watthana-kasetr, S., Sirinavin, S., Ruangkanchanasetr, S., Hotrakitya, S., Wasi, C., and Puthavathana, P. (1990). A study of nonbacterial agents of acute lower respiratory tract infection in Thai children. *Rev Infect Dis.* 12(Suppl 8): S923–S928.

Suwanjutha, S., Sunakorn, P., Chantarojanasiri, T., Siritantikorn, S., Nawanoparatkul, S., Rattanadilok Na Bhuket, T., Teeyapaiboonsilpa, P., Preutthipan, A., Sareebutr, W., and Puthavathana, P. (2002). Respiratory syncytial virus-associated lower respiratory tract infection in under-5-year-old children in a rural community of central Thailand, a population-based study. *J Med Assoc Thai.* 85(Suppl 4): S1111–119.

Tangcharoensathien, V., Laixuthai, A., Vasavid, J., Tantigate, N., Prajuabmoh-Ruffalo, W., Vimolkit,D., and Lertiendumrong, J. (1999). National Health Account Development: Lessons from Thailand. *Health Policy and Planning* 14(4): 342–353.

Tangcharoensathien, V., Harnvoravongchai, P., Pitayarangsarit, and S., Kasemsup, V., (2000). Health impacts of rapid economic changes in Thailand. *Social Science and Medicine* 51: 789–807.

Tangcharoesnathien, V., Srithamrongswat, S., and Pittayarangsarit, S. (2001). Overview of health insurance systems. In: Thammathat-aree, J. (ed). *Health Insurance Systems in Thailand.* Health Systems Research Institute, Desire Publishing, Bangkok.

Tangcharoensathien, V., Tantivess, S., Teerawattananon, Y., Auamkul, N., and Jongudoumsuk, P. (2002). Universal coverage and impact on reproductive health service in Thailand. *Reproductive Health Matters* 10(20): 59–69.

Tangcharoensathien, V., Teokul, W., Chanwongpaisal, L. (2003). Social Welfare System in Thailand: A challenge from targeting to universality. A paper presented at United Nations Research Institute for Social Development (UNRISD) workshop on Social Policy in a Development Context: Transforming the Developmental Welfare State in East Asia, 30 June–1 July 2003, Novotel, Bangkok, Thailand.

Tangkanakul, W. (2002). Leptospirosis. In: Department of Disease Control, Ministry of Public Health, Thailand (ed.), *Important Infectious Diseases 2001*, Agricultural Co-Operation Printing, pp. 53–56.

Tangkanakul, W., Tharmaphornpilm P., Plikaytis, B.D., Bragg, S., Poonsuksombat, D., Choomkasien, P., Kingnate, D., and Ashford, D.A. (2000). Risk factors associated with leptospirosis in northeastern Thailand, 1998. *Am J Trop Med Hyg.* 63(3-4): 204–208.

Tangkanakul, W., Siriarayaporn, P., Pool, T., Ungchusak, K., and Chunsuttiwat, S. (2001). Environmental and travel factors related to leptospirosis in Thailand. *J Med Assoc Thailand* 84(12): 1674–1680.

Thaikruea, L., Charearnsook, O., Reanphumkarnkit, S., Dissomboon, P., Phonjan, R., Ratchbud, S., Kounsang, Y., and Buranapiyawong, D. (1997). Chikungunya in Thailand: A re-emerging disease? *Southeast Asian J Trop Med Public Health* 28(2): 359–364.

Thainua, M. (1952). A case report of scrub typhus. *J Med Assoc Thai.* 35: 9–27.

Ungchusak, K., and Kunasol, P. (1987). Dengue haemorrhagic fever in Thailand, 1987. *Southeast Asian J Trop Med Public Health* 19(3): 487–490.

United Nations Development Program. (2003). Human Development Report. UNDP, New York.

Vathanophas, K., Sangchai, R., Raktham, S., Pariyanonda, A., Thangsuvan, J., Bunyaratabhandu, P., Athipanyakom, S., Suwanjutha, S., Jayanetra, P., Wasi, C., Vorachit, M., and Puthawatana, P. (1990). A community-based study of acute respiratory tract infection in Thai children. *Rev Infect Dis.* 12(Suppl 8): S957–S965.

Vaughn, D.W., Green, S., Kalayanarooj, S., Innis, B.L., Nimmannitya, S., Suntayakorn, S., Endy, T.P., Raengsakulrach, B., Rothman, A.L., Ennis, F.A., and Nisalak, A. (2000). Dengue viremia titer, antibody response pattern and virus serotype correlate with disease severity. *J Infect Dis.* 181(1): 2–9.

Vasavid, C., Tisayatikom, K., Patcharanarumol, W., and Tangcharoensathien, V. (2003). Thailand National Health Account. A research report. Ministry of Public Health, International Health Policy Program. Nonthaburi.

Wangroongsarb, P, Petkanchanapong, W., Yasaeng, S., Imvithaya, A., and Naigowit, P. (2002). Survey of leptospirosis among rodents in epidemic areas of Thailand. *J Trop Med Parasitol.* 25(2): 56–58.

Watt, G., and Jongsakul, K. (2003). Acute undifferentiated fever caused by infection with Japanese encephalitis virus. *Am J Trop Med Hyg.* 68(6): 704–706.

Watt, G., Chouriyagun,e C., Ruangweerayud, R., Watcharapichat, P., Phulsuksombati, D., Jongsakul, K., Teja-Isavadharm, P., Bhodhidatta, D., Corcoran, K.D., Dasch, G.A., and Strickman, D. (1996). Scrub typhus infections poorly responsive to antibiotics in northern Thailand. *Lancet* 348(9020): 86–89.

Watt, G., Kantipong, P., Jongsakul, K., Watcharapichat, P., and Phulsuksombati, D. (1999). Azithromycin activities against *Orientia tsutsugamushi* strains isolated in cases of scrub typhus in Northern Thailand. *Antimicrob. Agents Chemother.* 43(11): 2817–2818.

Wiwanitkit, V. (2002). High prevalence of malaria in Myanmar migrant workers in a rural district near the Thailand-Myanmar border. *Scand J Infect Dis.* 34(3): 236–237.

Wongsrichanalai, C., Pickard, A.L., Wernsdorfer, W.H., and Meshnickd, S.R. (2002). Epidemiology of drug-resistant malaria. *Lancet Infectious Diseases* 2(4): 209–218.

World Health Organization. (2002). National Health Expenditure, Thailand. WHO, Geneva.

Wright, A., and Breakspears, O.T. (1903). Twentieth Century Impressions of Siam. Health and Hospitals. Lloyd Greater Britain Publishing Company. pp. 128–134.

Yanai, H., Uthaivoravit, W., Panich, V., Sawanpanyalert, P., Chaimanee, B., Akarasewi, P., Limpakarnjanarat, K., Nieburg, P., and Mastro, T.D. (1996). Rapid increase in HIV-related tuberculosis, Chiang Rai, Thailand, 1990-1994. *AIDS* 10(5): 527–531.

Yanai, H., Uthaivoravit, W., Mastro, T.D., Limpakarnjanarat, K., Sawanpanyalert, P., Morrow, R.H. Jr., and Nieburg, P. (1997). Utility of tuberculin and anergy skin testing in predicting tuberculosis infection in human immunodeficiency virus-infected persons in Thailand. *Int J Tuberc Lung Dis.* 1(5): 427–434.

Yanai, H., Limpakarnjanarat, K., Uthaivoravit, W., Mastro, T.D., Mori, T., and Tappero, J.W. (2003). Risk of *Mycobacterium tuberculosis* infection and disease among health care workers, Chiang Rai, Thailand. *Int J Tuberc Lung Dis.* 7(1): 36–45.

Yoshiyama, T., Supawitkul, S., Kunyanone, N., Riengthong, D., Yanai, H., Abe, C., Ishikawa, N., Akarasewi, P., Payanandana, V., and Mori, T. (2001). Prevalence of drug-resistant tuberculosis in an HIV endemic area in northern Thailand. *Int J Tuberc Lung Dis.* 5(1): 32–39.

Yunibandu, J. (1943). First report of Weil's disease in Thailand. *J Med Assoc Thailand* 26: 83–139.

21

Infectious Diseases in China

Zeng Yi[1], Xu Hua[1], and Zhang Jiaxi[2]

[1] Chinese Foundation for Prevention of STD and AIDS, Beijing, China
[2] China Preventive Medicine Association, Beijing, China

HISTORY OF INFECTIOUS DISEASES

Before 1949, many epidemic diseases occurred in China due to corruption in the government, foreign invasions, and poor technologies. According to Chinese history, up to 305 years prior to the founding of the People's Republic of China (P.R.China), a plague epidemic affecting a total of 2.6 million people caused 2.4 million deaths. Smallpox epidemics occurred every year. Between 1933 and 1944, about 380,000 people contracted smallpox. In 1820, cholera was introduced into China; since then there have been about a hundred of serious cholera epidemics in China. Schistosomiasis once reached a two million square kilometer epidemic area, with 11 million people contracting the disease. There were hundreds of thousands of people who died or became disabled from measles, malaria, diphtheria, pertussis, meningococcal meningitis, and polio. Due to the lack of a basic infectious disease reporting system, statistics were very difficult to accurately obtain and monitor. Epidemics of sexually transmitted infections (STI) were rampant in both urban and rural areas; these were regarded as a social issue. In China's five thousand years of history, no governments have had the capability to control infectious epidemics and to establish a national epidemic preventive system.

In the early days of the founding of P.R.China, the Chinese government faced tough challenges. For example, in 1950, there were about 3400 human plague cases with 1200 deaths; 43,000 and 61,000 smallpox cases were reported respectively in 1951 and in 1952. In 1952, there were 1.04 million measles cases with 41,000 deaths, and 2.93 million malaria cases with 39,000 deaths reported (Ministry of Public Health, 1990; 2002). Pertussis, kala-azar, diphtheria, and relapsing fever were rampant. In 1951, a relapsing fever epidemic occurred, affecting 100,000 Chinese with relapsing fever and causing more than 10,000 deaths. STI epidemics were very severe; the incidence rate of syphilis in large cities was 3.8%–4.5%, and in some minority areas the rate reached from 21.7% to 48%. Among the female sex workers (FSW) in Beijing, Shanghai, Wuhan, and Guishui, the incidence rate of STI was between 89.3% and 100%. To confront these challenges, the Chinese government carried out a "Put prevention first" principle, established an anti-epidemic system nationwide, and concentrated its efforts to prevent and control severe and life threatening infectious diseases. With a focus on infectious disease prevention and treatment, the Chinese government developed a national health campaign, and enforced occupational health, food hygiene, school hygiene, and radiation protection regulations. Through these strategies, the sanitation situation in urban and rural areas has greatly changed, and citizens' health status has been greatly improved.

By the end of the 1950s, China had basically eliminated smallpox, plague, kala-azar, typhus, relapsing fever, and STI. By the end of 2002, the morbidity rate of notifiable infectious diseases had decreased from $20{,}000/10^5$ at the beginning of the founding of P.R.China to $180/10^5$ in 2002. The total incidence number for measles, pertussis, and diphtheria has decreased from 11.83 million to 56,252 (Ministry of Public Health, 1990; 2002). There have now been four consecutive years without a reported case of wild virus strain polio. The morbidity rates for schistosomiasis, filariasis, malaria, and leprosy have also decreased significantly. However, infectious diseases are key health issues within specific regions of China. In recent years, some infectious diseases have reemerged, such as tuberculosis, malaria, and STI. Other new diseases like AIDS and SARS have emerged to threaten the lives and health of the Chinese, as well as China's economic development.

HEALTH CARE INSTITUTIONS

Health care institutions in China originated in 1873 when the first health Quarantine institutions were constructed. In 1919, the first anti-epidemic department was started in the North of China.

In 1949, based on the experience and practices of the former USSR, a health anti-epidemic station was set up in the former Zhong Chang Railway Administration in the Northeast of China. After the founding of the P.R. China, according to the principle of the Chinese government "To put prevention first," health anti-epidemic stations were set up in several provinces and cities of China. By the end of 1952, there were 147 such stations, 188 special preventive and treatment services, with 20,504 health anti-epidemic workers, including 19,750 health technical personnel. By the end of 1956, the health anti-epidemic stations covered most of China, except the areas of minority nationalities and remote areas. The health anti-epidemic stations were also set up within the railway system, and in large factories, mines, and enterprises. In addition, preventive and care sections were set up in the county hospitals and the health anti-epidemic groups were set up in the township health institutions. By 1965, there were 2499 health anti-epidemic stations at all levels and 822 preventive and treatment institutions, with 63,879 health technical personnel throughout China. This represents a 16-fold increase compared with 1952 (Chinese Association of Preventive Medicine, 2003).

During the Cultural Revolution, the health anti-epidemic system and its services were seriously impacted. After the Cultural Revolution, the health anti-epidemic system and its services were resumed and further developed.

In 1983, in order to increase the capabilities of the health system, the National Preventive Medical Center was set up by the ministry of Health (it was changed to the Chinese Academy of Preventive Medicine in 1985, and changed to National Centers for Disease Prevention and Control in 2002). In 2002, there were 3580 Centers for Disease Prevention and Control, including 31 Centers at the provincial level, 383 at the prefecture level, 2519 at the county level, and 637 in other fields. There were a total of 204,444 personnel, including 156,838 health technical workers. China, in 2002, had as well 1839 special prevention and treatment institutions, and 571 health supervision services (Chinese Association of Preventive Medicine, 2003).

HIV/AIDS PREVENTION AND CONTROL

Epidemic Situation

In 1982, Clotting Factor VIII with HIV-1 was sent from the USA to China; during 1983–1985, four Hemophilia patients were infected with HIV-1 through the injection of this Factor VIII from the USA. In 1985 the first AIDS patient came to China from the USA and died in China.

The cumulative reported number of people living with HIV/AIDS (PLWHA) had reached 40,560 by the end of 2002, with a total of 2639 AIDS cases and 1216 AIDS-related deaths in the 31 provinces, autonomous regions, and municipal cities in China except Taiwan, HongKong and Macao (see Figure 1). In 2002, 9824 new HIV infections were reported; reflecting a 19.5% increase over the same period in 2001. The number of infections has increased in 26 provinces, autonomous regions, and municipal cities in China. Among these, Hainan, Guizhou, Chongqing, Hubei, Hunan, and Anhui provinces reported that the number of PLWHA had an increase compared to the figure reported in the same period of 2001. In 2002, 1045 AIDS cases were reported, with 363 AIDS-related deaths, another increase from the previous year. Among reported cases, 4928 were infected through intravenous drug use, accounting for 50.2% of infections; infection through blood and blood products accounted for 10% of infections; heterosexual contact for 11%; maternal-to-child transmission (MTCT) for 0.4%; and 28.3% of infections occurred through unknown transmission modes. Statistics also show that 78.4% of reported infections are among young people aged 20 to 39 (China HIV/AIDS Information Network, 2002).

Between 1985 and 2002, most HIV/AIDS cases were reported in the Yunnan province, followed by Xinjiang, Guangxi, Guangdong, Sichuan, and Henan provinces (see Figure 2). HIV/AIDS cases have been mainly distributed in the rural areas.

The proportion of male and female cases is 4:1 (see Figure 3).

HIV infection among different age groups is: 1% for age <15; 5.9% for ages 15–20; 51.1% for ages 20–29; 28.9% for ages 30–39; 10% for age >40; 3% unknown (see Figure 4).

The major modes of transmission for HIV/AIDS in China since 1985 have been: intravenous drug use (IDU), accounting for 63.7% of infections; infection through the whole blood supply accounted for 9.3% and blood products accounted for 1.6%; heterosexual contact for 8.1%; MTCT for 0.2%, and unknown for 17.1% (see Figure 5).

This year, according to a joint HIV/AIDS epidemiological survey conducted by China, WHO, and UNAIDS, China has an estimated 840,000 persons living with HIV/AIDS, including 80,000 AIDS cases. Experts estimate

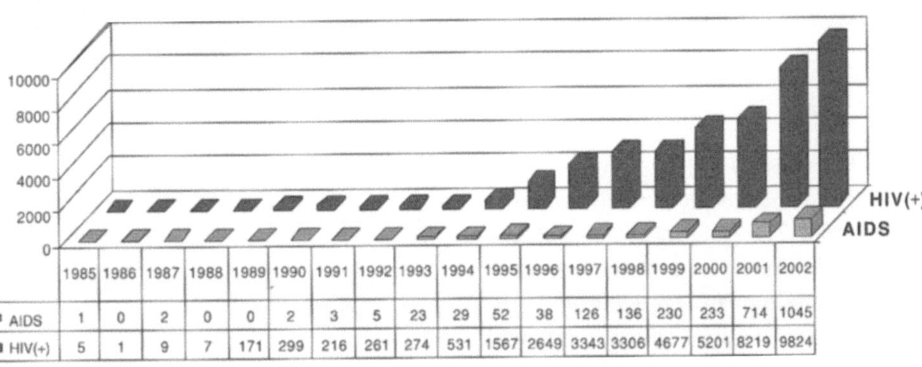

	1985	1986	1987	1988	1989	1990	1991	1992	1993	1994	1995	1996	1997	1998	1999	2000	2001	2002
AIDS	1	0	2	0	0	2	3	5	23	29	52	38	126	136	230	233	714	1045
HIV(+)	5	1	9	7	171	299	216	261	274	531	1567	2649	3343	3306	4677	5201	8219	9824

FIGURE 1. Annual Reported Number of HIV/AIDS Cases in China (1985–2002)

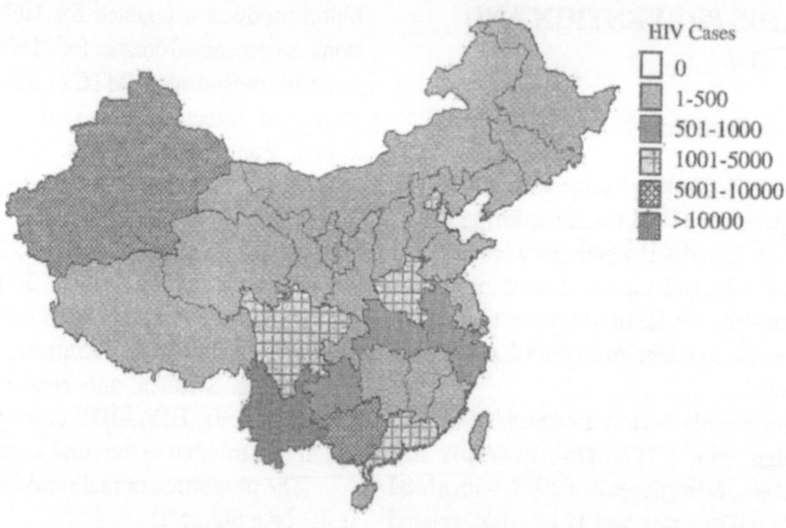

FIGURE 2. Geographic Distribution of HIV/AIDS in China (1985–2002)

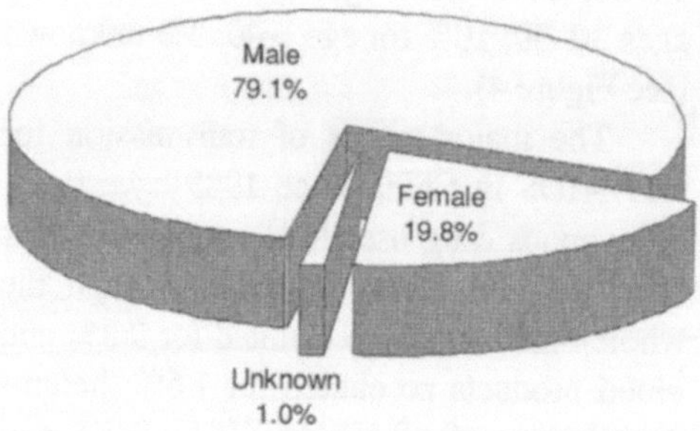

FIGURE 3. Gender Distribution of HIV Infection in China (1985–2002)

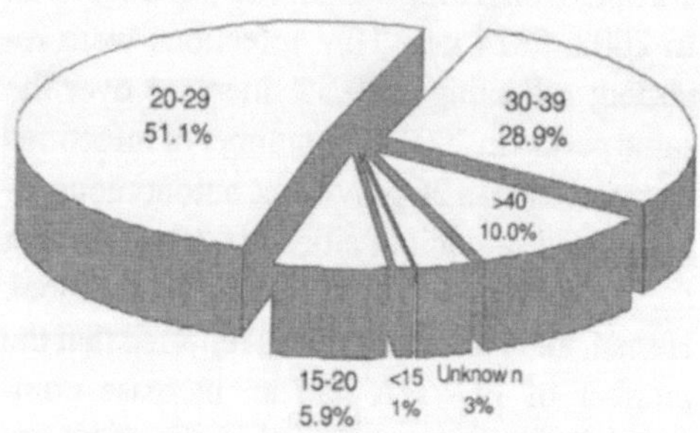

FIGURE 4. Age Distribution of HIV Infection in China (1985–2002)

there will be 10 million HIV/AIDS cases without effective control (see Figure 6).

Three Phases of the HIV Epidemic in China

The First Phase

The first phase, which began in 1985 and end in 1988 was marked by a small number of imported cases. The majority of infected persons during this time were foreigners or overseas Chinese, and the cases appeared only sporadically in coastal cities. Four hemophiliac patients infected with HIV through imported factor VIII were reported from Zhejiang.

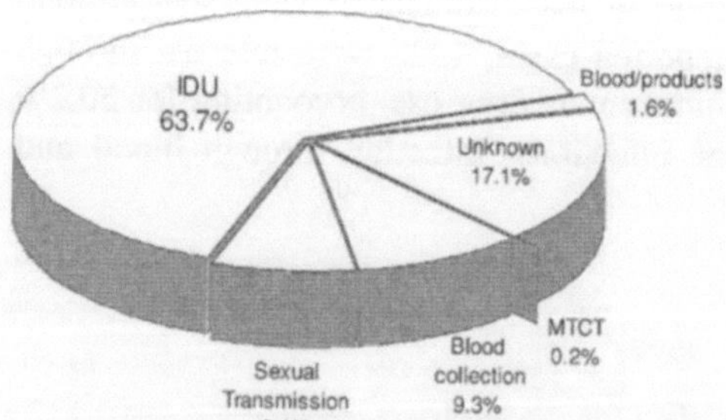

FIGURE 5. Reported HIV Infections in China by Transmission Route (1985–2002)

The Second Phase

The second phase, from 1989 to 1994, might be termed a limited epidemic. It began

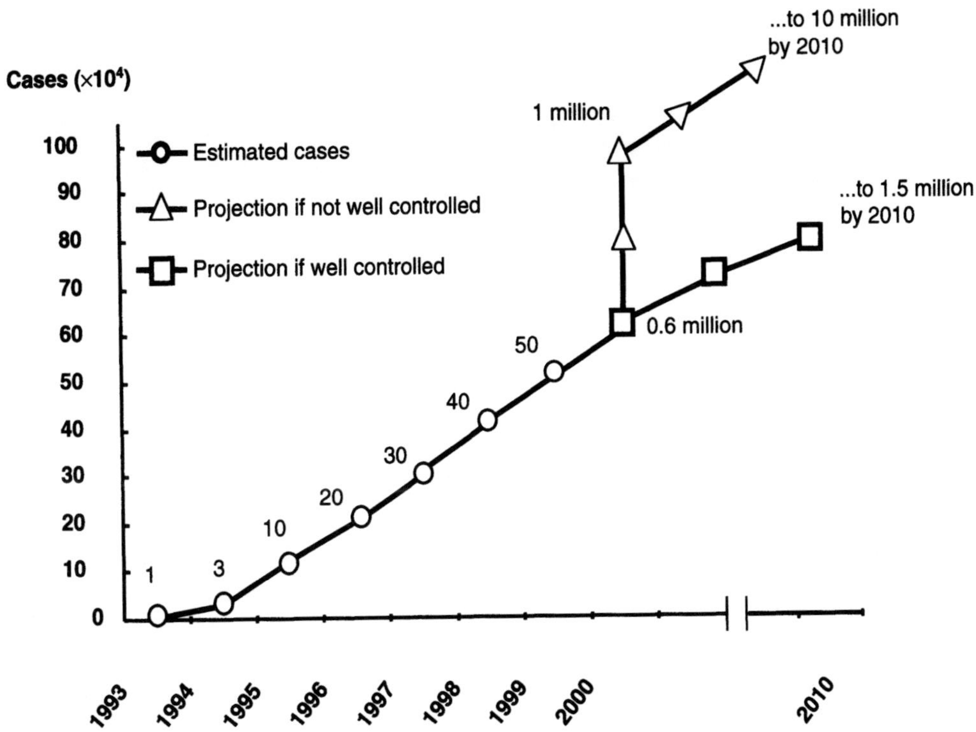

FIGURE 6. Estimated HIV/AIDS Cases, 1993–2000, and Predicted Cases, 2010

in October 1989 with the identification of HIV infection in 146 drug users in southwest Yunan (these were imported cases of HIV), and was followed by an epidemic in a few counties in Dehong prefecture. During this phase some HIV infections were also reported among IDU in other parts of China. At the same time, a small number of HIV infections were reported among laborers returning from abroad, STI patients, and FSW; the number of cases increased gradually during this time.

The Third Phase

The third phase began in 1995 when HIV transmission among IDU spread beyond one prefecture in Yunan province and into various regions such as Xinjiang, Guangxi, and Sichuan. Simultaneously, a large number of HIV infections were reported among blood/plasma donors in central China, mainly rural blood donors who moved frequently and were more likely to transmit HIV to different regions. Furthermore, cases of HIV infection among STI patients and FSW also increased.

Characteristics of the HIV Epidemic in China

The Epidemic is Increasing Dramatically

Currently, there is a low prevalence of HIV nationally but a high prevalence in specific populations and certain regions. The main transmission routes are through intravenous drug use and, in the past, through the sale of blood and plasma. In 2003, according to a China CDC survey supported by WHO, UNAIDS, and US CDC, China has 840,000 people living with HIV/AIDS, among which 80,000 are AIDS cases. Although the adult prevalence rate is less than 0.1%, the epidemic has spread to 31 provinces and the number of reported HIV/AIDS cases has increased significantly.

Increasing Number of AIDS Cases and AIDS-Related Deaths

According to the annual case reports on HIV/AIDS, there has been a significant increase in the cumulative number of HIV/AIDS cases reported. Since 2001, China has approached a peak of AIDS cases and AIDS related deaths. In the 15 years from 1985 to 2000, the cumulative number of AIDS cases reported was 880, with 496 deaths, while the number of AIDS cases and related deaths between 2001 and 2002 were 1742 and 716 respectively. The reported number of AIDS cases in 2002 increased by 44% compared with 2001. In some villages in counties of Henan and Anhui provinces where the HIV epidemic is acute, concentrations of AIDS cases and deaths have occurred since 2001.

The HIV/AIDS Epidemic Is Spreading from High-risk Populations to the General Population

Although sharing injection equipment among IDU is the main transmission route, the proportion of sexually transmitted HIV infections also increased from 5.5% in 1997 to 10.9% at the end of 2002. Data from sentinel surveillance indicated that the HIV prevalence among FSW is increasing, and Mother to Child Transmission (MTCT) has continued to increase since the first reported case in 1995.

Risk Factors Exist for a Generalized HIV Epidemic

High risk behaviors among IDU has increased, including sharing needles and syringes. There still is a low rate of condom use in China. There is a persistent lack of HIV/AIDS related knowledge among Chinese, coupled with severe social discrimination against PLWHA. A high reproductive tract infection (RTI) prevalence rate among rural women is increasing the risk of HIV transmission in some areas. There remains a risk of HIV infection through blood transfusions and iatrogenic infections. Significantly, there is an imbalance in economic development, which has produced poverty in different areas and increased the risk of HIV infections. If China is not able to address these risk factors, the HIV/AIDS epidemic will not be controlled and there will be both serious individual and socio-economic repercussions. The AIDS epidemic will become a serious problem threatening national security and prosperity, social stability, and economic development.

High Risk Factors

Migrant Population

The current internal movement of temporary and permanent migration across China is without precedent. Estimates suggest that the total number of migrants, both temporary and permanent, may be as high as 120 million; that is, some 15% of the total labor force. This number, while extremely large, is actually increasing. A number of additional factors make the migrant labor force particularly vulnerable to HIV infection.

The mere fact that they are mobile makes it extremely difficult to reach this population. Migrants easily escape efforts at education and health promotion. AIDS knowledge within the migrant population is, therefore, very low.

Second, migrants in China are often young and live for extended periods of time away from the social pressure of their families and communities. They are frequently unmarried or are living apart from their spouses and children. Nevertheless, they are still sexually active and often have casual sex, often with FSW, without protection.

Sexually Transmitted Infections (STI)

STIs have risen sharply from 23,534 reported cases in 1985 to a level of 859,040 reported cases in 2000 (see Figure 7). Again, experts estimate that the actual number of STI cases in the country is 6–8 million. In most

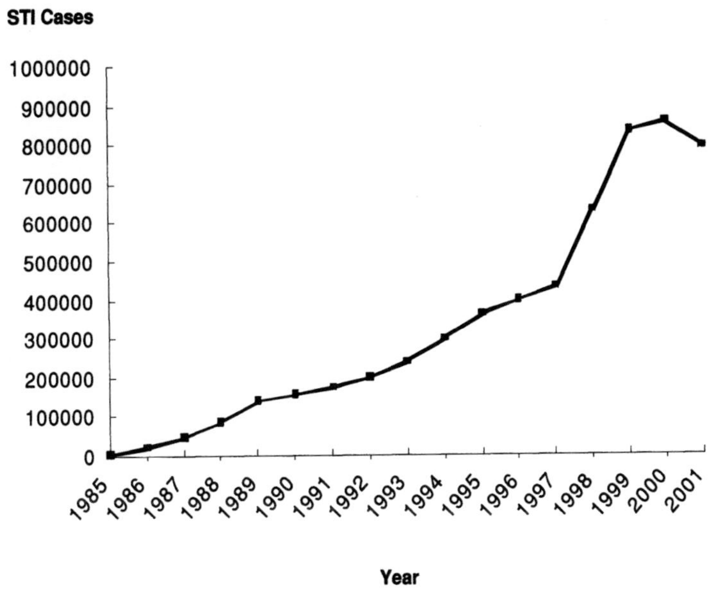

FIGURE 7. STI Cases in China by Year, 1985–2001

urban areas, the majority of STI patients come from within the nonresident population.

Drug Use

The most recent and severe increase in both drug trafficking and drug use in cities throughout China is closely connected with the migrant and nonresident population. There are some one million known drug users recorded by public security in Mainland China. The actual number is estimated to be between 3–5 million (Jianhua *et al.*, 2003).

Commercial Sex Work

Underground sex work is becoming a very serious issue. FSW working in most cities are often not permanent residents, but are migrants from distant regions. The number of FSW and clients arrested in 1985 was just 25,000, but in 1998 this number increased to 398,000 (see Figure 8). One estimate of the actual number of FSW in China is about six million (Jianhua *et al.*, 2003). Sexual transmission of HIV is expected to gradually increase and will likely become the major route of HIV transmission among the general population.

Men Who Have Sex with Men (MSM)

In China, homosexual activities are not illegal, but they are not acceptable in most of society. Most homosexual people are still under social pressure to hide their sexual orientation and to be married. Very few studies on homosexuality have been carried out in China. It is estimated that the total number of MSM in China is over 18 million. Because of high-risk behaviors and relatively little protection in this population, rates of HIV and STI infection among MSM are higher than in the general population. Based on one survey, the HIV infection rate in this population increased from 2.5% in 1998 to 5.5% in 2001 (Zeng, 2003).

Hazards Related to Blood and Blood Products

There are two main sources of donated blood in China: unpaid donations (either requested or voluntary donations), and paid donations. A small number of Chinese donate blood without being paid, but in general, people in China are reluctant to donate blood because of deep-rooted cultural beliefs. At

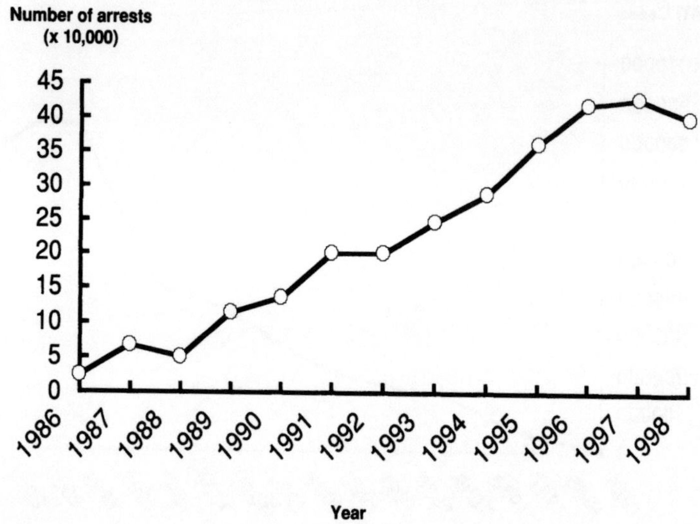

FIGURE 8. Female Sex Workers (FSW) and Their Clients Arrested in China (1986–1998)

present, there are about three million paid blood donors in China, many of them selling plasma during the 1990s. Most of these paid donors live in the poor provinces of central and southern China such as Henan, Hebei, Anhui, Shanxi and Guizhou. Some of them are migrants or are unemployed and rely on plasma sales for their primary income.

Inadequate Infection Control in Health Care Settings

In some rural and remote areas, hygiene is poor, and due to a lack of equipment and, in some cases, inadequate training, the sterilization of medical instruments is difficult. In addition, even in big cities disposable needles and syringes are often not destroyed, leaving the possibility that they will make their way into the larger community and be reused.

Challenges

With a population of 1.3 billion in China, the effective control of HIV/AIDS is not only a benefit to China but also to the world. The Chinese government has issued The Chinese Mid-long Term Plan for HIV/AIDS Prevention and Control (1998–2010) and The Five-Year Action Plan for HIV/AIDS Prevention and Control (2001–2005). Many provinces and ministries have carried out strategic planning and a great deal of practical work has been done. Now a comprehensive preventive and control system has been developed. The whole society has been mobilized and many sectors from central to local levels all have become involved in the related activities. In cooperation with the Chinese government, NGOs in China (especially the Chinese Foundation for Prevention of STD and AIDS, and the Chinese Association for STD and AIDS Prevention and Treatment) have played a very important role in HIV/AIDS prevention and control. Many effective efforts have been made, such as health education, community-based care, social mobilization, and high-risk population interventions. However, there are a lot of challenges and difficulties related to HIV/AIDS prevention and control in China. Support and assistance from various arenas both within China and abroad are seriously needed.

Countermeasures

It is critical to take strong action against this epidemic now, otherwise, this window of opportunity to control the HIV/AIDS epidemic in China will be lost. HIV/AIDS education interventions are the most important strategy for controlling the HIVAIDS epidemic. If countries fail to adopt education and intervention programs, about 46 million people, mostly in Sub-Saharan Africa, China, and India, would become infected (Zeng, 2003; Altman, 2002). A wider application of education and intervention programs would prevent 29 million people from becoming infected worldwide (Altman, 2002). This means that 70% of HIV infections in countries with rapidly growing epidemics (like China) would be prevented (Zeng, 2003). Thailand is a good example, where 5–6 million HIV infections have been prevented (Zeng, 2003). The cost of an aggressive prevention program would be USD$ 1000 for each infection prevented, much less than the cost of treating people once they have become infected (Zeng, 2003).

According to our experiences in the Shandong Weifang City, the cost of an HIV/AIDS education and intervention program would be RMB 2 yuans for each person in China, especially in counties and rural areas. Thus, the cost for carrying out an education and intervention program throughout China would be RMB 2.6 billion yuans for 3–5 years. Such a program may prevent 6 million people from becoming infected with HIV by 2010. Conquering HIV/AIDS requires a combination of prevention and treatment programs, yet aggressive efforts to prevent the spread of HIV/AIDS are far less expensive than treating those infected in an epidemic.

Recently, the Chinese government proclaimed that it would strengthen its efforts to fulfill the responsibility of containing and controlling the HIV/AIDS epidemic. The Chinese government has recognized HIV/AIDS prevention and treatment to be important tasks. The government will further define its goals in combating the disease, identify governmental responsibilities, and improve evaluation, supervision, and monitoring of activities. Accountability for the success or failure of prevention programs will be maintained and enforced.

Second, China is committed to providing free treatment and medicines to PLWHA who have economic difficulties. This health program will cover low-income PLWHA in urban areas, and all patients in rural areas. Moreover, central and local governments will invest more than 10 billion yuan to strengthen the medical assistance system for infectious diseases, and train professionals in comprehensive HIV/AIDS prevention and treatment modalities.

Thirdly, the Chinese government will improve its laws and regulations, and intensify interventions against dangerous behaviors that contribute to the spread of HIV/AIDS. Public awareness campaigns will be launched to educate the public and encourage citizens to participate in HIV/AIDS prevention and treatment efforts. Laws against illegal acts like drug trafficking, drug use, commercial sex work, and illegal blood collecting and distribution will be enforced, while drug-free communities and healthy sexual behaviors will be promoted.

The Chinese government will also work to protect the legitimate rights of PLWHA and oppose social discrimination. Throughout the 124 counties where the Chinese "care" project will be established, integrated measures including antiretroviral treatment, health care, and social programs will be adopted. The government will provide economic aid to PLWHA living in poverty, and their children will be able to attend school tuition-free.

Finally, the government will be more active in international cooperation relating to HIV/AIDS. The HIV/AIDS situation in China has caused both concern and commitment from the international community. China welcomes the continued financial and technical support from the governments of other nations and international organizations. Meanwhile, the Chinese government is ready to be active in the global fight against

HIV/AIDS and fulfill its responsibilities and obligations. The Chinese government has pledged USD$10 million to the Global Fund to Fight AIDS, Tuberculosis and Malaria. This money will support the HIV/AIDS prevention and treatment efforts of developing countries, fulfill the development goals of the UN Millennium Declaration, and contribute to the control of HIV/AIDS prevalence and the realization of global HIV/AIDS control objectives.

SARS EPIDEMIC AND CONTROL

SARS Epidemic in China and Worldwide

Severe acute respiratory syndrome (SARS) originated in November 2002 in the Guangdong Province of China and has subsequently spread to more than 30 countries and regions, including Hong Kong, Taiwan, Vietnam, Canada, and Singapore, infecting approximately 8459 patients and resulting in more than 800 deaths. In China alone, 5327 cases and 349 SARS-related deaths have been reported.

SARS is an emerging infectious disease, and an effective treatment remains unavailable. The underlying causes that led to the SARS epidemic in China are complicated, yet two critical factors are China's large transitory population and the unpreparedness of some Chinese agencies to recognize and fight the epidemic.

Although the transmission mechanism of the agent or agents causing SARS has yet to be fully understood, it is believed that SARS is transmitted probably mainly by droplet secretions, fomites, or close person-to-person contact. The incubation period of SARS ranges from one day to 12 days, with a median of four days. The SARS epidemic in China was characterized with both hospital clustering and family clustering. The disease affected people in all age groups, with patients aged between 2 months and 92 years. Nevertheless, 71% of patients were between 20 and 49 years old. The male-to-female ratio was 1:1.6. There was no statistically significant difference between men and women in the mortality rate; however, the mortality rate was associated with age and co-morbidities. According to WHO, the fatality rates are as follows: $<1\%$ for below age 24, 6% for ages 25–44; 15% for ages 45–64; $>50\%$ for above age 65 (Zheng, 2003).

SARS Epidemic Control in China

The outbreak and rapid spread of SARS in China caused fear and concern in ordinary citizens and caught the immediate attention of both the Chinese government and the world. The responses taken were as follows:

1. To protect people's health, the Chinese government set up a national command center to coordinate the efforts of disease treatment, control, and prevention. Thus, disease control became a national priority.
2. A massive nationwide campaign to educate people to take precautions was launched and decisive measures were mandated by all levels of the government to control the epidemic throughout China.
3. Both medical experts and the media played extremely important roles in disseminating scientific knowledge to the public, and raising awareness of SARS prevention.
4. Soon after the national command center was set up, effective strategies based on the experience in fighting against SARS epidemic in Guangdong Province were formulated and adopted.
5. Four effective principles against the outbreak were summarized and adopted: early identification and diagnosis, early reporting, early isolation, and early treatment. To prevent further cases, patients were treated locally and controls against nosocomial infection were instituted. Thus, in a surprisingly short period of time, SARS was controlled and daily normal life was restored.
6. During the SARS epidemic, public health professionals played an extremely important role in education and prevention. Epidemiologists worked very closely with physicians treating patients, helped identify local sources of the epidemic, and conducted outbreak investigations. These epidemiologists visited patients' families

and co-workers, and identified both suspected cases and super-spreaders. Numbers of identified cases were reported to the government daily, and the government then informed the public about the status of the outbreak. Under the leadership of the national command center, public health professionals helped government agencies strengthen the safety of public places by improving ventilation and reducing unnecessary activities. These professionals also educated people about how to minimize their risk of being infected, and how to enhance their immune system to fight SARS. Based on the information collected from hospitals and communities, public health professionals determined that both definite and suspected cases of SARS should be isolated for 12 to 14 days.

7. To control the epidemic, the Chinese government instituted scientific research on SARS etiology, treatment, and prevention, and encouraged international collaborations in these areas. On March 12, 2003, the WHO issued a global warning about the epidemic, and took unprecedented measures to effectively prevent the disease from spreading to unaffected countries and regions. The WHO dispatched a team of experts to China and set up a global disease control network in 10 countries including China. Chinese health professionals made important contributions toward identifying a novel coronavirus as the causal agent of SARS.

SARS and the Public Health System

The SARS epidemic has simultaneously evolved as both a significant challenge to humans' health, as well as a social and public health management problem. As an emergency crisis, the SARS epidemic has had at least the following 4 characteristics:

1. Unpredictability: SARS infections were unpredictable and, at least initially, the mode of transmission was in question.
2. Exigency: Swift attention to the infections, and quick treatment of cases was necessary to prevent further infections.
3. Social consequences: The SARS epidemic caused an imbalance in the social order, and damaged economic development, through rampant fear and anxiety. For a time, it was the most important issue facing China and overshadowed other priorities.
4. Worldwide implications: The SARS epidemic has spread from China and affected the entire world.

The SARS epidemic has created a significant challenge for the Chinese public health system. The Chinese government has responded by establishing and strengthening a prevention system to ensure an effective response to any future epidemic. Scientific studies on the origin of SARS, its pathogenesis and immunology, potential anti-SARS drugs and vaccines, and animal models are being conducted.

REFERENCES

Altman, L.A. (2002). *Modest Anti-AIDS Efforts Offer Huge Payoff, Studies Say*, New York Times. July 5, 2002.

China HIV/AIDS Information Network. (2002). Situation of HIV/AIDS Epidemic and Its Prevention and treatment in China in 2002. Beijing, China.

Chinese Association of Preventive Medicine. (1993). Review and Prospects for Chinese Health Anti-epidemic System.

Chinese Association of Preventive Medicine. (2003). Review and Prospects for Chinese Health Anti-epidemic System.

Jianhua, Y., Qi, X., Tao, J., and Houbao, X. (2003). Simulation of Impact of Policy and Law Environment on HV/AIDS Spreading in China. United Nations Development Program.

Ministry of Public Health. (1990). A Brief Introduction on China's Medical and Health Services. Beijing, China.

Ministry of Public Health. (2002). National Situation of Morbidity and Mortality of Infectious Diseases in China. Beijing, China.

Zeng, Yi. (2003). Health Education and Intervention Are Major Strategies for AIDS Control. *Chinese Journal of Health Education*. 11(19): 846–848.

Zheng, L. (2003). *SARS and Response to Emergency Public Health Events*. Sciences Publishing House, Beijing.

22

The History of HIV and Other Infectious Diseases in the Republic of Korea

Origin, Damage, and Control

June-Myung Kim[1], Jongkoo Lee[2], and Joo-Shil Lee[3]

[1] *Division of Infectious Diseases, Department of Internal Medicine, Yonsei University College of Medicine, Seoul, Korea*

[2] *Department of Infectious Disease Control, Korea Center for Disease Control and Prevention, Seoul, Korea*

[3] *Department of Virology, National Institute of Health, Seoul, Korea*

NATIONAL HISTORY AND CURRENT STATUS OF INFECTIOUS DISEASES IN KOREA

National History of Infectious Diseases

Historically, a great number of infectious diseases in Korea have been related to drought, flood damage, famine, natural disaster, and war. According to historical records predating the 14th century, smallpox, malaria, respiratory infections, and diarrheal diseases were the major infectious diseases in addition to dysentery, sexually transmitted diseases, dermatologic diseases, and tetanus.

At the end of the 14th century, numerous medical books were published and many medical institutions and schools were founded, which helped form a system of traditional medicine and patient care (Park, 1999). Infectious diseases such as cholera, dysentery, typhoid fever, relapsing fever, influenza, smallpox, chickenpox, measles, epidemic meningitis, malaria, tuberculosis, dermatologic diseases, leprosy, and syphilis had been major diseases before this system existed.

Horace Allen, an American missionary doctor, introduced Western medicine to Korea at the end of the 19th century. Kwanghaewon, the Royal hospital, built in 1885, was renamed Jejoongwon soon after the start of its service and played a great role in the development of modern medicine. The characteristics of infectious diseases in the Chosun dynasty (A.D. 1392–1910) were summarized in the report for the year of 1886 released by Jejoongwon (Park, 1999). The report makes special reference to smallpox, leprosy, syphilis, and malaria. Through efforts to control the cholera outbreaks, a systematic approach to the control of infectious disease was developed.

Koreans suffered from many infectious diseases along with syphilis and tuberculosis, according to the 1901 report from Jejoong-won. The government had started to give group syphilis examinations for prostitutes in the beginning of the 20th century. At that time, a guideline to control scarlet fever was recommended. Modernized management of infectious diseases, such as an establishment of sanatoria for patients with contagious diseases, was implemented. Some infectious diseases were designated by law as nationally notifiable diseases. Quarantine, sterilization, and traditional vaccination for smallpox were also introduced for the first time. The first statistics of infectious diseases were published around this time (Chen, 1975).

In 1945 Korea was divided into the Republic of Korea (ROK) and the Democratic People's Republic of Korea (DPRK), more commonly referred to as North Korea.

A national organization responsible for the control of infectious disease was established, and as a result, a new public health system for the control of infectious disease was founded during the mid-20th century (Chen, 1975). Many major infectious diseases were still prevalent, such as cholera, dysentery, typhoid fever, poliomyelitis, smallpox, scarlet fever, diphtheria, epidemic meningitis, measles, pertussis, relapsing fever, epidemic typhus, Japanese encephalitis, and malaria.

Korea began to achieve progressive economic development beginning in the mid 20th century. The epidemiologic trend of infectious diseases changed along with this economic development. Smallpox, relapsing fever, and epidemic typhus disappeared in the 1960s, while poliomyelitis, typhoid fever, paratyphoid fever, diphtheria, tetanus, malaria, and Japanese encephalitis were greatly decreased in their incidence. Up until the 1960s, infectious diseases such as pneumonia and tuberculosis were the main causes of death. However, in the 1970s, non-contagious diseases became the main causes of death (Chung, 1989).

The causative organisms for several diseases were identified through great improvement of diagnostic techniques and epidemiology of infectious diseases (Seo, 1999). For example, in 1976, H.W. Lee and his colleagues isolated the Hantaan virus, which is the causative organism of Korean hemorrhagic fever (Lee and Lee, 1976). Scientists also found *Leptospira interrogans*, the causative organism of a pneumonia-like disease, which spread through the central part of Korea (Cho *et al.*, 1984). They also identified *Orientia tsutsugamushi,* which led them to find the existence of scrub typhus in Korea. *Vibrio vulnificus* infection and legionellosis were also documented during the 1980s (Kim, 1984; Lee and Kim, 1989). Some of these diseases, such as Korean hemorrhagic fever, leptospirosis, and scrub typhus, continue to be important endemic febrile diseases in autumn.

Some infectious diseases continued to cause medical problems, although they appeared with different clinical characteristics. For example, the serotype of bacteria causing dysentery changed in 1990. The original bacteria, *Shigella sonnei*, which is mild in its clinical symptoms, had most frequently been isolated (Oh, 1999). The proportion of non-typhoidal salmonellosis had been increasing among the salmonellosis (NIH, Korea, 1997). The malaria, *Plasmodium vivax*, which had almost disappeared since the late 1970s appeared again in the early 1990s (Chai *et al.*, 1994).

About thirty thousand people caught the measles in Korea in 2000. As part of a strategy to control measles by 2005, which was designed by government authorities in collaboration with the United States Centers for Disease Control and Prevention (U.S. CDC) and the World Health Organization (WHO), 4.8 million students were vaccinated. The school entry requirement for children entering elementary school in 2001 was also enforced. These measures effectively prevented the further spread of measles.

It is difficult to know the current status of infectious diseases in North Korea (DPRK) because of limited information. However, based on current information from limited exchange and cooperation with North Korea, malaria, tuberculosis, and waterborne diseases seem to be serious problems in today's DPRK.

Current Status and Changing Trends

The statistics of nationally notifiable infectious diseases have been recorded in Korea since 1921. According to these records, incidence of acute infectious diseases decreased from 215 per 100,000 persons in 1962 to 14.9 in 1990 (MHSA, 1985; MHSA, 1991).

The Communicable Disease Prevention Act was established in 1954 to control infectious disease and to improve public health, and has since been revised according to changing infectious disease trends.

The pattern of infectious disease has changed remarkably. The infectious diseases with a high infectivity have either disappeared or reduced greatly while diseases caused by less virulent organisms have become more prevalent. Some infectious diseases which have had increased incidence have also had changing clinical patterns. Also, nosocomial infections have increased, and previously unrecognized infectious diseases have emerged. In order to cope with the rapid changes of infectious diseases, the government reestablished the Communicable Diseases Prevention Act, based on the advice and suggestions given by researchers, in 2000.

Current Problems of Infectious Diseases

Emerging and reemerging infectious diseases, microorganisms with resistance to antibiotics, and the increase of nosocomial infections have become major problems in Korea. The first patient with brucellosis, considered to be one of zoonosis, was reported (NIH, Korea, 2003).

Not only endemic infectious diseases, but also infectious diseases imported from other countries have increased in their incidence. Since the first AIDS patient was documented in Korea in 1985, the number of new HIV infections has increased each year. Fortunately, severe acute respiratory syndrome (SARS), which broke out in China and later spread worldwide in early 2003 only caused a few suspected and probable cases in Korea. Although many people are getting vaccinations every year, the risk of influenza and the potential for it to spread still exist.

A gradual increase in microorganisms resistant to antibiotics and nosocomial infections are currently important problems in Korea. The proportion of methicillin- resistant *Staphylococcus aureus* (MRSA) has increased seriously with a case of vancomycin-intermediate *Staphylococcus aureus* (VISA) (Kim *et al.*, 2000). Vancomycin-resistant *enterococcus* (VRE) and multi-drug resistant gram-negative microorganisms are also currently increasing (Seo, 1999).

COMMUNICABLE DISEASE CONTROL SYSTEMS IN KOREA

Disease Surveillance System

Disease Classification

Fifty-six communicable diseases or disease groups are designated as notifiable diseases, as stipulated by the Prevention of Contagious Disease Act. According to the revision of the Prevention of Communicable Disease Act on 12 January 2000, 29 communicable diseases or disease groups were newly added to the existing 27. Also, the categorization of these communicable diseases was changed and is now composed of Classes 1–4, designating communicable disease classes by the differences in prevention, reporting procedure, patient care, and the epidemiology of outbreaks. This was intended to handle with newly emerging or reemerging infectious diseases efficiently and effectively.

Class 1 consists of five diseases (e.g., cholera) which necessitate immediate isolation of patients. Class 2 consists of nine diseases, all preventable by vaccines. Class

3 consists of seventeen diseases (including HIV/AIDS) and one disease group, sexually transmitted diseases (STD), which are important to monitor consistently and to educate the public about preventing. Class 4 consists of twelve diseases, including yellow fever and dengue fever (new infectious diseases), and one syndrome (acute respiratory syndrome), as well as reemerging diseases or imported diseases. There are eight Class-5 or "designated" diseases, all of which are parasitic infectious diseases except viral hepatitis A and C and VRSA (vancomycin-resistant *staphylococcus aureus*).

Reporting System

A physician who clinically diagnoses a notifiable communicable disease in Class 1, 2, or 4 should report it immediately to the neighboring Community Health Center (CHC). A case of Class 3 or 5 diseases is to be reported within 7 days. The Korea Center for Disease Control and Prevention has published a weekly surveillance report, Communicable Disease Weekly Report (CDWR), which includes 23 diseases, but not newly added diseases, like STD and viral hepatitis BCJD. CDWR is planning to eventually include all notifiable diseases. Especially for designated diseases there is a surveillance system in which only the designated medical organizations or health institutes participate. In addition to the notification system, there is a laboratory surveillance system for diseases such as diarrheal diseases, respiratory diseases like influenza, bioterrorism, STD and HIV, antibiotic resistant microbes, acute febrile diseases, rodent-related, and newly emerging parasitic diseases. Epidemic or outbreak investigation is conducted on an ad hoc basis.

Information technology was introduced to the surveillance system in 1999. Through Web EDI (Electronic Data Interface) and RDBMS (Related Database Management System), the notifying and reporting system has become computerized, and all data of notified and reported cases are stored electronically. It is now possible for physicians and the CHC to access the notifying and reporting system (DisWeb, http://dis.mohw.go.kr) anywhere and anytime via the Internet.

Communicable Disease Control Program

Health Care Delivery System

The Korean health care system mainly depends upon the private sector. Private clinics and hospitals account for 92.6% of all medical facilities in terms of the number of facilities and 87.4% in terms of the number of beds. Most private facilities are concentrated in urban areas. In Korea, while about 79.7% of the population resides in urban areas, 90.7% of physicians and 91.8% of hospital beds are concentrated in cities, leading to disparities of access to healthcare services between urban and rural residents. There is a general preference for large hospitals in Korea and even slightly sick or injured patients favor large hospitals over small clinics, leading to the failure of the efficient division of the roles of medical institutions.

Traditional Vertical Control Program against Communicable Diseases

During the last few decades, infectious diseases have been continuing health problems for the Korean people, in spite of socio-economic development. Although most infectious diseases have been reduced by the modern healthcare system—through improved manpower, facility and equipment, organization, finance, management, and supplies (vaccines, antibiotics, etc)—some infectious diseases, such as tuberculosis, still rank among the leading ten causes of death (Figure 1).

To battle against infectious diseases, the Korean government has established the public health system, which delivers service through community health centers (243 units nationwide), sub-health centers (about 1200 units nationwide), and community nurse practitioners (about 2000 persons). They have played a major role in the Expanded Program of

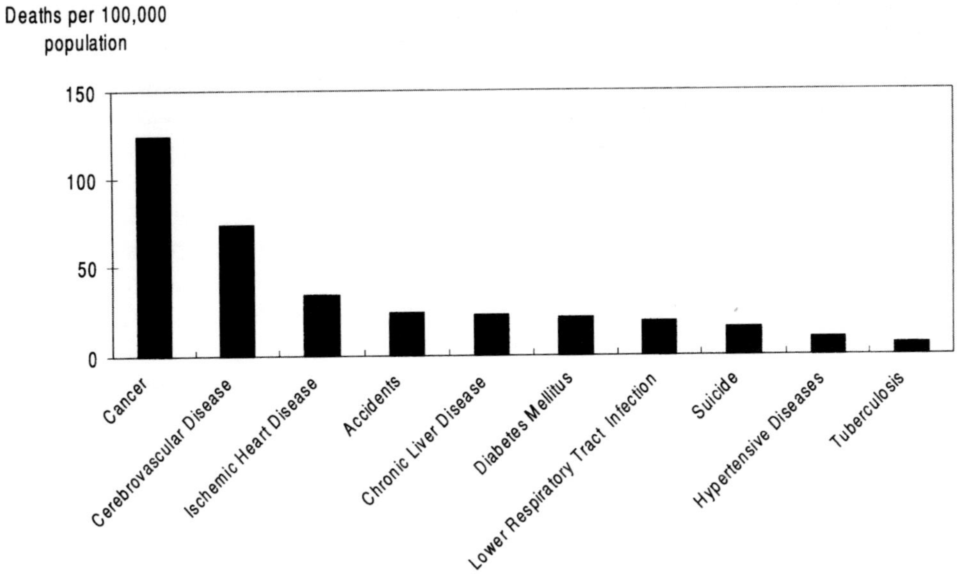

FIGURE 1. Major Causes of Death, Republic of Korea, 2000

Immunization (EPI), maternal-child health, family planning, and anti-tuberculosis programs, and have greatly contributed to a decrease in infant deaths from infection. As a result, the annual incidence rate of notifiable communicable diseases except tuberculosis, STD, Hansen's disease, and chronic viral hepatitis B has been at the level of about 10 per 100,000 populations since the early 1990s. But new infectious diseases, including HIV/AIDS, have also been detected. Furthermore, shigellosis, malaria, and even vaccine—preventable diseases like measles, mumps, and hepatitis A are recently reemerging. Investigations are underway to find out causes of infection. Due to the advent of re-emerging and emerging diseases, there exist disputes about whether to strengthen the public health system against infectious diseases in spite of current government downsizing.

New Strategies for Emerging and Reemerging Diseases

The plan for confronting emerging and reemerging infectious diseases has been prepared under the leadership of the Ministry of Health and Welfare (MOHW) and the National Institute of Health (NIH). Due to the shortage of manpower in government, many university researchers have been involved since 1995 in the epidemic investigation of cholera and the occurrence of vaccine injuries (death and encephalopathy) after immunization of inactivated Japanese Encephalitis vaccine. As a first step, the MOHW formed a task force to evaluate the monitoring system for infectious disease outbreaks and national immunization programs. During the last five years, the task force has expanded its role to develop strategies for the Emerging Infectious Disease (EID) control. Now the Korean government is implementing those strategies, including: reorganizing the public health infrastructure (Korea CDC), amending the Prevention of Contagious Disease Act, developing health manpower through the Field Epidemiology Training Program (FETP) and Field Management Training Program (FMTP), creating guidelines and field manuals for communicable disease control, developing an electronic reporting system, continuing research and development, building national stockpiles for antibioterrorism, and cooperating internationally with the WHO, U.S. CDC, Japan, and China.

THE HISTORY AND CURRENT STATUS OF HIV/AIDS IN KOREA

National Policy and Strategies for HIV/AIDS Prevention and Control

The Korean government launched an AIDS prevention program in June 1985 after the first report of a foreign AIDS patient in Korea. In March 1987, AIDS was classified as a Class 2 infectious disease to be controlled. Thereafter, on 28 November 1987, to establish a legal basis for AIDS management, the government proclaimed the Act for AIDS, which includes content on the duties of the national government, prefecture and district governments, and the general population for the prevention of AIDS. In 2000, the Communicable Disease Prevention Act was revised, and HIV/AIDS is now included as a Class 3 disease.

Even though details of the Act for AIDS have been revised according to changes in the high-risk groups and to social demand, the original goals were maintained. The first goal is the prevention of HIV infection and expansion. Education and advertising are the main means being used to prevent HIV transmission. Supply of safe blood, and blood products, is another means. Since 1987, all individual blood donors have been tested for HIV antibodies. The second goal is the care of patients with HIV infection and AIDS. All individuals identified with HIV/AIDS should be reported to the National Institute of Health, Korea. Public health centers not only educate and counsel infected individuals regularly, but also reimburse pharmaceutical drug payments to support health promotion and to prevent HIV transmission. To support these processes, and to assist the technical aspects of research and training, the Center for AIDS Research was established in the National Institute of Health in May 1987.

Participation by the private sector is indispensable to AIDS management, and is able to cover counseling and education for the target population, including homosexuals and sex workers who are not reached by the government. In addition, nongovernmental organizations (NGOs) play an important role in the care of AIDS patients. Several shelters have also been opened to support AIDS patients. In addition, the private sector may play a major role in achieving the aim of expanding knowledge of AIDS and in demonstrating a rational attitude towards infected individuals. Since 1994, five NGOs have been established, of which two, the Korean Anti-AIDS Federation and the Korean Alliance to Defeat AIDS, are involved entirely in HIV/AIDS prevention and patient care, in close cooperation with the government.

Epidemiology

Since the first report of HIV infection and AIDS in 1985, the number of HIV-infected individuals, including AIDS patients, has been increasing every year (Korean NIH report, 2003). About four million HIV tests are performed annually, in blood centers (two to 2.5 million tests), hospitals (about 0.8 million), and public health centers (about 0.5 million). The total reported number of cases of HIV/AIDS in Korea was 2259 by June of 2003 (Korean National Institute of Health, 2003). Newly reported HIV/AIDS cases have increased annually, and the increase in the rate has accelerated since 1998. Fortunately, the prevalence of HIV infection is still low (less than 0.1–0.01%), which is in the lowest prevalence group in the UNAIDS 2002 report. Estimated seroprevalence rates are 0.0003% among pregnant women, 0.002% among blood donors, 0.0375% among sex workers, and 0.083% among STD patients (Goh, 2001).

By June 2003, 89% of HIV/AIDS cases were male, and the sex ratio was about 9:1. The 20–39 age group constituted 61.9% of cases at the time of diagnosis. The main mode of transmission was sexual contact. Excluding unexamined and unknown cases, 97.5% of reported HIV/AIDS patients have been infected

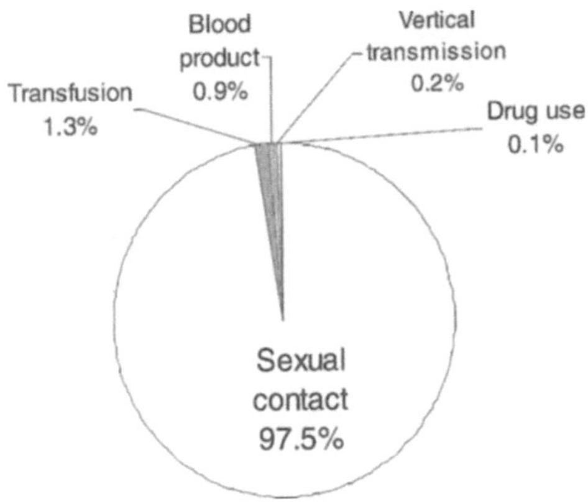

FIGURE 2. Modes of HIV Transmission in the Republic of Korea, June 2003 (Korean National Institute of Health, 2003)

with HIV through sexual contact (Figure 2) (Korean National Institute of Health, 2003). In addition to numbers of men who have sex with men (MSM), which was reported at about 20–45%, the high male sex ratio and the low seroprevalence rate of female sex workers indicate that homosexual activity might be underestimated as a transmission route, and may even be the main transmission route of HIV in Korea.

Molecular Epidemiology

Several Korean scientists have not only reported that subtype B of HIV-1 is prevalent in South Korea but also have constructed a distinct Korean subclade in phylogenetic trees (Kang *et al.*, 1998; Kim *et al.*, 1999). In unpublished Korean NIH data, among 277 subjects examined, 203 (73.3%) were subtype B and 74 (26.7%) were non-B subtypes (39A, 5C, 2D, 22E, 1F, 4G, 1H). The subtype B and non-B proportion was significantly different for all examined risk factors such as gender, transmission route, and infection place (table 1). The different migration of B and non-B viruses between men and women is distinguished primarily by year. The proportion of men infected with subtype B has increased from 38% in the late 1980s to over 90% after 1996. Conversely, the proportion of women infected with subtype B has decreased from 64% in the late 1980s to 44% in the early 2000s. These results suggest that HIV-1 subtype B predominates strongly within both homosexual and heterosexual men in Korea, while subtype B and non-B viruses have been transmitted among women in equal proportions. Collectively, the sex ratio and different prevalence of subtypes between men and women support the finding that HIV transmission is increasing rapidly in MSM but is limited in the general Korean population (Table 1).

Antiretroviral Treatment and Monitoring of Disease Progression

To care for HIV/AIDS patients, zidovudine was introduced into Korea in 1991 as monotherapy, and highly active antiretroviral therapy (HAART) was introduced in 1997. At present, two nucleoside analog reverse transcriptase inhibitors plus one protease inhibitor (zidovudine, didanosine and indinavir) is the most commonly used regimen for treating AIDS patients. Several sets of clinical data have reported that the most common AIDS-defining opportunistic diseases are tuberculosis and *Pneumocystis carinii* pneumonia (Kim *et al.*, 2003; Oh *et al.*, 1999). The type and frequency of opportunistic infections represent the prevalence of infection by the causative microorganism in Korea (Kim *et al.*, 2001). The most frequent adverse effects of HAART have been reported as bone marrow suppression, gastrointestinal intolerance and hyperbilirubinemia, respectively (Lee *et al.*, 2003). Genotypic resistance to antiviral drugs have been reported in naïve and treated patients (Cho *et al.*, 2002; Sung *et al.*, 2001). Also, numbers of CD4+ and CD8+ T cells have been counted every six months in all reported HIV/AIDS patients where possible. Other host genetic factors have also been studied, such as mutation of the CCR5 gene (Oh *et al.*, 2000), high frequencies of CCR2b-64I and SDF1–3'A mutations (Choi *et al.*, 2002), and HLA polymorphisms associated with HIV infection (Kim *et al.*, 1999).

TABLE 1. Distribution of HIV-1 Subtypes by Transmission Routes, Infection Places, and Gender in South Korea

			Male					Female				
Transmission Routes	Total	%	Subjects	Subtype B	Subtype B%	Non-B	Non-B%	Subjects	Subtype B	Subtype B%	Non-B	Non-B%
MSM												
Inside Korea	66		66	65	98.5%	1	1.5%					
Outside Korea	7		7	7	100.0%	0						
MSM Total	73	26.4%	73	72	98.6%	1	1.4%					
Heterosexuals												
Inside Korea	136		67	66	98.5%	1	1.5%	69	39	56.5%	30	43.5%
Outside Korea	62		61	21	34.4%	40	65.6%	1	1		0	
Unknown	2		2	1		1		0	0		0	
Heterosexuals Total	200	72.2%	130	88	67.7%	42	32.3%	70	40	57.1%	30	42.9%
Blood product related	1	0.4%	1	1		0		0	0		0	
Transfusion	2	0.7%	1	0		1		1	1		0	
Unidentified	1	0.4%	1	1		0		0	0		0	
TOTAL	277	100.0%	206	162	78.6%	44		71	41	57.7%	30	42.3%

Strategy on the Future Research of HIV/AIDS

It is very important that development of HIV prevention strategies is appropriate for the situation in each country. Through local or national progress, more effective worldwide HIV prevention and control strategies could be established. Until now, the prevalence of HIV infection in Korea has been low. However, the recent rapid increase tells us that we should prevent the transmission of HIV from unexposed high-risk groups into the general population. Therefore, we need various education strategies and estimations of population size according to target groups. In addition, future research will be focused on examining the differences between countries and ethnicities with regard to various scientific aspects such as HIV evolution, disease progression, and vaccine development.

REFERENCES

Chai, I.H., Lim, G.I., Yoon, S.N., Oh, W.I., Kim, S.J., Chai, J.Y.(1994). Occurrence of tertian malaria in a male patient who has never been abroad. *Korean Journal of Parasitology*. 32(3):195–200.

Chen, C.H. (1975) *General Perspectives of Infectious Diseases in Korea*, 3rd ed. New Edit Medicine Press, Seoul.

Cho, M.K., Paik, S.B., Oh, H.B., Song, C. (1984). Bacteriological Studies on Leptospirosis in Korea (1984). *Korean Journal of Epidemiology*, 6(1):16–35.

Cho Y.K., Sung H, Ahn S.H., Bae I.G., Woo J.H., Won Y.H., Kim D.G., and Kang M.W. (2002). Frequency of mutations conferring resistance to nucleotide reverse transcriptase inhibitors in human immunodeficiency virus type 1-infected patients in Korea. Journal of Clinical Microbiology 40(4):1319–1325.

Choi, B.S., Cha, S.H., Kim, S.S., Park, Y.K., Lee, J.S. (2002). High frequencies of the CCR2b-64I and SDF1–3'A Mutations with HIV Infection in Koreans. *Immune network*. 2(2): 86–90.

Chung, H.Y. (1989). Changes of Infectious Diseases in Korea. *The Journal of Catholic Medical College*, 42:19–30.

Goh, U.Y. (2001). Epidemiologic characteristics, estimation and prediction of HIV/AIDS epidemic in Korea. Ph.D. Thesis, Hanyang University Graduate School (unpublished paper).

Kang, M.R., Cho, Y.K., Chun, Y.S., Kim, Y.B., Lee, I.S., Lee, H.J., Kim, S.H., Kim, Y.K., Yoon, K.J., Yang, J.M., Kim, J.M., Shin, Y.O., Kang, C., Lee, J.S., Choi, K.W., Kim, D.G., Fitch, W.M., and Kim, S. (1998). Phylogeneic Analysis of the *nef* Gene Reveals a Distinctive Monophyletic Clade in Korean HIV-1 Cases. *J AIDS Human Retrovirol* 17:58–68.

Kim, E.Y., Cho, Y.S., Maeng, S.H., Kang, C., Nam, J.G., and Lee, J.S. (1999). Characterization of V3 loop sequences from HIV-1 subtype B in South Korea: Predominance of the GPGS motif. *AIDS Research and Human Retroviruses*, 15(7):681–686.

Kim, J.S. (1984). Epidemiologic Characteristics of Legionellosis. *Infection*. 16(2):1–12.

Kim, J.M., Cho, G.J., Hong, S.K., Chang, K.H., Chung, J.S., Choi, Y.H., Song, Y.G., Huh, A., Yeom, J.S., Lee, K.S., and Choi, J.Y. (2003). Epidemilogy and clinical features of HIV infection/AIDS in Korea. *Yonsei Medical Journal*, 44(3):363–370.

Kim, M.N., Pai, C.H., Woo, J.H., Ryu, J.S., Hiramatsu K. (2000). Vancomycin-Intermediate Staphylococcus aureus in Korea. *Journal of Clinical Microbiology*. 38(10):3879–3881.

Kim, O., Kim, S.S., Choi, B.S., Suh, S.D., Lee, M.W., Kim, K.S., Park, M.S., and Lee, J.S. (2001). Consistency of the low seroprevalence of Human Herpesvirus 8 and the rarity of Kaposi's Sarcoma in South Korea. *Journal of Bacteriology and Virology*, 31(3):275–279

Kim, T.G., Choi, H.B., Lee, J.S., Han, H. (1999). Effect of HLA Class II and HLA-DM alleles on HIV infection in Korean. *J Korean Soc Microbiol*. 34(1):37–43.

Korean National Institute of Health. (2003). Periodical report of HIV/AIDS (June 2003).

Lee, S.H., and Kim, S.J.(1989). Epidemiologic and Microbiologic Study in 64 Clinically Suspected Cases of V. Vulnificus Infections. *Korean Journal of Medicine*. 36(6):820–830.

Lee, H.W., and Lee, P.W. (1976). Korean Hemorrhagic Fever. *Korean Journal of Medicine*. 19:371–383.

Lee, K.S., Chang, K.H., Choi, J.Y., Park, Y.S., Han, S.H., Chin, B.S., Choi, S.H., Song, Y.G.., Kim, J.M. (2003). Adverse effects of antiretroviral drugs on HIV-infected Koreans. *Infection and Chemotherapy*, 35(2): 71–76.

Ministry of Health and Social Affairs.(1985). Yearbook of Health and Social Statistics. 31:11.

Ministry of Health and Social Affairs.(1991). Yearbook of Health and Social Statistics. 37:11

National Institute of Health, Korea. (1997). Yearly distribution of major *Salmonella* isolates serovar in Korea (1993–1996). *Communicable Diseases Monthly Report*. 8(4): 42–43.

National Institute of Health, Korea. (2003). Reported cases of national notifiable diseases by areas,

December 2002. *Communicable Diseases Monthly Report*. 14(1): 225–226.

Oh, M.D. (1999). Shigellosis. *J Korean Medical Association*. 42(7): 637–640.

Oh, M.D., Park, S.W., Kim, H.B., Kim, U.S., Kim, N.J., Choi, H.J., Shin, D.H., Lee, J.S., and Choe, K.W. (1999). Spectrum of opportunistic infections and malignancies in patients with human immunodeficiency virus infection in South Korea. *Clin Inf Dis*. 29(6):1524–1528.

Oh, M.D., Kim, S.S., Kim, E.Y., Lee, S., Kim, N., Park, K.Y., Kim, U., Kim, T., Kim, T.G., Choe, K.W., and Lee, J.S. (2000). The frequency of mutation in CCR5 gene among Koreans. *Int J STD AIDS*. 11:266–267.

Park, H.W. (1999). Infectious Diseases at the Chosun dynasty. *Infection*. 31:510–516.

Seo, H.J. (1999). Current Problems of Infectious Diseases (1975–1999). *Infection*. 31: 528–535.

Sung H., Foley B.T., Bae I.G., Chi H.S., and Cho Y.K. (2001). Phylogenetic analysis of reverse transcriptase in antiviral drug-naïve Korean HIV type 1 patients. *AIDS Res Hum Retroviruses*. 17(16):1549–1554.

UNAIDS. (2002) Report on the Global HIV/AIDS Epidemic 2002.

23

Transmission of HIV and Other Infections in Southeast Asia

Cultural and Genetic Factors

Chris Beyrer[1] and Henry Stephens[2]

[1]*Departments of Epidemiology and International Health, Johns Hopkins Bloomberg School of Public Health, Baltimore, Maryland, USA*

[2]*Institute of Urology and Nephrology, University College London, The Middlesex Hospital, London, UK*

INTRODUCTION

Southeast (SE) Asia is second only to Sub-Saharan Africa as the world's most heavily HIV/AIDS affected region in terms of number of infections (UNAIDS, 2002). While epidemic spread of HIV-1 began relatively late in the region, largely in the 1988–1990 period, the virus has spread widely and rapidly, and affected many millions in this densely populated, ethnically variable and politically diverse region. SE Asia includes some of the world's wealthier states (Singapore and Brunei), emerging economies (China, Thailand and Vietnam) and some of the poorest and most isolated nations (Burma and Laos). Its political spectrum spans emerging democracies, military dictatorships, Islamic Republics and three of the last five nominally communist states worldwide (China, Laos, and Vietnam). Also located in SE Asia are two of the world's leading heroin exporters, Burma and Laos (Beyrer, *et al.*, 2000). The ethnic and linguistic diversity of the region is extremely complex, as are the range of climates and ecologies—from rain forests and sparsely peopled mountains to overcrowded metropolises, with their associated socio-economic deprivations, poor housing and contaminated water supplies.

The range of infectious diseases affecting the peoples of SE Asia is as diverse as the peoples themselves: some parts of Burma and Laos are hyper-endemic zones for *P. falciparum* malaria, much of the region is affected by seasonal dengue outbreaks, and a wide array of other infectious pathogens cause endemic or epidemic diseases including scrub typhus, filariasis, hepatitis A, B and C viruses, typhoid, cholera, rabies, schistosomes, helminths, and mycoses. Understanding the dynamics of HIV and other disease spread across the region, and the ways HIV-1 interacts with the underlying human and biologic complexity is a challenge to epidemiology, virology, human and viral genetics, as well as to the political and social sciences. In a region as dynamic as SE Asia, attempting to understand these epidemics may yield vital insights into the future of HIV-1 spread, and the potential for vaccine induced control of this hyper-variable pathogen.

MAINLAND SE ASIA: LAND, POPULATIONS, LANGUAGES, ETHNICITY AND GENETICS

For the purposes of this exploration we can define mainland SE Asia as encompassing Burma, Thailand, Laos, Cambodia, Vietnam and Peninsular Malaysia; and three additional regions with close affinity to the mainland: Northeast India and Southeastern and Southwestern China. This area is often referred to as the Greater Mekong Subregion, for it is linked by the Mekong River and its tributaries (Figure 1). Geographic SE Asia is the tail end of the Himalayan mountain chain. It is cut by a series of great rivers, all of which come off the Tibetan Plateau to flow roughly South and East to the seas. The region can be seen as a series of these North–South running river valleys, which gradually fan out to highly fertile flood plains and deltas (Figure 1). These include the Irrawaddy, or Ayeyarwady, flood plain—the rice growing center of Burma; the Mekong, which supports the populations of Yunnan, Laos, Cambodia, and broadens to become the expansive Mekong Delta of South Vietnam; the Chao Phraya basin, the great central river system of Thailand; the Salween of Yunnan and the Shan States of Burma, and many other smaller bodies. These river valleys and lowland deltas have all been intensively cultivated for irrigated wet rice agriculture for millennia, and have long generated surpluses capable of supporting dense populations and advanced societies. The mountains above, however, have radically different climates and cultivation possibilities. Most of the chains are forested limestone Karsts, infertile and rugged. Because the valleys run north-south, each of the mountain ridges tends to be isolated from its neighbors, and little connection has ever been made by the mountain peoples across these ranges. While the dominant Burman, Thai, Lao, Vietnamese and Khmer rice growers of the lowlands built the great early civilizations of Pagan, Ayuthia and Angkor, the ethnically distinct and predominantly Sino-Tibetan mountain peoples still subsist on slash and burn agriculture and live in small shifting settlements little different from archaic times (Coedes, 1975). Only dry rice will grow in many of these mountain regions, and most are rainfall reliant. In the harshest zones, such as the stony Wa hill tracts of Burma, and the Karsts of northern Laos, the opium poppy, *Papaver somnifera*, has long been one of the few crops these tribal farmers could grow profitably (Beyrer, 1998).

The overall population in mainland SE Asia is estimated to be 344 million persons. This number includes the populations of the mainland states, an estimated 100 million Chinese in Yunnan and Guangxi Provinces combined, and the roughly 10 million residents of the Northeast Indian States of Manipur, Mizoram, and Nagaland on the India-Burma borders. It does not include the population of the Philippines, whose HIV epidemic appears to be unlinked epidemiologically to mainland SE Asia (UNAIDS, 2002). The rational for the inclusion of the Indian and Chinese regions becomes clear if we look beyond modern political boundaries to the ethnic and historical relationships of these regions. For example, the Manipuri people, the predominant ethnic group in Manipur State on the India–Burma border, are close linguistic and ethnic cousins of the Burmese, and their language is in the same sub-group of Tibeto-Burman as modern Burmese. In like manner, the formal name for Guangxi Province in Southeastern China, is the Guangxi Zhaung People's Autonomous Region. The Zhaung are a Daic people whose language is part of the same family which includes modern Thai, Lao, and Shan (the language of the Shan States of Eastern Burma) and which is unrelated to the Sino-Tibetan family to which modern

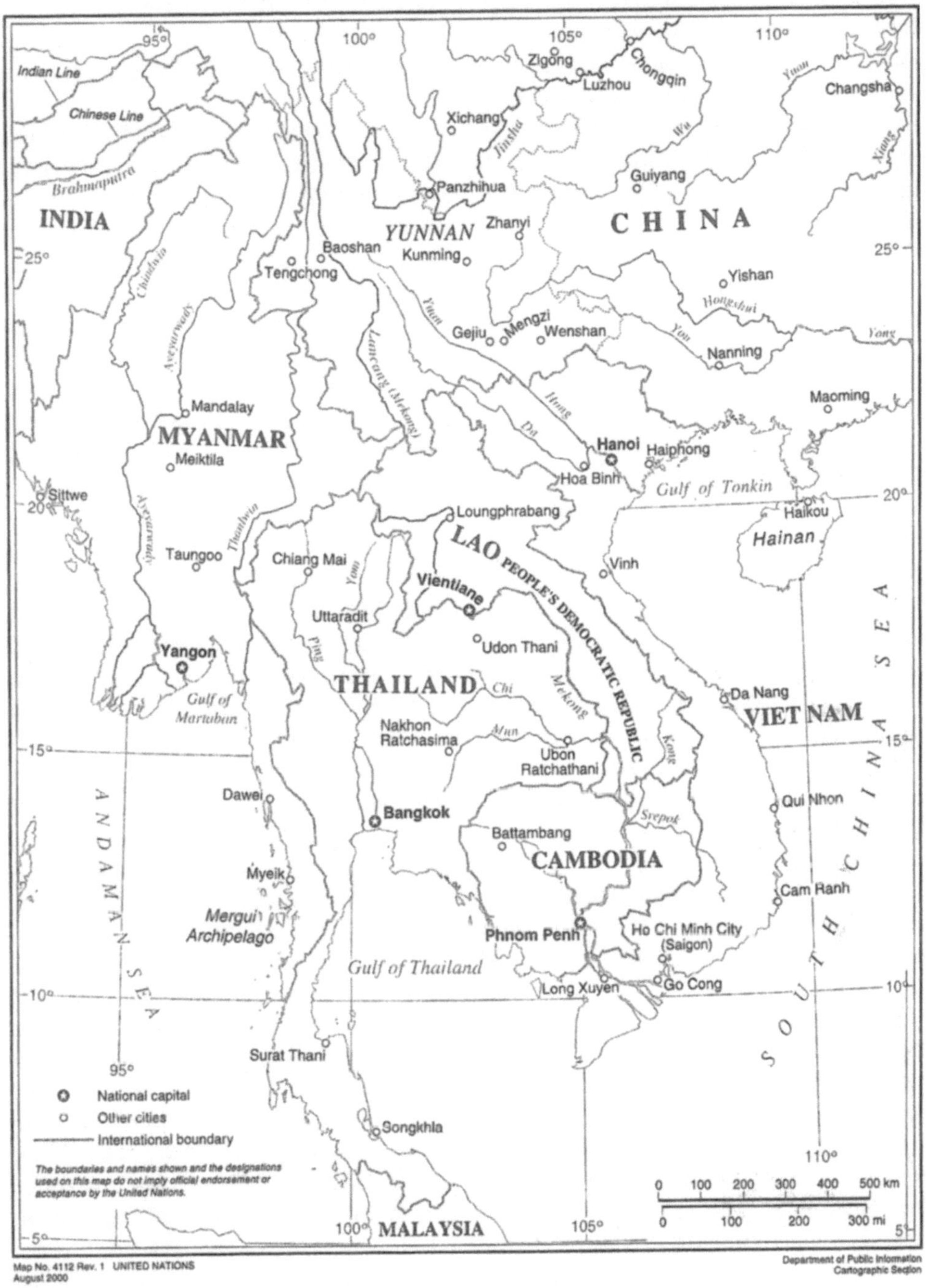

FIGURE 1. The Greater Mekong Subregion: Mainland Southeast Asia, Yunnan and Guangxi Provinces of China, and Northeast India.

Chinese belongs (Schliesinger, 2000). These linguistic relationships are recognized to be parallel markers of human genetic relationships (Cavalli-Sforza *et al.*, 1988), and hence immunogenetic relationships which may play important roles in host components of infectious disease resistance and spread in the region.

The emerging field of human genetic history is yielding a wide range of insights into this complex area. It is increasingly clear that SE Asia was one of the first areas inhabited by ancestral populations after leaving Africa. Early inhabitants of mainland and insular SE Asia were in turn ancestral to the peoples of Australia, China, and Polynesia as far east as Hawaii. Remnant populations, such as the Andaman Islanders off the Burma coast and the Semang (a negrito pygmy tribal people) of southern Thailand, appear to be virtually direct descendants of some of the first modern humans to have left Africa (Schliesinger, 2000). While the earliest human population spread was most likely north into mainland Asia, the movement of peoples in historical times has nearly always been south, out of the huge and populous mainland of East Asia into peninsular SE Asia. The Burmans of Burma moved south from Tibet to conquer the ancient Mon peoples. The Thais (Daic speakers) came out of their homelands in what is now Yunnan Province, China to populate the major river valleys of the region such as the Mekong, the Chao Phraya and the upper reaches of the Red River in north Vietnam. This led to the domination by the Thais of the indigenous Lawa peoples of modern day Thailand, Shan State in Burma, and Laos. The Vietnamese from the north (the Red River Delta) eventually conquered the Chams of Central Vietnam and the Khmers of the Mekong River Delta in the South to unify Vietnam. Among the mainland SE Asian States, Cambodia, with her majority population of Mon-Khmer people, may be somewhat unique in being peopled predominately by an indigenous ethnic group.

NARCOTICS AND HIV-1 DIVERSITY IN THE TRANSMISSION "HOT-ZONES"

The confluence of southwest China, Burma, Thailand, and Laos is known as the Golden Triangle, and it has long been one of the world's major opium poppy cultivation zones. As with other regions of high narcotic production, the insurgent wars between various ethnic groups and armed forces that have raged for the last 60 years in the Golden Triangle have exacerbated heroin production, trafficking, and its use in SE Asia (Lintner, 1994). Given the centrality of injecting drug use to the early spread of HIV in SE Asia, it is clear that we cannot understand HIV-1 spread in the region without an examination of the role of heroin and injection drug use (Beyrer, *et al.*, 2000). China, India, Burma, Thailand, Malaysia, and Vietnam have all had severe HIV-1 epidemics among injecting drug users (IDU) (Crofts *et al.*, 1998). In China, Malaysia and Vietnam, IDU account for the majority of reported infections; over 70% in all three countries. And across the region, IDU inject heroin, the refined product of opium poppy base. More than 90% of the region's heroin is from Burma, where the drug is exported as a highly pure injectable grade white powder called #4, for its four stage refinement (U.S. Department of State, 2003). In 2000, we reported on the relationship of overland trafficking of heroin from Burma and Laos on the HIV epidemics of the region (Beyrer *et al.*, 2000). Genetic analyses of HIV-1 sequence data from IDU along the regional heroin trafficking routes proved a powerful tool to understanding both HIV spread and the movement of narcotics and injection networks (Piyasirisilip *et al.*, 2000; McCutchan *et al.*, 2002 ; Takebe *et al.*, 2003). For example, we would assume that since the major heroin route north out of Vietnam into China followed the principal road and train route from Hanoi to the border crossing point at Pingxiang City in Guangxi Province (Figure 2), the HIV-1 subtype found in Pingxiang IDU would

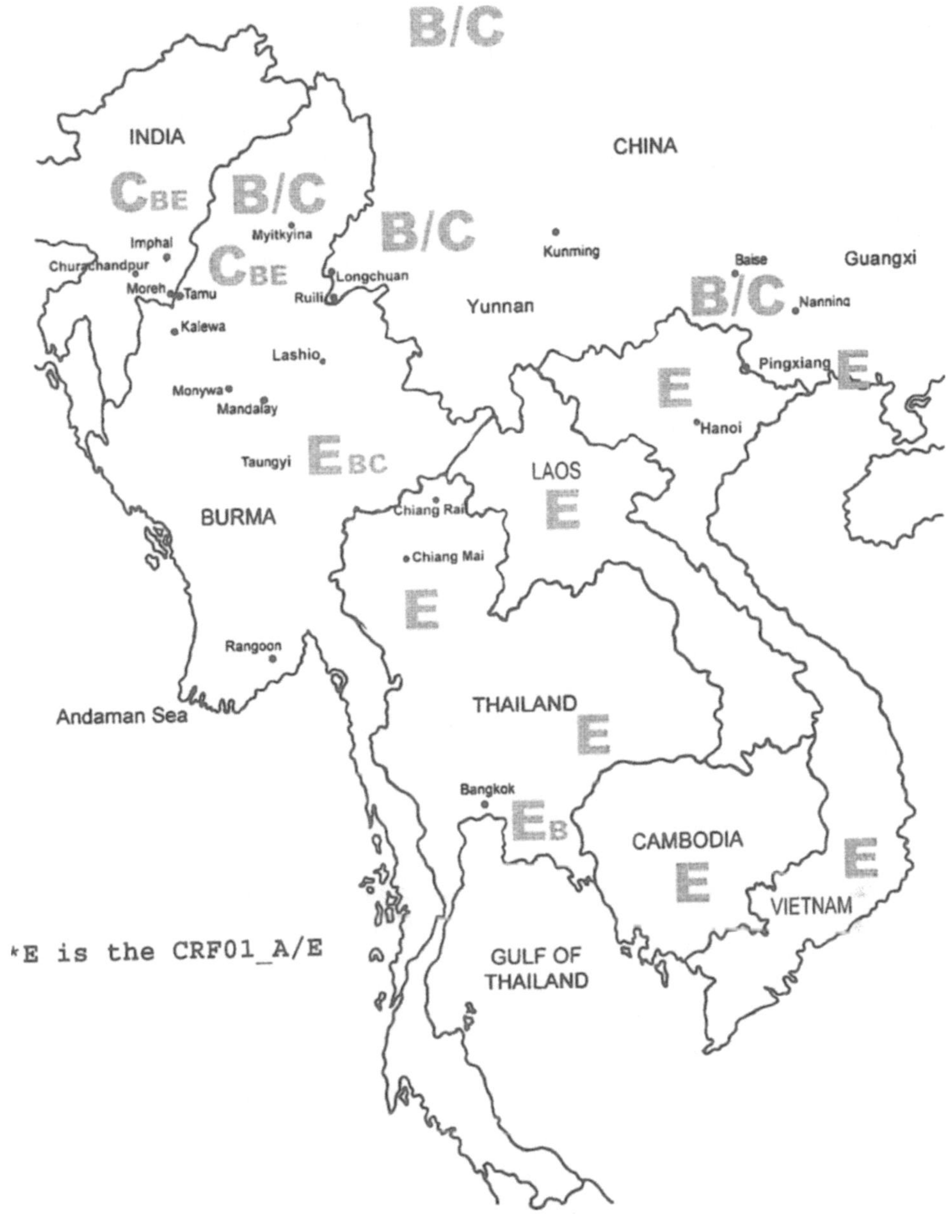

FIGURE 2. HIV-1 variants in the Greater Mekong Subregion, 2003. The B/C variants shown here are CRF07_B/C and CRF08_B/C and related recombinant forms. E is used for simplicity but always refers to the recombinant CRF01_A/E.

be similar to that found in HIV-infected IDU in northern Vietnam (Kato *et al.*, 1999). This was indeed the case—both were highly homogenous outbreaks of HIV-1 CRF01_A/E, generally referred to as subtype E (Yu *et al.*, 1999). But this subtype did not spread widely after its introduction into Guangxi Province. This is not because there are not IDU populations inland from the Vietnamese border—IDU are found throughout the Province, and indeed, another subtype of HIV-1 *has* spread widely among the drug users of central and northern Guangxi, a B/C recombinant virus that probably originated in upper Burma (Yu *et al.*, 1999; Piyasirisilip *et al.*, 2000; McCutchan *et al.*, 2002; Takebe *et al.*, 2003). A possible explanation may lie in the genetic make-up of the Guangxi Zhaung People's Autonomous Region. Before exploring this relationship, we must consider some host-viral interactions which may be relevant to disease spread.

HIV-1 MEETS HLA IN THE EAST

Trade routes facilitating the distribution of "black" economy products such as narcotics, together with the high-risk practices of IDU and limited prevention programs, act respectively as networks of transmission and nodes of amplification of HIV-1, in the large and vulnerable populations of mainland SE Asia. However, the observed segregation of HIV-1 CRF01_A/E in the ethnic Thais, Khmer, and Vietnamese, and HIV-1 B/C recombinants in the Han remains a paradox, as these populations intermix and share high-risk activities in the transmission hot zones of northern Vietnam and south-west China, Burma proper, and almost certainly in the Burma-Yunnan border zones, where all the viruses discussed here have been found in varying relative frequency (Yu *et al.*, 1999; McCutchan *et al.*, 2002; Takebe *et al.*, 2003). This segregation suggests a possible biological explanation for the population-based divergence of HIV-1 clades in SE Asians. Such a segregation could have an impact on future vaccine programs in the region, but could have wider impacts as well, as the relationship of population genetics to the spread of HIV-1 subtypes is little understood globally, and may become clearer, unfortunately, as HIV-1 continues to diversify as the pandemic reaches ever more human populations.

How might such population-pathogen interactions be mediated? Within the human genome, lies a dense cluster of genes on the short arm of chromosome 6, called the major histocompatibility complex or MHC, which spans some 3.6 megabases of DNA (Aguado *et al.*, 1999). At least 51, or 40% of the expressed MHC genes encode proteins that are involved in both acquired and innate immune responses to microbes (Aguado *et al.*, 1999). These include the classical class I and II human leukocyte antigens (HLA), which are transmembrane glycoproteins, whose biological function is to present endogenous (viral) and exogenous (bacterial) peptides to the antigen-specific T cell receptors of CD8+ cytolytic and CD4+ helper T cells, respectively. HLA class I molecules are also recognized by another group of receptors, that determine whether cells with innate natural killer (NK) activity spontaneously lyse virally infected cells (Parham, 2003). Thus, HLA class I molecules are essential recognition elements of both the acquired and innate immune responses to viruses.

The classical HLA class I (HLA-A, -B, -C) and class II (HLA-DR, DQ and DP) gene loci are highly polymorphic and each locus encodes hundreds of alleles, making these loci the most polymorphic loci in the human genome. The HLA-B locus is the most variable, encoding over 500 distinct alleles (see www.ebi.ac.uk/imgt/hla). This polymorphism is evident in different populations, as many alleles are detected at different frequencies, both within and between ethnic groups, be they African, Asian or Caucasoid in origin. Another feature of HLA class I and II genes is the phenomenon of linkage disequilibrium, where certain combinations of alleles encoded by different loci, tend to form stable haplotypes, which are inherited from one generation to another in a Mendelian fashion. Again, the composition and frequency of HLA haplotypes also varies between different ethnic groups. Thus, HLA class I and II alleles are recognized to be excellent markers of ethnicity, and the analysis of these genes has proved to be highly informative in anthropological studies (Cavalli-Sforza *et al.*, 1988).

However, the extreme polymorphism of HLA class I and II genes has a huge influence on the biological function of their products. Most of the polymorphism of these genes results in significant amino-acid changes in the first and second extracellular protein domains of HLA molecules, which affect the binding and subsequent presentation of microbial peptides to antigen-specific T cells. This has led to the concept that there are groups of HLA class I alleles or *supertypes,* with similar preferences for short antigenic peptides or *supermotifs* that share a similar structure (Sidney *et al.*, 1996). Our current understanding of HLA class I and II binding preferences, in terms of the size and composition of their bound peptides, contributes to the rational selection of target antigens in modern vaccines.

Fortunately, considerable information is available on the phenotypic and genetic diversity of HLA class I and II alleles and haplotypes in mainland SE Asian populations (Chandanayingyong *et al.*, 1994 and 1997; Stephens *et al.*, 2000). This is largely because high quality HLA typing was set up in Bangkok, Thailand, in the early 1970s and such work has further developed since. Ethnic Thais residing in Thailand and the related Dai, Dai Lue, Shan, Lao Loum, Black Tai, White Tai, and Red Tai ethnic groups in Burma, Yunnan and Guangxi Provinces of Southwest China, Laos, Cambodia, and Vietnam, comprise some 70 million people sharing a common language, spoken dialects, religion (Therevada Buddhism), architecture, agricultural practices, and culture (Chandanayinyong *et al.*, 1994). Ethnic Thais in Thailand proper are relatively homogeneous, probably because Thailand, unlike its neighboring countries, avoided European colonization in the 19th century. There is clear evidence from the analysis of HLA allele and haplotype profiles that Thai populations are highly representative of the genetic pool present in the large populations of this region (Chandanayingyong *et al.*, 1994 and 1997; Stephens *et al.*, 2000). For example, certain HLA-DR2 related class II allele and haplotype profiles that are characteristic of Thais (Stephens *et al.*, 2000), are also detected at similar frequencies in the dominant Vietnamese Kinh population of Vietnam (Vu-Trieu *et al.*, 1997), the Khmers of Cambodia (Goldfield *et al.*, 1998) and Indonesians from Java (Gao *et al.*, 1991). This is entirely consistent with the ethno-linguistic similarities and historic migrations between populations of the SE Asian mainland and the Indonesian archipelago (Stephens *et al.*, 2000). However, the same common DR2-related haplotypes, such as DRB1*1502, DRB5*0101, DQA1*0102, DQB1*0501, are rare in the dominant Han Chinese (non-Thai) populations of SW China (Stephens *et al.*, 2000, Gao *et al.*, 1991). Thus Thai-like genetic profiles dominate in much of SE Asia, and Han profiles dominate in China proper. The "mixing zone" of these two ethno-lingusitic branches is the southern China border regions with Burma, Laos, and Vietnam, which corresponds to the Chinese Provinces of Yunnan and Guangxi, precisely where the two major recombinant forms of HIV-1, CRF01_A/E and the group of B/C recombinants, are in circulation.

There is also evidence for inverse north-south gradients or clines of HLA allele and haplotype frequencies across the populations of SE Asia (Chandanayingyong *et al.*, 1994 and 1997; Stephens *et al.*, 2000). For example, the HLA-B22 group of class I alleles (HLA-B54, B55, B56), which have been associated with fast progression of HIV/AIDS in Caucasoids (Hendel *et al.*, 1999), is far more common in the Han groups of SW China than in ethnic Thais (Chandanayingyong *et al.*, 1997). Conversely, other major HLA class I and II alleles such as HLA-A33, B44 and DR7, which together can form a stable haplotype, are clearly more frequent in Thais and Vietnamese than in the southern Han of SW China (Chandanayingyong *et al.*, 1997). Herein lies a possible explanation for the apparent divergence of HIV-1 B/C variants into the more northerly Han populations of SW China and Burma, in contrast to

HIV-1 CRF01_A/E disseminating through the more southerly Thais and their HLA compatible Vietnamese Kinh and Cambodian Khmer populations. Namely, the current separation of HIV-1 clades in the large and diverse populations of SE Asia appears to correlate with major divisions within the immunogenetic profiles of those populations currently at risk of HIV-1 exposure.

THE HLA-A11 CONNECTION IN THAILAND

Detailed analyses of HIV-1 seroconverters have clearly shown that the presence or absence of certain HLA class I alleles correlates with the rate of developing AIDS in North American Caucasoids and African-Americans (Carrington *et al.*, 1999; Gao *et al.*, 2001). A similar picture has emerged from studies performed on HIV-1 infected cohorts identified in Africa (MacDonald *et al.*, 2000) and Western Europe (Hendel *et al.*, 1999; Flores-Villanueva *et al.*, 2003). There is also evidence that genes encoding certain HLA class I alleles and NK receptors are acting together to influence survival in the North American HIV-1 seroconverters (Martin *et al.*, 2002). By contrast, very little information is available on the influence of HLA gene and allele profiles on the development of AIDS in Asian HIV-1 seroconverters. However, a variety of studies involving cohorts of HIV-1 exposed ethnic Thais (Beyrer *et al.*, 1999; Sriwanathana *et al.*, 2001) are worth further review in the context of what may be the genetic basis of protective immune responses to HIV-1 infection in mainland SE Asians.

At the Berlin International AIDS conference of 1993, the first reports were revealed of HLA class I alleles associating with an apparent resistance to HIV-1 infection in a group of East African female sex workers (FSW) (Plummer *et al.,* 1993). These women had been highly exposed to HIV-1 but remained persistently seronegative (HEPS). Soon after, HLA class I restricted CTL responses to a variety of immunogenic peptides derived from HIV-1 Gag, Pol and Nef proteins, were also described in a similar cohort of West African HEPS FSW (Rowland-Jones *et al.*, 1995). Around the same period, a small but highly informative cohort of ethnic Thai HEPS FSW were identified in Chiang Mai and Chiang Rai in Northern Thailand (Beyrer *et al.,* 1999; Sriwanathana *et al.*, 2001), a region where the first introduction of HIV-1 clade CRF01_A/E had occurred some 10 years previously. It quickly became clear through HLA typing of these Northern Thai HEPS FSW that a significant proportion of these women were carrying the HLA-A11 antigen, as identified by classical serotyping in Bangkok (Beyrer *et al.*, 1999; Sriwanathana *et al.*, 2001). Molecular confirmation of alleles encoding HLA-A11 antigens, using a variety of PCR-based techniques including direct sequencing, has demonstrated a preponderance of HLA-A*1101 in these HEPS FSW (Stephens and Chanadanayingyong, unpublished observations). Given that HLA-A11 is a prevalent class I antigen in SE Asian populations (Chandanayingyong *et al.*, 1997), the presence of the A*1101 allele in the Northern Thai HEPS FSW came as no surprise, at least to the HLA researchers in Bangkok. However, the frequency was substantially higher when compared to the known Northern Thai population frequency for HLA-A11 (Beyrer *et al.*, 1999; Sriwanathana *et al.*, 2001). This suggested that a common host cytolytic mechanism, directed against HIV-1 and utilizing the HLA-A11 molecule, was occurring in the Northern Thai HEPS FSW.

HIV-1 *NEF*—A SUITABLE CANDIDATE FOR PRESENTATION BY HLA-A11 IN ETHNIC THAIS

By the mid-1990s, the Los Almos database had already accrued considerable information on HIV-1 immunogenic peptides, known to drive HLA class I allele- restricted antigen-specific CTL and proliferative responses in different populations (Korber *et al.*, 1996). From this database, it was reasonably easy for researchers in Bangkok to predict which potential peptides were likely to be driving HLA–A11 restricted CTL responses in ethnic Thais. The HIV-1 Nef protein came under close scrutiny, as this product was known to down-regulate HLA expression on HIV-1 infected cells, a molecular mechanism used by a variety of viruses to evade immune recognition, and it also acted as early infectivity factor for the virus (Collins *et al.*, 1998). One particular HIV-1 Nef-derived peptide, QVPLRPMTYK (positions 73–82), came under particular attention in Bangkok. This peptide had already been used to demonstrate HLA-A11 restricted CTL activity against HIV-1 in asymptomatic HIV-negative partners in discordant Caucasoid couples (Langlade-Demoyen *et al.*, 1994) and in asymptomatic HIV-positive Caucasoids (Coullin *et al.*, 1994), as well as CTL activity in West African HEPS FSW (Rowland-Jones *et al.*, 1995). In turn, the same HIV-1 Nef 73–82 peptide also proved to be a target of HLA-A11-restricted CTL activity in some of the Northern Thai HEPS FSW (Sriwanathana *et al.*, 2001).

It was also apparent, by the mid-1990s, that HIV-1 Nef pos 73–82 was under direct immunological pressure. Sequencing of HIV-1 clade E isolates from infected Thais had shown a variety of mutations in this peptide (Artenstein *et al.*, 1996), which had probably occurred within the 10 years since the introduction of HIV-1 clade CRF01_A/E into this population. However, the mutations do not appear to affect positions 74 and 82 of the HIV-1 Nef 73-82 peptide (Artenstein *et al.*, 1996), which are thought to be the critical anchor positions of the HLA-A11 binding antigen *supermotif,* recognized by the HLA-A3 *supertype* of HLA class I alleles (HLA-A*0301, A*1101, A*3101. A*3301 and A*6801), which share common preferences in the types of peptides they bind (Sidney *et al.*, 1996). Indeed, the putative HLA-A11 *supermotif* anchor residues Val74 and Lys82 present in Nef 73-82 peptide appear to be highly conserved in all clades of HIV-1, as well as HIV-2, SIVmac and SIVcpz (Korber *et al.*, 2002), suggesting that they are biologically necessary for productive infection. Furthermore, the region of HIV-1 *nef* containing the 73-82 peptide is saturated with overlapping CTL epitopes, recognized by a variety of class I alleles, such as HLA-A2, -A3, -A11, -B7, -B8, -B27, -B35 and -B60 (Korber *et al.*, 2002), which are common in many populations, including SE Asians (Chandanayingyong *et al.*, 1997). Taken together, this CTL epitope-dense region of the HIV-1 Nef protein, may be a strong contender for inclusion in future vaccines designed to reduce viraemia and induce protection against HIV-1 exposure.

HLA-A11—A SUITABLE CANDIDATE FOR NK RECOGNITION

Our current understanding of mature, circulating, cytolytic T cells is that they express a variety of receptors that mediate the lysis of virally infected cells (Ugloni and Vivier, 2001). Many of these receptors facilitate innate NK lysis of target cells. There are two major groups of NK receptors, the killer immunoglobulin-like receptors (KIR) and the lectin like receptors (NKG2), encoded on chromosomes 12 and 19, respectively (Middleton *et al.*, 2002). Depending on the structure of their cytoplasmic domains, NK KIRs can either functionally activate or inhibit NK lysis after interacting with their ligands, which are HLA class I molecules (Middleton *et al.*, 2002). Some NK KIR gene loci are ubiquitous and present in all individuals, while other loci are polygenic and can be either present or absent in certain individuals (Norman *et al.*, 2001 and 2002). NK KIR gene loci are also highly polymorphic (Carrington and Norman, 2003; Marsh *et al.*, 2003), and at least one locus (3DS1) has been associated with AIDS survival (Martin *et al.*, 2002).

One of the ubiquitous NK KIR gene loci, called 3DL2, encodes an inhibitory receptor that only recognizes the HLA-A3 *supertype* of class I alleles, including HLA-A11 (Pende *et al.*, 1996; Middleton *et al.*, 2002). Under normal circumstances, when 3DL2 interacts with HLA-A11, an inhibitory signal is transmitted to the NK cell, and lysis of the target cell is prevented. However, there is evidence that when HLA-A11 molecules are loaded with viral peptides *in vitro*, inhibitory signaling is curtailed and NK lysis of targets resumes (Gavioli *et al.*, 1996). The KIR-3DL2 locus has been detected in all individuals tested so far, including ethnic Thais (Norman *et al.*, 2001 and 2002). KIR-3DL2 would also appear to be the most polymorphic of the KIR receptors (Marsh *et al.*, 2003) and it forms dimers on the surface of NK cells (Pende *et al.*, 1996). Thus, we have a highly polymorphic NK receptor, probably expressed as a dimer in all ethnic Thais, which specifically recognizes HLA-A11 that can also dimerize (Li *et al.*, 2002). The overall outcome of this interaction, in terms of NK lysis, may depend on whether HLA-A11 is loaded with viral peptides. Could this be pure coincidence with the prevalence of HLA-A11 in the Northern Thai HEPS FSW? Or is it a serendipitous correlation with resistance to HIV-1 infection? Such issues may be resolved by further analysis of NK receptor gene and allele profiles in this unique cohort of HIV-1 exposed but uninfected mainland SE Asians. At present, the biological relevance of NK KIR polymorphism is unclear, but there are certainly allelic variations between different ethnic groups (Norman *et al.*, 2001 and 2002), which, in turn, may correlate with the known population variations of NK activity in HIV-1 infected individuals, including ethnic Thais (De Souza *et al.*, 2000).

RELEVANCE TO OTHER ENDEMIC INFECTIONS—TUBERCULOSIS, MALARIA, DENGUE, HEPATITIS B AND C

Tuberculosis

The analysis of HLA allele associations with infectious diseases in SE Asian populations remained a relatively neglected field until the early 1990's. However, considerable evidence has since accumulated suggesting that HLA alleles associate with the severity of dengue virus infections, (Stephens *et al.*, 2002), typhoid fever (Dunstan *et al.*, 2001), hepatitis C (Vejbaeysa *et al.*, 2000), meliodosis (Darakul *et al.*, 1998), malaria (Stephens *et al.*, 1995; Hirayama *et al.*, 1996; Buson *et al.*, 2002), and tuberculosis (Goldfield *et al.*, 1998; Vejbaeysa *et al.*, 2002), which are all endemic in mainland SE Asia. Much concern has developed over the inevitable occurrence of co-infections of HIV-1 with malaria or tuberculosis. Throughout the region, tuberculosis is the most common opportunistic infection seen in clinical AIDS, and TB rates among young adults have expanded dramatically in Thailand, Burma, and Cambodia (Chariyalertsak *et al.*, 2001). Re-activation of previous exposure to *Mycobacterium tuberculosis* is well documented in HIV-1 infected Northern Thais (Yanai *et al.*, 1996). Worldwide there is considerable evidence that HLA-DR2 related alleles and haplotypes, which are very common and diverse in SE Asians (Gao *et al.*, 1991; Chandanayingyong *et al.*, 1997; Stephens *et al.*, 2000), also associate with susceptibility to developing tuberculosis (Khomenko *et al.*, 1990). However, immunogenetic studies testing for associations between HLA alleles and the development of latent TB infections in

HIV-1 exposed individuals have yet to be performed.

Malaria

Malaria is an important pathogen with a strikingly uneven distribution in the region. Malaria morbidity and mortality rates are highly variable across the region, and correlate with the vector's preferred habitat of mountain forests and their resident ethnic groups. Malaria death rates are low in Southern China, most of Thailand, and most of Vietnam (Kidson *et al.*, 1999). By contrast, malaria disease and death rates are very high, in the 50–150/100,000 population range, in forest and mountain parts of Burma, most of Laos, and some parts of Cambodia (Nihei *et al.*, 2002). Labor-intensive forest encroachment for the logging of hard woods and mining of natural resources has increased the risk of exposure to malaria and co-infection with HIV-1, as co-infection among Burmese migrant workers in these zones is not uncommon. Chaotic and under-funded essential drug programs in Burma, Laos and Cambodia appear to have contributed to multi-drug resistant *P. falciparum* malaria outbreaks, and *P. falciparum* strains from these states are commonly resistant to chloroquine, antifolates, quinine, and mefloquine. (Wongsrichanalai *et al.*, 2002). Resistance to artesunate and artemisinin has also been found among *P. falciparum* isolates from the region (Picard *et al.*, 2003). For Thailand, malaria is virtually synonymous with border areas: her cases come largely from the forest/mountain regions on her western border with Burma, and her eastern border with Cambodia (Kidson, 1999). The ongoing civil conflict in Burma contributes substantially to the malaria disease burden: urban Burmese continue to flee east to Thailand through the dense malaria zones of the Thai–Burma border, many encountering forest malaria for the first time in adult life. Much of the malaria morbidity and mortality in this region occurs among Burmese migrants and refugees (Chareonviriyaphap *et al.*, 2001). While malaria disease rates are highest in Burma, Laos and Cambodia, the mortality differences also likely reflect much more limited health services and hence, death rates from cerebral malaria, renal failure, and the like. Clearly, this will be true for AIDS mortality as it is for malaria deaths: Thai citizens already have some access to anti-virals, while Burmese and Laotians, particularly in the mountain zones, cannot access HIV testing, much less AIDS care (Cohen, 2003). While Laos remains a very low prevalence country for HIV-1, Burma has among the most severe epidemics in the region, with a population prevalence estimated at 3.46% of reproductive age adults (Beyrer *et al.*, 2003b). Cambodia has the second highest HIV rate in the region, and high malaria morbidity and mortality as well. HIV-1 and malaria interactions are, therefore, likely to be problematic, mainly in Burma and Cambodia: both countries with multi-drug resistant *P. falciparum.*

Dengue Virus

Dengue virus infections in SE Asia appear to follow a very different pattern from malaria or HIV-1. The primary vector for this acute virus infection is the *Aedes aegypti* mosquito. This mosquito thrives in both the sprawling tropical capitals of the region and in rural environments. Dengue virus attack rates do not track disturbances in civil society or heroin trafficking routes through mountain ranges. However, outbreaks of dengue have been increasing in frequency and severity in the region. This phenomenon is little understood, but seems to correlate with temperature fluctuations associated with recent climatic changes, such as the "*El Nino*" phenomenon. Primary and secondary infections can occur with all four of the major dengue virus serotypes, which are in seasonal circulation in SE Asia. Exposure to dengue virus can result in either asymptomatic infections, clinical dengue fever (DF), or the more severe dengue hemorrhagic fever (DHF). Both DF and DHF are essentially untreatable except for supportive therapy in the case of DHF. In secondary dengue virus exposures, a memory immune response is induced that can both clear the infecting virus and contribute to disease pathology. There is clear evidence in ethnic Thais that certain HLA class I alleles associate with clinical outcome of secondary dengue exposure and the infecting virus serotype in previously exposed and immunologically primed individuals (Stephens *et al.*, 2002). Furthermore, the analysis of HLA-A11 restricted responses to dengue during the acute viraemic phase of infection in ethnic Thais has indicated that some CTL responses may be stunned or ineffective in secondary infections (Mongkolsapaya *et al.*, 2003). However, HLA-A11 would only appear to associate with susceptibility to severe secondary infections with one particular dengue serotype (Stephens *et al.*, 2002), and a detailed analysis of CTL responses driven by HLA class I alleles that associate with resistance to severe disease has yet to be performed. Nevertheless, the possibility that stunned cross-reactive CTL responses occur after secondary or multiple exposures to different clades of HIV-1 in SE Asians remains unexplored, although this possibility may have an impact on the efficacy of future HIV-1 vaccines in this region.

Hepatitis B and C Virus

East Asian populations have long been known to have high endemic rates of Hepatitis B virus (Nelson and Thomas, 2001). Indeed, field trials of HBV vaccines were conducted in Taiwan in the 1980s due to the exceptionally high population prevalence among reproductive age adults there (Beasley *et al.*, 1981). These HBV rates appear to play a role in making hepatocellular carcinoma one of the leading causes of cancer death in China and SE Asia. HCV in these populations is distinctly different. While population rates of HBV have long been high, HCV has seen explosive spread through injecting drug use, and hence has moved along the same heroin-IDU pathway in the region as HIV-1. HCV rates in IDU are very high in the region wherever they have been assessed. Indeed, in cohort studies among drug users in Chiang Mai, rates were so high (over 90%), that an analysis comparing HCV positive and negative IDU was impossible due to a classic "ceiling effect" (Razak *et al.*, 2003). Similar rates have been found in Chinese populations, though many fewer studies, relative to the scale of the epidemic, have been done. Preliminary disease association studies of HCV in ethnic Thais have indicated that certain HLA class II alleles associate with both transient and persistent HCV infection, as well as overall protection against disease (Vejbaeysa *et al.*, 2000). Since HCV, like HIV, has multiple subtypes, it may be that HLA and ethno-linguistic associations with this virus would help elucidate HCV epidemiology in the region.

PUBLIC HEALTH AND THE PROSPECTS FOR HIV PREVENTION AND CONTROL

Whatever the genetic relationships between HIV variants and human populations, two things are abundantly clear: preventive measures can work, and they are currently underused. HIV-1 epidemics among drug users have been contained and reduced in a number of countries including Australia, Brazil, the Netherlands and the UK (Des Jarlais and Friedman, 1998). Provision of those tools known to have efficacy for prevention of IDU transmission, including harm reduction, needle and syringe exchange, and drug treatment (methadone and buprenorphine on demand) can have major impacts on reducing the spread of blood-borne pathogens among injectors and their sex partners (Des Jarlais and Friedman, 1998). When we look across SE Asia, China, and India, however, the use of these tools is limited or absent (Crofts *et al.*, 1998). Among Asian nations, only Hong Kong provides both harm reduction and modern drug treatment on demand.

If prevention services are lacking for drug users in Asian communities, they are even more severely limited in Asia's prison systems. While very little information is available from many such prisons, it is clear in the case of the Thai epidemic that the Bangkok prison system played a key role in the early spread of HIV in the country (Choopanya *et al.*, 1991). In the Thai prison system, drug treatment is limited, needles and syringes are unavailable, but heroin is available, at least in some settings. This means that needle and equipment sharing is the norm for incarcerated drug users, and time in prison has been shown to be causally linked to HIV seroconversion among incarcerated drug users (Choopanya *et al.*, 2002). In the Choopanya study, the HIV infection rate among incarcerated drug users was over 30% per year, as opposed to less than 4% per year among those out of prison. Such high transmission prison settings may both concentrate and mix IDU from diverse networks and regions, and may play a crucial, but little understood, role in the dissemination of HIV subtypes.

Where sexual spread predominates, in Cambodia, Thailand, and parts of Burma, prevention has been strikingly more successful for those at sexual risk than among IDU. Both Thailand and Cambodia have seen substantial declines in HIV infection rates among pregnant women, indicating a general decline in new infections among sexually active adults (UNAIDS, 2002). Early on, Vietnam embraced and adapted the Thai prevention model (the 100% Condom Campaign for commercial sex venues) and may have largely prevented heterosexual spread. Unfortunately, however, the limitations on prevention for IDU means that ongoing sexual spread from IDU to their wives and girlfriends will continue in most SE Asian states. This may allow for further study of the host–viral pathogen interactions we have discussed.

In many respects, the immunological stage is now well set in terms of the HIV-1 epidemic in mainland SE Asian populations. Concurrent epidemics of HIV-1 CRF01_A/E and B/C variants are moving rapidly through some of the most densely populated regions of the world. The size and homogeneity of SE Asian populations contrast starkly with the relatively lower density but extreme genetic diversity of African populations at risk of HIV-1 exposure. There is already good evidence that the HIV-1 viruses, emerging after circulating for many years in Caucasoid HIV-1 seroconverters, are assiduously mutating in the key immunogenic regions or epitopes that are recognized by the prevalent HLA alleles in these populations (Moore *et al.*, 2002). If HLA is molding the HIV-1 virus in Caucasoids, then it is reasonable to assume that a similar phenomenon is occurring in SE Asians, as indicated by sequencing studies of viruses derived from infected ethnic Thais (Artenstein *et al.*, 1996), the original seed population of the SE Asian epidemic. The extensive information already available on immune response (HLA) gene and allele profiles in SE Asians will enable and facilitate further large-scale population-based investigations, with the power to make meaningful regional extrapolations on the genetic basis of susceptibility and resistance to HIV/AIDS. This can be achieved by utilizing local expertise and knowledge through establishing regional networks of collaborations, which could contribute to the rational design of future vaccines.

SE Asia will likely remain a region of sharp contrasts. While the modern Thai state is an emerging democracy and a regional economic power, Laos remains on the United Nations list of the world's 10 least developed nations. Malaria deaths are tragically common along the Thai–Burma border, while almost unheard-of in urban Bangkok. The regional narcotics economy shows no sign of abating, and HIV-1 spread continues apace in Southern China, threatening an enormous population. While these are challenges for individuals, communities, and countries, they are also regional challenges, and are likely to require regional solutions. This is well understood by public health authorities in the region, and increasingly by international donors. HIV/AIDS and malaria efforts are increasingly managed under a Greater Mekong Subregion framework within WHO and UNDP, for example. And the regional political body, ASEAN (The Association of Southeast Asian Nations) has public health task forces working on HIV/AIDS, tropical diseases, and increasing partnership across political borders. Such collaborations may be the key to addressing these regional challenges to the health of the people of SE Asia. It would not be the first time that public health has led the way in regional cooperation and improved relations. The peoples of the region certainly deserve no less.

REFERENCES

Aguado, B., Bahram, S., Beck, S., Campbell, R.D., Forbes, S.A., Geraghty, D., Guillaudeux, T., Hood, L., Horton, R., Inoko, H., Janer, M., Jasoni, C., Madan, A., Milne, S., Neville, M., Oka, A., Qin, S., Ribas-Despuig, G., Rogers, J., Rowen, L., Shiina, T., Spies, T., Tamiya, G., Tashiro, H., Trowsdale, J., Vu, Q., Williams, L., and Yamazaki, M. (1999). Complete sequence and gene map of a human major histocompatibility complex. *Nature* 401:921–923.

Artenstein, A.W., Hegerich, P.A., Beyrer, C., Rungruengthanakit, K., Michael, N.L., and Natrapan, C. (1996). Sequences and phylogenetic analysis of the *nef* gene from Thai subjects harboring subtype E HIV-1. *AIDS Res Hum Retroviruses* 12:557–560.

Beasley, R.P., Hwang, L.-Y., Lin, C.-C., and Chien, C.-S. (1981). Hepatocellular carcinoma and hepatitis B viru s: A prospective study of 22,707 men in Taiwan. *Lancet* 2:1129–1133.

Beyrer, C. (1998). *War in the Blood: Sex, Politics, and AIDS in Southeast Asia.* Zed Books, London. (Second Edition, 2000. Thai Language Edition, "*Songkram Nai Luat,*" Chulalongkorn University Press, Bangkok, 2002).)

Beyrer, C., Artenstein, A., Rungpao, S., Stephens, H., VanCott, T., Robb, M., Rinkaew, M., Birx, D., Khamboonruang, C., Zimmerman, P., Nelson, K.E., and Natpratan, C. (1999). Epidemiologic and biologic characterization of a cohort of HIV-1 highly exposed, persistently seronegative commercial sex workers in Northern Thailand. *JID* 179:59–67.

Beyrer, C., Razak, MH., Lisam, K., Wei, L., Chen, J., and Yu, X.F. (2000). Overland heroin trafficking routes and HIV spread in South and SE Asia. *AIDS* 14:1–9.

Beyrer, C., Juttiwutikarn, J., Teokul, W., Razak, M.H., Suriyanon, V., Srirak, N., Pripaipan, T., Vonchuk, T., Tovanabutra, S., Sripaipan, T., and Celentano, D.D. (2003a). Drug use, increasing incarceration rates, and prison associated HIV risks in Thailand. *AIDS & Behavior* 2(7):153–161.

Beyrer, C., Razak, M.H., Labrique, A., and Brookmeyer, R. (2003b). Assessing the magnitude of the HIV/AIDS epidemic in Burma. *J AIDS* 32:311–317.

Buson, M., Vu Trieu, A., Labelle, P., Phan-Van, K., Ho-Quang, H., Bouteiller, A.M., Bieux, H., Charron, D., and Hors, J. (2002). HLA-DRB1 and DQB1 allele distribution in the Muong population exposed to malaria in Vietnam. *Tissue Antigens* 59:470–474.

Carrington, M. and Norman, P. (2003). The KIR gene Cluster. 1 ed. National Library of Medicine, National Center for Biotechnology Information, Vol. 2003.

Carrington, M., Nelson, G.W., Martin, M.P., Kissner, T., Vlahov, D., Goedert, J.J., Kaslow, R., Buchbinder, S., Hoots, K., and O'Brien, S.J. (1999). HLA and HIV-1: Heterozgote advantage and B*35-Cw*04 disadvantage. *Science* 283:1748–1752.

Cavalli-Sforza, L.L. (2000). *Genes, Peoples, and Languages.* North Point Press, New York.

Cavalli-Sforza, L.L., Piazza, A., Menozzi, M., and Mountain, J. (1988). Reconstruction of human evolution: Bringing together genetic, archeological, and linguistic data. *Proc Natl Acad Sci. USA* 85:6002–6006.

Chandanayingyong, D., Stephens, H.A.F., Fan. L.A., Sirkong, M., Longta, P., Vangseratthana, R., Lekmak, S., Longta, K., Bejrachandra, S., and Rungruang, E. (1994). HLA-DP polymorphism in the Thais of Southeast Asia. *Hum Immunol.* 40:20–24.

Chandanayingyong, D., Stephens, H.A.F., Klaythong, R., Sirkong, M., Udee, S., Longta, P., Chantangpol, R., Bejrachandra, S., and Runruang, E. (1997). HLA-A, -B, -DRB1, -DQA1 and DQB1 polymorphism in Thais. *Hum Immunol.* 53:174–182.

Chareonviriyaphap, T., Bangs, M.J., and Ratanatham, S. (2001). Status of malaria in Thailand. *Southeast Asian J. Trop. Med. & Public Health* 31:225–235.

Chariyalertsak, S., Sirisanthana, T., Saengwonloey, O., and Nelson, K.E. (2001). Clinical presentation and risk behaviors of AIDS patients in Thailand, 1994–1998: Regional variation and temporal trends. *Clinical Infect Dis.* 32(6):955–962.

Chazee', L. (1999). *The Peoples of Laos: Rural and Ethnic Diversities.* White Lotus Press, Bangkok.

Choopanya, K., Vanichseni, S., Des Jarlais, D.J., Plangsringgarm, K., Sonchai, W., Carballo, M.,

Friedmann, P., and Friedman, S.R. (1991). Risk factors and HIV seropositivity among injecting drug users in Bangkok. *AIDS* 5:1509–1513.

Choopanya, K., Des Jarlais, D.C., Vanichseni, S., Kitayaporn, D., Mock, P.A., Raktham, S., Hireanras, K., Heyward, W.L., Sujarita, S., and Mastro, T.D. (2002). Incarceration and risk for HIV infection among injection drug users in Bangkok. *J AIDS* 29:86–94.

Chu J.Y., Huang W, Kuang S.Q, (et al)?. (1998). Genetic relationship of populations in China. *Proc Natl Acad Sci.* 95:11763–11768.

Coedes, G. (1975). *The Indianized States of Southeast Asia*. University of Hawaii Press, Honolulu.

Cohen, J. (2003). AIDS In Asia. *Science* 301(5640):1613–1796.

Collins, K. L., Chen, B.K., Kalams, S.A., Walker, B.D., and Baltimore, D. (1998). HIV-1 Nef protein protects infected primary cells against killing by cytotoxic T lymphocytes. *Nature* 391:397–401.

Coullin, I., Culmann-Penciolelli, B., Gomard, E., Choppin, J., Levy, J.-P., Guillet, J.-G., and Saragosti, S. (1994). Impaired cytotoxic T lymphocyte recognition due to genetic variations in the main immunogenic region of the human immunodeficiency virus 1 NEF protein. *J Exp Med.* 180:1129–1134.

Crofts, N., Reid, G., and Deany, P. (1998). Injecting drug use and HIV infection in Asia.
The Asian Harm Reduction Network. *AIDS* 12 Suppl B:S69–78.

Darakul, T., Vejbaeysa, S., Chaowagul, W., Luangtrakool, P., Stephens, H.A. F., and Sirirurg, S. (1998). HLA-DR and DQ associations with Meliodosis. *Hum Immunol.* 59: 580–586.

Des Jarlais, D.C., and Friedman, S.R. (1998). Fifteen years of research on preventing HIV infection among injecting drug users: What we have learned, what we have not learned, what we have done, what we have not done. *Public Health Rep.* 113 Suppl 1:182–188.

De Souza, M.S., Karnasuta, C., Brown A.E., Markowitz, L.E., Nitayaphan, S., Garner, R.P., McNeil, J.G., Birx, D.L., and Cox, J.H. (2000). A comparative study of the impact of HIV infection on natural killer cell number and function in Thais and North Americans *AIDS Res Hum Retroviruses* 16:1061–1066.

Dunstan, S.J., Stephens, H.A.F., Blackwell J.M., Duc, C.M., Lanh, M. N., Dudbridge, F., Phuong, C.X.T., Luxemberger, C., Wain, J., Ho V.A., Hien, T.T., Farrar, J., and Dougan, G. (2001). Genes of the Class II and Class III Major Histocompatibility Complex are associated with typhoid fever in Vietnam. *J. Inf. Dis.* 183:261–268.

Flores-Villanueva, P.O., Hendel, H., Caillat-Zucman, S., Rappaport, J., Burgos-Tiburcio, A., Bertin-Maghit, S., Ruiz-Morales, J.A., Teran, M.E., Rodriguez-Tafur, J., and Zagury, J.-F. (2003). Associations of MHC ancestral haplotypes with resistance/susceptibility to AIDS disease development. *J Immunol.* 170:1925–1929.

Gao, F., Bailes, E., Robertson, D.L., Chen Y., Rodenburg, C.M., Michael, S., Cummins, L.B., Arthur, L.O., Peeters, M., Shaw, G.M., Sharp, P.M., and Hahn, B. (1999). Origin of HIV-1 in the chimpanzee *Pan trogolodytes trogolodytes. Nature* 397:436–441.

Gao, X., and Serjeantson, S.W. (1991). Heterogeneity of HLA-DR2-related DR, DQ haplotypes in eight populations of Asia-Oceania. *Immunogenetics* 34:401–407.

Gao, X., Nelson, G.W., Karacki, P., Martin, M., P., Phair, J., Kaslow, R., Goedert, J.J., Buchbinder, S., Hoots, K., Vlahov, D., O'Brien, S.J., and Carrington, M. (2001). Effect of a single amino acid change in MHC class I molecules on the rate of progession of AIDS *N Engl J Med.* 344:1668–1675.

Gavioli, R., Zhang, Q-J., and Masucci, M.G. (1996). HLA-A11-mediated protection from NK cell-mediated lysis. Role of HLA-A11-presented peptides. *Hum Immunol* 49:1–12.

Goldfield, A.E., Delgado, J.C., Thim, S., Bozon, M.V., Uglialoro, A.M., Turbay, D., Cohen, C., and Yunis, E.J. (1998). Association of an HLA-DQ allele with clinical tuberculosis. *J A M A.* 279:226–228.

Hendel, H., Caillat-Zucman, S., Lebuanec, H., Carrington, M., O'Brien, S., Andrieu, J.M., Schachter, F., Zagury, D., Rappaport, J., Winkler, C., Nelson, G.W., and Zagury, J.-F. (1999). New class I and II HLA alleles strongly associated with opposite patterns of progression to AIDS. *J Immunol.* 162:6942–6946.

Hirayama, K., Zaidi, A.S., Lokman Hakim, S., Kimura, A., Ong, K.J., Kikuchi, M., Nasuruddin, H.A., Kojima, S., and Mak, J W. (1996). Molecular analysis of HLA-B in Malaysian aborigines. *Tissue Antigens* 48:692–697.

Kato, K., Shiino, T., and Kusagawa, S. (1999). Genetic similarity of HIV-1 subtype E in a recent outbreak among injecting drug users in Northern Vietnam to strains in Guangxi Province of Southern China. *AIDS Res & Hum Retroviruses* 15(13):1157–1168.

Khomenko, A.G., Litvinov, V.I., Chukanova, V.P., and Pospelov, L.E. (1990). Tuberculosis in patients with various HLA phenotypes. *Tubercle* 71:187–192.

Kidson, C., Singhasivanon, P., Supavey, S. (eds.). (1999). Mekong Malaria. Malaria, multi-drug resistance and economic development in the Greater Mekong subregion of Southeast Asia. *SE Asian J Trop Med Public Health*, 30 (Suppl.).

Korber, B., Brander, B., Moore, J., D'Souza, P., Walker, B., Koup, R., Haynes, B., and Myers, G. (eds.). (1996). *HIV Molecular Immunology Database 1996.* Los Alamos National Laboratory, Theoretical

Biology and Biophysics, Los Alamos, New Mexico. LA-UR 97-1150.

Korber, B.T.M., Brander, B., Haynes, B.F., Koup, R., Kuiken, C., Moore, J.P., Walker, B.D., and Watkins, D.I. (eds.). (2002). *HIV Molecular Immunology 2002*. Los Alamos National Laboratory, Theoretical Biology and Biophysics, Los Alamos, New Mexico. LA-UR 03-5816.

Langlade-Demoyen, P., Ngo-Giang-Huong, N., Ferchal., F., and Oksenhendler, E. (1994). Human immunodeficiency virus (HIV) *nef*-specific cytotoxic T lymphocytes in noninfected heterosexual contact of HIV-infected patients. *J Clin Invest.* 93:1293–1297.

Lawlor, D., Ward, F., Ennis, P., Jackson, A., and Parham, P. (1988). HLA-A and B polymorphisms predate the divergence of humans and chimpanzees. *Nature* 335:268–271.

Li, L., Promadej, N., McNicholl, J.M., and Bouvier, J. (2002). Crystallization and preliminary X-ray crystallographic studies of HLA-A*1101 complexed with an HIV-1 decapeptide. *Acta Cryst.* D58:1195–1197.

Lintner, B. (1994). *Burma in Revolt: Opium and Insurgency since 1948*. Westview Press, Boulder, CO.

MacDonald, K.S., Fowke, K.R., Kimani, J., Dunand, V.A., Nagelkerte, N.J. D., Ball.T., B., Oyugi, J., Njagi, E., Gaur, L.K., Brunham, R.C., Wade, J., Luscher, M.A., Kraus, P., Rowland-Jones, S., Ngugi, E., Bwayo, J.J., and Plummer, F.A. (2000). Influence of HLA supertypes on susceptibility and resistance to human immunodeficiency virus type 1 infection. *J Inf Dis.* 181:1581–1589.

Marsh, S.G.E., Parham, P., Dupont, B., Geraghty, D.E., Trowsdale, J., Middleton, D., Vilches, C., Carrington, M., Witt, C., Guethlein, L.A., Shilling, H., Garcia, C.A., Hsu, K.C., and Wain, H. (2003). Killer-cell immunoglobulin-like receptor (KIR) nomenclature report, 2002. *Tissue Antigens* 62:79–86.

Martin, M.P., Gao, X., Lee, J-H, Nelson G.W., Detels, R., Goedert, J.J., Buchbinder, S., Hoots, K., Vlahov, D., Trowsdale, J., Wilson, M., O'Brien, S.J., and Carrington, M. (2002). Epistatic interaction between KIR3DS1 and HLA-B delays the progression to AIDS. *Nature Genetics* 31:429–434.

McCutchan, F.E., Carr, J.K., Murphy, D., Piyasirisilp, S., Gao, F., Hahn, B., Yu, X.F., Beyrer, C., and Birx, D.L. (2002). Precise mapping of recombination breakpoints suggests a common parent of two BC recombinant HIV type 1 strains circulating in China. *AIDS Res Hum Retroviruses.* 18(15):1135–40.

Middleton, D., Curran, M., and Maxwell, L. (2002). Natural killer cells and their receptors. *Transplant Immunology* 10:147–164.

Mongkolsapaya, J., Dejinirattisai, W., Xu, X., Vasanawathana, S., Tangthawornchaikul, N., Chairunsri, A., Sawasdivorn, S., Duangchinda, T., Dong, T., Rowland-Jones, S., Yenchitsomanus, P., McMichael, A., Malasit, P., and Screaton, G. (2003). Original antigenic sin and apoptosis in the pathogenesis of dengue hemorrhagic fever. *Nature Medicine* 9:921–927.

Moore, C.B., John, M., James, I.R., Christiansen, F.T. Witt, C., and Mallal, S.A. (2002). Evidence of HIV-1 adaptation to HLA-restricted immune responses at a population level. *Science* 296:1439–1443.

Nelson, K.E., and Thomas, D.L. (2001). Viral Hepatitis: In Nelson, Williams, and Graham. *Infectious Disease Epidemiology*. Aspen Publishers, Gaithersberg, pp. 582–588.

Nihei, N., Hashida, Y., Kobayashi, M., and Ishii, A. (2002). Analysis of malaria endemic areas on the Indochinese Peninsula using remote sensing. *Jpn J Infect Dis.* 55:160–166.

Norman, P.J., Stephens, H.A.F., Verity, D.H., Chandanayingyong, D., and Vaughan R.W. (2001). Distribution of natural killer cell immunoglobulin-like receptor sequences in three ethnic groups. *Immunogenetics* 52:195–205.

Norman, P.J. Carrington, C.V.F., Byng, M., Curran, M.D., Stephens, H.A. F., Chandanayingyong, D., Verity, D.H., Hameed, K., Ramdath, D.D. and Vaughan, R.W. (2002). Natural killer cell immunoglobulin-like receptor (KIR) locus profiles in African and South Asian populations. *Genes and Immunity* 3:86–95.

Owens, K., and King, M.-C. (1999). Genomic views of human history. *Science* 286:451–453.

Parham, P. (2003). Immunogenetics of killer-cell immunoglobulin-like receptors. *Tissue Antigens* 62:194–200.

Pende, D., Biassoni, R., Cantoni, C., Verdiani, S., Falco, M., di Donato, C., Accame, L., Bottino, C., Moretta, A., and Moretta, L. (1996). The natural killer cell receptor specific for HLA-A allotypes: A novel memeber of the p58/p70 family of inhibitory receptors that is characterized by three immunoglobulin-like domains and is expressed as a 140-kD disulphide-linked dimer. *J. Exp. Med.* 184:505–515.

Piazza A. (1998). Human evolution: Towards a genetic history of China. *Nature* 395:636–639.

Picard, A.L., Wongsrichanalai, C., Purfeild, A., Kamwendo, D., Emery, K., Zalewski, C., Kawamoto, F., Miller, R.S., Meshnick, S.R. (2003). Resistance to antimalarials in SE Asia and genetic polymorphisms in *pfmdr1*. *Antimicrob. Agnts. & Chemother.* 47(8):2418–2423.

Piriyasilip, S., McCutchan, F., Carr, J.K., Sanders-Buell, E., Liu, W., Chen, J., Wagner, R., Wolf, H., Shao, Y., Lai, S., Beyrer, C., and Yu, X.-F. (2000). A recent outbreak of HIV-1 infection in Southern China was initiated by two highly homogenous, geographically separated strains: Circulating recombinant for AE and a novel BC recombinant. *J Virology* 74(23):11286–11295.

Plummer, F.A., Fowke, K., Nagelkerke, N.J.D., Simonsen, J.N., Bwayo, J., and Ngugi, E. (1993). Evidence of resistance to HIV among continuously exposed prostitutes in Nairobi, Kenya [Abstract WS-A07-3]. In: Program and abstracts: IX International Conference on AIDS/IV World STD Congress,Berlin. London: Wellcome Foundation, p. 23.

Razak, M.H., Jittiwutikarn, J., Suriyanon, V., Vongchak, T., Srirak, N., Beyrer, C., Kawichai, S., Tovanabutra, S., Rungruengthanakit, K., Sawanpanyalert, P., and Celentano, D.D. (2003). HIV prevalence and risks among injection and non-injection drug users in Northern Thailand: Need for comprehensive HIV prevention programs. *J AIDS* 33(2):259–266.

Rowland-Jones, S., Sutton, J., Ariyoshi, K., Dong, T., Gotch, F., McAdam, S., Whitby, D., Sabally, S.S., Gallimore, A., Corrah, T., Takiguchi, M., Schultz, T., McMichael, A., and Whittle, H. (1995). HIV-specific cytotoxic T-cells in HIV-exposed but uninfected Gambian women. *Nat Med.* 1:59–64.

Schliesinger, J. (2000). *Ethnic Groups of Thailand: Non-Tai-Speaking Peoples.* White Lotus Press, Bangkok.

Sidney, J., Grey, H.M., Kubo, R.T., and Sette, A. (1996). Practical, biochemical and evolutionary implications of the discovery of HLA class I supermotifs. *Immunology Today* 17:261–266.

Sriwanthana, B., Hodge, T., Mastro, T.D., Dezzutti, C.S. Bond, K., Stephens, H.A.F., Kostrikis, L.G., Limpakarnjanarat, K., Young, N.L., Qari, S.H., Lal, R.B., Chandanayingyong, D., and McNicholl, J.M. (2001). HIV-specific cytotoxic T lymphocytes, HLA-A11 and chemokine related factors may act synergistically to determine HIV resistance in CCR5 delta-32 negative female sex workers in Chiang Rai, northern Thailand. *AIDS Res Hum Retroviruses* 17:719–734.

Stephens, H.A.F., Brown, A.E., Chandanayingyong, D., Webster, H.K., Sirikong, M., Longta, P., Vangseratthana, R., Gordon, D.M., Lekmak, S., and Rungruang, E. (1995). The presence of the HLA class II allele DPB1*0501 in ethnic Thais correlates with an enhanced vaccine-induced antibody response to a malaria sporozoite vaccine. *Eur J Immuol.* 25:3142–3147.

Stephens, H.A.F., Kunachiwa, W., Sirikong, M., Longta, K., Maneemaroj, R., Wongkuttiya, D., Rungruang, E., Sittisombut, N., and Chandanayingyong, D. (2000). A comparison of molecular HLA-DR and DQ allele profiles forming DR51, DR52 and DR53-related haplotypes in five ethnic Thai populations from mainland Southeast Asia. *Hum Immunol.* 61:1039–1047.

Stephens, H.A.F., Klaythong R., Sirikong, M., Vaughn, D.W., Green, S., Kalayanarooj, S., Endy, T.P., Libraty, D.H., Nisalak, A., Innis, B. L., Rothman, A.L., Ennis, F.A., and Chandanayingyong, D. (2002). Class I HLA-A and B allele associations with secondary infections, correlate with disease severity and the infecting dengue virus serotype in ethnic Thais. *Tissue Antigens* 60:309–318.

Takebe, Y., Motomura, K., Tatsumi, M., Lwin, H.H., Zaw, M., and Kusagawa, S. (2003). High prevalence of diverse forms of HIV-1 intersubtype recombinants in Central Myanmar: Geographical hot spot of extensive recombination. *AIDS* 17(14):2077–2087.

Ugoloni, S., and Vivier, E. (2001). Mutifaceted roles of MHC class I and MHC class I-like molecules in T cell activation. *Nature Immunol.* 2:198–200.

UNAIDS. (2002). Report on the Global HIV/AIDS Epidemic, 2002. UNAIDS, Geneva.

United States Department of State. (2003). International Narcotics Strategy Control Report, 2002. U.S. Dept. of State, Washington, DC.

Vejbaesya, S., Songsivilai, S., Tanawandee, T., Rachaibun, S., Chantangpol, R., and Dharakul, T. (2000). HLA association with hepatitis C virus infection. *Hum Immunol.* 61:348–353.

Vejbaesya, S., Chierakul, N., Luangtrakool, K., and Stephens, H.A.F. (2002). Associations of HLA class II alleles with pulmonary tuberculosis in Thais. *Eur J Immunogenet.* 29:431–434.

Vu-Trieu, A., Djoulah, S., Tran-Thi, C., Ngyuyen-Thanh, T., Le Monnier de Gouville, I., Hors, J., and Sanchez-Mazas, A. (1997). HLA-DR and—DQB1 DNA polymorphisms in a Vietnamese Kinh population from Hanoi. *Eur J Immunogenet.* 24:345–356.

Wongsrichanalai, C., Pickard, A.L., Wernsdorfer, W.H., and Meshnick, S.R. (2002). Epidemiology of drug-resistant malaria. *Lancet Infect Dis.* 2:209–218.

Yanai, H., Uthaivoravit, W., Panich, V., Sawanpanyalert, P., Chaimanee, B., Akarasewi, P., Limpakarnjanarat, K., Nieburg, P., and Mastro, T.D. (1996). Rapid increase in HIV-related tuberculosis, Chiang Rai, Thailand, 1990–1994. *AIDS* 10:527–531.

Yu X.F., Chen J., Shao Y, Beyrer C., Wang Z., Liu B., Wang Z., Liu W., Yang J., Liang S., Viscidi R.P., Gu J., Gurri-Glass G., and Lai S. (1999). Emerging HIV infections with distinct subtypes of HIV-1 among injection drug users from geographically separated locations in Guangxi Province, China. *JAIDS* 22:180–188.

III

Diagnosis, Surveillance, and Projected Scenarios

24

Estimating Rates of HIV/AIDS in India

Shruti H. Mehta[1] and Robert C. Bollinger[2,3]

[1]*Department of Epidemiology, Johns Hopkins Bloomberg School of Public Health, Baltimore, Maryland, USA*
[2]*Division of Infectious Diseases and* [3]*Department of International Health, Johns Hopkins Bloomberg School of Public Health Baltimore, Maryland, USA*

INTRODUCTION

India has the world's 2nd largest population and is the 7th largest country geographically, sharing land borders with Bangladesh, Bhutan, China, Myanmar, Nepal and Pakistan. In recent years India has seen significant advancements in its economy and the health and well-being of its people; however poverty remains widespread and India's gross national product (GNP) is still one of the lowest in the world. Seventy five percent of the Indian population currently resides in rural areas.

Since 1986 when the first case of HIV was observed in Chennai, the spread of HIV in India has been rapid. Estimating the burden of HIV/AIDS in India and tracking patterns over time have been serious challenges, in part due to India's size, diversity, traditions and cultural myths on sex and sexuality. Although recent estimates of the prevalence of HIV infection from different sources are fairly consistent, estimates of the number of AIDS cases and projections for the future have been drastically different, depending on the source (Table 1). Estimates have come from the National AIDS Control Organization (NACO) of India, the Joint United Nations Programme on HIV/AIDS (UNAIDS), the World Health Organization (WHO) and the National Intelligence Council (NIC).

Getting an accurate picture of the epidemic in India is important for a number of reasons. All prevention and intervention strategies as well as policies and decisions about allocation of resources are based on epidemiologic estimates of the burden of disease. Numbers that are inflated may take resources and efforts away from competing priorities in a country where tropical diseases and nutritional deficiencies are endemic. On the other hand, numbers that are grossly underestimated can lead to complacency and might impair a strong political commitment which is necessary to adequately curtail the epidemic. It is important to note that even if one considers the lowest prevalence estimates, India is the country with the largest number of HIV infected adults globally, except for South Africa. Ninety percent of AIDS cases in India occur in adults between the ages of 15 and 44, the most sexually active and

TABLE 1. Estimates of HIV Prevalence, AIDS Cases and Future Projections

	NACO[a]	UNAIDS/WHO[a]	NIC[a]
HIV Prevalence			
Year	2002	2002	2002
Number of Cases	3.82–4.58 million	3.97 million (range, 2.6–5.4 million)	5–8 million
Population Prevalence	0.8%	0.8%	0.9–1.4%
Cumulative AIDS Cases			
Year	2003	2000	N/A
Number of Cases	55,764[b]	2.8 million[c]	N/A
Projected HIV Prevalence			
Year of Projection		1999	2002
Number of Cases		37 million by 2005	20–25 million by 2010

[a] NACO (National AIDS Control Organization), UNAIDS (Joint United Nations Programme on HIV/AIDS), WHO (World Health Organization), NIC (National Intelligence Council)
[b] Represents cumulative AIDS cases *reported* to NACO.
[c] Represents *estimated* AIDS cases

economically productive group. Even if the epidemic continues on the current trajectory, it could have serious ramifications for India's economic growth and political stability.

CURRENT HIV PREVALENCE ESTIMATES IN INDIA

Current HIV prevalence estimates range from 0.8 to 1.4%. However, because the total population of India exceeds one billion, the estimated number of persons living with HIV/AIDS (PLWHA) is as high as four to eight million persons (NACO, 2000; UNAIDS/WHO, 2002a; NIC, 2000). Moreover, in India, even a small increase in prevalence (0.1%) could reflect a dramatic increase in the number of PLWHA (one million).

HIV Prevalence Estimates from NACO

The official estimates in India come from NACO. In July of 2003, NACO estimated that between 3.82 million and 4.58 million Indians were living with HIV in 2002, reflecting a population prevalence of approximately 0.8%. The HIV prevalence estimates have been highly variable across India's 35 states, ranging from near zero in some states to more than 2% in others. Based on prevalence rates greater than 1% among women attending antenatal clinics (ANC), NACO classified six states: Andhra Pradesh, Karnataka, Maharashtra, Manipur, Nagaland, and Tamil Nadu as "high" prevalence states (Figure 1). States such as Goa, Gujarat and Pondicherry, were classified as "moderate" prevalence states because fewer than 1% of women attending ANC, but greater than 5% of high-risk groups were HIV-infected. All other states were classified into the "low" prevalence category with less than 1% of the women attending ANC and less than 5% of the high-risk groups HIV-infected. (NACO, 2001b). Given these geographic differences, it may be inappropriate to consider national averages to describe the HIV epidemic in India.

The National HIV Sentinel Surveillance System: History and Description

NACO HIV prevalence estimates are based exclusively on sentinel surveillance, which is primarily used to monitor trends in HIV among high risk groups. Surveillance

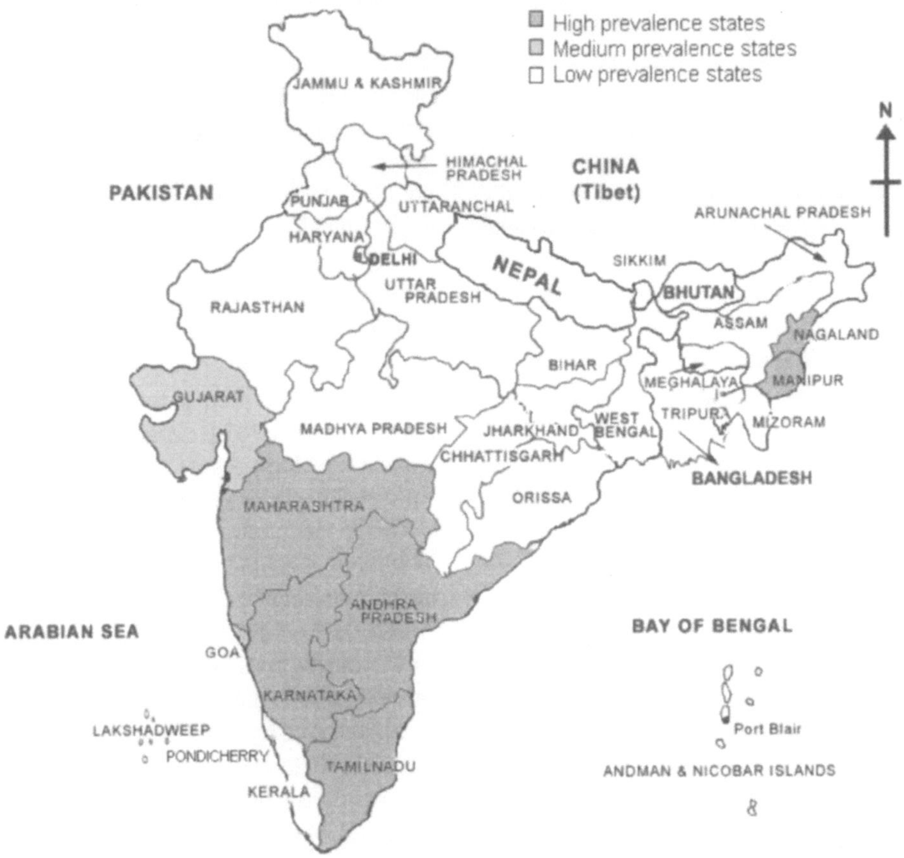

FIGURE 1. Adult HIV prevalence in India, 2002. Adapted from NACO, 2001.

began in India soon after the first case was discovered in 1986 at the Madras Medical College in Chennai, Tamil Nadu (Simoes *et al.*, 1993; Simoes *et al.*, 1987). The initial program, which began in 1987, included surveillance activities in 62 public health centers and nine referral centers (NACO, 2001b). With the formation of the National AIDS Control Organization (NACO) in 1992, HIV sentinel surveillance was also expanded (NACO, 2001). The number of sites increased from 55 in 1994 to 180 in 1998, 232 in 2000, and finally 320 in 2001. In 2001, the distribution of sentinel sites was as follows: 135 (42%) in sexually transmitted infection (STI) clinics, 170 (53%) in ANC, 13 (4%) for injection drug users (IDU) and 2 (1%) for men who have sex with men (MSM) (NACO, 2001; WHO, 2001c). Surveys are conducted each year from August to October at the designated sentinel sites and data collected is used to estimate the local and national HIV prevalence (NACO, 2000; NACO, 2001c).

Trends in HIV prevalence within specific groups over time have been tracked through the sentinel surveillance system. Initially in India, HIV was concentrated in urban poor and marginalized populations including female sex workers (FSW) and their clients, truck drivers, migrant laborers, MSM and IDU. By 1990, the prevalence of HIV among these high risk groups in urban centers of certain states (e.g. Maharashtra and Manipur) had already surpassed 5% (UNDP, 2003). Eventually, the line between the high risk/low risk and urban/rural became blurred and HIV began to move from the populations at the margins of society to the mainstream including middle class individuals and housewives and from urban to rural settings (Gangakhedkar *et al.*, 1997, UNDP, 2003; World Bank, 1999). This pattern was first observed in 1994 by detection of HIV among women attending ANC in Maharashtra and then subsequently in the southern states. By 1999, the prevalence of HIV among women attending ANC was as high as 6.5% in some cities, the prevalence of HIV among FSW in Mumbai had approached 60%, the prevalence of HIV among IDU in Manipur was 76% and the prevalence of HIV among STI patients was 30% in Andhra Pradesh and 14 to 60% in Maharashtra (UNDP, 2003).

Limitations of Sentinel Surveillance

The efforts put forth by NACO to conduct sentinel surveillance in a country as vast and diverse as India should be commended. The improvements in the system over the years and the ongoing addition of sites, especially those for IDU and MSM have all contributed to improving the accuracy of HIV prevalence estimates. However, there are a number of limitations associated with using sentinel surveillance which might impact HIV prevalence estimates.

The accuracy of prevalence estimates from sentinel surveillance is inherently dependent upon the representativeness of the sentinel populations. In general, it may be inappropriate to apply data from subpopulations such as pregnant women, IDU and STI clinic attendees to the whole population. For example, application of data from specific behavioral risk groups requires knowledge of the size of those risk groups in the population and the assumption that there is no selection bias (WHO, 2001c). Because of the stigma associated with these high risk behaviors, people might be reluctant to identify themselves as MSM or IDU, so it is difficult to estimate the actual size of these risk groups. If the size of the risk groups is underestimated then the population prevalence would also be underestimated. There is also potential for selection bias because there is heterogeneity in risk behavior within behavioral risk groups. For example, if persons within a specific risk group who practice the riskiest behavior do not come to the sentinel sites, prevalence estimates would be underestimated.

Even estimates of HIV prevalence among women attending ANC, which are thought to reflect the general population prevalence, may be biased (Medical Research Council, 1998). Women who attend ANC represent only a small subgroup of pregnant women who have access to the maternal and child health services of government hospitals. UNICEF estimates that only 34% of births in India are actually attended by a trained health professional (Ratnathicam, 2001; UNAIDS, 2002). Thus, there is a large group of poor women, particularly those in rural areas, who do not have access to antenatal services, and consequently would not be represented in these estimates. Similarly, women who use private nursing home services would not be included (Shreedhar, 1998). Since the prevalence of HIV may be different among these women, these exclusions could overestimate or underestimate the HIV prevalence in these settings. Additionally, application of HIV prevalence from ANC to estimate general population prevalence requires adjustment for the estimated male to female HIV prevalence ratio. NACO's estimates are adjusted for the male to female HIV prevalence ratio, which is assumed to be higher in low prevalence states (3:1) than in high prevalence states (1.2:1) (NACO, 2001b). However if the margin of error associated with this ratio is high, prevalence estimates may be affected.

Prevalence estimates would also be affected by other groups of people who might inadvertently be excluded from sentinel surveillance. Persons who are too ill to come to hospitals or sentinel sites for testing would not be included in these estimates. Many patients who die of opportunistic infections would have never made it to a testing site. There are also other pockets of people (e.g., tuberculosis patients) who are infected but do not get tested. People may not want to go for testing because of denial, fear, stigma, or discrimination. Moreover, some individuals from high risk groups (e.g., IDU and MSM) might be reluctant to identify themselves (Solomon and Ganesh, 2002; NIC, 2002). Failure of the sentinel surveillance system to capture these types of individuals would underestimate HIV prevalence.

Prevalence estimates would also be affected by the restriction of sentinel surveillance to public/government health institutions. The sentinel surveillance system in India does not collect any HIV testing information from clinical laboratories in the private sector (Solomon and Ganesh, 2002). In India, the private sector provides more than 80% of the health care in the country. In 2000, private health expenditures accounted for 4% of GDP, whereas public health spending accounted for less than 1% (UNDP, 2003). In general, the perception is that individuals who use private health services tend to be wealthier and thus at lower risk for HIV infection compared with those using government services (Uplekar and Rangan, 1993; Uplekar *et al.*, 2001). So by not including the private sector in sentinel surveillance, NACO might actually be overestimating the HIV prevalence. This trend may be changing as it has been suggested that the private sector is becoming a source of care even for poor people (Uplekar *et al.*, 2001). Within the sentinel sites, there are also a limited number of rural sites. Prevalence estimates are adjusted for the estimated urban to rural HIV prevalence ratio which is assumed to be higher in low prevalence states (8:1) than in high prevalence states (3:1) (NACO, 2001b). However, since little data has been collected from rural populations, there may be a high margin of error associated with these estimates as well.

Another issue that would affect HIV prevalence estimates is the quality of HIV testing, which has been questioned in India. Solomon and Ganesh have suggested that the majority of the laboratories in India do not participate in quality assurance and quality control activities for HIV testing. They have suggested that poor techniques are often used and that HIV testing could be inaccurate for a number of reasons, including tests being used after the expiration date, testing kits not stored at the correct temperatures, problems with electricity outages and air-condition, the use of poor-quality water, the use of recycled equipment and results given based on only a single rapid test (Solomon and Ganesh, 2002). These inadequacies in testing quality could result in overestimation or underestimation of HIV prevalence depending on the dynamics of the misclassification. It is imperative that all testing sites have quality assurance and quality control strategies in place and that these are standardized across the states.

Finally, NACO's estimates suggest that there is substantial geographic variability in the prevalence of HIV. On the one hand, this geographic variability could reflect real differences between the states with respect to risk behaviors or migration patterns. For example, commercial sex work, which contributed to the more rapid spread of HIV in states such as Maharashtra and Tamil Nadu, may not be as widespread in some of the low prevalence states. Migration from rural to urban areas might also be less common in some of the low prevalence states. If fewer men are migrating to urban areas for work, a practice which, in some of the high prevalence states, has contributed to the spread of HIV because of the increased frequency of extramarital relationships among men and reliance on commercial sex work among women, the spread of HIV might also be slower. Finally, if there is little sexual mixing between states in India, perhaps there have been limited opportunities for HIV to be introduced into the populations of certain states.

On the other hand, the observed geographic variability in HIV prevalence could be also explained by differential surveillance systems and testing capabilities. On average, there are seven sentinel sites per state, but the actual number of sites per state is variable. For the most part, it appears that the number of sites per state is dependent upon the population size of that state. The most populous states have the highest number of sentinel sites. However, there are a number of states with only one to four sentinel sites, which seems to be too few when the population size is near one million. Additionally, there are some exceptions whereby states such as Manipur and Nagaland, estimated to be high HIV prevalence states, have more sentinel sites than lower prevalence states with larger populations (e.g., Jammu and Kashmir, Kerala and Assam) (NACO, 2001c). In these cases, whether the number of sites is a reflection of the low prevalence of HIV in the state or the low prevalence is a function of the number of sites is unknown. However, since the accuracy of the prevalence estimates are entirely dependent on the representativeness of the sentinel sites, the generalizability of sentinel site prevalence rates is of special concern in states where there are very few sentinel sites.

Community-Based Prevalence Studies

An effective way to obtain unbiased estimates of HIV prevalence in the general population would be to conduct large-scale, population-based surveys. However, these studies can be difficult to undertake because of cost, sampling difficulties and the sensitive nature of HIV. In India, a USAID-funded study in Tamil Nadu state was conducted to ascertain the HIV prevalence in the community (Thomas *et al.*, 2002). In this study, the probability proportional to size cluster sampling technique was used to obtain a representative sample of the state of Tamil Nadu. Samples were taken from clusters selected from urban and rural areas of the major districts in Tamil Nadu. The prevalence of HIV infection was 1.8% overall. The prevalence was estimated to be higher in rural (2.2%) compared to urban sites (0.8%), among women (2.1%) than men (1.5%) and among older individuals (2.3%) compared to younger ones (1.9%) (Thomas *et al.*, 2002). Some of these differences were surprising, in particular the male vs. female and the urban vs. rural prevalence estimates. These differences could be indicative of selection bias, which occurred even after random sampling techniques were used. The authors stated that some of the rural sites were actually semi-urban so the prevalence of HIV in rural sites might have been overestimated (Thomas *et al.*, 2002).

It is important to note that all of these estimates (with the exception of those in urban sites) were double that of NACO's estimates for Tamil Nadu, (NACO, 2001b) suggesting that prevalence rates from antenatal clinics might underestimate the underlying HIV prevalence in the general population. The data also suggested that prevalence rates were highest in older individuals who are probably not adequately represented in antenatal clinics. The differences might be even more substantial in states where fewer sentinel sites have been included. It is unlikely that large scale population-based studies can be conducted in each state and probable that antenatal surveillance, which is much easier to conduct than population-based surveillance, will continue to be used as the primary mode for HIV surveillance. Thus, it is important to take into account the potential for underestimation when using this data.

HIV Prevalence Estimates from UNAIDS/WHO

At the end of 2001, UNAIDS estimated that 3.97 million adults and children (range, 2.6 million to 5.4 million) were living with HIV/AIDS in India. Of those infected, approximately 3.8 million were estimated to be adults between ages 15 to 49, translating into an adult prevalence of 0.8% (UNAIDS, 2002).

These HIV prevalence estimates come from a joint effort by UNAIDS and WHO. As part of the UNAIDS/WHO Working group on Global HIV/AIDS and STI Surveillance, a group of experts arrive at HIV prevalence estimates by applying a demographic and HIV projection model to in-country surveillance data (Stover *et al.*, 2002; UNAIDS/WHO, 2002a). Since these estimates rely on official government statistics from India, the estimates are very similar to those from NACO and are subject to the same limitations discussed above.

HIV Prevalence Estimates from NIC

In September 2002, the United States National Intelligence Council (NIC) released a controversial report titled, "The Next Wave of HIV/AIDS: Nigeria, Ethiopia, Russia, India and China." In this report, the NIC suggested that the HIV/AIDS epidemic in the next decade would be fueled by the spread in five countries. They estimated that in 2002, between 5 and 8 million Indians were living with HIV/AIDS (NIC, 2002).

The NIC estimate was based on a combination of government of India statistics and assessments from academic institutions and non-governmental organizations (NGOs). The NIC report criticized the Indian government estimates of HIV prevalence, suggesting that they were underestimated due to inadequacies in the sentinel surveillance system and chronic underreporting. The NIC report further criticized the UNAIDS estimates as being underestimated because of their reliance on official government statistics. Using data from the additional sources who would not have been included in the NACO estimates might explain the difference between the NIC estimates and the NACO and UNAIDS/WHO estimates. However, it is difficult to interpret the NIC estimates, because a detailed description of their estimation process is not available. The NIC report even qualified their numbers as rough estimates whose purpose was to give a general sense of the magnitude of HIV infection in India within a relatively high margin of error. Moreover, the data used to generate this report were not declassified (NIC, 2002). The government of India has questioned the NIC estimates (Mehta, 2003; Thomas *et al.*, 2002).

CURRENT AIDS ESTIMATES IN INDIA

Whereas the estimates of HIV prevalence are not strikingly different between all agencies, the estimates of India's AIDS cases are. The number of AIDS cases reported to NACO is substantially lower than those estimated by WHO and UNAIDS. No AIDS estimates were available from the NIC.

AIDS Estimates from NACO

In September 2003, NACO released the most recent figures on reported AIDS cases in India. The cumulative reported total at the end of 2002 was 55,764 cases. The proportion of AIDS cases was greatest in the states with the highest estimated HIV prevalence. In fact, 75% of AIDS cases occurred in only five states: Andhra Pradesh, Karnataka, Maharashtra, Manipur and Tamil Nadu (NACO, 2003). Of the AIDS cases reported in 2003, 39% occurred among women. Based on the cumulative number of reported AIDS cases from 1986 to 2003, NACO estimated that 85% of AIDS cases (and by translation, HIV infections) were associated with sexual transmission. Perinatal transmission, injection drug use and unsafe blood and blood products accounted for 2.7%. 2.4% and 2.7% AIDS cases, respectively. Transmission mode was unknown in approximately 7.0% of AIDS cases (NACO, 2001a). Transmission routes also varied substantially by geographic location. Whereas heterosexual transmission drives the epidemic in the "high" prevalence states of Maharasthra, Tamil Nadu, Karnataka and Andhra Pradesh, injection drug use drives the epidemic in the northeastern "high" prevalence states of Manipur and Nagaland (NACO, 2001c).

In India, all medical institutions are required to report suspected and confirmed AIDS cases to NACO. However, the reporting process is very cumbersome and it is acknowledged even by NACO that many AIDS cases go unreported (Mudur, 2000; Sharma, 2000; Solomon and Ganesh, 2002). In addition to the cases that are not reported by physicians, many patients die without ever having been diagnosed with AIDS and often the cause of death is attributed to the opportunistic infection rather than to AIDS. It is not uncommon in India for families of patients to request that the doctor not list HIV/AIDS as the cause of death and doctors often oblige (Solomon and Ganesh, 2002).

AIDS Estimates from UNAIDS/WHO

It is difficult to get consistent information on estimated AIDS cases even from UNAIDS and WHO. At one time, UNAIDS estimated that there had been 310,000 AIDS deaths in 1999 alone (Ratnathicam, 2001). WHO later estimated that there had been 350,000 AIDS deaths among individuals between 15–49 years of age in 2000 and projected that there would be 500,000 AIDS deaths in India in 2005 (WHO, 2001b). Cumulative estimates from the United Nations population division have suggested that there have been 2.8 million AIDS deaths in India through 2000. The United Nations further projected that between 2000 and 2015, there would be 12.3 million AIDS deaths in India and that by 2050, India's population would be 5% smaller than it would have been without AIDS (Population Division of the Department of Economic and Social Affairs of the United Nations Secretariat, 2003).

AIDS case reporting in most developing countries is carried out at the request of WHO and UNAIDS. In most countries, data on AIDS cases is collected at the national level and sent to WHO for further analysis. However, reporting of AIDS cases is highly variable between countries and even between states within countries. AIDS definitions may be different, and underreporting is common especially in developing countries where there may be weaknesses in health care infrastructure (UNAIDS/WHO, 2002a). The limitations of AIDS case reporting forces UNAIDS and WHO and other organizations to rely on estimates of AIDS deaths rather than actual data on reported AIDS cases in developing countries. In 1995, WHO suggested that the estimated to reported (E:R) AIDS case ratio in India was 36.6:1, which was substantially higher than any African or other Asian country at the time. By comparison, the E:R ratio in sub-Saharan Africa ranged from 5–10:1 and was 2:1 in Mexico and Brazil (WHO, 1995). Since AIDS reporting does not appear to have substantially improved over time in India, this ratio may have narrowed but most likely remains high.

The data from NACO described above deals only with reported AIDS cases, thus explaining the discrepancy between the UNAIDS/WHO estimates and the NACO figures. However, even though NACO would admit that there is underreporting of AIDS deaths, they have often criticized the UNAIDS/WHO estimates as being too high (Sharma, 2000). In 2000, NACO criticized estimates of AIDS deaths from both UNAIDS and WHO, suggesting that it would have been difficult for UNAIDS to make estimates on AIDS deaths when the Indian government itself did not have any data on deaths. They further suggested that since NACO was the only organization actually collecting field data through sentinel surveillance, UNAIDS should stop making its own projections and instead rely on the Indian statistics as the only *official* estimates for India (Sharma, 2000).

PROJECTED HIV INFECTION ESTIMATES IN INDIA

Year 2000 projections for the number of HIV-infected persons in India ranged from 5 million cases (Bollinger *et al.*, 1995) to 12 million cases (The World Bank Group, 1991). Actual estimates for the year 2000 were closer to the lower of the two estimates. Since then, there has continued to be a wide range of projections for the future of the HIV epidemic in India.

Projected Estimates from NACO

According to NACO, the estimated number of adults living with HIV was 3.5 million in 1998, 3.7 million in 1999, 3.86 million in 2000 and 3.97 million in 2001. Based on the assumption that the number of HIV-associated deaths was uniform over time, an estimated 0.2 million new infections occurred between 1998–1999, 0.16 million between 1999–2000 and 0.11 million between 2000–2001. Although NACO has not made any numeric future projections, based on this data, NACO suggested that over time, the number of new infections was likely to reduce to a negligible number which would indicate a plateauing of the epidemic (NACO, 2001; Srinivasan, 2003). However, the most recent statistics from 2002 suggest that the trend may be changing. In 2002, some reports have suggested that there were 0.61 million new infections suggesting that the incidence was once again increasing (Kumar, 2003). Based on these figures, India accounted for nearly 87% (n = 610,000) of all HIV infections (n = 700,000) that occurred during 2002 in South and Southeast Asia (UNAIDS/WHO, 2002a).

There is very little data to estimate the incidence of HIV infection in India. Future projections of the magnitude of the HIV epidemic, which should be based on incidence data, are based predominately on serial seroprevalence data. However, estimates of incidence from serial seroprevalence data can be biased because of changes in the population due to migration, mortality due to HIV and other causes, differential inclusion of people screened, and changing selection biases (Brookmeyer and Quinn, 1995). Moreover, previous studies in some African populations have suggested that HIV prevalence may decline even in the presence of a stable or increasing incidence (Batter *et al.*, 1994; Peterman *et al.*, 1995; Wawer *et al.*, 1997). Thus, it may not always be appropriate to estimate trends in incidence from trends in prevalence.

Projected Estimates from UNAIDS/WHO

In 1991, WHO predicted that by the year 2000, there would be 12 million persons living with HIV in India and a cumulative total of 1 million AIDS cases (The World Bank Group, 1991). In 1999, the World Bank warned that there would be 37 million cases of HIV infection in India by 2005 if successful preventive measures were not implemented (World Bank, 1999). The basis for these calculations has not been described. However, based on even the highest current estimates of HIV infection in India, these projections do not reflect the current situation.

Projected Estimates from NIC

The NIC report projected that India will have 20–25 million HIV cases by 2010, the highest estimate for any one country. India was considered to be one of five "second wave" countries, along with Nigeria, Ethiopia, Russia and China, on the verge of a "breakout," or transmission of the epidemic from "high risk" groups to the general population (NIC, 2002). Again, the procedures behind these estimates have not been disclosed and the data has not been declassified.

The NIC projections parallel others which have suggested that the HIV/AIDS epidemic in India may follow the same pattern as Africa. Like sub-Saharen Africa, the early patterns of HIV in India were characterized by a sharp increase in the seroprevalence among high risk groups followed by a more gradual spread to the general population (Shreedhar, 1998). The epidemic in many African countries is now a generalized one that is not contained within specific subgroups of the population. The overall prevalence of HIV in sub-Saharan Africa is 10% and some countries like Botswana and Zimbabwe have prevalence rates that exceed 20%. The dissemination of the epidemic in Africa is also illustrated through movement from urban to rural areas. Early on in Africa, there was a marked urban-to-rural differential (10:1) in the prevalence of HIV infection. Over time, this differential has decreased as well, and currently is only 2:1 (UNAIDS, 2003).

It is not clear whether the epidemic in India will follow the African trajectory. In general, it is difficult to apply the African experience to India when making projections because one needs to take into account differences between the African and the Indian settings with respect to social norms, sexual behavior, living standards and customs. For example, whereas in many African countries, both men and women may have multiple sexual partners (Hartung *et al.*, 2002; Kelly *et al.*, 2003), this is not the case in India. In India, it is not uncommon for men to have premarital and extramarital sex and multiple sexual partners. However, this is not the case for women, who tend to have only one sexual partner throughout their lifetime (Gangakhedkar *et al.*, 2003). This difference between the two epidemics is reflected in the male to female ratio of HIV prevalence, which is less than one in Africa and greater than one in India.

There are some data that are suggestive of the HIV epidemic transitioning into the general population in India the same way it did in Africa. Based on HIV prevalence estimates within risk groups, it has been suggested that there has been a decline in HIV transmission attributable to contaminated blood and blood products (from 6.1% of all HIV infections in 1999 to 3.0% in 2002) and that attributable to injection drug use (from 5.2% of all HIV infections in 1999 to 2.9% in 2002). By contrast, the proportion of HIV infections attributable to perinatal transmission has increased (from 0.3% in 1999 to 2.6% in 2002). Some have argued that the increase in infections attributable to perinatal transmission suggests a shift of the epidemic from high risk groups to the general population. On the other hand, these large changes in a relatively short period of time could also be interpreted as reporting bias. Earlier in the epidemic, most of the HIV cases were detected in the high risk groups (e.g., injecting drug users) and captive populations (e.g., blood donors) who were more likely than others to be tested for HIV. So these trends could also reflect improved detection of HIV in lower risk groups rather than an actual shift in the epidemic.

There is additional evidence to suggest that the epidemic in India is on a different trajectory than the one in Africa. The low overall population prevalence in India despite high prevalence estimates in specific risk groups suggests that the epidemic may be more contained within certain risk groups. Whereas in Africa, the population at risk for HIV infection is essentially the total population, the population at risk in India may be a smaller one. There is little data on HIV prevalence from rural sites, but it appears that the penetration of HIV into rural populations has not been as rapid as it was in Africa.

HIV SURVEILLANCE IN NEIGHBORING COUNTRIES

Many of the countries bordering India have lower rates of HIV infection than India, although data collection and surveillance is problematic in all of these countries. Overall, HIV prevalence rates appear to be lower in the bordering countries of Pakistan, Bangladesh, Nepal and Sri Lanka (Mehta, 2003; WHO, 2001a). Since the epidemics are young in these countries, the governments have the opportunity to effectively deal with HIV/AIDS early before it becomes more prevalent, but all of these countries face similar challenges as India.

Other countries in South and Southeast Asia that do not directly border India actually have higher HIV prevalence, including Cambodia (2.8%), Myanmar (2%) and Thailand (1.9%) (WHO, 2001). Despite the higher HIV prevalence in these countries, India actually has more HIV-infected individuals than all of these countries combined. In general, the sentinel surveillance system in Thailand has been hailed as the best in the developing world. Thailand's system analyzes annual samples (formerly biannual) from high risk groups: IDU, FSW and men attending STI clinics as well as low risk groups: women attending

ANC and blood donors. Thailand also conducts routine HIV testing among young men entering the Royal Thai Army. Information from all of these sources is routinely gathered for all provinces in Thailand and used to make local and national HIV prevalence estimates. Prevalence estimates are derived from mathematical models that incorporate data from the sentinel surveillance program, the Royal Thai Army, regional surveys and reported AIDS cases and deaths. General population estimates are based on data from the ANC, blood donors and military conscripts. Whereas the accuracy of HIV estimates from other developing countries have been questioned, those from Thailand are considered to be among the best available and have been used to promote public awareness and to guide prevention programs and interventions (Saengwonloey *et al.*, 2003).

The success of the surveillance system in Thailand is also a product of the unique role played by the Thai government, a role that has often been sighted as an example for other developing countries. Initially in Thailand, the response to HIV was not unlike that of other countries. There was denial and the perception that HIV was a problem of "foreigners," IDU, and homosexuals, and government activities specifically targeted these marginalized groups. However, when data from sentinel surveillance began to suggest that HIV/AIDS was moving into the general population, the attitude of the Thai government shifted towards more open acknowledgement and combating HIV became a priority for the government. HIV/AIDS programs and policies in Thailand have since then been a joint effort of governmental officials and NGOs and even the media (FHI, 2003).

RECOMMENDATIONS

Estimating HIV Prevalence

Estimates of HIV prevalence in India from different organizations vary from approximately four million infections to eight million infections. Estimates from NACO and UNAIDS/WHO are fairly similar while those from the NIC are substantially higher. All estimates of HIV prevalence rely, to some extent, on the sentinel surveillance data, so limitations of this system would affect all estimates. The sentinel surveillance system in India has been expanded over the years to include additional sites. However, efforts should be made to continue to increase the number of sites, especially in states that have only one to four sites. The number of sites should be directly proportional to the population size of the state. The number of sites specifically for IDU and MSM should be increased as well. Currently, there are only two sites for MSM, so HIV prevalence estimates in this population are not likely to be very accurate.

It is also possible to expand the surveillance system to include other types of populations. Potential sentinel sites that might be useful in estimating the prevalence of HIV in the general population include primary health centers, general practitioners' offices, or outpatient departments of hospitals. Specific efforts to include private health care settings would be useful, since the private sector delivers the majority of health care in India. Since rates of HIV infection are estimated to be very high among tuberculosis patients in India, inclusion of tuberculosis clinics as sentinel sites could also be considered.

Combining other information with sentinel surveillance data, such as population-based surveys or screening of military recruits, as is done in Thailand, would also improve the accuracy of prevalence estimates, especially those of the general population. Population-based surveys are difficult and expensive to perform if initiated on a large scale, but perhaps smaller-scale surveys in specific urban and rural centers would be possible.

Estimating the Number of AIDS Cases

There remains a large gap between the number of reported AIDS cases to NACO and the estimated number of AIDS cases in India. Although physicians are supposed to report all AIDS cases to NACO, it does not appear that this is happening. Perhaps the system for AIDS case reporting needs to be simplified to ensure that clinicians report all AIDS cases. Improvements in AIDS case reporting should especially be integrated into places which would be expected to have high numbers of AIDS cases (e.g. tuberculosis clinics and hospitalized patients).

Projected Estimates of HIV Infection

There is a range of projections for the future of the HIV epidemic in India. The most dramatic projections suggest that India will follow the experience of sub-Saharan Africa and have the highest number of HIV infections in any one country by 2010. However, without data on trends in incidence over time, it is difficult to make definitive conclusions. Large scale cohort studies to determine incidence are not feasible. Thus, strategies to estimate incidence using cross-sectional data need to be explored in this population. One option is to use the detuned ELISA assay. The main limitation of this strategy is cost. Another option, which has already been applied to some Indian settings, is screening for viral core protein (p24 antigen), which is detectable several weeks prior to seroconversion (Bollinger *et al.*, 1997; Brookmeyer and Quinn, 1995). However, testing for p24 antigen can be expensive as well. Another approach utilizes a multistage pooling method for the detection of HIV RNA. Initially specimens can be divided into pools of approximately 100. Pools that are positive for HIV RNA are subsequently subdivided into smaller and smaller pools until pools of size 10 are reached. The estimate of incidence is based on the number positive for HIV RNA in the smallest pool size. Incidence estimates from this method have been shown to be comparable to those derived from p24 antigen testing and the method was 5-fold less expensive. Thus, pooled PCR testing represents a cost-effective method of estimating incidence when only cross-sectional data is available (Quinn *et al.*, 2000).

CONCLUSIONS

Based on current estimates, between four and eight million Indians may be infected with HIV. Although the overall population prevalence remains low, there appears to be considerable geographic variation, so overall prevalence estimates may not be as informative as state-specific prevalence estimates. The number of AIDS cases cannot be accurately estimated from available data; however there may have been as many as three million AIDS deaths in India since the start of the epidemic. Future projections for the epidemic are variable, but there is little doubt that HIV/AIDS will continue to be a major public health problem. The surveillance system has been improved over the past several years, but it needs to be further expanded and combined with other strategies to improve estimates and projections of HIV/AIDS in India. Accurate estimates of the HIV/AIDS epidemic in India are needed to guide future prevention and intervention strategies as well as policies and decisions about allocation of resources.

REFERENCES

Batter, V., Matela, B., Nsuami, M., Manzila, T., Kamenga, M., Behets, F., Ryder, R.W., Heyward, W.L., Karon, J.M., and St Louis, M.E. (1994). High HIV-1 incidence in young women masked by stable overall seroprevalence among childbearing women in Kinshasa, Zaire: Estimating incidence from serial seroprevalence data. *AIDS* 8:811–817.

Bollinger, R.C., Tripathy, S.P., and Quinn, T.C. (1995). The human immunodeficiency virus epidemic in India: Current magnitude and future projections. *Medicine* 74:97–106.

Bollinger, R.C., Brookmeyer, R.S., Mehendale, S.M., Paranjape, R.S., Shepherd, M.E., Gadkari, D.A., and Quinn, T.C. (1997). Risk factors and clinical presentation of acute primary HIV infection in India. *JAMA* 278:2085–2089.

Brookmeyer, R. and Quinn, T.C. (1995). Estimation of current human immunodeficiency virus incidence rates from a cross-sectional survey using early diagnostic tests. *Am J Epidemiol.* 141:166–172.

FHI. (2003). Policy Profile: HIV/AIDS Policy Lessons: Learning from Thailand. Available:www.fhi.org/en/

HIVAIDS/Publications/Archive/articles/ AIDScaptions/volume3no3/LearnFromThailand.htm. Accessed on 11-01-2003.

Gangakhedkar, R.R., Bentley, M.E., Divekar, A.D., Gadkari, D., Mehendale, S.M., Shepherd, M.E., Bollinger, R.C., and Quinn, T.C. (1997). Spread of HIV infection in married monogamous women in India. *JAMA*. 278:2090–2092.

Hartung, T.K., Nash, J., Ngubane, N., and Fredlund, V.G. (2002). AIDS awareness and sexual behaviour in a high HIV prevalence area in rural northern Kwazulu-Natal, South Africa. *Int. J. STD AIDS* 13:829–832.

Kelly, R.J., Gray, R.H., Sewankambo, N.K., Serwadda, D., Wabwire-Mangen, F., Lutalo, T., and Wawer, M.J. (2003). Age differences in sexual partners and risk of HIV-1 infection in rural Uganda. *J Acquir. Immune Defic. Syndr.* 32:446–451.

Kumar, S. (2003). HIV cases rising sharply in India. *BMJ* 327:245.

Medical Research Council. (1998). STD/HIV/AIDS Surveillance Project: Draft outline of a national STD/HIV/AIDS surveillance strategy. Available: http://www.wpro.who.int/pdf/sti/aids2001/annex 7.pdf. Accessed on 11-10-2003.

Mehta, M. (2003). The HIV/AIDS Crisis in India. *South Asian Monitor*. 58. Center for Strategic and International Studies. (May 1, 2003). Available: http://www.csis.org/saprog/sam58.pdf. Accessed on 20-1-2004.

Mudur, G. (2000). Indian agency admits publishing "wrong" HIV figures. *BMJ* 321:402.

NACO. (2000). Indian scenario: Estimation of HIV infection among adult population. Available:http://www.naco.nic.in/indianscene/ country.htm. Accessed on 10-01-2003.

NACO. (2001a). National Baseline General Population Behavioral Surveillance Survey. New Delhi. Available: http://www.naco.nic.in/nacp/ publctn.htm. Accessed on 11-10-2003.

NACO. (2001b). Combating HIV/AIDS in India, 2000–2001. Revised, 8-12-2003. Available:http://www.naco.nic.in/indianscene/country.htm. Accessed on 10-28-2003.

NACO. (2001c). HIV Estimates for Year 2001. Available:http://naco.nic.in/indianscene/esthiv.htm. Accessed on 10-28-2003.

NACO. (2003) HIV/AIDS Indian Scenario: HIV/AIDS Surveillance in India, as reported to NACO as on 31, September 2003. Available: http://www.naco.nic.in/indianscene.overv.htm. Accessed on 11-10-2003.

NIC. (2002). The next wave of HIV/AIDS: Nigeria, Ethiopia, Russia, India and China. ICA 2002-04D. Available: http://www.cia.gov/nic/pubs/other_products/ICA%20HIV-AIDS%20unclassified%20092302POSTGERBER.htm. Accessed on 10-15-2003.

Peterman, T.A., Zaidi, A.A., and Wroten, J. (1995). Decreasing prevalence hides a high HIV incidence: Miami. *AIDS* 9:965–970.

Population Division of the Department of Economic and Social Affairs of the United Nations Secretariat. World Population Prospects: the 2002 Revision. Highlights (2003). Available: http://www.um.org/esa/population/publications/wpp2002/wpp2002 annextables.PDF. Accessed on 11-10-2003.

Quinn, T.C., Brookmeyer, R., Kline, R., Shepherd, M., Paranjape, R., Mehendale, S., Gadkari, D.A., and Bollinger, R. (2000). Feasibility of pooling sera for HIV-1 viral RNA to diagnose acute primary HIV-1 infection and estimate HIV incidence. *AIDS* 14:2751–2757.

Ratnathicam, A. (2001). AIDS in India: Incidence, prevalence, and prevention. *AIDS Patient Care STDS* 15:255–261.

Saengwonloey, O., Jiraphongsa, C., and Foy, H. (2003). Thailand report: HIV/AIDS surveillance 1998. *J. Acquir. Immune Defic. Syndr.* 32 Suppl 1: S63–S67.

Sharma, D.C. (2000). India challenges UN agencies' estimates of HIV prevalence. *Lancet* 356:662.

Shreedhar, J. (1998). Beyond the numbers. Frontline. Available: http://www.flonnet.com/fl1522/15220890.htm. Accessed on 11-01-2003.

Simoes, E.A., Babu, P.G., John, T.J., Nirmala, S., Solomon, S., Lakshminarayana, C.S., and Quinn, T.C. (1987). Evidence for HTLV-III infection in prostitutes in Tamil Nadu (India). *Indian J Med Res* 85:335–338.

Simoes, E.A., Babu, P.G., Jeyakumari, H.M., and John, T.J. (1993). The initial detection of human immunodeficiency virus 1 and its subsequent spread in prostitutes in Tamil Nadu, India. *J Acquir Immune Defic. Syndr.* 6:1030–1034.

Solomon, S., and Ganesh, A.K. (2002). HIV in India. *International AIDS Society—USA Topics in HIV Medicine*. 10:19–24.

Srinivasan, S. (2003). HIV: The Numbers Controversy. Available: http://www.infochangeindia.org/features97print. jsp. Accessed on 10-30-2003.

Stover, J., Stanecki, K.A., and The UNAIDS Reference Group on Models, Estimates and Projections. (2002). Estimating and projecting the size and impact of the HIV/AIDS epidemic in generalized epidemics: The UNAIDS reference group approach (2002). Available: http://www.futuresgroup.com/Documents/PAAStover02.pdf. Accessed on 11-15-2003.

The World Bank Group. (1991). Project Update: South Asia Region-India. Yielding Results: Early Response to HIV/AIDS in India. Available: http://lnweb18.worldbank.org/sar/sa.nsf/Attachments/india1/$File/InHIV1.pdf. Accessed on 11-01-2003.

Thomas, K., Thyagarajan, S.P., Jeyaseelan, L., Varghese, J.C., Krishnamurthy, P., Bai, L., Hira, S., Sudhakar, K., and Peedicayil, A. (2002). Community prevalence of sexually transmitted diseases and human immunodeficiency virus infection in Tamil Nadu, India: A probability proportional to size cluster survey. *Natl Med J India* 15:135–40.

UNAIDS. (2002). Report on the Global HIV/AIDS Epidemic. Geneva. Available: http://www.naco.nic.in/indiascene/esthiv.htm. Accessed on 1-02-2003.

UNAIDS. (2003). HIV/AIDS in Sub-Saharan Africa: Fact Sheet. Available: http://www.unaids.org/html/pub/Publications/Fact-Sheets03/FS_AIDS_in_Africa_2003_en.doc.htm. Accessed on 11-15-2003.

UNAIDS/WHO. (2002a). AIDS Epidemic Update. Available: http://www.unaids.org/worldaidsday/2002/press/update/epiupdate2002_en.doc. Accessed on 1-02-2003.

UNAIDS/WHO. (2002b). India: Epidemiological Fact Sheet on HIV/AIDS and Sexually Transmitted Infections, 2002 Update.

UNDP. (2003). Human Development Report. New York. Avaiable: http://www.undp.org. Accessed on 11-01-2003.

UNDP, UNAIDS. (2003). HIV/AIDS Portal for Asia Pacific. Available: http://www.youandaids.org/ AsiaPacific/ India.asp. Accessed on 11-01-2003.

Uplekar, M., Pathania, V., and Raviglione, M. (2001). Private practitioners and public health: Weak links in tuberculosis control. *Lancet* 358:912–916.

Uplekar, M.W., and Rangan, S. (1993). Private doctors and tuberculosis control in India. *Tuber Lung Dis.* 74:332–337.

Wawer, M.J., Serwadda, D., Gray, R.H., Sewankambo, N.K., Li, C., Nalugoda, F., Lutalo,T., and Konde-Lule, J.K. (1997). Trends in HIV-1 prevalence may not reflect trends in incidence in mature epidemics: Data from the Rakai population-based cohort, Uganda. *AIDS* 11:1023–1030.

WHO. (1995). Estimated to Reported AIDS Case Ratios. Available: http://www.cdpc.com/ratio.htm. Accessed on 10-15-2003.

WHO. (2001a). HIV/AIDS in Asia and the Pacific Region 2001. ISBN 929061 158 8. Available: http://www.who.int/ hiv/strategic/ pubwpraids00/en. Accessed on 10-20-2003.

WHO. (2001b). HIV/AIDS in Asia and the Pacific Region: 2001, Group II- Moderate HIV prevalence countries: India. Available: http://www.who.int/hiv/strategic/pubwpraids00.en. Accessedon 10-20-2003.

WHO. (2001c). HIV/AIDS in Asia and the Pacific Region: 2001, Methods for estimation/projection of HIV infection and AIDS cases/deaths.

World Bank. (1999). India-Second National HIV/AIDS Control Project. Project Appraisal Document. 18918. Washington, DC.

25

Current HIV/AIDS Diagnosis, Reporting, and Surveillance in China

Yiming Shao and Fan Lv

National Center for AIDS and STD Prevention and Control, Chinese Center for Disease Control and Prevention, Beijing, China

BACKGROUND

Since the first case of HIV infection was identified in China in 1985 (Zeng, *et al.*, 1988; Zheng, *et al.*, 1989), the HIV spread in China has undergone three phases: an introduction phase, from 1985 to 1988, an expansion phase, from 1989 to 1994, and a rapid transmission phase since 1995 (Ministry of Health (MOH) and NCAIDS, China, 1998; Lv, *et al.*, 2002). In the introduction phase, only a few cases of HIV/AIDS were reported each year, mostly in big cities. These HIV infected people were either hemophiliac patients who had been transfused with imported plasma, foreigners, or Chinese who had returned from overseas. The first outbreak of HIV infection in the country was found among injecting drug users (IDU) in a border area between China and Myanmar in 1989 (Ma, *et al.*, 1990). One year earlier, Thailand reported an outbreak of HIV among IDU (Wongkhomthong, *et al.*, 1995).

China has experienced a different HIV/AIDS epidemic compared with most other developing countries. China's epidemic of HIV infection began among IDU in border areas of Yunnan Province, spread steadily among IDU in the nearby regions of Guangxi and Guangdong (Cheng, *et al.*, 1997; Shao, *et al.*, 1991; Shao, *et al.*, 1994; Shao, *et al.*, 1996a, b, c; Zhang, *et al.*, 1999; Graf, *et al.*, 1998) and then followed a major drug trafficking route to Sichuan, Gansu, Qinghai and Xinjiang (Yin, 1998; Shao, *et al.*, 1996a, 1999a; Su, *et al.*, 2000; Wang, 1998; Wu, 1999; Zheng, 1999; Zheng, 2000; (MOH) and NCAIDS, China, 2001). The spread of HIV through infected IDU and illegal plasma collection activities converged in central China during the early 1990s and caused the outbreaks of HIV infection among commercial plasma donors in rural communities in several provinces (Wu, *et al.*, 1995; Shao, *et al.*, 1998; Shao, *et al.*, 2001; Yan, J.Y. *et al.*, 2000; Zheng, *et al.*, 2000; Liu, *et al.*, 2000; Wu *et al.*,

2001; Wang *et al.*, 2001; Liu *et al.*, 2001; US Embassy, 2001). HIV infection through sexual transmission has become a steadily increasing trend since the mid-1990s. The sexual transmission of HIV is expected to continue in the future.

HIV/AIDS testing and surveillance work in China started at the central disease control institution immediately after the first case was found in 1985. Due to the lack of reagents, very limited testing capabilities, and few pick-up cases, no meaningful epidemiology data could be collected in the first five years. Beginning in the early 1990s, more efforts were made by the Chinese Ministry of Health (MOH) to build an HIV testing laboratory and surveillance infrastructure, and HIV-diagnostic reagents were produced by the domestic pharmaceutical industry. After the HIV outbreak in plasma donors was discovered, nationwide HIV-testing laboratory networks and surveillance systems were gradually established. The domestic HIV diagnostic reagents industry developed into the major player in the domestic HIV testing market.

In responding to the alarming nationwide HIV/AIDS epidemic, the Medium- and Long-Term National Plan for AIDS Prevention and Control (1998–2010) was issued by the State Council in 1998 (MOH, *et al.*, 1998). In the same year, as part of the national AIDS control effort, the National Center for AIDS Prevention and Control (NCAIDS) was founded by the central government in the Chinese Academy of Preventive Medicine (CAPM). In an effort to strengthen China's capability for disease control and to improve the public health service, CAPM was restructured and named the Chinese Center for Disease Control and Prevention (China CDC) in January 2002. NCAIDS was renamed to National Center for AIDS/STD Control and Prevention (NCAIDS) as part of the China CDC. Since its founding, NCAIDS has been a major national AIDS control and research force and has played a central coordinating and technical supporting role in the national AIDS prevention and control effort under the leadership of the Ministry of Health and China CDC. In the area of HIV testing and surveillance, NCAIDS is the national center for both the HIV testing laboratory network and the epidemiology survey and surveillance database. This article will attempt to provide a brief review of the infrastructure and developments in these areas in the past and an overview of future activities and challenges.

CHINA'S HIV TESTING LABORATORY NETWORK AND TESTING ACTIVITY

Development of HIV Testing Laboratory Network

HIV testing activity in China began with a few research laboratories in the CAPM in the early to mid-1980s. When the first cases of HIV infection and AIDS were found in 1985, the MOH authorized CAPM to organize a series of training courses in the disease control and prevention system, the provincial Epidemic Prevention Stations (EPSs). HIV testing laboratories began to develop in most provinces. When large numbers of HIV infections were discovered in the early 1990s by the HIV testing laboratories of the EPS system in illegal or unregulated plasma collection banks, HIV laboratories were set-up in all blood banks and plasma collection banks. In the beginning of the nationwide HIV/AIDS epidemic driven by IDU and triggered by the blood contamination events, one of the top priorities of the Ministry of Health was to establish a network of HIV testing laboratories throughout China. To meet the ever-increasing demand for HIV tests, the HIV testing laboratory networks in China have been growing steadily from several hundred in the mid-1990s, to over 1000 in the late 1990s, and up to the current number of over 3000 (Table 1).

TABLE 1. Organizational Structure and Responsibilities of HIV Network Laboratories in China

Level	Number	Type of Laboratory	Responsibility
Level I	1	National AIDS Reference Laboratory (NARL, NCAIDS, China CDC)	• Provide guidance and technical assistance to the network • Organize annual external quality assessment of Level II and III laboratories • Organize biannual clinical evaluation of commercial HIV diagnostic kits • Provide comprehensive training together with EEGHCL, to examine Level II and III labs
Level II	31	Provincial HIV confirmatory lab	• Provide technical assistance to Level IV and V labs • Organize annual external quality assessment to Level IV and V labs • Participate in clinical evaluation of commercial HIV diagnostic kits • Provide reliable HIV confirmatory test results and report to higher labs and China CDC
Level III	18	Confirmatory labs in hospitals, medical schools and entry-exit inspection and quarantine bureaus	• To provide reliable HIV confirmatory testing results • To report testing results to higher labs
Level IV	400–500	Central screening labs, mainly in blood banks and city CDC	• To screen a large scale number of samples and provide reliable results • To report testing results to higher labs
Level V	3000	HIV screening labs in hospitals, clinics, and county CDC	• To screen samples and provide reliable results • To report test results to higher labs

Management and Quality Control of the HIV-Testing Laboratory Network

In 1997, the MOH issued the 'National Regulation on HIV Testing and Management' (NRHTM) to strengthen the HIV testing laboratories and their quality control (MOH, 1997). The MOH set up the "Expert Examination Group on HIV Confirmatory Laboratory" (EEGHCL) and authorized the National AIDS Reference Laboratory (NARL) in NCAIDS to work together with the national experts panel to provide training, supervision and quality control of the nationwide HIV testing laboratory networks. Following the NRHTM, the HIV testing laboratory network in China has been designed with five levels, including two layers of management systems (Table 1). NARL, together with EEGHCL, are authorized by the MOH to provide supervision and quality control (QC) for the level II and III laboratories. The provincial HIV confirmatory laboratory at level II is authorized by Provincial Health Bureau (PHB) to provide supervision and QC for the level IV and V laboratories.

For a level II or III laboratory to be opened, the PHB will send a request to the MOH. The MOH will inform NARL to start the examination process. The EEGHCL members will pay a site visit to check the hardware and software of the candidate lab, and its staff members have to pass a quality examination including correctly performing and issuing a report on a panel of samples prepared by NARL. The examination report is then sent back to MOH who authorize the laboratory's opening through PHB. The level II and III laboratories have to pass annual QC tests run by NARL and EEGHCL to gain a work permit for the next year. The labs that receive consecutive, excellent QC scores will be issued a 3-year work permit. Similar lab opening check-ups and annual QC programs are conducted by the provincial HIV confirmatory laboratory and the provincial expert groups authorized by the PHB, in the level IV and V labs in the provinces.

NARL, together with EEGHCL, have drafted national regulations on HIV laboratory examination and guidelines on laboratory QC and safety performance. The above regulations and guidelines have been issued by the MOH and CAPM to guide and standardize the HIV testing activities in the network. Each year, dozens of inspection and site visits are conducted by the NARL and EEGHCL in the level II and III laboratories and hundreds of visits and inspections are performed by the provincial central labs in the level IV and V laboratories. More than 95% of HIV testing laboratories at different levels pass the inspection with an excellent score rate of over 85%. A small percentage of laboratories which failed to pass the inspection or had problems with their internal QC procedures were shut down or required revisions and improvement within a given time (NCAIDS, 2003). Steady improvements have been seen throughout the HIV laboratory networks.

HIV Testing Activity Conducted by the Network

The major tasks of the HIV testing laboratory network include epidemiological study and surveillance, clinical diagnostic services, and blood screening to safeguard blood supplies. Of the total number of HIV tests, about three-fourths were conducted by the HIV testing labs in the blood banks, 10% by labs in the CDC system, and 15% by labs in hospitals and clinics. The majority of HIV tests were screening assays using EIA (enzyme immune assay) reagents performed in the level IV and level V HIV testing labs described above. EIA and Western blot (WB) tests form the primary screening and confirmatory tests for HIV laboratory diagnosis. Schematic flow diagrams of HIV screening and confirmatory tests are illustrated in Figures 1 and 2 (NCAIDS, 2003). In HIV screening, if the sample is positive in the primary screening test, then it should be retested with the original kit and another kit in using a different principle or from a different manufacturer. The repeated positive or indeterminate samples should then be sent to the confirmatory laboratories to conduct a confirmation test using Western blot reagents under the guidance described in Figure 2. The HIV antigen tests and nucleic acid tests are also used to help diagnose samples in the early stage of HIV infection.

A small number of tests were done in HIV testing sites using HIV rapid test reagents. These HIV testing sites were usually located in very small hospitals in remote areas far from blood banks, and used blood only in rare cases of medical emergency. In the current revision of the 1997 NRHTM, it has been recommended that the level IV and V laboratories be merged to make room for the HIV testing sites to become the level V laboratories in the network.

According to the national HIV surveillance database and estimations of the amount of plasma collection, around 30 million HIV tests were performed in China in 2002. About 75% of the tests were done for blood screening and the rest in epidemic study, surveillance, and clinical diagnostic works. The latter includes both high-risk groups and the general population. In 2002, more than 23,000 positive screening results were reported, in which more than 22,000 confirmatory tests were performed (NCAIDS, unpublished data). The HIV-testing lab network finally found more than 5500 confirmed HIV infections and reported them to the national HIV surveillance database.

Training and Network Building

Training is an important component of continuous education in the HIV testing lab

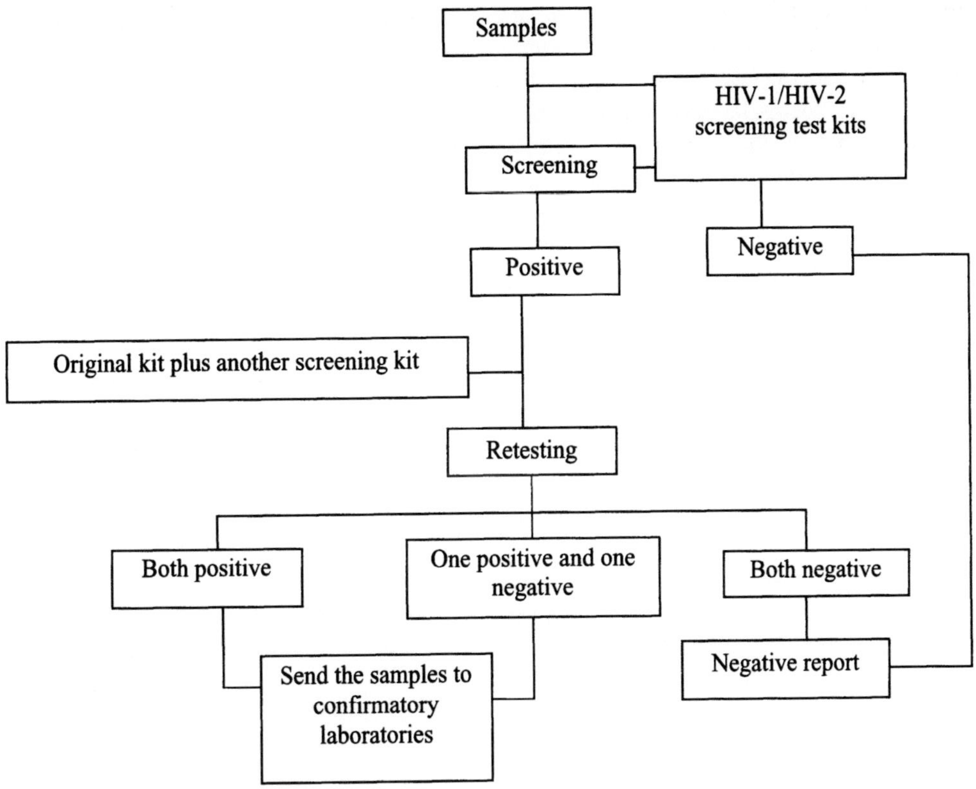

FIGURE 1. Schematic flow diagram of HIV screening test.

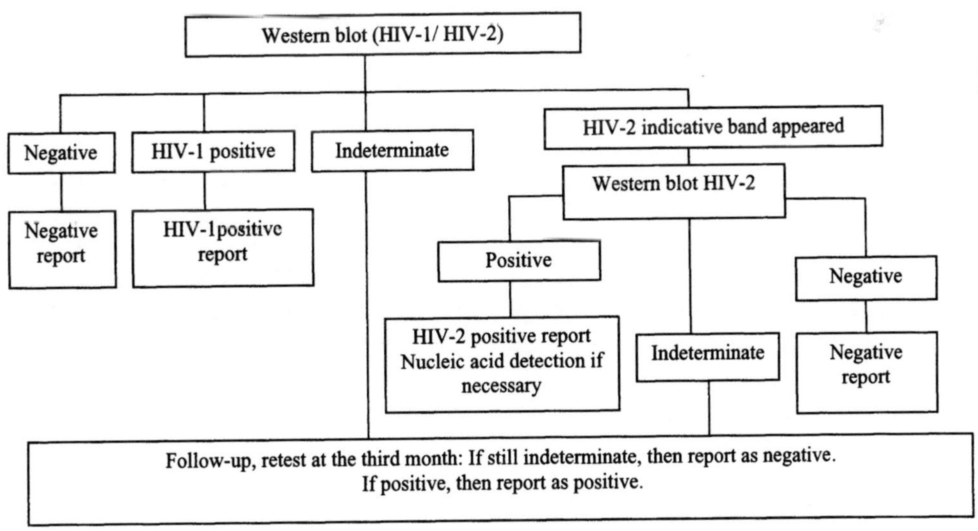

FIGURE 2. Schematic flow diagram of HIV confirmatory test.

network. Each year, many training courses are conducted in the network. The training topics include various diagnostic techniques, quality control protocols, laboratory safety procedures, counseling skills, as well as informed consent and confidentiality. In collaboration with the World Health Organization (WHO) and international institutions in the HIV diagnostic field, NARL and NCAIDS organize several training courses for the staff from the level II and III HIV testing labs each year. The level II provincial central lab conducts several training courses for the staff from Level IV and V HIV testing labs in their provinces every year. More than 3300 lab personnel in the network were trained in 2001, and over 6000 in 2002.

Another frequently used training module is to send lower level lab staff to upper level laboratories for one to three months of on-the-job training. It has been shown that this is a very efficient training method across different levels of the network, especially for newly established labs or staff who have limited experiences in the viral diagnostic field.

In order to provide post exposure prophylaxis (PEP) services to the nationwide HIV lab networks when no anti-HIV drugs were available in China, NARL established PEP programs throughout the network. Eight regional anti-HIV drug stocks were instituted, with a renewable mechanism, available contact persons, and telephone hot lines. This PEP service infrastructure can provide anti-HIV drugs to any laboratory within 24 hours of an exposure (MOH and NCAIDS, 2002). The PEP program is currently expending. All provincial central laboratories are required to develop their own anti-HIV drug stocks and provide independent PEP service within their provinces. Any laboratory that has nearby highly active antiretroviral therapy (HAART) treatment programs should also have their own anti-HIV drug stocks, and provide services to its staff according to the national PEP guidelines.

Clinical Evaluation of HIV Diagnostic Reagents by the Network

Another responsibility of the HIV testing lab network is the evaluation of the HIV diagnostic kits on the Chinese market. NARL and EEGHCL have developed guidelines for clinical evaluation of HIV diagnostic reagents. According to these guidelines, 15 to 20 provincial central labs with excellent QC scores participate in this work. All the licensed HIV diagnostic kits are sampled and tested against 200 sera panel, of which 50 are prepared by NARL, 50 prepared by each participating lab, and 100 random clinical samples from each region. The total 30,000 to 40,000 units of test data are collected and analyzed. The final results rank evaluated kits by their specificity, sensitivity, and Youden's index (Youden's Index (J) is a measure of the probability of correct classifications which is invariant to prevalence. It is used to study the overall performance of a test. The J takes on the value 1 if a diagnostic test discriminates perfectly and without making any mistakes. It is established using Sensitivity (Se) and Specificity (Sp) as $J = Se + Sp - 1$). Tables 2 and 3 list one of the evaluation results as an example. (NARL and NCAIDS, 2003).

The clinical evaluation work on HIV diagnostic kits is organized by NARL twice a year. The evaluation results are published for the public, and circulated within the HIV lab network. The technical data on the HIV diagnostic kit's performance in the market has been used by both the Chinese State Food and Drug Administration (SFDA) and HIV labs as an important reference for regulating work, and for choosing good quality products from the market. This work has always been welcomed by the pharmaceutical industry since it provides an objective indicator of the quality of their products. Clinical evaluation has also helped to shift the competition in the field from a former price war to one of quality improvement. One can clearly see this trend in the steady improvement of the domestic HIV

TABLE 2. Quality Evaluation of HIV-1/HIV-2 ELISA Screening Test Kits, November, 2003

Manufacturer and type of reagent	Sensitivity y%	Specificity y%	False negative rate %	False positive rate %	Youden's index
Lizhu, China ELISA Double antigen sandwich	100	99.10	0	0.90	99.1
BioMerieux, France ELISA Double antigen sandwich	99.21	98.73	0.79	1.27	97.94
Wantai, China ELISA Double antigen sandwich	100	98.22	0	1.78	98.22
Abbott/Murex, USA HIV 1/2gO ELISA Double antigen sandwich	100	98.09	0	1.91	98.09
Lvke, China ELISA Double antigen sandwich	100	97.96	0	2.04	97.96
Yonghua, China ELISA Double antigen sandwich	99.70	97.12	0.30	2.88	96.82
Jinhao, China ELISA Double antigen sandwich	99.67	96.98	0.33	3.02	96.65
Kehua, China ELISA Double antigen sandwich	99.35	96.87	0.65	3.13	96.22
Xinchuang, China ELISA Double antigen sandwich	99.58	96.67	0.42	3.33	96.25
Pusheng, China ELISA Double antigen sandwich	98.98	96.01	1.02	3.99	94.99
Zhongshan, China ELISA Double antigen sandwich	100	95.21	0	4.79	95.21
Huamei, China ELISA Double antigen sandwich	100	94.98	0	5.02	94.98
GBI, China ELISA Double antigen sandwich	100	94.82	0	5.18	94.82

TABLE 3. Quality Evaluation of HIV-1/HIV-2 Rapid Test Kits, November 2003

Manufacturer	Type of reagent	Sensitivity y%	Specificity y%	False negative %	False positive %	Youden's index
Kehua, China	Gold colloid conjugate	94.29	99.77	5.71	0.23	94.06
Xinchuang, China	Gold colloid conjugate	96.77	98.58	3.23	1.42	95.35
FujiRebio, Japan	Passive particle agglutination	99.15	97.93	0.85	2.07	97.08
Abbott, USA	Determine, Selenium colloid conjugate	96.71	98.61	3.29	1.39	95.32
EY, Hongkong, China	Gold colloid conjugate	99.07	97.77	0.93	2.23	96.84
Aikang, China	Gold colloid conjugate	91.48	97.85	8.52	2.15	89.33
Wantai, China	Gold colloid conjugation	94.93	94.68	5.07	5.32	89.61

diagnostic kits. More domestic HIV diagnostic kits receive top rankings in the evaluation list, which was previously dominated by imported kits.

Other Research Conducted by the Networks

In addition to the main task of performing HIV testing and control activities in the country, the HIV laboratory network also conducts various research projects using the resources of the extensive infrastructure. One example of this research is the HIV molecular epidemiology study. The HIV testing lab network conducted the first national HIV molecular epidemiology surveys (NHMES) from 1996 to1998. This survey identified eight HIV subtypes in China: A, B, B', C, D, CRF01—AE, F and G (Shao, *et al.*, 2000; Shao, 2001; Xing,*et al.*, 1999; Pan, *et al*; 1999; Su, *et al.*, 1997). The most prevalent strains are Thailand B', followed by C, and CRF01—AE. In addition to HIV-1 strains, HIV-2 strains have also been found in China (Shao, *et al.*, 1999b; Yan, Y.S. *et al.*, 2000; Xing, *et al.*, 2000). These findings suggest that China is one of the countries with the most HIV-1 subtypes in the world. During the study, a circulating recombinant HIV-1 strain, the B'/C strain was found in southwest and northwest China (Shao, *et al.*, 1999a). It was later found that at least three recombinant events occurred between the B' and C HIV strains and generated two circulating recombinant HIV-1 strains, CRF07—BC and CRF08—BC (Piyasirisilp, *et al.*, 2000; Su, *et al.*, 2000). The CRF07—BC strain from Yunnan traveled through northwestern Sichuan, Gansu, Ninxia, and Xinjiang provinces and across the border into Kazakhstan; while CRF07—BC spread from Myanmar across the border into Yunnan and then through Guangxi and Hong Kong to western countries (Shao, *et al.*, 1996a; Shao, 2001; Yu, *et al.*, 1998; Yu, *et al.*, 1999; Piyasirisilp, *et al.*, 2000; Su, *et al.*, 2000).

The HIV lab network conducted the second NHMES study between 2001 and 2003. A new profile of the HIV-1 subtypes and the pattern of transmission in different risk populations was observed (Shao, 2003). The two surveys created a national HIV database with thousands of Chinese HIV sequences, sera, genomic DNA, and PBMC samples from HIV-positive patients as well as hundreds of

HIV isolates and clones. The database has provided support to both the HIV testing activities in the network and to HIV/AIDS research within China and abroad. The resources and experience accumulated from these studies are not only useful for vaccine design but are also valuable for evaluation of future vaccine trials.

CHINA HIV/AIDS SURVEILLANCE SYSTEM

Based on the concept of 'Secondary Generation of HIV/AIDS Surveillance,' HIV/AIDS surveillance in China currently consists of comprehensive surveillance, including case reporting, sentinel surveillance, behavioral surveillance, and special epidemiological survey.

Case Reporting

An HIV/AIDS case reporting system has been in place since 1985 when HIV was first reported in China. Currently, HIV is reportable through two separate surveillance systems. The first is the HIV/AIDS reporting system that is coordinated by the Division of Epidemiology in NCAIDS, China CDC. The second is the Communicable Diseases Reporting system that is coordinated by the Division of Epidemiology, the Institute of Infectious Disease Control and Prevention, China CDC; this system collects data on 35 infectious diseases, including HIV.

The HIV/AIDS reporting system is the main channel for information regarding HIV/AIDS case reporting in China. At present, according to the 'National Criterion for HIV/AIDS Surveillance' published by the Chinese Ministry of Health in 2002 and the 'National Protocol for HIV/AIDS Case Reporting' published by the China Center for Disease Control and Prevention (China CDC, 2002), confirmed HIV infections and AIDS cases are reported to NCAIDS by provincial CDC (or epidemic preventive station, EPS). An updated summary on the HIV/AIDS epidemic situation, with brief interpretation, is then reported to the MOH and made available to provincial CDC, and provincial health bureaus, quarterly by NCAIDS (Figure 3).

HIV/AIDS case reporting is laboratory-based. HIV infected cases are diagnosed with a laboratory confirmation test. AIDS cases are diagnosed following the 'Diagnosis Criteria and Treatment Principles of HIV Infected Person/AIDS Patient' published in 1995 by the Ministry of Health.

Provincial CDCs are responsible for reporting HIV/AIDS case databases quarterly, and statistic forms annually to the National Center for AIDS/STD Control and Prevention, China CDC, which is responsible for the China HIV/AIDS epidemic situation analysis. CDCs at county levels send HIV/AIDS cases monthly, and statistic forms quarterly and annually to provincial CDCs. In the quarterly and annual forms, a brief epidemic analysis and work overview are attached, including cumulative case numbers, numbers of new tested cases, the number of deaths, the constitution of case categories, distribution characteristics, and other related information.

Sentinel Surveillance

Sentinel surveillance is a rapid and cost effective epidemiological monitoring method, and includes the continuous collection of the HIV/AIDS epidemic data and related information of targeted populations in a fixed place and time. This then elucidates the local epidemic trend of HIV/AIDS, and acts as a reference for the evaluation of HIV/AIDS prevention and control, and the efficacy of these measures.

China's HIV sentinel surveillance program was first established in 1995 in collaboration with WHO. At the national level, the program is coordinated by NCAIDS, and at the provincial level by the Provincial Center for HIV/AIDS Prevention and Control, located within the provincial CDC. Within

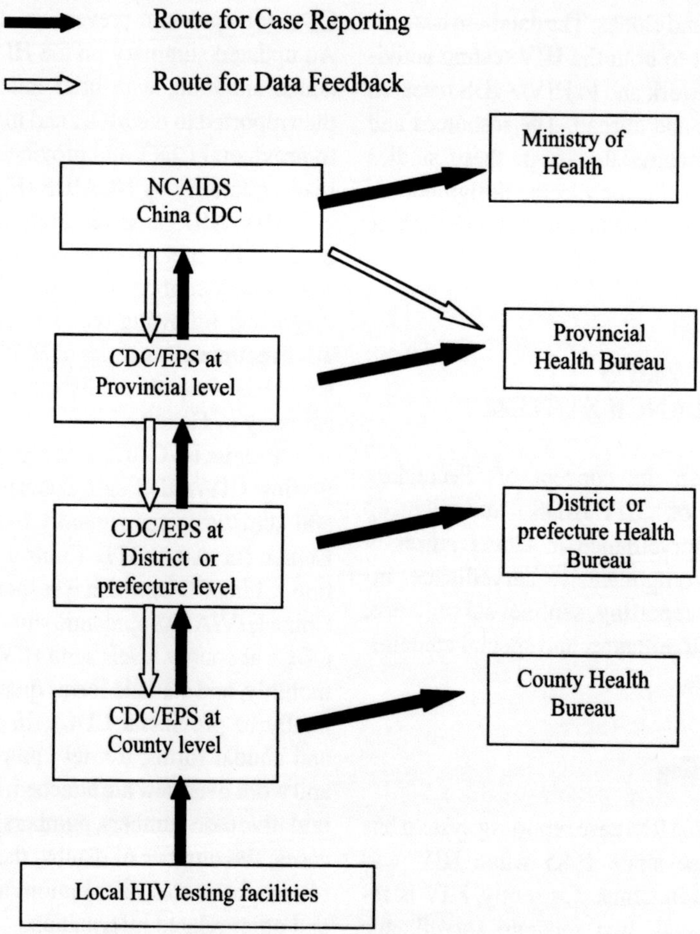

FIGURE 3. Flow chart on HIV/AIDS case reporting system.

NCAIDS, the Division of Epidemiology is responsible for the sentinel surveillance program.

A standardized operational protocol for sentinel surveillance was developed by NCAIDS. The protocol includes directives for data and specimen collection, data management, and transfer of data to China CDC. Staff from NCAIDS of China CDC are also responsible for providing the necessary training, data management software (including predesigned data entry programs), and support for the oversight of operations. The Division of Epidemiology of NCAIDS organizes an annual surveillance conference at which provincial level coordinators meet to review the previous year's surveillance results and discuss operations for the upcoming round of serosurveys. Thus, national level staff members collaborate with provincial CDC staff who in turn work with prefecture and county-level staff as well as site-specific clinic staff. In addition to coordinating the sentinel surveillance program, staff from China CDC have also conducted and/or assisted with small-scale, community-based behavioral surveys among men who have sex with men (MSM), IDU, and female sex workers (FSW) in a few of the provinces outside of Beijing.

In 2002, the number of national HIV sentinel surveillance sites increased to 158. Although there are sites in all 31 provinces, most are in the Eastern and Southern regions of the country (Figure 4). Sentinel surveillance

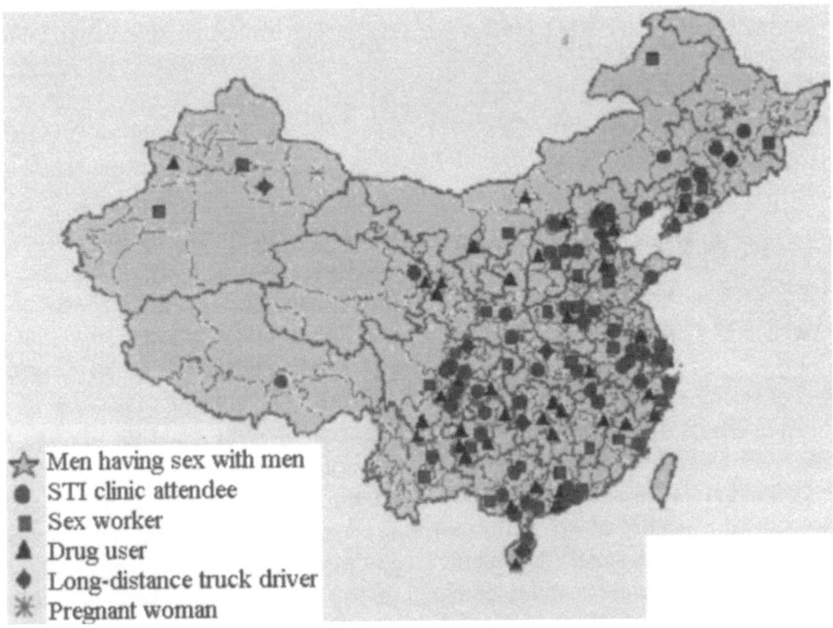

FIGURE 4. Geographical distribution of national sentinel sites in China, 2002.

is conducted among public sexually transmitted infection (STI) clinic attendees, FSW in detention, IDU in detention, long-distance truck drivers, and prenatal clinic attendees. All surveys are facility-based and are conducted in STI clinics, IDU detoxification and FSW re-education centers, trucking company clinics, and maternal-child health clinics. The national sentinel surveys are conducted twice yearly (April–May and October–November), and each survey lasts between two and three months. In principle, blood samples and data are collected from consecutive attendees with a target sample size of 250–400 persons per site. Provincial CDC staff are responsible for providing oversight and ensuring the quality assurance of site-specific data collection operations. As specified by the national protocol, sites collect blood specimens as well as demographic and limited behavioral data on a standard data collection form. For example, among attendees of STI clinics, collected data elements include gender, year of birth, marital status, residential status, limited behavioral data on condom use and number of sexual partners, and STI diagnosis.

In 2002, there were 411 such provincial sentinel sites. However, except for limited studies, all province-led surveillance of IDU and FSW occurs in institutional settings, and there is great variation between provincial sites in the operation of provincial sentinel surveillance.

Behavioral Surveillance

The concept of "HIV/AIDS Behavioral Surveillance Survey" (BSS) was introduced into China in 1998 (Zeng, 1998). In order to collect high risk behavioral data to warn of the HIV/AIDS epidemic and to evaluate the efficacy of prevention efforts, BSSs targeting high risk groups, such as IDU, FSW, and the general population including college students, have been conducted since 1999 within the provinces of World Bank Health IX project and the UK Department for International Development's (DFID) "China Cooperation HIV/AIDS Prevention and Care Project." Data was collected, directed by the "National Protocol for BSS" developed by NCAIDS, to create core indicators, including information on condom use for FSW, and needle sharing for IDU. By 2002, BSS were practiced in about 26 provinces. These surveys will be an essential component of comprehensive HIV/AIDS surveillance in China (Lv, 2002).

CHINA'S EXPERIENCES, CHALLENGES, AND OPPORTUNITIES

Due to strong government support and the concerted efforts of professional personnel, China has established nationwide HIV laboratory and surveillance networks. These two networks have functioned well in the past decade; they provide both an HIV testing service to China's huge population, and epidemic surveillance data to various levels of the government for organizing control measures. The networks' two-tiered (national and provincial) management structure, supported by central and provincial government, conforms to Chinese technical and economic capabilities, and the local environment. Past experience has proven that this is the most practical and cost effective way of managing a large infrastructure in resource-limited settings.

The major challenges posed to the two networks are a result of the rapid evolving HIV/AIDS epidemic in the country. The national management arm has always been the predominant force in the two-level management structure of the networks. This arrangement was able to meet most of the demands to the two networks when the HIV/AIDS epidemic was in its early stage, with localized epidemics. Now that the epidemic is spreading rapidly in most parts of the country, more responsibilities and resources should be given to the provincial level in order to organize timely responses and services as well as sizable control measures.

Examples of new strategies and reform within the old system can be seen in several areas. The new version of the national regulation on HIV testing and management currently being drafted will give the approval power over HIV confirmatory laboratories to the provincial health authorities and provincial central labs instead of MOH and NCAIDS. Hospitals will be encouraged to build more HIV confirmatory laboratories to provide direct testing and counseling to patients instead of sending screening results to HIV confirmatory labs in the public health system for confirmation. How to integrate the various sentinel surveillance sites owned by the provinces into the national sentinel surveillance system is a challenge to the HIV surveillance network. Methods of collection of all the HIV-testing results and the sharing of the surveillance data outside the public health infrastructure should be studied and formulated as soon as possible. Thus, more power at the provincial level will not weaken the responsibility at the national level but will require greater coordination capability and management powers. The governmental reform underway will grant more authority to the national and provincial CDCs. This change will definitely strengthen the management capability of the two networks at the national level and provincial levels.

Most of the progress achieved thus far in the development of the networks has been through team building, including training and research, and international collaboration and support from abroad. Through participation in different research projects and international programs, the capacity of the two networks has been greatly strengthened, and their staff members have received additional training in various skills. The Chinese HIV testing and surveillance networks should be united with more partners and research teams, both at home and abroad, in their future work in order to meet the challenges of the HIV/AIDS epidemic and seize the opportunities of growth and development.

REFERENCES

Cheng, H.H., Zhang, J.P., Kou, J.D., Zhang, Y., Zhang, X.B., Jia, M.H., Bi, X.Q., Ma, Y.L., Liang, Y.B., Yang, C.J., Pan, S.F., and An, X.J. (1997). The overgrowing epidemic of HIV infection in Yunnan Province. *Chinese Journal of Prevention and Control of STD & AIDS* 2(2):54–57.

China Center for Disease Control (CDC). (2002). National Protocol of HIV/AIDS Comprehensive Surveillance. April, 2002.

Graf, M., Shao, Y., Zhao, Q.B., Seidl, T., Kostler, J., Wolf, H., and Wagner, R. (1998). Cloning and characterization of a virtually full-length HIV-1 genome from a subtype B'-Thai strain representing the most prevalent B-Clade isolate in China. *AIDS Res Hum Retroviruses* 14(3):285–288.

Liu, S.Z., Zheng, X.W., Fu, J.H., Yan, J.Y., Xing, H., Kang, D.M., and Wang, S.J. (2001). HIV prevalence and subtypes among paid blood donors in Shandong and Hubei Provinces, China. *China Preventive Medicine* 2:8–11.

Liu, Z.F., Mei, Z.Q., Zheng, X.W., Zhang, W.J., Wang, F.X., Zhou, Y., Mao, Y.R., and Qu, S.X. (2000). Investigation of HIV infection among plasma donors in three illegal plasma collection places in middle China. *Chinese Journal of Epidemiology* 21(6): 466–467.

Lv, F., and Zeng, G. (1999). Introduction to the second generation of surveillance of AIDS/HIV. *Chinese Journal of Epidemiology* 20(6):387–389.

Lv, F., Liu, Z.F., and Sun, X.H. (2002). Chinese current situation of HIV/AIDS surveillance and the working emphasis in the near future. *Chinese Journal of Prevention and Control of STD & AIDS* 8(6):321–324.

Ma, Y., Li, Z., and Zhang, K. (1990). HIV was first discovered among IDU in China. *Chinese Journal Epidemiology* 11:184–185.

Ministry of Health, China. (1997). National Regulation on HIV testing and Management. Beijing.

Ministry of Health and National Center for AIDS Prevention and Control (NCAIDS). (1998). Characteristics of HIV/AIDS in China 1985–1997. *Chinese Journal of Prevention and Control of STD & AIDS* 4(3):141–143.

Ministry of Health and NCAIDS. (2001). HIV/AIDS in China Update to 2000. National Center for AIDS Prevention and Control. Beijing.

Ministry of Health and NCAIDS. (2002). Executive plan of anti-HIV drug stock set-up for post exposure prophylaxis. http:// www.chinaids.org.cn

Ministry of Health, NCAIDS and Collaboration Group for National HIV Sentinel Surveillance Program. (2000). HIV Sentinel Surveillance in China 1995–1998. *Chinese Journal of Epidemiology* 21(1): 7–9.

Ministry of Health, State Development Planning Commission, Ministry of Science and Technology, Ministry of Finance. (1998). China's Medium- and Long-Term Program for the Prevention and Control of AIDS (1998–2010). State Council, Beijing.

National AIDS Reference Laboratory (NARL) and NCAIDS. (2003). Clinical quality evaluation of HIV serological diagnostic kits in 2003. http:// www.chinaids.org.cn

NCAIDS and China CDC. (2003). Standardization of National HIV testing. May, 2003.

Pan, P.L., Zeng, C.H., Fan, X.J., Yao, J., Xing, H., Feng, Y., and Shao, Y. (1999). Identification and characterization of human immunodeficiency virus type 1 subtype F *env* gene in China. *Chinese Journal of Virology* 15(2):97–101.

Piyasirisilp, S., McCutchan, F.E., Carr, J.K., Sanders-Buell, E., Liu, W., Chen, J., Wagner, R., Wolf, H., Shao, Y., Lai, S.H., Beyrer, C., and Yu, X.F. (2000). A recent outbreak of human immunodeficiency virus type 1 infection in southern China was initiated by two highly homogeneous, geographically separated strains, circulating recombinant from AE and a novel BC recombinant. *J Virol* 74(23):11286–11295.

Shao, Y. (2001). HIV/AIDS: perspective on China. *AIDS Patient Care STDS* 15(8):431–432.

Shao, Y. (2003). National Molecular Epidemiology survey of HIV infection in China. Research Project 973 report. Beijing. (Unpublished report).

Shao, Y., Zeng, Y., Chen, Z., and Zhao, Q.B. (1991). Isolation of human immunodeficiency virus (HIV) in epidemic area of HIV infection in Yunnan Province. *Chinese Journal of Epidemiology* 12(3):129–135.

Shao, Y., Zhao, Q.B., Wang, B.,Chen, Z., Su, L., Zeng, Y., and Wolf, H. (1994). Sequence analysis of HIV *env* gene among HIV infection IDU in Yunnan epidemic area of China. *Chinese Journal of Virology* 10(4):291–299.

Shao, Y., Zhao, Q.B., and Guan, Y.J. (1996a). Follow-up studies on molecular epidemiology of HIV-1strains in region of southwest China. XI International Conference on AIDS, Vancouver, Canada. p. 38.

Shao, Y., Zhao, Q.B., and Guo, Y. (1996b). Molecular epidemiology and diversity of HIV-1 strains in Dehong region of Yunnan in Southwest Chain, Xth International Congress of Virology, Jerusalem, Israel, w62.

Shao, Y., Guan, Y.J., Zhao, Q.B., Zeng, Y., Zhang, J.P., Zhang, Y., Duan, Y.J., Yang, G.L., Kostler, J., and Wolf, H. (1996c). Genetic variation and molecular epidemiology of the Ruily HIV-1 strains of Yunnan in 1995. *Chinese Journal of Virology* 12(1): 9–17.

Shao, Y., Su, L., Sun, X.H., Xing, H., Pan, P.L., Wolf, H., and Shen, J. (1998). Molecular epidemiology of HIV infection in China. XII International Conference on AIDS. Geneva, Switzerland. June 1998 [abstract 13132]. (Unpublished paper).

Shao, Y., Zhao, F., Yang, W.Z., Zhang, Y.Z., and Gong, X.C. (1999a). The identification of recombinant HIV-1 strains in IDU in southwest and northwest China. *Chinese Journal of Experimental and Clinical Virology* 13(2):109–112.

Shao, Y., Dai, Y.L., Xing, H., Pan, P.L., and Feng, Y. (1999b). Demonstration of the first HIV-1 and HIV-2 dual infection found in China. *Chinese Journal of Experimental and Clinical Virology* 13(4): 383–385.

Shao, Y.M., Xing, H., Pan, P., Feng, Y., Shen, T., Zhang, Y., Yang, W., Zhang, J., and Lu, B. (2000). The evolution of subtype C HIV-1 and its recombinant forms among IDU in China. XIII International conference on AIDS. Durban, July 2000 [abstract A167]. (Unpublished paper).

Shao, Y. et al. (2001). National Molecular Epidemiology survey of HIV infection in China. Research Project 973 report. Beijing. (Unpublished report).

Su, L., Xing, H., Yang, H.T., Luo, X.G., and Shao, Y.M. (1997). Identification and characterization of HIV-1 subtype A in China. *Chinese Journal of Virology* 13(3):265–268.

Su, L., Graf, M., Zhang, Y.Z., Briesen, H.V., Xing, H., Kostler, J., Melzi, H., Wolf, H., Shao, Y., and Wagner, R. (2000). Characterization of a virtually full-length human immunodeficiency virus type 1 genome of a prevalent intesubtype (C/B') recombinant strain in China. *J Virol.* 74(23):11367–11376.

U.S. Embassy, Beijing. (2001). Shaanxi Province Blood Donor HIV. Environment, Science, Technology, and Health (ESTH) Section. (March 19, 2001); http://www.usembassy-china.org.cn/english/sandt/hivartic.html.

Wang, L., Zheng, X.W., Li, D.M., Xiao, Y., and Yan, J.Y. (2001). A study of HIV infection among children aged 0–7 years in three villages in a rural county of Central China. *Chinese Journal of Epidemiology* 22(1):38–39.

Wang, Z. (1998). Current epidemics of STDs and HIV/AIDS and control strategies and programs in China. *Chinese Journal of Prevention and Control of STD & AIDS* Supplement:1–4.

Wongkhomthong, S., Kaime-Atterhog, W., and Ono, K. (1995). AIDS in the developing world: A case study of Thailand. ASEAN Institute for Health Development, Mahidol University, Bangkok.

Wu, Z.Y. (1999). Epidemics of HIV/AIDS in China. In: Wu, Z., Qi, G., and Zhang, J. (eds.), *Epidemiology and Intervention of AIDS in China*. Science Press, Beijing, pp. 39–56.

Wu, Z.Y., Liu, Z.Y., Detels, R. (1995). HIV-1 infection in commercial plasma in China. *Lancet* 364:61–62.

Wu, Z.Y., Rou, K.M., and Detels, R. (2001). Prevalence of HIV infection among former commercial plasma donors in rural eastern China. *Health Policy and Planning* 16(1):41–46.

Xing, H., Qin, G.M., Feng, Y., Liu, G., Pan, P.L., Fan, X.J., and Shao, Y.M. (1999). Identification and characterization of HIV-1 subtype D strain in China. *Chinese Journal of Experimental and Clinical Virology* 13(2):157–162.

Xing, H., Pan, P.L., Feng, Y., Lin, X.D., Yu, J.S., Gong, X.C., Dai, Y.L., and Shao, Y.M. (2000). Viral sequence analysis of HIV-1 and HIV-2 dual infection firstly found in China. *Chinese Journal of Virology.* 16(2):111–115.

Yan, J.Y., Zheng, X.W., Zhang, X.F., Liu, S.Z., Zhang, Y., Wang, C.L., and Liu, S.L. (2000). The survey of prevalence of HIV infection among paid blood donors in one county in China. *Chinese Journal of Epidemiology* 21(1):10–12.

Yan, Y.S., Zhen, Y.S., Chen, G., Zhen, J., Yan, P.P., and Shao, Y.M. (2000). Confirmation of the first HIV-2 case in China. *Chinese Journal of Prevention and Control of STD & AIDS* 6(1):16–18.

Yin, D.K. (1998). Epidemics of and responses to HIV/AIDS in China. *Chinese Journal of Prevention and Control of STD & AIDS* 4(4):145–147.

Yu, X.F., Chen, J., Shao, Y.M., Beyrer, C., and Lai, S.H. (1998). Two subtypes of HIV-1 among injection-drug users in southern China. *Lancet* 351(9111):1250.

Yu, X.F., Chen, J., Shao, Y.M., Beyrer, C., Liu, B., Wang, Z., Liu, W., Yang, J., Liang, S., Viscidi, R.P., Gu, J., Gurri-Glass, G., and Lai, S. (1999). Emerging HIV infections with distinct subtypes of HIV-1 infection among injection drug users from geographically separate locations in Guangxi Province, China. *J Acquir Immune Defic Syndr.* 22(2):180–188.

Zeng, G. (1998). Second generation of HIV/AIDS surveillance. *Chinese Journal of Prevention and Control of STD & AIDS* 4(1):49–50.

Zeng, Y., Wang, B.C., and Zheng, X.W. (1988). Serological screening of HIV antibody in China. *Chinese Journal of Epidemiology* 9:138–140.

Zhang, J.P., Chen, H.H., Jia, M.H., and Zhang, Y. (1999). Epidemic of HIV infection and prevention researches in Yunnan 1989–1998. *Chinese Journal of Epidemiology* 20(6):377–380.

Zheng, X.W. (1999). Epidemiology of HIV infection, prevention efforts and achievement in China. *Chinese Journal of Epidemiology*. 20(3):131–134.

Zheng, X.W. (2000). Control the epidemic of AIDS by the route of drug use and blood donation in China. *Chinese Journal of Epidemiology* 21(1):6–7.

Zheng, X.W., Zhu, L., Yang, G.H., and Zhang, G.Y. (1989). HIV/AIDS Surveillance in China, 1985–1988. *Chinese Journal of Epidemiology* 10:65–67.

Zheng, X.W., Wang, Z., Xu, J., Huang, S., Wang, C.J., Li, Z.Z., Wang, L., Zhang, G.Y., Gao, M., Li, H., Qu, S.Q., Cui, W.G., Li, X.G., and Wei, W. (2000). The epidemiological study of HIV infection among paid blood donors in one county of China. *Chinese Journal of Epidemiology* 21(4):253–255.

26

Men Who Have Sex with Men and HIV/AIDS Prevention in China

Wu Yu-Hua, Bai Li-Shi, Liu Yan-Cheng, and Zhao Zhong-Hou

Heilongjiang Provincial Center for Disease Control and Prevention, Harbin, China

INTRODUCTION

Men who have sex with men (MSM) worldwide are among the most vulnerable groups that are at high risk for HIV infection. Between 1989 and 1992, three nationwide studies found that 8% to 16% of university students in Beijing and Shanghai had had various homosexual experiences (Zhang, 2003), and another large-scale study from 1998 to 2001 showed that 10% to 15% of male adults reported homosexual behavior (Zhang, 2003). Based on the data from these studies, the number of homosexuals in China is estimated to be between 30 and 48 million (Li, 1998).

Although openly homosexual lifestyles are possible in China, and there have even been a few same-sex marriages, most Chinese homosexuals are living secret lives. Many, particularly in cities, marry someone of the opposite sex and pretend to be heterosexual in their public life, but then engage in extramarital homosexual relationships. According to Chinese traditional values, saving face and continuing a family line is much more important than self-realization. However, as shown in other countries, this type of concealed bisexuality can create an effective bridge to spread HIV/AIDS from MSM, a specific high-risk group, to others in the general population. Furthermore, the secretive nature of this type of lifestyle presents a challenge for HIV surveillance, reporting, prevention and treatment efforts. This chapter provides a brief review of MSM and HIV/AIDS in China and our epidemiological studies and interventions in Heilongjiang province.

MSM AND HIV/AIDS IN CHINA

HIV Infection among MSM

Men who have sex with men have been one of the groups at high risk for HIV infection since the epidemic began. This is primarily due to the transmission risks associated with anal intercourse and to the practice of having multiple sexual partners. In China the first case of HIV infection found to be transmitted by sexual intercourse, was discovered at the end of 1989 in a man who had had sexual relationships with several men. At the end of 1996, 48% of the HIV carriers found in Beijing were MSM. Some experts estimated that 10% to 20% of the people who were infected with HIV in Chinese cities were MSM. However, Beijing was the only place in China to have reported cases of HIV infection among MSM by the end of 1998. In sharp contrast, investigations led by Zhang Beichuan in 2001 indicated that there were 29 provinces or cities throughout China in which there were HIV-infected MSM (Zhang, 2003). Results from this series of investigations also showed that the positivity rate among MSM who had had HIV antibody testing varied greatly over years. In 1998, the positive rate was 2.5%, it was 1.7% in 1999, the rate increased to 4.9% in 2000, and to 5.5% in 2001 (Zhang, 2003). Researchers from the University of California, San Francisco reported in 2003 that 3.1% of 481 MSM were HIV-positive in Beijing; nearly half of them had engaged in anal intercourse without protection in the previous six months, and about 22% of them had engaged in sexual intercourse with women in the previous six months. Among them, the HIV-positive rate of those whose age was above 39 was 4.5 times higher than those who were age 39 and younger (Zhang, 2003).

The investigations led by Zhang Beichuan (Zhang, 2003) also indicated that MSM living in large cities as white-collar workers whose average age was 30 had accumulated about 30 sexual partners on average (in their lifetimes), and the median number was 10. About half had had sexual intercourse with men they did not know in public bath houses and public parks. More than 90% had engaged in oral intercourse, and 60% to 80% of them had engaged in anal intercourse. Nearly one-third to one-half had engaged in oral–anal intercourse. Around one-third had had group intercourse at least once. About 10% of them had paid for sex in the past, and 3% had been paid for sex. About 50% had engaged in sexual intercourse with females. About one-third of them had been married, and more than 70% to 80% of adult MSM were married to a woman at the time of the survey. During marriage, almost all of them maintained a sex life with their wives and also had sexual relationships with other men.

Six to seven percent of Chinese MSM are reported to be infected with sexually transmitted infections (STI) every year (Zhang, 2003). In recent years, condom use, especially among people who have anal intercourse, has greatly increased because of health education and behavioral interventions. However, the rate of condom use at each sexual act is still not high, and the possibility for rapid spread of HIV among MSM still exists. Controlling the spread of HIV in this group is difficult because public awareness and acceptance of homosexuality is low, resulting in difficulties for homosexuals in establishing steady sexual relationships. Most MSM are involved in multiple, short-term sexual relationships. If HIV spreads among MSM, this practice will facilitate its spread to more heterosexual women (the wives or girlfriends of MSM). With changes in the social acceptability of homosexuality, and the loosening of policies that were previously very restrictive, the population of active homosexuals in China is likely to grow, bringing new challenges to HIV prevention and control efforts.

HIV/AIDS Interventions for MSM

In the 1980s, discussions about homosexuality began to appear in popular magazines, dealing with social, psychological, and medical issues. By 1991, some researchers began to focus on HIV/AIDS health interventions for homosexuals (Chen, 1993). In 1994, the monograph *Homoerotism: a comprehensive introduction to homoerotic phenomena*, was published by Zhang Beichuan (Zhang, 1994). In the same year, Qiu Renzong organized experts and volunteers to hold a seminar focusing on homosexuality and HIV/AIDS issues. Since the mid 1990s, HIV infection in the whole nation, including among MSM, has sharply increased, and health interventions have received more attention. In 1995, *The Current Sexual Situation in China* was published by Pan Suiming (Pan, 1995). His survey of more than 180 male homosexuals in four large cities revealed that many MSM were very active and that a high risk of HIV transmission existed in this group.

Combating AIDS: Report on the Situation and Needs in China (Joint Team, 1997) was published at the end of 1997 with the cooperation of the Chinese Ministry of Public Health and the Chinese AIDS special team of the United Nations. It included key statements such as: "homosexuals come from all ranks in society;" "homosexual behavior is not illegal in China, however, it is not accepted by the majority of common people;" "most homosexuals are forced by social pressure to conceal their sexual orientation and get married;" and "we need to pay more attention to this group susceptible to AIDS, find better ways to reach them, provide them with information and support, and improve their ability to self-protect against HIV infection and sexually transmitted infection."

The Textbook of the National AIDS Prevention and Control Program, compiled by the Ministry of Public Health points out: "It is particularly significant to eliminate social discriminations during the ongoing health promotion process, for social discriminations increase the chances for people to be exposed to HIV, decrease the chances for them to access medical care and decrease the possibilities for prioritizing AIDS research to address their needs. Therefore, discrimination can be regarded as a social risk factor. Prevention of social discriminations should be the priority of the prevention, health care and research efforts in the AIDS prevention and treatment program".

In 1998, a health intervention program called "Friends" was launched and began to carry out activities geared towards increasing understanding of homosexuality and HIV/AIDS. This program was sponsored by the Ford Foundation and the Belly-Martin Fund. Nearly 20 authoritative scholars specialized in different subjects, and homosexuals participated in this program directly. In more than 10 large cities all over the country, such as Harbin, Shenyang, Beijing, Wuhan, Nanjing, and Chengdu, hot lines were set up to provide psychological health and HIV/AIDS intervention services. The psychological support aspect of the program has mainly relied on volunteers' efforts, and education interventions have been implemented in places like bars. For example, the team in Chongqing installed condom dispensers in bars. This initiative received the approval of the chief of the HIV/AIDS and STD Prevention Section in the Chongqing government, the cooperation of the police, and the support of homosexuals. The Chongqing team also organized a seminar on Homosexuality and HIV/AIDS Issues, and the Friends Program in 2001. It was the first equal and active communication and cooperation between Chinese nongovernmental organizations (NGOs) and the homosexual community. A Sexual Orientation and Health Workshop was held in August 2003. Most participants came from intervention teams; some famous experts, homosexuals, and CDC staff working in HIV prevention among MSM also took part. They reached an agreement that people from all walks of life should be mobilized to combat HIV/AIDS, and that controlling the prevalence of HIV in MSM was urgent. They also discussed mental health issues for MSM, cooperation with the mass media, and the elimination of discrimination against MSM.

The Friends Program, as an NGO backed by international organizations and government agencies, is actively promoting psychological support and health interventions for MSM. It has set up intervention groups in more than ten provinces. Through hot line consultation, regular distribution of the Friends Newsletter, and frequent epidemiologic surveys, it has improved psychological health for many MSM, promoted social understanding of homosexuality, and taught safer sexual behaviors, in order to reduce the risk of HIV transmission and combat discrimination.

The 5-year Sino-Britain Joint Program of STD/AIDS Prevention and Control was launched in 2000. This project sponsored HIV/AIDS prevention and behavioral intervention for MSM in the cities of Qing Dao, Beijing, Chengdu and Kunming from 2001 to 2002. It distributed materials on HIV/AIDS health education, provided educational lectures, and established close relationships with homosexuals. Through in-depth interviews, this program also discovered information on the background of and reasons for high-risk behavior among MSM.

The National Center for HIV/AIDS/STD Prevention and Control established the first national sentinel surveillance site for MSM at the Heilongjiang Provincial CDC in 2002, to conduct HIV antibody tests and behavioral surveys annually. The China CDC system has recognized HIV/AIDS prevention and control among MSM as key to controlling the overall HIV epidemic in China. Prevention efforts and their impacts have significantly increased. In 2003, with the sponsorship of the Health Department, the China CDC and the Heilongjiang CDC cooperated in the launch of a study to estimate MSM population size and analyze trends in the HIV epidemic among MSM. Internationally used methods were employed to quantify the MSM population, and basic data on the conditions of the epidemic were collected. The purpose of collecting this information was to be able to better select and carry out appropriate interventions.

As an NGO, the Chinese Association of AIDS & STD Prevention and Control established close relationships with MSM several years ago and held a training on HIV/AIDS prevention for more than 40 homosexuals in 2002 with the cooperation of international organizations and domestic HIV/AIDS prevention. Thus, a great number of volunteers were trained and recruited into this program, and communication and understanding between MSM and government agencies were greatly improved.

Many organizations, including NGOs and public health departments have devoted their efforts to HIV prevention and control, formed a powerful team focused on health intervention, and found an effective intervention model. Important elements of this model included adapting responses to the specific situation in China, depending heavily on NGOs, using multisectoral collaboration, including experts and volunteers of different sexual orientations, and employing modern means of communication to reduce high-risk behavior and promote safer sexual practices, such as decreasing the number of sex partners and 100% use of condoms.

Challenges for HIV/AIDS Prevention Programs

Insufficient Social Support and Few Intervention Programs

Health interventions targeted towards MSM require broad social support and understanding. Currently, there is still a great gap in understanding between scientific circles and the public. A majority of people still hold a prejudice against homosexuals. Many believe that AIDS is the curse of homosexuals and that they get what they deserve if they become infected with HIV. As a result, intervention programs are often hindered by these and other forces. For example, staff are barred or interrogated if their sexual behavior survey is considered pornographic or immoral; the legal status of homosexual websites is obscure and their development is limited. We should utilize the coordinating mechanism of multisectoral departments in the HIV/AIDS prevention and control system, and encourage the participation and support of related sections such as the press, police and civil administration. In the long term, it is necessary to incorporate scientific knowledge about homosexuality into sex education across the country, so that homosexuality will be more widely accepted and homosexuals will be equitably treated as members of the society. It is in our common interest to work together; to protect homosexual people from HIV infection is to protect the whole society. Currently there are only a few provinces, such as Sichuan, Yunnan, and Heilongjiang, where there are homosexual intervention programs carried out on a large scale and with significant influence. The problems, in general, are the insufficient knowledge related to this kind of program, the difficulties in establishing them, and the lack of financial support. The most accessible targets for interventions are MSM who socialize in public sites in big cities. However, MSM in medium- and small-sized cities and rural areas are more hidden and less organized, so it is difficult to reach them.

Young MSM frequently visit the "comrade" websites, which makes the internet an effective way to promote AIDS health interventions and to popularize AIDS-related knowledge among people who seldom go to public places and those living in remote and small towns. We should make full use of these network resources, set up targetted health columns and teach safer sexual behavior. Intervention programs are critical, as they can promote communication, improve the psychological health and quality of life of MSM and others affected by HIV/AIDS, and enhance the awareness of HIV/AIDS prevention and the adoption of safer sexual behaviors. In the future, we should mobilize academic circles, try to gain more support from leaders in different sectors of society, and include more geographic areas in intervention efforts. In addition, we should make great efforts to leverage international cooperation and adopt best practices proven in other countries.

Misperceptions among MSM and the Need for More Education

MSM often avoid HIV tests because of fear. They may be unwilling to visit doctors in public medical centers for fear of being identified as MSM. MSM must be able to access appropriate medical services and psychological support and care from medical professionals and doctors who understand them and are familiar with the complex issues surrounding their health care.

Peer education can be used to support psychological health and as a main teaching method for strengthening MSM skills for coping in an unfavorable environment. At the same time, the energy and insight of peer teams can aid professionals involved in intervention design. We should recruit homosexuals who are good advocates and provide them with training and the necessary support so that they can participate in the design, implementation, and evaluation of programs, and play a central role in program decision-making. We should recruit volunteers to work in more areas and set up a volunteer network led by NGOs to coordinate intervention efforts.

Strengthening Communication, Eliminating Estrangement, and Developing Additional Activities

Some MSM are alienated by medical workers carrying out interventions. They may feel they are treated as laboratory specimens for research purposes, and consequently refuse to cooperate. The active participation of MSM in interventions and surveys should be encouraged; the research environment must be made more accessible/comfortable and sensitivity trainings should be conducted among research staff. Only when potential research subjects consider the research setting safe and acceptable, may accurate information be collected, which is crucial for designing appropriate interventions. It is not enough to give lectures and distribute educational materials and condoms. Further knowledge of the economic, social and individual factors behind high-risk behavior is key to addressing the root causes of this behavior, and increasing the impact of STD interventions. The emphasis and objective of our work is to prevent and control HIV/AIDS. Therefore, we should base our work on disease surveillance, behavior intervention, transmission prevention, and epidemic control, rather than on moral judgment or prejudice.

We should also recognize the rapid progress China has made. More and more people are caring for underprivileged groups and their health, listening to their plight and protecting their rights. Meanwhile, we should appeal to the government to do its part to create a loving, caring and comfortable living environment for the many stigmatized groups, including MSM and HIV-infected people. This is a hallmark of a civilized society, and also the duty and responsibility of each citizen.

HIV/AIDS PREVENTION AND CONTROL AMONG MSM IN HARBIN, HEILONGJIANG PROVINCE

Heilongjiang CDC Efforts to Identify Local MSM and Prevent High-Risk Behavior and HIV Transmission

The Heilongjiang CDC is a provincial institution of health and disease prevention, to which the Heilongjiang AIDS Surveillance and Test Center is attached. It administers an authorized HIV confirmatory test laboratory. Before 2001, three MSM were found among the confirmed HIV-infected patients. But the concealment of most homosexual activity made our contact with MSM difficult. We did not get to know members of this group until the beginning of 2001, when the First National Conference of AIDS Prevention and Control was held with the help of the National Center for AIDS/STD Prevention and Control; here, we met some enthusiastic volunteers who were MSM. In the National AIDS Prevention and Control Technical Training Seminar held by the Heilongjiang CDC in July 2001, 11 MSM volunteers were admitted as formal trainees. In later trainings and seminars, we admitted more homosexual volunteers into HIV/AIDS prevention and control efforts, providing them with educational opportunities and welcoming their ideas and input. On December 1st each year, homosexual activists are invited to join in our public procession with a "volunteer" sash on their chest. We have already introduced more than 20 volunteers, committed to HIV/AIDS prevention and control, into the National Center for AIDS/STD Prevention and Control. These collaborative efforts have developed relationships between AIDS prevention staff and the homosexual community, harmonized mutual goals, and enhanced trust. Our work has been recognized by officials from the public health department under the provincial government, and supported and assisted by the National Center for AIDS/STD Prevention and Control. Our efforts have bridged the communication gap between the homosexual population and mainstream society.

In order to reinforce open communication with homosexuals, we have officially registered a health consulting website for homosexuals, or "comrades" in China, called "aixinsky.com & xiaobie.com". This website aims to provide information and resources for the general public as well as high-risk groups more directly and rapidly, and to develop behavioral interventions among the specific groups.

MSM HIV Sentinel Surveillance

Establishing and Conducting MSM Sentinel Surveillance in Harbin

The first and only MSM HIV sentinel surveillance site was set up in the Heilongjiang CDC in 2002, to measure the HIV infection rate and high-risk behavior of MSM in the area of Harbin. As the capital city of Heilongjiang Province, Harbin is more progressive, and the homosexual lifestyle is more active and open than in other cities. The primary identified meeting places for MSM are public bath houses, bars, parks, public toilets, and the Internet. Presently, the MSM HIV sentinel surveillance site can only target those who are active in these public places.

In 2001, we assisted the China CDC and the National Center for AIDS/STD Prevention and Control in conducting an investigation into the prevalence of HIV infection among

MSM in the city of Harbin. The results were as follows: 153 MSM were tested, with five HIV-antibody-positive after the first screening and two confirmed positive later. In 2002, 30 blood samples from 30 individuals were collected in a bar, with 1 HIV-antibody-positive. One hundred-forty blood samples from 140 individuals were collected from January to October of 2003, with 2 HIV-antibody-positive. The positive rate of screening was 1.38%.

The sentinel surveillance strategy uses two ELISA antibody tests on samples collected from fixed places in a fixed time period. Sample quantity must be consistent. Two rounds are conducted annually, starting from April 1 and October 1, respectively. Each round lasts four to eight weeks, surveying 250–400 individuals. Standard questionnaires and behavioral surveillance are also administered. The biggest problem in MSM HIV sentinel surveillance is that many have no desire to have blood tests due to fear of being exposed publicly and fear of positive test results. Thus, it is often difficult to collect sufficient numbers of samples in the prescribed time limit.

Social Support and Coordination

The first step to improving MSM HIV sentinel surveillance is to establish a safe environment and keep the locations of the sites confidential. It is very difficult to establish a gathering place where MSM HIV surveillance and behavioral interventions can be carried out, particularly because of stigma and the possibility of police bans. It should be emphasized that HIV/AIDS control is the responsibility of the whole society, and necessitates the coordination and support of each section of the government. The Ministry of Public Security has issued an official document, stating that education regarding safer sexual behavior and HIV/AIDS prevention activities are allowed to be carried out in public bars.

We must continue to gather information and experience and to advocate our policies to people of influence across the country, in order to gain the recognition of leaders. At the same time, we should promote public awareness of homosexuality. In this way, we can create a more tolerant social atmosphere in which to expand HIV/AIDS surveillance, prevention and control among MSM.

During HIV testing, MSM often ask what they should do if the result is positive. What they actually fear is not HIV/AIDS, but the reaction the people in their life will have if they are known as HIV- infected. Will their loved ones and peers treat them differently? Will they be rejected by the people in their life? Therefore, the elimination of stigma and the development of a culture of compassion for people living with HIV/AIDS (PLWHA) is very important.

High-Risk Behavior and HIV Epidemic Trends among MSM in One City in Heilongjiang Province

With Chinese political reform, and the loosening of social mores, homosexuality has gradually become a more public issue. The MSM population has been growing and they report having more sexual partners and changing partners more frequently than before. In order to learn more about the risk behaviors and HIV status of MSM, several epidemiological studies were done among MSM in public places in one city in Heilongjiang Province in 2001 and 2003. The results of this research are outlined below.

Objectives and Methods

The target population: MSM in public places in one city in Heilongjiang. All the people in this group had engaged in homosexual activity. In 2001, 215 urine samples were collected from this group, and 140 blood samples were collected in 2003.

The on-site survey. With the help of MSM volunteers, the MSM who often appeared in bars, baths or other public places were interviewed with a questionnaire, and blood and urine samples (5ml) were collected at the same time for HIV antibody testing.

After going over the informed consent form with a potential participant, the investigator began filling out the study requirements portion of the survey form. If potential survey participants met the requirements, the survey form would be completed. If not, the investigator would express their thanks to the person and end the survey. This process was helped by key MSM volunteers. The principles of respect, voluntary participation, confidentiality and strict quality control were adopted to ensure the success of the study.

ELISA kits made by two different companies were used to make screening assays. If the test results using the two kinds of kits both indicated positive, Western blot kits were used for a confirmatory test. When urine samples were tested, the same kits were used to make both screening assays and confirmatory tests. EPI6.04 (US Centers for Disease Control and Prevention software) was used to input the data and analyze the results statistically. The significance of the statistical results were determined by the T test.

Results

The median age of the 215 MSM surveyed in 2001 was 29; ages ranged from 16 to 67. The percentage of those who were younger than 25 was about 33.8%. The degree of literacy in the study population was generally high: 2.8% had only elementary school education or were illiterate; 14% went to junior high school; 40.5% went to high school or secondary technical school; and 42.7% obtained college education or higher. In terms of marital status, 49.8% were unmarried; 26.5% were married; 9.3% were divorced; and 14% were cohabitating. Of these, 26 cohabitated with males, four with females. No participants were separated or widowed. In terms of self-identified sexual orientation, 57.5% regarded themselves as homosexuals, while 3.3% considered themselves heterosexual and 34% considered themselves bisexual; 4.1% were uncertain of how to answer, and 0.9% refused to answer. Questions were also asked about openness about homosexual behavior: 12.1% (25/207) of the group had once talked about their own homosexual behavior with their mothers; 9.9% (20/203) had talked with their fathers; and 9.4% (19/203) had talked with doctors. Among the 57 persons who were married, 12 participants (about 21.1%) reported that their wives knew about their homosexual behavior.

Participants' understanding of HIV risk was also assessed: 52.8% considered their risk of HIV infection to be zero; 34.1% thought the risk was very low; and 3.7% thought the risk was relatively high. Only 4.2% thought that the risk of HIV infection was very high.

Data were collected about participants' source of HIV/AIDS information and knowledge of HIV/AIDS: 76.3% had gained knowledge related to HIV/AIDS through television and radio; 80.5% through newspaper and magazines; and 16.3% from healthcare workers. The proportion of participants who were aware of HIV transmission risks through injection drug use, and mother-to-child transmission were high: 90.0% and 85.8%, respectively. About one-third (50/211) believed that withdrawing the penis before ejaculation would avoid the risk of being infected with HIV. One-fourth of the participants thought that asymptomatic HIV-infected people would not transmit HIV to others. Fifty participants (23.7%) thought they would not be infected with HIV if they had sex with a person who could be trusted, while 19.4% believed they would be infected with HIV if they had sex with foreigners. The percentage of those who knew the correct usage of condoms was low: 55% mistakenly thought that Vaseline or cooking oil could be used as a condom lubricant. The pass rate (scoring ≥60% correct) was 77.2%.

Among study participants, the ratio of using a condom "every time" was low, 14.4%, while the ratio of no condom usage was quite high. The rate of condom use every time for insertive anal intercourse was 16.2% while

TABLE 1. Use of Condoms in Different Modes of Sexual Intercourse, 2001

Mode of sexual intercourse	Number of respondents	Never use (%)	Use each time (%)
Vaginal	86	62.8	10.5
Anal (with female partner)	10	60.0	10.0
Insertive anal (MSM)	173	41.6	16.2
Receptive anal (MSM)	131	45.0	13.3
Prostitution	43	53.5	14.0

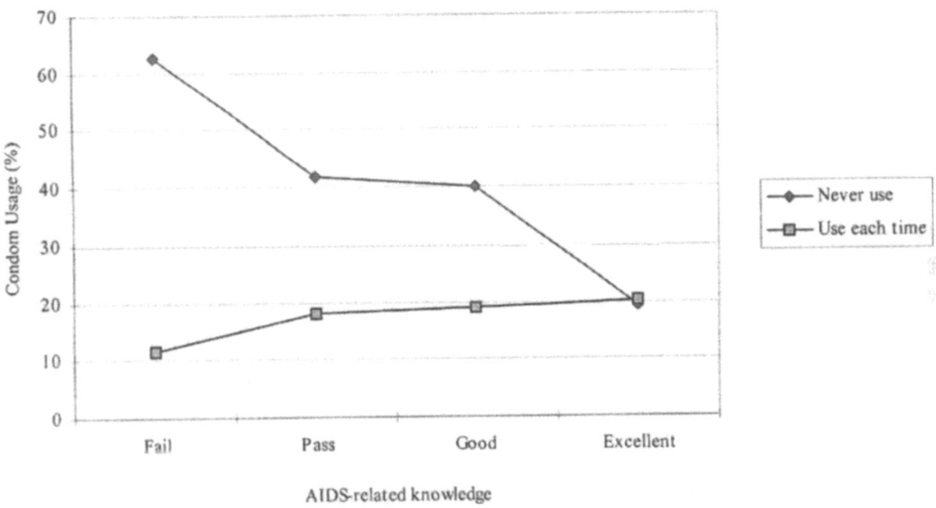

FIGURE 1. Relationship between condom usage and AIDS-related knowledge.

for receptive anal intercourse this reduced to 13.3% (Table 1). Reason for not using condoms included personal dislike of condoms (63.3%), partner's dislike of condoms (51.6%), lack of condoms (41%), fear that carrying condoms would lead to being regarded as a prostitute by the police (32.4%), concerns that condoms were of low quality (9.6%), and lack of money (5.9%).

The relationship between condom use and HIV/AIDS-related knowledge was also assessed in this study (Figure 1). Participants were categorized into four levels according to their HIV/AIDS related knowledge: fail (score <60), pass (60–70), good (71–85) and excellent (>85). Condom use fell into 3 categories: "never using," "sometimes using," and "using each time." With the accumulation of AIDS-related knowledge, the percentage of participants who "never use condoms" fell remarkably and the percentage of using a condom "each time" increased. Among those who failed in the AIDS-related knowledge section, 62.8% never used condoms and 11.6% used condoms each time. Among those who were excellent in AIDS-related knowledge, 19.4% never used condoms and 22.2% used a condom each time.

Median age at first sexual intercourse among the participants was 18. The youngest was 12, and the oldest 32. Among the participants, 69.6% experienced first sexual intercourse with a male and 29.5% with a female partner; 0.9% refused to answer this question.

About two-thirds of participants (143/213) had ever had sex with a female partner; 70.6% (101/143) had had one to five female sexual partners; 29.4% (42/143), six or more female sexual partners; and eight (3.8%) of them had had more than 50 female sexual partners. Eighty-five (40.5%) of the participants had had female sexual partners within the last six months, and the average number of female sexual partners was about 1.1.

All participants had had male sexual partners: 31.9% had had one to 10 male sexual partners; 36.1% (77/213) had had 11–50 male sexual partners; 6.6% had 51–100 male sexual partners; 22.1% (47/213) had had more than 100 male sexual partners; and 3.3% refused to answer this question. Most, 96.6% (200/217), had had male sexual partners within the last six months. The average number of male sexual partners was 10.3, with a median of 5 and a highest reported number of 100.

History of anal intercourse data were collected: 79.8% (166/208) of participants had insertive anal intercourse within the last six months, and 58.7% had had receptive anal intercourse. Many, 89.9% (187/208), had once had anal intercourse in the last six months; 84.5% had anal intercourse without a condom within the last six months.

All survey participants had heard of AIDS. Study results indicated that 45.5% of them decreased their risk of infection by reducing their number of sexual partners, and 42.3% by avoiding anal intercourse. 40.2% began to use condoms to reduce the risk of infection and 27.% began to use condoms at each act of sexual intercourse. However, the percentage of those who said they used a condom each time in the last six months was higher than that reported from the behavioral investigation (16.4%). This indicates that participants may not have fully understood this question.

Twenty-five participants 11.7% had already had an HIV test. Among them, the average number of times they had been tested was 3.2, and no one had received a positive result. Among the 158 participants who had never been tested for HIV, 78.5% gave "low possibility of infection" as the reason they had not been tested; 51.9% thought themselves negative; and 42.4% did not want to think about it. 40.5% had not had an HIV test for fear of exposing their homosexuality.

Comparing the Results of the First Investigation to the Second Investigation

The median ages in the two surveys were very close. The percentage of divorced and cohabiting people dropped significantly and that of single people increased. The age of this group tended to be younger.

In the second study in 2003, the numbers of female and male sexual partners dropped markedly compared with the 2001 data (Table 2). In the first investigation, most homosexuals had between one and 20 female sexual partners, and some had more than 50. In the 2003 survey, the majority did not report having female sexual partners (72%), and many reported five female sexual partners at most. In the first investigation, most homosexuals had between one and 20 male sexual partners, and some had more than 50. In the 2003 survey, most people (88%) reported one to five male sexual partners, and many had 15 at most.

It is clear that all indices dropped in the 2003 investigation, with the most obvious drop in the average number of sexual partners. The rate of unprotected sexual behavior changed little, revealing that condom use remained unsatisfactory. The reasons were varied, but the major one was low awareness of HIV prevention. Most people are able to use a condom sometimes, but not consistently, suggesting that condom use should be re-emphasized in future interventions and efforts should be stepped up to raise awareness of HIV prevention methods. Because the risk of HIV transmission during unprotected anal intercourse is two to three times higher than in vaginal intercourse, it is important that we educational interventions incorporate information on reducing risk for MSM.

In 2003, the rate of sexual activity with females rose, while the rate of condom use "each time" decreased from 10.5% to 5% (Table 3). The rate of "never using condoms" fell sharply from 60% to 20%, indicating that

TABLE 2. Distribution of MSM Sexual Partners Reported in 2001 Compared to 2003

2001				2003			
Number of female sexual partners	%	Number of male sexual partners	%	Number of female sexual partners	%	Number of male sexual partners	%
0	28.2	0	0	0	72	0	6.4
1–20	58.2	1–20	55.2	1–5	25.8	1–5	88
21–50	5.2	21–50	13.1	Over 6	0	6–15	4.2
Over 50	3.8	Over 50	28.7	No response	2.2	Over 15	0
No response	4.7	No response	3.3			No response	1.4

TABLE 3. 2001–2003 Comparison of Reported Sexual Activity with Females

Year	Average number of female sexual partners	Reported sexual activity with females within six months (%)	Use condom each time (%)	Never use condom (%)
2001	1.1	40.5	10.5	60
2003	0.46	45	5	20

most people realized the importance of using condoms. However, they were not always able to do it consistently. Therefore, it is necessary to provide education on condom-use techniques for this group to increase the rate of consistent condom use.

Because of the current ease of networking among MSM, sexual behavior in this group is apt to be frequent, and an active sex trade has developed. In the 2001 investigation, 26.3% of participants surveyed had sold sex, and 85.7% had bought sex. In the 2003 investigation, the two figures were 31% and 38%, respectively. The number of people buying sex decreased markedly in the second study.

In the 2001 investigation, 153 urine samples were collected, of which two were confirmed positive using an ELISA antibody test and a Western Blot confirmatory test, resulting in a prevalence of 1.31%. In the 2003 investigation, two out of a total of 140 blood samples (1.4%) were HIV-1 antibody positive. There was no significant difference in the infection rate between the two studies.

Discussion

Although homosexual behavior is not prohibited by law in China, it is not well accepted by society in general. Many homosexuals in China marry women and have children despite their sexual orientation, enduring heavy psychological strain. Studies show that depression and lack of social support will lead to increased high-risk behavior among homosexuals.

The surveys also discovered that 67.1% of study participants had had sex with both males and females, many had bought sex, and some maintained sexual relationships with their wives. This bisexual behavior sets up a bridge between two high-risk groups, MSM and sex workers, and the general population. Therefore, providing help for members of these high risk groups will not only protect them, but will also protect the general population.

The rate of HIV transmission through sexual behavior is mainly determined by the transmission risk during each instance of sexual intercourse, and by the number of different sexual partners. The risk of transmission during sex is related to many factors, the major one being condom use. The infection rate of the receiver of anal intercourse is 0.5%–3%, if his partner is HIV-positive and they do not use a condom. The results of the 2001 investigation indicated that HIV high-risk behavior was relatively frequent in this group. For example, the rate of those who use a condom in each instance of anal intercourse is low (15.5%), and the added risk of having multiple sexual partners may result in the potential for rapid HIV spread. If we do not adopt effective measures to control this situation immediately, the HIV/AIDS epidemic in this group may follow the same path it has taken among injection drug users. However, the investigation in 2003 showed that HIV prevalence had not risen significantly among MSM. There are several possible reasons for this. First, the average number of male sexual partners had dropped significantly, from 10.3 to 2.8, and the average number of female sexual partners also dropped. Second, the rate of participants who reported using condoms some of the time increased dramatically.

Currently, there are not many systematic studies focused on MSM in China, and only a few small-scale studies have been done and reported. Throughout this investigation we were cognizant of the fact that high-risk behavior among MSM is apt to decline because of the ongoing reinforcement of HIV/AIDS education and prevention in China. But as the sample size was limited in these studies, and the participant group might not represent the most susceptible to HIV infection, the level of risk and the rate of infection among MSM in general might have been underestimated. Therefore, it is necessary to conduct more epidemiological studies to obtain results that better reflect the reality of the epidemic in this population. At the same time, the HIV prevention efforts targeted towards MSM are still important and urgent.

SUGGESTIONS FOR THE FUTURE

Development of an Overall Strategy for Preventing HIV Transmission among MSM

By the end of 2001, there were 40 million PLWHA globally, among whom about three-fourths were infected through heterosexual transmission and one-fourth through male–male sexual transmission. Two studies on HIV infection among MSM in Heilongjiang Province (2001–2003) reported the HIV infection rate to be about 1.5% in general. The actual HIV infection rate was probably higher than this figure, since some people known to be or suspected of being HIV-positive avoided participation in the study. This suggests that HIV prevalence among MSM has already reached a relatively high level in China. For many complex reasons, the health problems of MSM do not get enough attention. To date, there is no mid- or long-term strategy concerning HIV/AIDS prevention and control among MSM in China. It is very difficult to control HIV prevalence in this group without any strategies or definite goals. MSM participating in our studies had little knowledge about HIV infection risk and prevention. Printed materials are not sufficient for the education of this group, and existing educational activities are only held on a small scale at MSM gathering places by the nearby disease control organizations or hospitals. There have been no systematic intervention programs targeting MSM. It is urgent that we expand epidemiological research in the MSM population and launch extensive prevention interventions in order to prevent the further spread of HIV among MSM, and the subsequent spread to the general population.

Collaboration with MSM

Our work has taught us that it is not as difficult to launch HIV/AIDS prevention programs targeting MSM as had been expected. As long as we abandon our prejudices, and approach our work with MSM with professionalism and respect, we can reach our public health objectives. We found working with MSM different from working with some other high-risk groups, in that many of them were eager to collaborate with us in our work, and approached the prevention and control of HIV actively, and with a sense of responsibility and passion. Their help is fundamental to our work.

Cooperation with Other Government Sections

The development of our work relies on the support of MSM volunteers and the cooperation of the managers of MSM gathering places. Homosexuality is a reality, not only in big cities like Beijing, Shanghai, and Dalian, but also in very remote places in Heilongjiang Province. Even in these remote areas, there are many gathering places for MSM. As we have observed, most come to these places for social activities and to build a sense of community. As with heterosexuals, a sex trade has developed among MSM, and we should try our best to control its expansion through behavioral interventions and education. However, many MSM and managers of MSM gathering places, whose cooperation and trust is essential to the success of our efforts, fear that the prevention education materials and condoms we distribute will become evidence for police action against them. This fear greatly hampers our efforts. Therefore, we must work toward true collaboration with various sections of government, such as public security officials, so that we are all working towards the same objective.

Further Research and Collaboration

We should collaborate with research institutions in the area of social sciences, so that we can enhance the efficacy of HIV/AIDS prevention and control measures with knowledge gained from sociological research on homosexuality and sexual behavior. We should work to establish contacts within the MSM community, capture the attention and support of political leaders, and secure more funding for HIV/AIDS prevention efforts. Meanwhile, we should also strengthen the exchange of information, and leverage international cooperation and support, as we further develop research and interventions for HIV/AIDS prevention and control among MSM.

ACKNOWLEDGEMENTS. Thanks are due to Ellen Stiefvater and Dr. Yichen Lu of Harvard University, and to Kou Yang, Chong Jing, and Luo Ling of Nankai University for their many long hours of translation of this paper.

REFERENCES

Chen, B.Z. (1993). AIDS, homosexuality, and health education. *Chinese Health Education* 9:9–16.

Joint Team of the Chinese Ministry of Health and the UNAIDS China Team. (1997). Combating AIDS: Report on the Situation and Needs in China. Beijing, 11–12.

Li, Y.H. (1998). *Subculture of Homosexuality* (1st edition). Beijing: Today's China Press, 334–349.

Ministry of Public Health. (1997). The Textbook of the National AIDS Prevention and Control Program.

Pan, S.M. (1995). The Current Sexual Situation in China. Beijing: China People's University Press.

Zhang, B.C. (1994). Homosexuality. Jinan: Shandong Science and Technology Press, 644.

Zhang, B.C. (2003). Homosexuality. *Friends Newsletter* Qingdao February; 25–31.

27

Trends in Injection Drug Use and the HIV Epidemic in Southern China

Rebecca J. Garten[1], Shenghan Lai[2], Wei Liu[3], Jie Chen[3], and Xiao-Fang Yu[1]

[1] *Department of Molecular Microbiology and Immunology, Johns Hopkins Bloomberg School of Public Health, Baltimore, Maryland, USA*

[2] *Department of Epidemiology, Johns Hopkins University Bloomberg School of Public Health, Baltimore, Maryland, USA*

[3] *Guangxi Centers for Disease Control and Prevention, Guangxi Province, China*

DRUG ABUSE IN CHINA

The history of drug abuse in China can be traced back several centuries. China, along with Southeast Asia, has suffered through a long epidemic of opium addiction. By the early nineteenth century, smoking opium was commonplace within the region. Besides recreational and social use, many individuals used opium for medicinal relief of illness or physical and mental stress (Suwanwela and Poshyachinda, 1986). By the 1900s, the northern mountainous regions of Laos had begun opium poppy cultivation (Poshyachinda, 1993). Opium production spread throughout Southeast Asia, creating the Golden Triangle of opium production, including parts of Myanmar, Laos, Thailand, China and India. The high availability of opium in this area likely led to an increase of drug users (McCoy *et al.*, 2001).

By the end of the 1940s, an estimated 5% of the Chinese population were opium users (McCoy *et al.*, 2001). After the founding of the People's Republic of China in 1949, the new government took strong action to crack down on opium trafficking and abuse. As a result of these changes, drug abuse would be considered practically non-existent in China over the next few decades. Meanwhile, other Southeast Asian countries also began to pass laws restricting the sale and use of opium. In order to circumvent the authorities, drug dealers needed a more compact, highly pure drug that would be easier to distribute. Heroin fit these specifications. Through the 1960s and 1970s, smoking heroin largely replaced opium use in Southeast Asia (Poshyachinda, 1993).

The 1980s saw the beginning of dramatic changes in China's economic market structure. China eased border restrictions to increase trade with the west. Opium and heroin began trafficking once again from the Golden Triangle into southern China on roads once used by smugglers for gold and silver (Lai *et al.*, 2000). With the new wide availability of opium and heroin, China's history of drug abuse was reborn. To address this rise in drug abuse, the government developed a framework for drug control. Penalties for ingesting or injecting narcotics included detention, hefty fines, and forced treatment (China Ministry of Health, 2003). Drug users who were unable to control their addiction underwent further rehabilitation through labor. The punishment for drug manufacturing, dealing or trafficking included harsh penalties, even death. If an individual possessed over 50 grams of heroin, the penalty was seven years to life imprisonment. By 2000, the Chinese government reported approximately 800,000 documented drug users, while the actual number could be many times higher (UNAIDS Task Force, 2000).

ADOPTION OF INJECTION DRUG USE IN CHINA

The 1980s brought an important change in the method of heroin administration; shifting from smoking to injecting. The formerly common method of smoking heroin, known as "Chasing the dragon" originated in Shanghai in the 1920s (Strang *et al.*, 1997). "Chasing the dragon" refers to inhaling the vapors of heroin that has been heated in tin foil over a flame. This method of drug administration spread across Southeast Asia and eventually into the west. In response to rises in drug abuse, countries in Southeast Asia again stepped up anti-drug enforcement efforts, leading to an increase in heroin prices. Higher prices of heroin led to the change of abuse from smoking to injection. In Thailand, heroin users saw injection as a way to achieve a better high for less cost (Des Jarlais *et al.*, 1992).

Studies of drug use patterns in heroin users in the mid-1990s from the southern Chinese Provinces of Yunnan (Zhou and Li, 1999) and Guangxi (Lai *et al.*, 2000) found injection drug use on the rise. Heroin users were predominantly young (<40 years old), uneducated, single, and relatively new drug users (<3 years). Drug users initiated heroin use through smoking or snorting the drug. Over 80% had injected heroin at least once. Injectors are more likely to have friends or family members who are heroin users. Therefore, initiation of injection drug use is likely to occur through social networks. New injectors often are taught injection techniques by more experienced peers. Drug users who injected heroin were more likely to use a larger quantity of drug and use heroin longer than non-injectors (Lai *et al.*, 2000). Newer heroin users were more rapidly changing over from smoking to injection drug use than older heroin users. This has effectively shortened the time span between initiation of heroin use and injection drug use. Individuals cited a better high or a lower cost as the reason they switched from smoking to injection.

Additional studies in Guangxi heroin users found over 50% of injectors used a needle more than once (Garten *et al.*, 2004). It is not illegal in China to be in possession of needles, and they are available for purchase at local stores at a small cost, but many users prefer to recycle needles. In between needle uses, 90% of injectors rinse the needle with water or boil them in an attempt to sterilize their equipment. Over 50% of injectors share needles and potentially share other injection paraphernalia. In addition, most injectors share needles occasionally, but approximately 10% share on a daily basis. Some injectors do not share the same needle for injecting, but use each others' needles to dissolve and share the drug, called "backloading". Backloading, like sharing needles, helps decrease the overall cost of the drug. Since 1999, the percentage of injection drug users (IDU) who share drug equipment has been steadily increasing (UNAIDS/WHO, 2002).

HIV SURVEILLANCE PROGRAMS IN CHINA

Surveillance programs within IDU in Southeast Asia began to see a rise in HIV-1 prevalence (hereafter referred to simply as HIV) in the late 1980s. The first epidemic of HIV among Chinese IDU arose in cities along the Myanmar border of Yunnan Province in 1989 (Zheng *et al.*, 1994). Frequent traveling of Yunnan IDU across the border to purchase or share drugs/paraphernalia may have introduced HIV strains from Myanmese IDU. Heroin trafficking across the border was also on the rise and HIV may have been brought into China by infected drug dealers. Re-using and sharing of needles among social networks of IDU resulted in a HIV seroprevalence of over 80% among injectors by 1992 (Zheng *et al.*, 1994). The epidemic was spreading in neighboring counties along the Myanmar border within Yunnan Province.

The introduction of HIV into the IDU population in Yunnan sent out a warning signal that the HIV epidemic in China was beginning (China Ministry of Health, 1997). The Chinese government set-up HIV surveillance programs within IDU populations, female sex workers (FSW), blood donors, and sexually transmitted infection (STI) clinic visitors. As of 2002, there were 158 national surveillance sites in 31 provinces in China, as well as additional provincial surveillance sites within high-risk groups (China Ministry of Health, 2003).

EPIDEMIOLOGY OF HIV IN CHINESE IDU

Statistics

HIV cases among IDU have been reported in all 31 provinces. HIV prevalence in IDU from Yunnan, Xinjiang, Sichuan, Guangxi, and Guangdong continues to be over 10%; in some areas rates are as high as 80% (China Ministry of Health, 2003). As of June 2003, over 45,092 HIV-positive cases have been reported to the Chinese government. Although the total number of HIV/AIDS cases remains unknown, it is estimated over one million individuals have contracted HIV in China. The number of estimated AIDS patients exceeds 80,000, although only 3532 have been reported. Injection drug use was responsible for HIV transmission in approximately 70% of the cases.

HIV Clades and Circulating Recombinant Forms (CRF) in Chinese IDU

The initial HIV subtype epidemics within Yunnan were predominately a mixture of clade B viruses found circulating in Myanmar, Laos, and Thailand (Graf *et al.*, 1998).

From 1994 to1995, the addition and shift from clade B to clade C viruses, likely from Indian IDU, occurred (Xia *et al.*, 1994; Luo *et al.*, 1995). At some point between 1994 and 1996, there were multiple recombination events between clades B and C within Yunnan IDU to create several B/C recombinants (Su *et al.*, 2000; Piyasirisilp *et al.*, 2000; Rodenburg *et al.*, 2001). From these recombinants sprang two circulating recombinant forms (CRF07_BC and CRF08_BC) which likely shared a common ancestor that was an initial BC recombinant (McCutchan *et al.*, 2002). The majority of the genome in these viruses consists of clade C, with small clade B segments. After originating in Yunnan, the CRFs have spread out into neighboring provinces of Sichuan and Guangxi, and to the northwestern province of Xinjiang, leading new HIV-1 epidemics there (Piyasirisilp *et al.*, 2000; Su *et al.*, 2000; Rodenburg *et al.*, 2001). Another notable clade circulating within IDU populations in China is CRF01_AE, which likely entered from Vietnam. CRF01_AE is a recombinant from a clade A and an extinct clade virus. Transmission of CRF01_AE was initially through injection drug use, but it established a significant sexually transmitted epidemic throughout Southeast Asia (Kaldor *et al.*, 1994).

FOCUS ON IDU IN GUANGXI PROVINCE

HIV sentinel studies at drug detoxification clinics were established in border cities within Guangxi. HIV was first detected in two separate border cities in late 1996–early 1997 (Yu *et al.*, 1998). An HIV CRF01_AE epidemic was found in the southern city of Pingxiang, a major border city into Vietnam. Data from molecular sequencing and heroin trafficking routes suggests that the HIV epidemic flowed from Laos through Vietnam (Beyrer *et al.*, 2000). In addition, the AE subtype in Pingxiang has been linked to HIV from the Lang Son Province in Vietnam (Yu *et al.*, 1999; Kato *et al.*, 1999). Unlike Pingxiang, the AE epidemic in Southeast Asia has been spread efficiently and predominately by sexual transmission (Kaldor *et al.*, 1994). Information from IDU in Pingxiang suggests that many cross the forested border on foot to buy cheaper heroin in Vietnam (Beyrer *et al.*, 2000). Buying practices included using the dealer's needle to test the purity of drug. Pingxiang IDU have also admitted to sharing needles and drugs with Vietnamese users.

At nearly the same time, another HIV epidemic surfaced in the city of Baise near the western border to Yunnan Province. Initial partial *env* sequencing identified this outbreak to be clade C (Yu *et al.*, 1998). Full-length sequencing of the subtype C found in Baise confirmed it was a BC recombinant (CRF08_BC) similar to, yet distinguishable from, another BC recombinant (CRF07_BC) which had spread into the northwestern provinces of Sicuan and Xinjiang (Piyasirisilp *et al.*, 2000). Again, the initial spread of HIV in Baise IDU likely occurred by sharing needles with local dealers during the buying process. Due to these initial case studies, sites throughout Guangxi were established to track and hopefully prevent the further spread of HIV.

By 2001, Guangxi Province had the third largest reported population of HIV-positive individuals in China (Yu *et al.*, 2001). Injection drug use continued to be the major mode of HIV transmission in the Province, but other modes of transmission, such as heterosexual contact, were occurring. The two strains of HIV were introduced in Guangxi at the same time, but have had vastly different expansion patterns. The HIV BC recombinant strains have rapidly expanded from Yunnan to IDU in the cities of Baise, Tianyang, Tiandong, Nanning, Binyang, Liuzhou, and Guilin (Yu *et al* ., 2001; Yu, X.F., unpublished data). Conversely, the HIV AE was largely confined to Pingxiang, near the Vietnam border. Molecular epidemiology data traced the HIV epidemic spreading throughout the province following major highway routes (see Figure 1). Since the two strains stem from separate drug trafficking routes, the route from Yunnan Province may be more active. Alternatively, the drug users on this route may have more interaction with each other than those in Pingxiang.

Sequence analysis continues to find a low genetic diversity within the *env* region of the HIV genome between study subjects in geographically separated cities throughout Guangxi (<1% difference for BC and <2% for AE) (Yu *et al.*, 1998; Piyasirisilp *et al.*, 2000; Yu *et al.*, 2001; Yu *et al.*, 2002; Yu, X.F., unpublished data). The mechanism driving the low diversity is unknown. It is plausible each subtype epidemic is the result of a single introduction into networks of IDU with high transmission rates, therefore creating a strong founder effect. Additionally, the rapid spread of HIV during acute infection may lead to decreased HIV diversification. Within the CRF08_BC virus, there is a remarkable, well-conserved (<0.1% difference) V3 region of the *env* gene, while the V4 region is

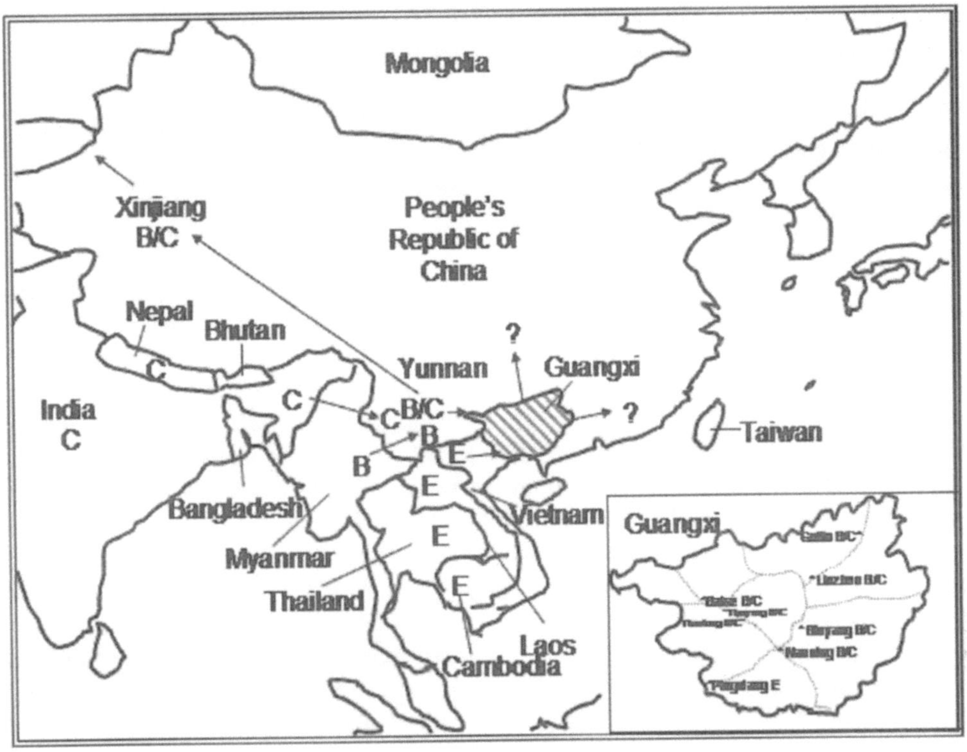

FIGURE 1. Introduction and spread of HIV clades in Southern China through injection drug use. E refers to CRF01_AE. B/C refers to either CRF07_BC or CRF08_BC. Insert: Mapping of HIV-1 subtypes along major highways in Guangxi Province.

considerably less conserved (>4.0% difference) (Yu *et al.*, 2002). It is not yet known whether there is any intrinsic advantage to the virus to maintain such a homogenous *env* sequence.

Approximately 20% of heroin users in Guangxi Province are HIV-positive, while over 70% are Hepatitis C (HCV) antibody positive (Garten *et al.*, 2004). In addition, 15% were Hepatitis B virus surface antigen positive. Nearly all HIV-positive individuals were HCV positive (98%). HIV continues to spread in IDU at an incidence rate of around 7.0 per 100 person years. The HCV incidence rate was found to be extremely high, at 37.6 per 100 person years. Seroprevalence by years of injecting heroin, found that with one year of injection drug use history, over 80% were HCV antibody prevalent. HCV prevalence continued to climb, reaching a maximum of over 90% in individuals with five years of injection drug use. HCV is rapidly acquired after onset of injection drug use through high-risk injection behaviors. The HIV virus, presumably less infections than HCV, had a gradual increase in seroprevalence with increasing lengths of injection drug use. Differences in infectiousness alone may explain the dissimilarity in HIV and HCV seroprevalence, or perhaps high-risk injection practices, i.e. sharing cookers, cotton, or rinse water, may affect the transmissibility of the two viruses.

PREVENTION METHODS

Heroin users who enroll in HIV surveillance programs receive education on the ways in which HIV and HCV can be transmitted, behaviors in which the study subject engages that could put him/her at risk, as well as ways to reduce further risk. The participants are counseled on the ways to reduce the risk of HIV and HCV infection in the future, such as (1) using condoms with all sexual partners; (2) reducing the number of partners; (3) not sharing injection equipment with others; (4) using bleach when cleaning needles. Public health teams have worked extensively on counseling not only the participants but also their peers on the consequences of injection drug use and sharing needles. Needle exchange programs are not available in China. However, needles are freely and inexpensively available for purchase from the local stores. In addition, pilot programs in Guangxi and Guangdong encouraged IDU to purchase new needles and syringes by offering discounts at local pharmacies (China Ministry of Health, 2003). Participants may also receive condoms.

All drug users arrested by the Chinese authorities are sent to compulsory treatment centers. Drug users identified through surveillance programs are not reported to the authorities but instead encouraged to join voluntary drug cessation programs. Treatment and rehabilitation centers have increased their capacities to treat drug users over the last five years (UNAIDS Task Force, 2000). Methadone for maintenance is not routinely practiced in China, although patients are treated for detoxification using western and traditional Chinese medicines.

The current prevention methods are not sufficient to prevent the spread of HIV, and are especially insufficient in preventing the spread of HCV. Education on the harms of re-using needles and sharing any type of injection paraphernalia is currently ineffective and needs to be strongly re-addressed. Additional programs that focus on reducing the transition from oral to injection drug use and promote primary substance abuse prevention are urgently needed. IDU in China are developing faster than before and HIV/AIDS prevention methods must target youth. But only targeting high-risk populations, such as young IDU, is insufficient. Individuals at high-risk for HIV will likely not identify themselves as part of this group, therefore prevention strategies must include the entire population.

PROJECTED SCENARIOS

HIV is likely to continue to spread throughout China through heroin trafficking and as IDU move throughout the country. The future of HIV subtypes in Chinese IDU will likely include the formation of further recombinant strains, both within and between clades or CRFs, as already seen in Yunnan Province (Yang *et al.*, 2002). It will be of interest to watch whether the fitness of the emerging recombinants will match the widespread CRF07_BC and CRF08_BC strains. The BC recombinant has spread mainly through injection drug use. With the increasing possibilities of sexual transmission, the recombinant may reach outside the IDU community.

Along with sweeping changes in the economic structure, China is also undergoing social restructuring (Wang *et al.*, 2000). The creation of a self-employed class has led to newer social structures divergent from the government-employed class. The social structures of the self-employed class have resulted in increased risks for sexually transmitted infections. By 2002, over 10% of HIV infections were due to sexual transmission (China Ministry of Health, 2003). In addition, HIV prevalence in FSW in Guangxi rose from 0% in 1996 to over 10% by 2000, due to continued low condom usage (UNAIDS/WHO, 2003). In order to prevent an explosion of HIV sexual transmission, prevention programs must identify and relate to the newer social structures evolving within China.

The HIV epidemic has been present for just over a decade within the majority of Chinese IDU. With each passing year, the number of HIV/AIDS patients will undoubtedly rise. Many heroin users may not know their current HIV status, or how to prevent spreading the virus to others. In addition to diagnosis and treatment, the government will be responsible for the majority of health care costs for heroin users, since the majority live in rural areas and are at the very low end of the economic scale. The public health infrastructure in China currently lacks expertise in diagnosing, monitoring and treating the looming numbers of people with HIV/AIDS.

REFERENCES

Beyrer, C., Razak, M.H., Lisam, K., Chen, J., Lui, W., and Yu, X.F. (2000). Overland heroin trafficking routes and HIV-1 spread in south and south-east Asia. *AIDS* 14(1):75–83.

China Ministry of Health and UN Theme Group on HIV/AIDS. (1997). *China responds to AIDS: HIV/AIDS situation and needs assessment report.* Chinese Ministry of Health, Beijing, China.

China Ministry of Health and UN Theme Group on HIV/AIDS in China. (2003). *A Joint Assessment of HIV/AIDS Prevention, Treatment and Care in China.* UNAIDS/World Health Organization, Geneva, Switzerland.

Des Jarlais, D.C., Friedman, S.R., Choopanya, K., Vanichseni, S., and Ward, T.P. (1992). International epidemiology of HIV and AIDS among injecting drug users. *AIDS* 6(10):1053–1068.

Garten, R.J., Zhang, J., Lai, L., Liu, W., Chen, J., Vlahov, D., and Yu, X.F. (2004). Rapid transmission of hepatitis C virus among young injecting heroin users in southern China. *International Journal of Epidemiology* (accepted, in press early 2004).

Graf, M., Shao, Y., Zhao, Q., Seidl, T., Kostler, J., Wolf, H., and Wagner, R. (1998). Cloning and characterization of a virtually full-length HIV type 1 genome from a subtype B'-Thai strain representing the most prevalent B-clade isolate in China. *AIDS Res. Hum. Retroviruses* 14(3): 285–288.

Kaldor, J.M., Effler, P., Sarda, R., Petersen, G., Gertig, D.M., and Narain, J.P. (1994). HIV and AIDS in Asia and the Pacific: An epidemiological overview. *AIDS* 8 Suppl 2: S165–S172.

Kato, K., Shiino, T., Kusagawa, S., Sato, H., Nohtomi, K., Shibamura, K., Nguyen, T.H., Pham, K.C., Truong, X.L., Mai, H.A., Hoang, T.L., Bunyaraksyotin, G., Fukushima, Y., Honda, M., Wasi, C., Yamazaki, S., Nagai, Y., and Takebe, Y. (1999). Genetic similarity of HIV type 1 subtype E in a recent outbreak among injecting drug users in northern Vietnam to strains in Guangxi Province of southern China. *AIDS Res Hum Retroviruses* 15(13):1157–1168.

Lai, S., Chen, J., Celentano, D., Page, J.B., Lai, H., Yang, J., Liu, W., McCoy, C.B., and Yu, X.F. (2000). Adoption of injection practices in heroin users in Guangxi Province, China. *J Psychoactive Drugs* 32(3):285–292.

Luo, C.C., Tian, C., Hu, D.J., Kai, M., Dondero, T., and Zheng, X. (1995). HIV-1 subtype C in China. *Lancet* 345(8956):1051–1052.

McCoy, C.B., McCoy, H.V., Lai, S., Yu, Z., Wang, X., and Meng, J. (2001). Reawakening the dragon: Changing patterns of opiate use in Asia, with particular emphasis on China's Yunnan province. *Subst Use Misuse* 36(1–2): 49–69.

McCutchan, F.E., Carr, J.K., Murphy, D., Piyasirisilp, S., Gao, F., Hahn, B., Yu, X.F., Beyrer, C., and Birx, D.L. (2002). Precise mapping of recombination breakpoints suggests a common parent of two BC recombinant HIV type 1 strains circulating in China. *AIDS Res Hum Retroviruses* 18(15): 1135–1140.

Piyasirisilp, S., McCutchan, F.E., Carr, J.K., Sanders-Buell, E., Liu, W., Chen, J., Wagner, R., Wolf, H., Shao, Y., Lai, S., Beyrer, C., and Yu, X.F. (2000). A recent outbreak of human immunodeficiency virus type 1 infection in southern China was initiated by two highly homogeneous, geographically separated strains, circulating recombinant form AE and a novel BC recombinant. *J Virol* 74(23): 11286–11295.

Poshyachinda, V. (1993). Drug injecting and HIV infection among the population of drug abusers in Asia. *Bull Narc.* 45(1):77–90.

Rodenburg, C.M., Li, Y., Trask, S.A., Chen, Y., Decker, J., Robertson, D. L., Kalish, M.L., Shaw, G.M., Allen, S., Hahn, B.H., and Gao F. (2001). Near full-length clones and reference sequences for subtype C isolates of HIV type 1 from three different continents. *AIDS Res Hum Retroviruses* 17(2):161–168.

Strang, J., Griffiths, P., and Gossop, M. (1997). Heroin smoking by 'chasing the dragon': Origins and history. *Addiction* 92(6): 673–683; discussion 685–695.

Su, L., Graf, M., Zhang, Y., von Briesen, H., Xing, H., Kostler, J., Melzl, H., Wolf, H., Shao, Y., and Wagner, R. (2000). Characterization of a virtually full-length human immunodeficiency virus type 1 genome of a prevalent intersubtype (C/B') recombinant strain in China. *J Virol* 74(23): 11367–11376.

Suwanwela, C., and Poshyachinda, V. (1986). Drug abuse in Asia. *Bull Narc.* 38(1–2):41–53.

UNAIDS Task Force on Drug Use and HIV. (2000). *Drug Use and HIV Vulnerability: Policy Research Study in Asia.* UNAIDS Asia Pacific Intercountry Team, Bangkok, Thailand.

UNAIDS/WHO. (2002). *China Epidemiological Facts Sheets on HIV/AIDS and Sexually Transmitted Infections 2002 Update.* UNAIDS/World Health Organization, Geneva, Switzerland.

UNAIDS/WHO. (2003). *AIDS epidemic update December 2003.* UNAIDS/World Health Organization, Geneva, Switzerland.

Wang, S.M., and Gao, M.Y. (2000). Employment and contextual impact of safe and unsafe sexual practices for STI and HIV: The situation in China. *Int J STD AIDS* 11(8):536–544.

Xia, M., Kreiss, J.K., and Holmes, K.K. (1994). Risk factors for HIV infection among drug users in Yunnan province, China: Association with intravenous drug use and protective effect of boiling reusable needles and syringes. *AIDS* 8(12):1701–1706.

Yang, R., Xia, X., Kusagawa, S., Zhang, C., Ben, K., and Takebe, Y. (2002). On-going generation of multiple forms of HIV-1 intersubtype recombinants in the Yunnan Province of China. *AIDS* 16(10):1401–1407.

Yu, X.F., Chen, J., Shao, Y., Beyrer, C., and Lai, S. (1998). Two subtypes of HIV-1 among injection-drug users in southern China. *Lancet* 351(9111):1250.

Yu, X.F., Chen, J., Shao, Y., Beyrer, C., Liu, B., Wang, Z., Liu, W., Yang, J., Liang, S., Viscidi, R.P., Gu, J., Gurri-Glass, G., and Lai, S. (1999). Emerging HIV infections with distinct subtypes of HIV-1 infection among injection drug users from geographically separate locations in Guangxi Province, China. *J. AIDS* 22(2):180–188.

Yu, X.F., Liu, W., Chen, J., Kong, W., Liu, B., Yang, J., Liang, F., McCutchan, F., Piyasirisilp, S., and Lai, S. (2001). Rapid dissemination of a novel B/C recombinant HIV-1 among injection drug users in southern China. *AIDS* 15(4): 523–525.

Yu, X.F., Liu, W., Chen, J., Kong, W., Liu, B., Zhu, Q., Liang, F., McCutchan, F., Piyasirisilp, S., and Lai, S. (2002). Maintaining low HIV type 1 *env* genetic diversity among injection drug users infected with a B/C recombinant and CRF01_AE HIV type 1 in southern China. *AIDS Res Hum Retroviruses* 18(2):167–170.

Zheng, X., C. Tian, K.H. Choi, J. Zhang, H. Cheng, X. Yang, D. Li, J. Lin, S. Qu, X. Sun and et al. (1994). Injecting drug use and HIV infection in southwest China. *AIDS* 8(8):1141–1147.

Zhou, Y., and Li, X. (1999). Demographic characteristics and illegal drug use patterns among attendees of drug cessation programs in China. *Subst Use Misuse.* 34(6): 907–920.

28

Infectious Diseases in Asia

Implications for Global Health

Bryan Roberts[1] and Yichen Lu[2,3]

[1] *Parallel Solutions, Inc., Cambridge, Massachusetts USA*
[2] *The Harvard AIDS Institute, Boston, Massachusetts USA*
[3] *Nankai University Vaccine Laboratory, Tianjin, China*

INTRODUCTION

This chapter examines the vulnerability of Asian countries to the current AIDS crisis in the context of social, economic and environmental factors that facilitate the emergence and global spread of new infectious diseases. As half of the world population and the majority of the poor people in the world live in Asia, the status of emerging and re-emerging infectious diseases in this part of the world has profound implications for global public health. This chapter argues that the new wave of economic globalization should be accompanied by an improvement in global public health. The imbalance of wealth and resource distribution in the world has been a critical source of concern for international security and stability, yet the potentially disastrous consequence of the imbalance in global public health has not received adequate attention from the world community. If the current AIDS crisis in Asia is not rapidly resolved, it could lead to an unparalleled social and economic disaster. Following a brief review of the current status of infectious disease, this chapter focuses on the analysis of public and private efforts to prevent and control their global spread. It suggests actions and organizations that could address the imbalance in global health and outlines the logic for global vaccine development by which both developed and developing countries collaborate to mutual benefit.

EMERGING INFECTIOUS DISEASES AND THEIR GEOGRAPHIC EPICENTERS

Over the past three decades, more than 30 previously unrecognized human infectious diseases have been identified, including AIDS, Lyme disease, Legonnaire's disease, toxic shock syndrome, Hantavirus, Pulmonary Syndrome, West Nile fever, and SARS. This significant increase of new infectious diseases can be attributed to two important factors. First, many new medical detection methods have been invented during the same time period, thus making it possible to rapidly identify the causative pathogens of new infectious diseases. These new methods include various immunological based techniques, Polymerase Chain Reaction (PCR) assays, automated DNA sequencing, and DNA chips, which collectively permit the unambiguous identification of pathogens that cause new disease outbreaks. Historically, diseases were defined by medical symptoms such as respiratory distress, fever or diarrhea, which alone are insufficient parameters for the identification of the causative agents of disease. Many of these newly identified pathogens may have co-existed with humans for a long time, and their associated diseases are now identified due to the enhanced sensitivity of new detection methods. Second, the unprecedented increase of the global population and international trade and travel in recent years has provided a favorable environment for regional outbreaks of infectious diseases to spread rapidly and effectively around the world. For example, HIV-1 virus may have infected human hosts and caused AIDS long before the 1980s, when it was first discovered, but it was in the past two decades that the AIDS epidemic spread globally and became one of the major infectious diseases in human history.

In order to illustrate the trend of emergence of infectious diseases and the level of difficulty in controlling them, this chapter divided them into two main classes, emerging viral diseases and emerging bacterial and parasitic diseases. Such a classification also helps to describe different public health strategies for prevention and treatment of these diseases.

Emerging Viral Diseases

In recent times, the predominant groups of microorganisms that have contributed to emerging infectious diseases are viruses, in particular those containing RNA genomes. This can be attributed to their enormous replicative capacity with high mutation rate due to the lack of efficient proofreading and mismatch repair systems, or high frequency of recombination between different members of a virus family, and re-assortment of viral gene segments among viruses from different hosts. In recent times, the retrovirus HIV, the causative agent of AIDS, and the flavivirus HCV, which causes Hepatitis C, both RNA viruses that mutate rapidly, have emerged as major global diseases. A recent dramatic example of the emergence and rapid establishment of another flavivirus, West Nile Virus (WNV), occurred in the USA and Europe. This virus was originally isolated from a patient in Uganda in 1937, and subsequently found to be widespread in Africa and Eurasia. In 1999, WNV was introduced into New York and was efficiently disseminated across the entire country within three years, due to the presence of numerous mosquito vectors and an efficient zoonosis with wild birds (Petersen and Roehrig, 2001). A similar pattern of emergence of WNV occurred in Europe with sporadic outbreaks in Russia in1962, the Ukraine in the 1970s and 1980s, Romania in 1996, and Italy in 1998 (Hubalek and Halouzka, 1999). The outbreak in Romania in 1996 involved 500 clinical cases, with a 10% fatality rate (Hubalek and Halouzka, 1999). The rate of spread in the US and Europe are differentiated by ecological factors, such as the number and frequency of different mosquito vectors and the distribution of animals in which WNV is epizootic.

In 2003, a new human disease called Severe Acute Respiratory Syndrome (SARS) emerged. It is a positive sense RNA virus belonging to the coronavirus family. The virus appears resident in wild animals in Southern China and upon transfer to humans induces a lethal respiratory infection. The virus spread within the human population by direct transfer and assumed a global distribution within months due to international airline travel. The establishment of SARS as a persistent threat to humans will require that the virus develop either a human reservoir or become epizootic by establishing effective animal reservoirs. Currently, the spread of the SARS virus between humans is relatively inefficient; however, the selection of variants that exhibit improved transmission characteristics will enhance its threat to the human population.

The myxovirus group are negative strand RNA viruses, from which have emerged serious human diseases during the last century and which remain ongoing threats to global health. This group of RNA viruses contains two virus families: the orthomyxoviruses, which include influenza virus, and the paramyxoviruses, which contain measles, mumps and human respiratory syncytial virus.

The RNA genomes of influenza viruses are comprised of eight gene segments, which exhibit continuous mutational changes called "drift" that result in the annual global emergence of new epidemic strains of influenza that infect humans and transmit efficiently within the human population. On three occasions (1918, 1957, and 1968), pandemic influenza viruses emerged in which there was a "shift" that is a complete replacement of the gene segment encoding the surface protein, haemagglutinin. Molecular analysis of these pandemic strains suggested that the new gene segment in 1918 originated from swine influenza and those in 1957 and 1968 originated from avian viruses. The global deaths were approximately 40 million in 1918, five million in 1957 and 2.5 million in 1968. In each case, the pandemic virus combined a new surface antigen with internal proteins that were well adapted to growth in humans. It is assumed that the viruses arose due to the simultaneous infection of swine with both swine and human viruses to form the 1918 strain, and the co-infection of swine with avian and human viruses to generate the 1957 and the 1968 strains (Horimoto and Kawaoka, 2001).

Recently, a number of highly virulent avian influenza viruses were shown to directly transmit from birds to humans, inducing a highly lethal disease in the recipients. Fortunately, these viruses have not evolved the capacity to transmit infections between humans and, to date; their spread has been controlled by quarantine and mass slaughter of avian populations. In Southern China, the avian influenza, H5N1 in 1997 and H9N2 in 1999, were shown to directly transmit from domestic birds to humans and cause high morbidity infections (Mounts *et al.*, 1999; Uyeki *et al.*, 2002). In both cases, human infections were contained by the lack of effective transmission between humans and the large-scale destruction of infected domestic chicken flocks. Phylogenetic studies established that both viruses contained eight gene segments of avian origin (Horimoto and Kawaoka, 2001), thus suggesting that avian viruses can cause serious infections of humans without reassortment with human viruses in mammalian hosts such as swine. Furthermore, avian influenza viruses, whether virulent or not, represent an enormous reservoir of viruses that can rapidly evolve into lethal pandemic influenza virus, either directly in humans or by reassortment with human viruses, either in pigs or humans. This indicates that the large-scale domestication of chickens and swine that occurs throughout the globe represents an efficient breeding ground for the evolution of new influenza viruses, which could pose a significant threat to public health worldwide. For example, a highly pathogenic avian influenza (H5N2), found in poultry farms in Pennsylvania in 1983, was eradicated by the slaughter of 17 million birds (Webster, 1998). In 1993, a H5N2 influenza virus emerged in domestic chickens in Mexico and within months evolved from an avirulent strain into a highly pathogenic strain, which was finally eradicated by quarantine and vaccination (Webster, 1998).

The advent of a pandemic influenza virus with pathogenicity equivalent to that of the 1918 pandemic strain would result in rapid worldwide human infection and morbidity to an extent that would overrun public health prevention and treatment modalities and overwhelm routine societal function.

A pattern of newly emerging diseases is also observed in paramyxoviruses, which are epizootic in bats and cause lethal human infections that currently are not transmitted between humans. In Australia, in 1994, the Hendra virus caused severe respiratory infections, killing a number of horses and a trainer; and in 1996, the Menangle virus induced stillbirths in pigs and mild flu like symptoms in piggery workers (Mackenzie, 1999). In Malaysia, the Nippah virus infected pigs and caused 265 human cases of encephalitis, which was 50% lethal; further spread was controlled by quarantine and the culling of over one million pigs (Wang *et al.*, 2001). These paramyxovirus infections in humans are lethal, and if these agents evolve efficient human transmission characteristics, possessed by other members of this group such as measles, the resultant pandemic strains would pose a major threat to the human population.

In 1993, a previously unknown group of hantaviruses emerged in southwestern USA due to environmental factors favoring their natural rodent reservoir. Although a member of this group of negative-sense RNA viruses (Hantaan virus) was previously associated with hemorrhagic fever with renal syndrome, the new hantaviruses (Sin Nombre virus) present in rodent excrement infect humans and induce a lethal pulmonary syndrome. Fortunately, the establishment and spread of these human pathogens was limited by lack of human-to-human transmission and limitations in the annual growth cycle of the rodent reservoir.

Among all these new viral infectious diseases that emerged in recent decades, HIV/AIDS has become a major threat to global public health.

Emerging Bacterial and Parasitic Diseases

The gram-negative bacterium *Vibrio cholera* is the agent defined by Koch as causing the human diarrheal disease, cholera. The microorganism is endemic to the Indian sub-continent where the disease cholera has been recorded for centuries. Global traffic initiated the first of six global epidemics in 1812, finally receding in the middle of the twentieth century. In 1991, a new strain called *V. cholera 0139* emerged in Bangladesh and quickly spread to 11 countries in Southeast Asia. This strain was antigenically distinct from the classical strain, and immunity to the classical strain offered no protection against infection by *V. cholera 0139*. This new strain acquired resistance to numerous antibiotics and continued to spread in Asia. Shipping was responsible for its dissemination to Peru and it subsequent spread throughout South and Central America. Between 1991 and 1994, the Pan-America Health Organization (PANO) reported approximately one million infections and 10,000 deaths.

Other new bacterial diseases, such as Toxic shock syndrome, caused by *Staphylococcus aureus* contaminated tampons, or *Legionellosis*, caused by the contamination of water in plumbing systems like cooling systems and large air conditioners by the bacterium *Legionella*, are sporadic, and were controlled by simple preventative and sanitary measures. The largest recorded outbreak of the waterborne parasite *Cryptosporidium parvum* occurred in 1993 in Milwaukee, where contaminated drinking water infected more than 370,000 individuals with 47 deaths. In 1996, over 850 cases of intestinal infection by the food-borne parasite *Cyclospora cayetanensis* occurred in the US and Canada caused by the importation of contaminated raspberries from Guatemala.

In general, bacteria and parasites make a smaller contribution than viruses to newly emerging diseases, yet due to the development of multi-drug resistance, they are the major pathogen types in re-emerging diseases. Diseases like tuberculosis, malaria, and numerous bacterial diseases represent syndromes in which a degree of control had been achieved, but, due to drug resistance, they have resumed spreading in the population. For example, resistance to fluoroquinolones, the effective treatment for gonorrhea, developed in Southeast Asia in 1990, and is spreading globally. Nosocomial infections are demonstrating alarming antibiotic resistance; for example, *Staphylococcus aureus* developed methicillin resistance, and the only remaining treatment is vancomycin, for which resistant strains have been identified in Japan. Another serious nosocomial infection is *Enterococcus faecalis*, for which the only available treatment is the antibiotic, vancomycin. In 2000, however, vancomycin resistant strains were discovered to be spreading with high fatality rates in patients maintained on supportive care.

The increasing emergence of antibiotic-resistant bacterial pathogens in Asia is especially worrisome. In many Asian countries, various antibiotics are widely available and affordable without proper medical prescription and supervision. As opportunistic infections are the major causes of mortality in AIDS patients, these drug-resistant bacterial pathogens will make AIDS treatment much more difficult, if not impossible. Moreover, the increased number of immunocomprimised AIDS patients in the area will further facilitate the spread of these untreatable bacterial infections, and support their re-emergence.

Geographic Epicenters for Disease Emergence and Spread

There are global epicenters that foster the emergence and spread of new human infectious diseases, which occur when new pathogens expand from animals into the human population, with a corresponding increase in disease incidence. An epicenter has three main characteristics. First, the density of a human population and its close interface with domestic and wild animal populations enhances the rate at which new infectious diseases emerge. Second, the process by which new infectious diseases emerge is further facilitated by dramatic changes of social environment and population migrations associated with regional imbalance of economic development and urbanization. Third, a global spread of new infectious disease is made possible by the lack of regional disease surveillance and control and its close proximity to international or national trade and travel centers.

For example, many areas in the tropics and subtropics are some of the most highly populated regions on the globe, sustaining two thirds of the world's people. These include a contiguous area that comprises India, Southeast Asia, China, the Western Pacific, and smaller, highly-populated regions in sub-Saharan Africa and South America. The majority of these populations live in poverty, under conditions of poor nutrition and sanitation, with substandard public health services. On one hand, the geographic, climatic, and ecological conditions in these areas have supported the evolution of the greatest diversity of animal species on the globe. These extensive animal populations serve as reservoirs for an equivalent diversity of microorganisms, which propagate throughout the year in the conductive tropical and subtropical climate (Shope, 1999). On the other hand, the conditions in these regions are apparently ideal for the emergence and spread of new diseases, and this is supported by the recent emergence of diseases including AIDS, West Nile fever, Ebola hemorrhagic fever, Rift Valley fever, and SARS.

For the same reasons that make these epicenters focal points for the emergence of new infectious diseases, these areas are also vulnerable to the establishment and spread of new infectious diseases that originated elsewhere. AIDS in Asia is an example. The initial epicenter for AIDS emergence was in Africa, where the causative agent HIV was probably derived from a primate virus that infected humans and continued human to human spread by sexual transmission and blood contact. Whereas AIDS continues to spread in Africa and western countries, it emerged in Asia in the late 1980s and poses an enormous threat to one of the poorest and most populated regions in the world.

GLOBAL SPREAD OF INFECTIOUS DISEASES

The spread of an emerging infectious disease within the human population is determined by multiple factors, the most important of which is the route of disease transmission. For example, in the spring of 2003, the world witnessed how a regional infectious disease outbreak, SARS, could be spread globally in a matter of days by air travel. Fortunately, the relatively short period of SARS disease incubation and easily identifiable disease symptoms made it possible to use quarantine as an effective tool to control the spread of the disease. As described in the following sections, HIV/AIDS is a totally different case.

Routes of Disease Transmission

The mode of transmission of pathogens between humans determines the rate of disease spread in both space and time in the human population. Pathogen transmission between humans can occur by means of respiratory aerosols, sexual contact, exchange of bodily fluids, insect vectors, or by contact with contaminated materials, water or food. Respiratory aerosols, including influenza, measles and tuberculosis, spread some of the highly transmissible infectious diseases. The indiscriminate infection profile of respiratory diseases causes extreme public concern. In the absence of preventative vaccines, public health officials control disease spread by enforced quarantine; this old public health measure still remains the most effective way to control the aerosol transmission of infectious disease. This approach, combined with the timely onset of identifiable clinical symptoms, allows the control of these diseases in an effective manner.

Sexual transmission, on the other hand, results in a slower but progressive spread of disease. The global spread of AIDS within three decades has resulted in the infection of 42 million people. The directional transmission of this disease has also resulted in the efficient extinction of that specific age segment of the population that is sexually active. The societal consequence is devastating, due to the high disease incidence in the child-rearing age group, resulting in a spiraling increase in the number of orphaned children. In sub-Saharan Africa, the AIDS epidemic is most advanced, and by 2002 there were already more than 11 million orphans, a number that is expected to exceed 20 million by 2010. This predictable and horrific outcome, unlike any other disease in history, results in the erosion of family structure and orthodoxy, thus subjecting the children to possible societal anarchy, coercion, and sexual abuse. As described in more detail by other chapters in this book, sexual transmission is also a major route of transmission for HIV/AIDS in Asia. Unlike the diseases transmitted by aerosols, HIV/AIDS has a much longer asymptomatic period, measured not in weeks and days, but in years. Consequently, infected individuals can effectively and unknowingly transmit the virus to their contacts.

The exchange of bodily fluids has catalyzed the efficient transmission of blood-borne infections such as HBV, HCV, and HIV, which collectively have chronically infected enormous numbers of the world's population. This is especially true in Asia, where blood supply for medical use was collected commercially in many countries. Retrospective analysis indicates that the exchange of body fluids incurred in childhood vaccinations and the delivery of injectable medicines by contaminated needles and syringes in China caused an unprecedented spread of HBV. This iatrogenic dissemination of disease has been estimated to account for 60% of the more than 100 million chronic HBV infections in China (Sun *et al.*, 2002). Intravenous drug use has also facilitated the efficient global distribution of blood-borne infections including HBV, HCV, and HIV.

Insect vectored diseases are transmitted either directly between humans, as in malaria, or between animal reservoirs and humans in zoonotic infections. Diseases spread by insects are limited by the geographic distribution of the vector. For example, dengue fever is caused by a flavivirus, which is transmitted by the mosquito, *Aedes aegypti*, and has been resident in Asia, Africa, South America and the Caribbean since the 1800s (Gubler,1988). The spread of Dengue into southern US and northern Australia has been limited by the range of this mosquito vector. In contrast, diseases can rapidly expand into new geographic areas if their insect vectors are endemic in these areas. An excellent example is the rapid spread of West Nile Virus (WNV) throughout the USA within three years.

Pathogens that spread via contaminated materials (fomites), food, or water cause sporadic disease outbreaks that can be controlled by standard public health approaches, including quarantine and sanitation. Examples of diseases caused by fomitic transfer include smallpox and Ebola hemorrhagic fever, water-borne infections such as cholera and shigella and *Cryptosporidium parvum* and food-borne diseases caused by *E. coli 0157*, *Cyclospora cayetanensis* and *Salmonella enteritidis*.

Standard public health approaches to improving sanitation control the spread of infectious diseases that are transmitted by contaminated food or water. Increasing the level of living standards usually results in significant reduction of the scale and frequency of these kinds of disease outbreaks. Similarly, transmission efficiency of insect vectored infectious diseases also reduces significantly with the improvement of urban housing environments accompanied by economic development. Ironically, the increasing prosperity in most Asian countries in recent decades has translated into better prevention and control of water- and food-borne diseases, whereas blood-borne and sexually transmitted diseases have significantly increased in incidence. For example, the economic advances in China since the 1980s have been accompanied by an annual 20% increase in reported cases of sexually transmitted diseases. Similar trends have been observed in India, Thailand, and Vietnam and are described in more detail in other chapters in this book. In these cases, an increase of disposable incomes for men has apparently driven the expansion of the commercial sex market to a new height, facilitating the explosive spread of sexually transmitted diseases such as HIV/AIDS. Similarly, the high profit margin for plasma-derived biological products and high market demand for such products in China and neighboring countries during the 1990s has created local economies where large amounts of human plasma were collected from farmers in countryside and rural areas. The failure to enforce proper sanitary processes during blood collection has not only failed to bring long-term prosperity to these impoverished areas, but has resulted in the spread of blood-borne diseases, including HIV/AIDS and hepatitis. Intravenous drug use (IDU) in Asia is prevalent in developed areas, where the average income has increased significantly in past decades. The practice of IDU is responsible for a significant increase in a number of blood borne infections, including HCV, HIV and Hepatitis B.

The Spread of Infectious Disease by Global Trade and Travel

The establishment of trade between nations led to an early appreciation of the hazards of the import and export of disease causing pathogens. Prior to the middle of the nineteenth century, this problem was resolved by national governance methods established by individual trading countries without international cooperation. By 1851, however, the volume and speed of international travel and trade demanded international governance of infectious diseases, which was implemented at the International Sanitary Conference. The International Sanitary Conventions were adopted until they were modified in 1951 by the World Health Organization (WHO) and renamed the International Health Regulations (IHR). These regulations only covered three infectious diseases, Cholera, Yellow Fever, and Plague, and they supported the mandate *"to ensure the maximum protection against the international spread of disease with minimum interference with world traffic."* The focus of these rules was on the transmission of diseases across borders. They required an individual country to notify other countries of outbreaks of specific diseases in their territories and to maintain adequate public health capabilities of disease control at points of entry or exit. They further required countries to exercise disease prevention measures restricting international trade and travel based on scientific evidence and public health principles (WHO, 1983; Fidler, 2003). Problems associated with IHR have been recognized since the late nineteenth century, and the ability of the WHO to enforce the legal implementation of these regulations has always been limited.

In recent decades, the progressive growth of marine and air transportation for business and pleasure has introduced a manmade transmission route for pathogens and their vectors that greatly facilitates their global spread. Estimates of travel volume are vast, with one million people crossing national boundaries daily and the same number commuting between developed and developing countries each week (Garrett, 1994). As described in other chapters in this book, the current global trade and travel volume are capable of spreading new infectious diseases in a matter of days and weeks, thus making it impossible to build national barriers to prevent the incoming infectious diseases. Examples of the role of trade and travel in the global spread of disease include *V. cholera 0139* from Bangladesh in 1991, West Nile Fever from Africa in 1999, and SARS from Southern China in 2003. The problem of the control of infectious disease spread with increasing globalization of trade and travel has long been recognized. In 1995, the WHO acknowledged the failure of IHR to control the global spread of disease (WHO, 1995). There are no IHR provisions for an international organization to take action against states that fail to comply. Despite the failure of the IHR to adequately meet international health needs, WHO mandated extensive revisions of these regulations, an effort which was widely criticized and eroded the credibility of the Organization (WHO, 2002).

Meanwhile, the General Agreement on Tariffs and Trade (GATT), established in 1947, was providing an international forum for 110 countries to encourage free trade and the orderly resolution of trade disputes. This organization encouraged liberalizing international trade, while still recognizing that states may need to restrict trade to protect international health and the environment. In 1995, the World Trade Organization (WTO) replaced GATT, and has a membership of 146 countries (as of 2003), which administers trade agreements and negotiations and resolves trade disputes. WTO has established the Agreement on Trade Related Aspects of Intellectual Property Rights (TRIPS) and the Application of Sanitary and Phytosanitary Measures (SPS Agreement). The adoption, in 2001, of the Declaration on the TRIPS Agreement placed public health objectives above the trade-related goal of increasing pharmaceutical patent protection. In 2003, the WTO demonstrated its commitment to public health by implementing legal changes in intellectual property protection so that poor countries can import cheap generic drugs to treat diseases, including HIV/AIDS and malaria. These achievements, along with its powerful dispute resolution mechanisms indicate that the WTO could play a pivotal role in the future of global health.

VACCINES AND GLOBAL HEALTH

Vaccines are universally regarded as the most successful medical intervention to date. The deaths of three million children per year due to serious childhood diseases was avoided by the development in the middle of the twentieth century of vaccines against measles, poliomyelitis, tuberculosis and diphtheria, pertussis, and tetanus. In fact, the efficacy of vaccines in blocking the growth of pathogens has resulted in the eradication of smallpox, and has nearly completed the global elimination of poliomyelitis. Large-scale immunization protects vaccinated individuals, but also confers benefit to the population as a whole. Vaccines are the most effective approach for the control of infectious diseases and the overall improvement in global health. However, the emergence of serious pandemics like HIV and HCV indicate that the process of new vaccine development is flawed and is in need of complete reevaluation and revision in order to reverse the continued deterioration in global health. The following sections analyze these problems with the intent of evaluating appropriate solutions.

Undervalued Social and Economic Benefits of Vaccines

The population benefit of vaccines is difficult to personalize, and vaccines are seriously undervalued at the social and political level. Despite the value they provide to society, vaccines are of negligible economic value when compared to pharmaceuticals. The global vaccine market is estimated to be approximately $6.5 billion, which is the equivalent of 2% of that of the pharmaceutical market (Greco, 2002). Furthermore, as vaccines progressively eliminate disease and dissipate the threat to society, the success of vaccine products will also ultimately erode their own market demand. However, economists have evaluated vaccines for benefits beyond prevention of infectious diseases, as their cost is significantly lower than the cost of disease treatment and loss of working days. Calculations indicate that the combination vaccines for measles, mumps and rubella saves $16.34 dollars in direct medical costs for every dollar spent and the diphtheria, tetanus and pertussis vaccine saves $6.21 dollars for every dollar spent (CDC, 1999). Rappuoli and colleagues deduce that avoiding disease altogether would enhance the current value of vaccines between 10 to 100 fold (Rappuoli *et al.*, 2002). The World Bank suggested in 1983 that poor health was a major impediment to economic growth of developing countries, and that vaccination could help improve their economy (Bloom and Channing, 2000). Although it is apparent that successful globalization will rely on improving health worldwide to allow economies to thrive in developing countries, the control of infectious diseases that disrupt international travel and trade and the development of relevant new vaccines remains a low priority issue to international political and industrial leaders. In fact, international discussions and new initiatives about vaccine development are usually viewed in the category of international charity or philanthropic issues, rather than pivotal issues that are as important as peace treaties, trade barriers and balance, or currency exchanges and monetary policies.

Lack of Incentives to Produce New Vaccines for Developing Countries

The global vaccine market is dominated by five major manufacturers; Aventis Pasteur (23%), Glaxo Smith Kline (23%), Wyeth (19%), Merck (17%), Chiron (7%), and the remaining 11% is comprised of small manufactures distributed around the globe. In fact, the low return on investment and legal liability associated with vaccines resulted in a reduction in companies manufacturing vaccines in the US from 37 to 10 since 1967, with a similar trend in Europe (Rappuoli *et al.*, 2002). This reduction in vaccine production capacity has impacted the availability of low margin vaccines, both in the US and in developing countries. An Institute of Medicine (IOM) report on "*Immunization Finance Policies and Practices*" in 2000 warns that vaccine-preventable diseases may recur, due to declines in national vaccine coverage (IOM, 2000). However, despite this consolidation of the vaccine industry, the annual vaccine market has grown from $2 billion in 1982 to $5.4 billion in 2000, with a projected annual increase of 12%. This is due to the development of high-priced vaccines for major markets in the developed world, which include HBV and the conjugate vaccines for *Haemophilus influenzae* type b and the heptavalent Pneumococcal conjugate vaccine. This focus on high value vaccines for lucrative markets has polarized vaccine development to diseases of significance in the developed world, with little serious effort being expended on addressing important diseases in the rest of the world. This is reflected by the fact that only a small portion of global vaccine research and development is dedicated to diseases that are a major burden in low and middle-income countries. This purely financial approach to preventing infectious diseases has proven to be shortsighted, since a number of serious diseases that emerged in the developing world have assumed global distribution: AIDS, Hepatitis B and C, West Nile Fever, and SARS, to name only a few.

Currently, the cost of the development of a new vaccine is approximately $350 to $500 million, which includes pre-clinical research, toxicology and clinical evaluation. Major vaccine manufacturers undertake this kind of substantial investment only when research has defined a viable development candidate that will command a large market, supporting a price per dose that ensures a return on investment and a substantial annual profit. Despite the enormous public health demand for vaccines in the developing world, there is little financial incentive for vaccine companies to make vaccines for this market. This reluctance is due to a combination of factors, which includes the scientific risk of preclinical studies, development costs, the lack of assurance of a lucrative market for new vaccines, and deficits in the local infrastructure for vaccine distribution in the developing countries. This situation would change if the public sector could make funds available to assure manufacturers of a reasonable price per vaccine dose and a commitment to a specified annual purchase of vaccines. Other incentives for vaccine company participation could include the direct financing of vaccine development, sponsorship of clinical trials, investment in improving clinical trial infrastructure, the establishment of regulatory and manufacturing reciprocity between the US, EU and Japan, and capital loans for the development of infrastructure and scale up in specific developing countries. The appropriate commitment to these incentives would make the production of vaccines for the developing world an attractive opportunity for all vaccine manufacturers. This would result in the active participation of public and commercial entities in establishing a rational agenda for preventing diseases like HIV-AIDS, hepatitis C, malaria, tuberculosis and newly emerging diseases that threaten global health.

In addition, there are two organizations that focus on making new vaccines for the developing world, the International Vaccine Institute (IVI) in Seoul, Korea established in 1969 and the International AIDS Vaccine Initiative (IAVI) founded in 1996 and head quartered in New York. Both interact with government and international agencies, academic and commercial organizations to facilitate the development of vaccines for enteric diseases (IVI) and AIDS (IAVI). They support preclinical studies and early stage vaccine clinical development, yet in both cases the budget for costly Phase III studies and large-scale vaccine manufacture and distribution remains an issue. Both organizations have highlighted the need for specific vaccines and have made seminal contributions to initiating their development.

The Public Sector's Inability to Develop New Vaccines

The public sectors in most countries, especially in the developed world, traditionally are expert in raising large funds to support basic research, implement policies and programs at the country level, impact international laws, and support international public health initiatives. They are not, however, capable of conducting applied research such as vaccine development as effectively as private vaccine manufacturers. The public sector funds academic research institutions and universities to expand our fundamental understanding of biology and to spearhead new approaches in medicine and human health. Recently, progress in the understanding of immunology and the composition of both human and pathogen genomes has been outstanding; yet, to date, its application to the understanding of protective immunity and vaccine development is minimal. During the last three decades of the twentieth century, traditional empirical approaches to early vaccine development were replaced by thought leaders in both scientific and commercial settings guessing as to the types of protective immune responses required for new vaccines. This misplaced concept, combined with a fear of failure, impeded the use of clinical studies to rapidly evaluate the efficacy or lack thereof of vaccine formulations and delivery methodologies. As a consequence, the development of vaccines for a number of serious diseases including HIV, HCV, malaria, dengue fever and tuberculosis, has stagnated. A more effective means of harnessing information from basic science and its productive application towards applied scientific goals such as vaccine development is required. This was exemplified recently in the role of the public sector in trying to advance experimental HIV vaccines into clinical evaluation. Public funding, since the early 1990s, has become the major driving force in HIV vaccine development. An analysis showed that the average probability of advancing candidate vaccines, excluding HIV-1 vaccines, from Phase I to Phase II human trials was about 72%, and from Phase II to Phase III was approximately 79% (Struck, 1996). In contrast, during the same period (1983–1994), only 20% of the HIV-1 vaccine candidates in Phase I human trials entered Phase II evaluation, and none of these advanced into phase III human trials. A detailed analysis of this unique phenomenon is discussed elsewhere (Lu, 1997).

To hasten HIV vaccine development, the US government, in 1998, established the Vaccine Research Center (VRC) within the National Institutes of Health (NIH) with a mandate, a designated facility, and a budget to develop an effective HIV vaccine. The successful clinical development of an HIV vaccine would establish the VRC as a model for other countries for follow.

Vaccines for Developing Countries

The World Bank divides the 208 world economies into high, middle and low groups based on gross national income per capita (GNI). There are 45 high-income countries with GNI above $9076, followed by 82 middle-income countries with GNI between $736 and $9075, and 81 low-income countries with GNI below $735. The 45 high-income economies are developed countries located in North America, Western Europe, Australia, New Zealand, and Japan, with highly industrialized economies and productive agricultural systems. The 163 middle- and low-income economies make up the developing countries located in Asia, Africa, Latin America, and various islands where agriculture is the predominant source of income.

The developed world is the major research and industrial base for the development of new preventative vaccines, but with a focus predominantly on diseases relevant to industrial societies. The developing world, on the other hand, is the major focal point for the emergence and spread of infectious diseases. Their inability to develop affordable vaccines has resulted in enormous annual loss of life and productivity. Moreover, the rapid global spread of diseases originating in developing countries by international trade and travel poses an ever-growing threat to developed societies. When the developed world population faces the threat of an infectious disease for which new vaccines are needed, the necessary national resources and expertise can be quickly assembled to research and develop such vaccines in the shortest time possible. The development of the polio vaccine in the US in the 1940s and 1950s is a good example of a streamlined approach to vaccine development. Recently, during the 1980s, a new infectious disease, Lyme disease, created significant public concerns in the northeastern US, where people living in the affluent suburbs were at high risk of being infected. This public health threat quickly resulted in dedication of the best of vaccine research facilities in the country to develop a Lyme vaccine. Within a few years, an effective vaccine product was developed and made available in the country. In comparison, the middle and low-income developing countries are completely reliant on donors for the supply of basic childhood vaccines and lack the resources to conduct research and development of new vaccines. A number of middle-income countries, such as China, India, Indonesia, Cuba, Brazil, and Mexico, have the capacity to manufacture existing vaccines. In fact, more than half of the low profit margin vaccines currently administered in the Extended Program for Immunization (EPI) are manufactured in these developing country facilities. There has been an effort to improve the infrastructure for vaccine evaluation and manufacture in developing countries by capital investment and appropriate technology transfer, so that domestic vaccine production in developing countries can be supported. In 1999, however, a Children's Vaccine Initiative Task Force cautioned that there were a number of drawbacks to local production in the developing countries. These drawbacks included concerns about objective oversight of reliable and consistent vaccine production, the maintenance of long term stability and viability of production facilities, and doubts about cost effective vaccine production in developing countries, since vaccines are capital intensive and may require costly technology transfer (Blanc and Brewer, 1999).

The current HIV/AIDS crisis in Africa and Asia further demonstrates a serious problem with the process of new vaccine development. The rampant spread of AIDS created a sense of national urgency in many southern African countries, yet they lacked the ability and resources to develop an effective HIV vaccine on their own. Now, Asia faces the same crisis and it remains to be seen whether countries such as China, India, and Indonesia, which comprise more than half the world's population and have considerable resources and expertise in vaccine production, will depend on the developed world to produce an HIV vaccine. Alternatively, Asian countries could devote their national resources and expertise to collaborating with international initiatives to develop HIV vaccines on their own timetable. Based on the African experience, a nation with its own resources, like China, should coordinate a campaign to integrate national and international resources in an attempt to develop an HIV vaccine, and not depend entirely on industrial nations. It would be better to attempt HIV vaccine development and fail than to await the inevitable social and economic disaster of a widespread HIV infection of the population, as occurred in Africa. The chapter, in this book, on the Chinese vaccine industry, outlines the capacity of this industry to apply new technologies and manufacture cost-effective vaccines for a vast population within a developing country, and outlines the well-established Chinese public health infrastructure that is necessary for vaccine evaluation and distribution.

GLOBAL CONTROL OF INFECTIOUS DISEASES

By the middle of the last century, there were significant improvements in urban sanitation and water quality, and vaccines had been developed that afforded protection against numerous childhood diseases, including polio, measles, mumps, rubella, diphtheria, tetanus, and pertussis. The discovery of antibiotics had resulted in the treatment of a broad range of bacterial diseases, including tuberculosis and typhoid fever, and small molecule drugs were effective against malaria, one of the major parasitic diseases.

These successes fostered a spirit of optimism so that WHO promoted the concept of "Health for All by the Year 2000." In 1969, the US Surgeon General stated "time to close the book on infectious diseases, declare the war on pestilence won and shift national resources to such chronic problems as heart disease" (Mayer, 2000). However, contrary to these optimistic predictions and conclusions, infectious diseases at the start of the 21st century are responsible for 13 million annual deaths, of which two thirds are children, mainly in the developing world. Approximately 50% of these childhood deaths are preventable by existing vaccines. Tuberculosis is currently estimated to infect about two billion people, nearly a third of the world population. WHO estimates that between 2002 and 2020, one billion (1,000,000,000) new TB infections will occur, with 150 million people becoming sick and 36 million deaths. WHO data indicates that malaria affects approximately 300 million people worldwide predominantly in Africa, Asia and Latin America, resulting in 1–1.5 million deaths annually. 80% of malarial cases occur in Africa, where it is the primary cause of mortality in children under five years of age. Also, during the second half of the 20th century, chronic viral diseases achieved worldwide distribution and infect over half a billion of the world's population, including 300 million with HBV, 170 million with HCV, and 42 million HIV cases. In 2002, AIDS, malaria, and tuberculosis alone were responsible for six million deaths. The immune deficiency caused by HIV is accelerating the spread and pathogenicity of a broad spectrum of infectious diseases including tuberculosis and malaria. Vaccine development for each of the three major diseases, tuberculosis, malaria and AIDS, is only in the early stages of clinical evaluation.

The current global efforts to thwart infectious disease are apparently inadequate, and require a comprehensive reorganization. The following sections focus on review of the current system and possible future improvements.

Recent History of the Global Public Health Effort

Following World War II, the United Nations was established, and a number of its affiliated organizations contribute to global health. These include the WHO, the United Nations Children's Fund (UNICEF), United Nations Development Fund (UNDP), and the World Bank (WB). The WHO's mission is the attainment of physical, mental, and social well-being of all peoples, and a major focus is providing advice and guidance to countries on communicable and non-communicable diseases. UNICEF's focus is on children's rights and survival, UNDP facilitates the dissemination of knowledge and technologies for countries to build a better life, and the WB is dedicated to the eradication of global poverty. Each organization contributes different expertise relevant to global health. In 1981, WHO and UNICEF established the Expanded Program of Immunization (EPI) to assure the distribution of childhood vaccines to more than 80% of the world's children. The US Agency for International Development (USAID) is a significant contributor to the purchase and distribution of vaccines for developing countries. National public health agencies including the CDC (Centers for Disease Control and Prevention) and NIH in the US, the MRC (Medical Research Council) in the UK, and CSIRO (Commonwealth Scientific and Industrial Research Organisation) in Australia, contribute disease research and surveillance expertise to international agencies. The CDC has the most advanced disease surveillance and containment expertise, which together with the WHO, coordinates efforts to identify and contain infectious disease outbreaks. The expertise relevant to global health within these agencies is formidable and its coordinated contribution would be central to an organization with responsibility for global infectious disease prevention.

In 1990, the Children's Vaccine Initiative (CVI) was established through the sponsorship of WHO, UNICEF, WB, UNDP, and the Rockefeller Foundation. The CVI was an international collective of public and private entities, including UN and government agencies, academic scientists, industrial executives, and applied scientists, established to harness new technologies to improve vaccine design and delivery to protect the world's children. The mission of CVI was to develop combination vaccines that by a single mucosal administration could induce protective immunity against numerous childhood diseases. For various reasons, this ambitious goal did not come to fruition. Nevertheless, this initiative demonstrated that the health of the world's children could attract professionals with expertise in global health, vaccine research, development, production, and distribution to collaborate effectively and to consistently attend annual meetings.

In 1995, the Program for Appropriate Technology in Health (PATH) was established as an international nonprofit organization to improve the quality of life around the world. An emphasis is placed on improving the quality of reproductive health services and on preventing and reducing the impact of widespread communicable diseases. PATH works in partnership with governments, companies, organizations and funding agencies to identify and apply appropriate and innovative solutions to public health problems. PATH established the Malaria Vaccine Initiative (MVI), which is the recipient of $100 million dollars from the Bill & Melinda Gates Foundation. Currently, MVI is supporting the development of 15 malaria vaccine candidates, of which seven have advanced into 13 clinical trials.

In 1999, the Global Alliance for Vaccines and Immunization (GAVI) and its financial arm, the Vaccine Fund, were established; they represented a consolidation of public and private efforts dedicated to saving children's lives and people's health through the widespread use of existing vaccines. These objectives are shared by a partnership of international institutions, governments, vaccine companies, research institutions, and major philanthropists. GAVI is stimulating vaccine companies to develop and supply vaccines needed by developing countries, and the Fund raises money and motivates national governments to use vaccines to secure the health of their children. For example, GAVI and the Chinese government have equally contributed to a $75 million fund to vaccinate all children safely against Hepatitis B. WHO estimated that approximately 60% of HBV infections result from unsafe injections, administered, ironically, during routine childhood vaccinations (Sun *et al.*, 2002). This new fund will also supply 500 million auto-disable syringes for safe vaccination, and also boost the Chinese A-D syringe industry. The Bill and Melinda Gates Foundation donated $750 million to the Fund; that together with other donations exceeded $1.1 billion. Since its inception in 1999, GAVI has been very successful in achieving its vaccine supply goals using a rigorous business-like approach. GAVI serves as a model for the more ambitious Global Fund to Fight AIDS, Tuberculosis, and Malaria, and was subject to a critical evaluation by the London School of Hygiene and Tropical Health. This report identified a number of issues that must be addressed, including that the infrastructure in some countries could not effectively distribute the vaccines supplied, and that the data on population size and coverage was often unreliable. The local public health staff found the support of the GAVI initiative often too time consuming and there was variation in the ability of the personnel in different countries to coordinate the distribution of vaccines (Brugha *et al.*, 2002). These were minor issues compared with the overall achievements of the GAVI programs. However, the deficiencies in public health personnel and infrastructure required for vaccine evaluation and distribution in developing countries could pose serious problems for the broader and more complex task of the new Global Fund's efforts to control AIDS, tuberculosis, and malaria. The experience of GAVI and the Global Fund on disease prevention using vaccines in developing countries will be invaluable in defining the structure of a global entity exclusively dedicated to infectious disease prevention. It would be naive to assume that all barriers to the development and distribution of vaccines for the developing world can be readily resolved. For example, it is widely believed that in the development of an HIV vaccine, the major uncertainty is the scientific issue of whether an effective vaccine can be derived. But equally important is the issue recently confronted by GAVI, as to whether a functional infrastructure can be established in developing countries for the distribution and evaluation of vaccines in the field.

Global Infectious Disease Authority

The current HIV/AIDS crisis in Africa and Asia inevitably has profound political, social, and economic impact in the most populous countries in the world. This scenario seems to have attracted the attention of the world leaders. In 2002, the Security Council of the United Nations discussed the HIV/AIDS pandemic for the first time in history of this world body. However, unlike the Security Council's role in the world political affairs like peace and war, or the WTO's authority in dealing with international trade issues or disputes, WHO lacks the corresponding structure and authority to control the current and future spread of infectious diseases. SARS in the spring of 2003 was a convincing example. Considering the disastrous forecast for AIDS in Asia and Africa, and the increasing threats of global spread of new infectious diseases, a Global Infectious Disease Authority (GIDA) should be created, with a legally binding authority over individual member countries.

The structure of GIDA would follow the model of the Security Council of the United Nations, with a clear mandate and legal authority. GIDA should be given the responsibility and authority for worldwide infectious disease surveillance and reporting, the effective distribution of currently available vaccines, and the timely development of new vaccines. GIDA would closely coordinate its efforts with WTO and the Security Council for public health issues that have potential global consequences. Moreover, it should have the necessary authority to settle disputes and punish uncooperative members by political and economic means. GIDA would organize interactions with other partnerships in global health, including WHO and UN agencies, GAVI and PATH to avoid effort duplication and to collaborate in vaccine clinical evaluation and distribution in developing countries. The efforts of all participants will be unified by a clear mandate outlining their goals and responsibilities and supported by transparent and enforceable international laws. Resources would be raised from governments and private funds to adequately finance, over the long term, the research and development of new vaccines, their clinical evaluation, and reliable and reproducible manufacture and distribution. Incentives will be leveraged to assure the active participation of vaccine manufacturers and biotechnology companies in the development and manufacture of new vaccines. Developing countries with the appropriate infrastructure will be encouraged to support vaccine clinical development and manufacture so they become active participants in resolving regional public health problems.

Recently, there have been a number of positive indications that the developed world would directly contribute finances to improve global health. A UN commission suggested that "rich countries" make a major financial donation by contributing 0.1% of their gross national product towards the establishment of a fund to support health for the world's poor (Sachs, 2002). GIDA would be the focal point for this activity, and in order to attract the support of political leadership, the organization must produce a clear, well thought-out plan, which outlines a detailed timetable of activities and describes the responsibilities of both the public and private partners. The successful outcome would also be facilitated by the identification of political leaders of stature that would become actively involved in achieving the goals of GIDA and capable of articulating the positive attributes of the long-term goals of global health within the short frame of political horizons.

In exchange for full cooperation and active participation in standardizing infectious disease surveillance and transparent reporting in member countries from the developing world, GIDA would award qualified developing countries to support the process of vaccine evaluation and manufacture. These awards would include technology transfers, direct financing of vaccine development, sponsorship of clinical trials, investment in improving clinical trial infrastructure, the establishment of regulatory and manufacturing reciprocity with US, EU and Japan, and capital loans for the development of infrastructure and scale up.

Like the establishment of the Security Council after the World War II and the WTO in the global economy era, GIDA must be given the necessary authority to deal with the increasing threats of emerging infectious diseases to humanity and the world.

CONCLUSION

AIDS is becoming a global public health disaster of a scale that has no precedent in human history. Unfortunately, the vulnerability of Asian Countries to emerging infectious diseases will not be limited to HIV/AIDS only. The majority of the Asian population faces the continuing threats of new respiratory infectious diseases such as influenza and SARS, viral diseases that are transmitted by sex, IDU, and body fluids, and a growing number of bacterial diseases that cannot be treated by existing antibiotics. Compared with America and Europe, Asia appears much more vulnerable to new infectious diseases, regardless of their origin.

Vaccines prevent the establishment of infectious diseases and are regarded as the most successful medical intervention to date. Yet they are undervalued for financial reasons because, compared to pharmaceuticals, they generate less profit, and because of their efficacy, they progressively erode their own market segment. Vaccine development is costly, and a rapid return on investment is only achieved in lucrative markets. Consequently, vaccines have been predominantly focused on the diseases of concern to wealthy industrial countries. This imbalance has disregarded the loss of life in the developing world and permitted the emergence and global spread of many diseases from developing world epicenters. The recent establishment of a number of international organizations, reviewed in this chapter, envisages the development of vaccines for the global prevention of infectious disease with the active involvement of governments, industry, agencies, nonprofit organizations, and other public-private partnerships. Finally, a Global Infectious Disease Authority is proposed, with a legally binding mandate to control the development of vaccines for world health.

REFERENCES

Blanc, D. and Brewer, K. (1999). Issue Paper: Motivations for Local Vaccine Production. Children's Vaccine Initiative. Geneva, Switzerland.

Bloom, D. E., and Channing, D. (2000). The health and wealth of nations. *Science* 287:1207–1209.

Brugha, R., Starling, M., and Walt, G. (2002). GAVI, the first steps: Lessons for the Global Fund. Lancet 359:435–438.

Center for Disease Control (CDC). (1999). An Ounce of Prevention... What are the Returns? 2nd ed. CDC, Atlanta.

Fidler D.P. (2003). Emerging trends in international law concerning global infectious disease control. *Emerg Infect Dis.* 9(3):285–290.

Garrett, L. (1994). *In The Coming Plague: Newly emerging diseases in a World out of Balance.* Farrar, Strauss and Giroux, New York.

Greco, M. (2002). The future of vaccines: An industrial perspective. *Vaccine* 20(suppl1):S101–S103.

Gubler, D.J. (1988). Dengue. In: Monath, T. P. M. (ed.), *Epidemiology of Arthropod-borne Viral Disease.* CRC Press, Boca Raton, FL, pp. 223–260.

Horimoto, T. and Kawaoka, Y. (2001). Pandemic threat posed by avian influenza A viruses. *Clinical Microbiological Reviews* 14(1): 129–149.

Hubalek, Z., and Halouzka, J. (1999). West Nile Fever — A reemerging mosquito-borne viral disease in Europe. *Emerg Infect Dis.* 5(5):643–650.

Institute of Medicine (IOM). (2000). Calling the Shots. Immunization Finance Policies and Practices, National Academy Press, Washington, D.C.

Lu, Y. (1997). HIV-1 vaccine candidates evaluation in non-human primates. *Critical Review in Oncogenesis* 8:273–291.

Mackenzie, J. (1999). Emerging viral diseases: An Australian perspective. *Emerg Infect Dis.* 5(1): 1–8.

Mayer, J.D. (2000). Geography, ecology and emerging infectious diseases. *Social Sciences and Medicine* 50:937–952.

Mounts, A.W., Kwong, H., Izurieta, H.S., Ho, Y., Au, T., Lee, M., Bridges, C.B., Williams, S.W., Mak, K.H., Katz, J.M., Thompson, W.W., Cox, N.J., and Fukuda, K. (1999). Case—control study of risk factors for avian influenza A (H5N1) disease, Hong Kong, 1997. *J Infect Dis.* 180(2):505–508.

Petersen, L.R., and Roehrig, J.T. (2001). West Nile Virus: A reemerging global pathogen. *Emerg Infect Dis.* 7(4):611–614.

Rappuoli, R., Miller, H.I., and Falkow, S. (2002). The intangible value of vaccination. *Science* 297:937.

Sachs, J. (2002, January 6). Wage a global battle against epidemics. *San Francisco Chronicle*, D6.

Shope, R.E. (1999). Factors Influencing Geographic Distribution and Incidence of Tropical Infectious Diseases. In: Guerrant, R.L., Walker, D.H. and Weller, P.F. (eds.), *Tropical Infectious Diseases: Principles, Pathogens, & Practice* Volume1. Churchill-Livingstone (A division of Harcourt Brace & Co.)

Struck, M. (1996). Vaccine R&D success rates and development times. *Nature Biotechnology* 14:591–593.

Sun, Z., Ming, L., Zhu, X., and Lu, J. (2002). Prevention and control of hepatitis B in China. *J Med Virol.* 67:447–450.

Uyeki, T.M., Chong, Y., Katz, J.M., Lim, W., Ho, Y., Wang, S.S., Tsang, T.H.F., Au, W.W., Chan, S.T., Hu-Primmer, J., Bell, J.C., Thompson, W. W., Bridges, C.B., Cox, N.J., Mak, K., and Fukuda, K. (2002). Lack of evidence for human to human transmission of avian influenza A (H9N2) viruses in Hong Kong, China 1999. *Emerg Infect Dis.*8(3):154–159.

Wang, L., Harcourt, B., Yu, M., Tamin, A., Rota, P., Bellini, W., and Eaton, B. (2001). Molecular biology of Hendra and Nipah viruses. *Microbes Infect.* 3:279–287.

Webster, R.G. (1998). Influenza: An emerging disease. *Emerg Infect Dis.* 4(3):436–441.

World Health Organization (WHO). (1983). International Health Regulations. 3rd ed. [WHO, Geneva.]

World Health Organization (WHO). (1995). World Health Assembly resolution 48.7. WHO, Geneva.

World Health Organization (WHO). (2002). Doc. WHO/CDS/CSR/GAR/2002.4. WHO, Geneva.

IV

Prevention Efforts and Treatment Options

29

The Role of Antiretroviral Therapy in Asia

Bruce L. Gilliam, Anthony Amoroso, Charles E. Davis, and Robert R. Redfield

Division of Clinical Care and Research, Institute of Human Virology, University of Maryland, Baltimore, Maryland, USA

INTRODUCTION

The AIDS pandemic is the most important health problem facing the world today. More lives are lost to HIV/AIDS worldwide than malaria and tuberculosis combined. HIV/AIDS has caused a rapid decline in life expectancy in many African Nations. This has lead to the loss of teachers, workers, heads of households, and young parents throughout sub-Saharan Africa. Also as a direct result of premature death from HIV, many countries are experiencing an expanding epidemic of orphans whose parents have died from AIDS. As a consequence of these events, AIDS is the first disease that has transitioned from a global health challenge to an international geopolitical crisis whose impact may soon be measured by increasing economic and political instability throughout the world.

In the developed world, advances in antiretroviral (ARV) therapy have resulted in dramatic declines in hospitalizations and death rates, with concomitant steady increases in life expectancy. Unfortunately, these advances have not penetrated the developing world due in part to the cost of ARV therapy. Despite the fact that more than 40 million persons became HIV-infected in the developing world over the past decade, there is only limited availability of ARV therapy outside of Australia, Canada, Europe and the US. Today this treatment is available to only about 1 million people infected worldwide (Cochrane, 2000). As a consequence the global health care gap has widened despite unprecedented scientific discovery over the past twenty years.

Ultimately, an efficacious, preventative HIV vaccine will have the greatest impact on containing the HIV epidemic in Asia and Africa. However, it will most likely take ten years or more before an efficacious vaccine can be developed; the necessary clinical trials planned, implemented, evaluated, and global implementation initiated. By that time another 10 to 50 million people are projected to acquire HIV infection worldwide. Given the potentially catastrophic impact of HIV, and the unrelenting pace of new infections in many parts of the world, the development and implementation of sustainable and affordable therapies for the developing world has become a global priority.

Up until now, one major limitation of ARV therapy worldwide has been the lack of access to ARV drugs. Now, with the concessions on cost by major pharmaceutical firms, combined with investment by many Nations in the Global Fund for HIV, tuberculosis (TB) and malaria, and the historic commitment by President Bush and the President's Emergency Program for AIDS Relief, worldwide access to ARV therapy has become more plausible (Office of the Press Secretary, 2003).

It is important to recognize that despite the importance of these accomplishments, access to the ARV drugs is only the tip of the iceberg. Developing the infrastructure for drug delivery, drug procurement and tracking procedures, gaining the expertise in the management of ARV therapy, enhancing care and treatment infrastructure, training and augmenting in-country health care personnel, developing alternative treatment delivery models which lend themselves to rapid scalability, validating the safety and efficacy of optimal in-country ARV regimens, and establishing monitoring and evaluation capacity to ensure success in different settings and populations are just a few of the issues which must be addressed when developing an ARV treatment strategy for resource-limited countries (World Health Organization, 2002).

KEY CONCEPTS FOR IMPLEMENTATION OF ANTIRETROVIRAL PROGRAMS: ACCESS, DURABILITY, SCALABILITY, AND SUSTAINABILITY

Enormous progress has been made over the past 15 years in the treatment of HIV/AIDS and many patients are now able to live a normal life span if treated effectively. Clinicians in the US and Europe have learned much about the limitations of effective ARV chemotherapy. Recently, clinical trials of new ARV agents have demonstrated astounding success rates at ranges greater than 80% (Robbins *et al.*, 2003; Tavel *et al.*, 1999; de Truchis *et al.*, 2001; Staszewski *et al.*, 2003). In real life clinic settings however, the success rates have been much lower (Lucas, 2003). This has led to an increase in the prevalence of resistance mutations in both those on highly active antiretroviral therapy (HAART) and those who are newly infected. The potential for high failure rates and the spread of resistance within populations are important realities to consider when developing and managing ARV therapy programs worldwide. The proactive prevention of the emergence of ARV drug resistance in both the individual patient and the wider community is extremely important. How successfully this can be accomplished will determine the long-term sustainability of newly initiated national ARV programs.

Key concepts that will define treatment success and local and national programmatic goals are 1) access to treatment, 2) durability of treatment at the patient level, 3) scalability of treatment modalities, and 4) sustainability of the program at the community or national level. Central to each of these strategic variables is the definition of programmatic success.

Access to treatment is the ability of individuals or communities to obtain not only ARV treatment but also appropriate medical care and therapeutic management. Access to the medical care needed to administer high quality ARV treatment is also a major hurdle to the delivery of ARV in developing countries. Once ARV treatment is finally obtained there is then the challenge of appropriate management of these complex treatments including: drug toxicities, drug-to-drug interactions, adherence, and resistance. Despite the fact that only an estimated one million patients are on therapy in developed countries, access to ARV and to medical care with expertise in HIV treatment is still a recognized problem. Even in the United States, many individual states have waiting lists to obtain recommended ARV treatment. Some European countries limit access to ARV drugs until CD4 counts are 200 cells/mm^3 or symptomatic AIDS occurs (British HIV Association, 2001).

The durability of ARV treatment in the individual patient is extremely important. Durability of treatment can be defined as treatments that produce the desired effect, for example viral suppression, for an extended period of time. It is hoped that this period of time would be decades. In studies to date, this has been difficult to achieve in real life settings. The ramifications of a non-durable treatment regimen include disease progression, opportunistic infections, ARV drug resistance, and expanded diagnostic monitoring (such as frequent viral load testing and specialized viral resistance testing) as required components of routine clinical care. In countries where only one treatment regimen is available failure of that treatment regimen may lead to death for an individual who has no further options. In addition, a resistant virus may be transmitted leading to lack of efficacy of a given country's regimen in ARV-naïve patients. This would, in turn, limit therapeutic options for all HIV-infected individuals in that country.

Once access to a durable treatment regimen has been established, the ability of HIV treatment strategies to be "scaled up," to allow for the treatment of all HIV-infected individuals in a region, country, or worldwide, is critical to the long-term successful management of HIV disease. This can be termed scalability (World Health Organization, 2002; Joint United Nations Programme on HIV/AIDS, 2002). Without it, many who "on paper" have access to HIV drugs may not actually be able to obtain treatment due to lack of infrastructure, specialized lab tests, a certain level of education to administer the drugs, facilities to store temperature-sensitive drugs, or the resources to afford the care. The cost of providing care far exceeds the cost of the ARV medication. Each of these concepts is hopelessly intertwined and equally important in the consideration of ARV therapy in a country or region and worldwide.

After an ARV program is brought to scale and is able to provide ARV treatment to the people living with HIV in the community, it will become critical to sustain this capacity in order for the ARV program to negate the impact of HIV on its society. Two major prerequisites will be required for long-term sustainability. First, the development of ARV resistance must be successfully minimized during the course of implementation of the ARV program, so that the selected ARV regimen still retains antiviral efficacy once the program is scaled. Second, sustainability is dependent on the continued support of donor agencies to underwrite the cost of ARV programs for resource-limited countries. The investment required could easily exceed US$ 30–100 billion annually. National donors such as the G8 will need to see that these programs are effective in terms of globalization and relevant economic, social and humanitarian concerns to justify this sustained level of support.

The strategies created in each country to deliver ARV treatment are developed with the goal of "success." However, success is determined by one's outlook. For example, the implementation of ARV therapy in Brazil has been proclaimed as a success by some and a failure by others. Those who view it as a success point out the tremendous access to ARV treatment that the program has created and that the mortality rate of HIV-infected individuals has declined since the implementation of ARV treatment. However, others will look at the fact that in a short period of time, 6% of newly diagnosed patients in Brazil show evidence of drug resistance (Brindeiro *et al.*, 2003), and more than 40% of patients receiving treatment demonstrate evidence of viral resistance (Tanuri, 2003). This can be viewed as an early indicator that this country's treatment strategy will lead to increased costs and mortality downstream. Therefore, in order to determine the success or failure of a therapeutic strategy, the goals of this strategy must first be defined. Possible goals to attain or avoid could include: the number of people on therapy, the number of people with viral suppression on therapy initially and over time, the number of people with an immunologic response on therapy (increased CD4 count), and the percentage of people with HIV drug resistance. A decision has to be made as to the goals of therapy so that a successful treatment strategy can be implemented. Certain goals such as a decrease in AIDS mortality at three years, can be reached easily when treatment is initiated in symptomatic patients with AIDS. More complex goals such as decreasing rates of AIDS orphans, stabilizing a targeted work force, significantly increasing national life expectancy or reversing HIV/AIDS impact on economic and global security concerns, will require high levels of sustainable treatment response.

COMPLEXITIES OF ANTIRETROVIRAL THERAPY

Antiretroviral therapy began with the approval by the US Food and Drug Administration (FDA) of zidovudine (AZT) monotherapy in 1988. Prior to that, management of HIV/AIDS involved the prevention of opportunistic infections and expanded access to mental health and palliative health care services. A few years later, with the introduction of didanosine and zalcitabine, the concept of combination therapy with two agents began to evolve. With the introduction of the protease inhibitors in the mid 1990s, the concept of ARV therapy changed dramatically (Palella *et al.*, 1998). Morbidity and mortality due to HIV/AIDS declined rapidly. The term HAART was coined to indicate the ability of these new regimens to completely suppress viral replication. As newer agents have been added to this armamentarium, the durability of these regimens in clinical trials has increased. Currently, there are 20 available anti-HIV medications in four classes available in the United States and more in the developmental pipeline. Four new agents were approved by the FDA in the past year, including emtricitabine (FTC), T-20, and two new protease inhibitors, atazanavir and fosamprenavir. FTC is similar to 3TC, and T-20 is the first of a new class of entry inhibitors (Van Der Horst *et al.*, 2001), representing a new target for drug therapy, which includes chemokine coreceptor blockers (Lalezari *et al.*, 2001). With the development of entry inhibitors the future of HIV therapeutics may lay in pre-integration therapeutic strategies totally different from the current treatment paradigms.

In order to manage ARV therapy effectively, one must learn from the hard-learned lessons of the past 15 to 20 years of treatment. When therapy with AZT as a single drug initially began, there was an inadequate understanding of the importance of adherence, resistance, pharmacokinetics, and provider experience. Yet there was a perceived need of urgency. Without alternative options, the use of AZT and nucleoside reverse transcriptase inhibitor (NRTI) mono- and dual therapy was rapidly implemented and scaled up in the United States and Europe. It is now clear that sequential monotherapy or dual therapy as occurred with AZT or ddI therapy led to resistance and limitation of future treatment options. In retrospect, it may have been more prudent to optimize and validate issues related to ARV durability before wide-scale recommendations and implementation of treatment for persons with non-advanced HIV infection. These decisions have had significant impact on the lives of many of the men and women treated in the first decade of ARV treatment. In addition, although not intended, these early decisions served to enable viral resistance and further complicate HIV treatment at the national level. For example, a high prevalence of resistance in patients with primary or early HIV infection can inadvertently lead to monotherapy in a newly treated patient if resistance exists to one or two of the agents chosen for that person's initial ARV therapy regimen. Wide scale non-nucleoside reverse transcriptase inhibitor (NNRTI) resistance will likely impact the success of mother-to-child-transmission (MTCT) programs employing nevirapine. Inversely, wide-scale NNRTI resistance induced by "successful" MTCT programs could negatively impact, to a significant degree, the success of a National ARV program utilizing an NNRTI containing ARV regimen. These are just several examples of how early decisions may impact future ARV program options and add to the complexity of ARV therapy management.

Out of 20 drugs and multiple preparations, one must consider which agents to use, when to start them, when to switch them, and how to treat highly experienced patients with drug resistance. In addition, management includes dealing with the toxicities of these drugs (Carr *et al.*, 1998; Medina *et al.*, 1994; Brinkman *et al.*, 1998; Copeland *et al.*, 1992; Fortgang *et al.*, 1995; Sundar *et al.*, 1997), drug-to-drug interactions, difficulties with the need for 100% adherence (Paterson *et al.*, 2000;), lack of long-term efficacy of regimens in real life settings (Chaisson *et al.*, 2000; Casado *et al.*, 1998; Deeks *et al.*, 1999; Lucas *et al.*, 1999; Ledergerber *et al.*, 1999), cost, comorbid illnesses such as hepatitis and tuberculosis, opportunistic infections and their prophylaxis, substance abuse, mental illness, and the social situations of patients (housing, nutrition, stigma, family/reproductive counseling, secondary prevention, etc.). Adding to the complexity is the fact that there is no single answer for any of these issues. It is therefore not a surprise that numerous studies have demonstrated that the more experience a provider has in the care of HIV-infected patients the better the outcomes in terms of viral suppression, disease progression, and life span. New treatment strategies built on the hard-learned lesson from existing ARV programs can and should be developed in order to avoid the mistakes of the past.

BASIC PRINCIPLES OF ANTIRETROVIRAL THERAPY

Appropriate management of ARV therapy is a continually evolving process that changes as new data becomes available. There are a few major concepts that are important to consider when treating HIV-infected individuals. When considering the selection of an ARV regimen one must synthesize the issues of viral dynamics and pathogenesis (Chun *et al.*, 1997a; Chun *et al.*, 1997b; Finzi *et al.*, 1997; Wong *et al.*, 1997; Chun and Fauci, 1999), resistance, drug pharmacokinetics, drug toxicities, and drug durability. The critical question is when to start ARV therapy in an individual.

This is a much-debated question without a clear answer, as evidenced by the United States and Great Britain choosing different criterion after evaluating the same data. There is consensus that therapy should be initiated when a patient develops an opportunistic infection or has a CD4 cell count less than 200 (Hogg *et al.*, 2001); but there is a debate over the optimal starting CD4 cell count (Kaplan *et al.*, 2001; Opravil *et al.*, 2001; Sterling *et al.*, 2001). Data indicate a much higher morbidity and mortality rate if treatment is started at CD4 counts less than 200. However, the benefit of therapy to prevent disease progression is lower above a CD4 cell count of 200 while therapy has been demonstrated to have a greater efficacy and lower toxicity at these higher CD4 cell counts.

Lowering the potential to develop drug toxicities becomes a very important issue when ARV programs select one national regimen, which may include thymidine analogs (Medina *et al.*, 1994; Carr *et al.*, 1998) and nevirapine (Boehringer Ingelheim Pharmaceuticals Inc., 2003). This is balanced by accumulating toxicities of long-term therapy, increased cost, and potential for development of resistance prior to onset of symptomatic AIDS. Further data may help to elucidate the optimal starting point but one must weigh the above issues carefully for each individual, group, or country.

The issue of what regimen to start is also changing frequently with the development of new agents and the presentation of new data. The basic criteria for the choice of an ARV regimen include: high potency, high threshold of resistance, low toxicity, favorable pharmacokinetics (i.e., once or twice daily administration, co-formulation), similar half lives amongst drugs used, equal activity in different cellular growth cycles, few short term and long term side effects and few drug interactions, particularly with TB medications.

Consideration to switching or changing therapy is given when an individual does not have an appropriate initial response to therapy, has an increase in viral load following complete viral suppression, has a decreasing CD4 cell count, and/or toxicity or intolerability to therapy. Antiviral drug resistance and side effects are the major reasons to switch therapy. Resistance has become a significant problem in the United States, Europe and, more recently, Brazil. The high replication rate and low replication fidelity (high error rate) of HIV predisposes an individual to the development of resistance. In general, resistance develops on ARV therapy in the face of ongoing viral replication. Significant resistance can be occurring despite a stable or increasing CD4 count, thus treatment strategies which rely only on CD4 counts to determine treatment failure will likely see patients with accumulated resistance mutations at the time of recognized clinical failure. Some data also suggests that resistance may occur when initiating therapy and prior to complete viral suppression. This can be problematic when considering agents with a low mutation threshold such as lamivudine, efavirenz, and nevirapine. These are agents that have been chosen in developing countries due to their ease of administration, costs, and potency. Resistance to efavirenz and nevirapine has been shown to develop rapidly in clinical use and has been documented to occur in up to 15% of patients with primary/early HIV infection and no history of exposure to ARV therapy (Little *et al.*, 2002). In addition, we are recognizing the fact that high rates of resistance to NNRTIs occur after a single dose of nevirapine is given for prevention of mother-to-child transmission (PMTCT) (Eshleman *et al.*, 2001). What impact this resistance will have on new mothers seeking treatment with NNRTI based regimens is uncertain although there is no reason to suggest that developing resistance in this setting is any different than developing resistance in any other setting. It is now clear that significant cross-resistance occurs within each of the ARV drug classes, thus use of one or two agents in a given class may lead to resistance to the entire class of agents. Stated another way, if resistance to the initial treatment regimen occurs and is allowed to accumulate, future treatment options may be seriously limited not only for the individual but to the community if resistance occurs to a high degree amongst treated patients.

CREATING DURABLE ANTIRETROVIRAL REGIMENS

The key to successful treatment strategies in resource-limited countries is the concept of durability. A durable regimen can prevent the emergence of resistance, promote health, decrease the complexities of care, and save money in total health care costs. Durable regimens can be created with prudent, intelligent use of the ARV agents currently available.

Selecting treatment regimens and delivery strategies prior to validating durability of the selected regimen in the specific patient population could have long-term serious public health consequences particularly in countries where only one regimen is chosen or affordable for use. For example, recently it was found that certain combinations of reverse transcriptase inhibitors had unacceptable high rates of failure. These failure rates were observed in clinical trials using the combination ddI, abacavir, and 3TC; or ddI, tenofovir, 3TC; or abacavir, tenofovir, 3TC. Unfortunately these failure rates were recognized only after such regimens were used in clinical practice (Farthing *et al.*, 2003; Glaxo Smith Kline, 2003).

Recent clinical trials have demonstrated increased efficacy and durability with newer

TABLE 1. Principles for Creating Durable Treatment

1. Maximally suppress viral load (reduce viral load to as low as possible, <50 c/ml).
2. Use clinically proven triple combinations; avoid mono- or dual drug therapy.
3. Select highly potent drugs with proven efficacy in advanced disease and high viral loads.
4. Select regimens containing drugs with high mutational thresholds.
5. Select regimens that combine drugs with similar pharmacokinetic profiles.
6. Limit use of drugs with high gastrointestinal toxicity or increased toxicity in advanced disease.
7. Ensure adherence particularly at the time of inducing viral control through treatment preparation and adherence support.
8. Limit pill burden and food requirements.
9. Avoid adding a single drug to a "failing" regimen.

agents. This has not been translated into clinical practice even in the United States and Europe where the average initial HAART regimen is taken for only 1.6 years and is switched mainly for drug toxicities and treatment failure (Chen *et al.*, 2003).

Key principles for optimizing durable ARV drug therapy have emerged (Table 1). Central to these principles is to obtain maximal viral suppression to viral load thresholds of at least less than 50 HIV RNA copies per ml. Only clinically proven regimens of three or more primary ARV drugs should be used. Selected regimens should include drugs with high mutational thresholds. This is particularly important when considering the use of 3TC and NNRTI drugs which are very vulnerable to loss of activity due to an occurrence of a single point mutation. Because patients interrupt medication due to illness and non-adherence, it is also important to use medications with similar pharmacokinetic (PK) profiles.

As important as the regimen choice is, the care delivery structure used to deliver ARV treatment is equally as important. Treatment adherence is paramount to durable viral suppression. This is particularly important during the induction of viral control and periods when virus is actively detectable. Data is emerging that events during the initial induction of viral control will determine durability limitations not recognized until one to two years later. Thus, programs are developing intensive treatment preparation strategies to adequately prepare patients for treatment. ARV treatment preparation is then coupled with intensive treatment support, especially during the first three months after treatment initiation, to include a menu of observational ARV delivery strategies. Both treatment preparation and treatment support proactively incorporate family and community involvement into HIV care programs. All of this is intended to give the patient needed support to ensure adherence, particularly when patients are first placed on ARV treatment. Given that much remains to be learned about alternative ARV delivery models, it is important to create and validate new models for ARV treatment strategies for different settings and populations.

With the choice of potent regimens consistent with the principles highlighted in Table 1 and intensive treatment preparation and support, especially during the first three months of treatment initiation, durable ARV suppression should become the rule. Unlike the reality of today, virologic treatment failure could become the rare exception.

CREATING AN ANTIRETROVIRAL THERAPY PROGRAM

Understanding the strengths and weaknesses of current ARV therapy programs in resource-rich and resource-limited countries is important when developing new strategies for countries looking to implement a treatment program.

The United States government has a multi-pronged approach to funding HIV/AIDS treatment. The basis of treatment programs in the United State is the Ryan White Program, which supplies funding for the care and treatment of HIV-infected individuals, particularly the uninsured and the underinsured. Care is also provided through the Medical Assistance Program, which provides care for those with low incomes and/or chronic illnesses. This is supplemented by the AIDS Drug Assistance Program, which provides funding for the ARV drugs.

Although the US ARV treatment program has had enormous impact on decreasing morbidity and mortality from HIV/AIDS, between 1998 and 2000 major US cities detected a significant rise in the spread of ARV drug-resistant virus in newly HIV-infected individuals from 3.5% to 14% (Little et al., 2003). Today the sub-optimal use of ARV drugs by both physicians and patients has set the stage for a public health crisis—an epidemic of multi-drug resistant HIV infection. For the United States, the race is on. Fueled by the occurrence of cross-class drug resistance, the future success of ARV therapeutics is dependent on research, development and approval of newer ARV drugs with unique resistant mutation patterns. The use of antiretroviral therapy, beginning with AZT monotherapy, continues to evolve, moving through dual NRTI therapy, combination triple drug regimens (2 NRTI and 1 PI), combination triple drug regimens (NRTI, NNRTI, and a PI), combination PI with a NRTI or NNRTI, two NRTI and 1 NNRTI, three NRTIs, four-drug regimens, five-drug regimens and salvage therapy. This scenario of sequential treatment failure has been at the heart of the use of ARV drugs in resource-rich countries and, without intervention, could be at the heart of their use in resource-limited countries. As a consequence, major emphasis is being placed on increasing the therapeutic durability of the current programs and building on the remarkable achievements of the 1990s in order to advance treatment outcomes for the next generation of patients in the United States. This emphasis should now be applied to new programs developing in resource-limited settings.

To maintain state-of-the-art care, clinical research is federally funded through research networks including the Adult/Pediatric AIDS Clinical Trials Groups and the Community Programs for Clinical Research on AIDS (CPRCA). Additionally, research funding is provided through grant mechanisms from the US National Institute of Health (NIH). To ensure the expertise of the providers supplying this care, there is the AIDS Education and Training Center program that educates and trains HIV providers at all levels of experience to enhance the quality of care provided.

Outside of the United States, funding for HIV/AIDS treatment programs is provided through multiple pathways. The Global Fund for HIV, TB and Malaria, supported through contributions largely from G8 and developed countries, provides support to individual countries for ARV treatment programs. More recently, President Bush made an historic commitment and pledged a minimum of 15 billion dollars to support treatment care and prevention of HIV infection. The President's Emergency Program for AIDS Relief will support HIV treatment and care and include ARV procurement and treatment in 14 of the world's most severely affected resource-limited countries. Other operational treatment programs are funded through the United States Agency for International Development (USAID), the Centers for Disease Control (CDC), and the U.S. Military HIV Research Program. There are also numerous programs worldwide that work to prevent mother to child transmission.

Brazil has championed access to ARV therapy as a human right for its citizens. As such, Brazil's ARV therapy program is an extremely successful model for increased access to ARV treatment in a resource-limited setting. Brazil built the required capacity to manufacture generic drugs, and rapidly scaled up treatment to over 100,000 people in urgent need of treatment. There has been a rapid and dramatic decrease in short-term morbidity and mortality in those with AIDS. However rapid implementation of ARV treatment was done without emphasizing the need to develop alternative ARV delivery mechanisms to strongly enhance adherence. Instead, care delivery mimicked that used in Europe and the US. Unfortunately, as was the case in the US, this approach has led to significant viral drug resistance. In their first report of the program of Brazil, 6.6% of newly diagnosed patients (not newly infected) show evidence of drug resistance just two years after initiation of their treatment program (Brindeiro *et al.*, 2003). An additional cross sectional study in a limited number of patients have shown nearly 44% of patients on HAART have resistance to at least one class of drugs (Tanuri, 2003). Similar levels of resistance took nearly 15 years to develop in the U.S. and Europe. Fortunately Brazil has a strong health care infrastructure that combines the required diagnostic capabilities with access to 2nd and 3rd line ARV salvage regimens. As the level of resistance continues to increase, there will be significant limitations of future treatment options for not only those who are treatment-experienced but also for those who are newly and chronically infected.

Haiti developed a treatment program more suitable for many in severely resource-limited countries which do not have access to 2nd and 3rd line therapy or diagnostic capabilities. They implemented ARV therapy in a well-designed treatment support structure where every patient on therapy received directly observed therapy. This circumvented some of the limitations of Brazil's program, particularly, non-adherence. The treatment model was first validated and showed resistance not to be a significant problem. They have documented very high success rates (Farmer *et al.*, 2001). Although the Haitian model of ARV treatment delivery has not yet treated large numbers of patients, it has several key components to a scalable program.

THE CONCEPT OF "SCALABILITY"

The lynch pin for a scalable program is creating a durable treatment regimen and delivery model. If a therapeutic strategy can be validated to be successful in a very high percentage of patients on treatment, then the need for frequent viral load or CD4 cell count monitoring will be unnecessary. If the regimen selected has low rates of toxicity, and whatever effects do occur are predictable and easily recognized through symptomatic complaints, this could negate frequent medical visits and frequent safety laboratory work.

The current model of therapy in the US and Europe relies heavily on the frequent use of viral load measurements and resistance testing in order to optimally manage the treatment of HIV. Such an approach is necessary since the treatment model cannot ensure perfect adherence and significant resistance already exists in many patients. Medical personnel with extensive experience are needed to interpret resistance testing and select salvage regimens. This is not a scalable model for resource limited settings. Even frequent monitoring of CD4 counts could cost as much or more than the cost of the medications. For example, in Nigeria the drug costs per patient are approximately $300 per year, yet the monitoring requirements are approximately $1200 per year. Since the ability to monitor HIV therapy also requires laboratory infrastructure and technical staff support, treatment models that require even the simplest medical monitoring may not be an option for millions of patients. Although the optimal treatment strategies are not known, linking scalability to therapeutic outcomes should be a required step prior to plans for exponential scale up of a program.

There are a number of key variables that will determine the scalability of a selected ARV program. First, the selection of the regimen will dictate capacity to scale. For example, the regimens selected that do not require laboratory testing for toxicity monitoring will be easier to bring to scale. Second,

TABLE 2. Characteristics of a Scalable Program

1. Adequate local supply of antiretrovirals
2. No reliance on viral load testing and genotype
3. Minimal reliance on medical/hospital-based care
4. Ability to distribute antiretrovirals at the local community village level
5. Trained local community/village paramedical providers to deliver observed antiretroviral therapy and recognize toxicity
6. Selected regimen has predictable and easily recognized toxicities
7. Strong community-based educational programs for early diagnosis and treatment

the ARV treatment model selected will dictate capacity to scale. For example, a hospital or clinic-based ARV program will have limitations. Village, workplace, or parish centered ARV treatment programs lend themselves to rapid expansion. Third, systems needed to maintain an adequate supply of the necessary ARV must be in place. The logistical management required to ensure that the drug supply is maintained without interruption and that the drug is utilized prior to expiration is substantial. Fourth, development and implementation of strong community-based treatment education preparation programs that proactively engage community participation in a program promoting early diagnosis, early treatment and support of persons living with HIV infection will be crucial.

Scalability will be key to ultimately allowing persons living with HIV access to treatment. It is fundamental to reversing the declining life expectancy, now a reality in many resource-limited countries. Overall, it is important that from the initial vision of a national ARV program, these issues related to scalability are thought through (Table 2).

CLOSING COMMENTS

Over the past 25, years HIV/AIDS has emerged as an international crisis of catastrophic proportions that threatens the survival not just of individual persons living with HIV but also the nations in which they live. Today a person diagnosed with HIV infection in the United States or Western Europe can anticipate living a natural life time. Yet if one is diagnosed in Africa or Asia, premature death is the most likely outcome.

We live at an historic time in history. Science has provided the tools to confront HIV/AIDS and reverse its progressive destruction of individual patients, family, communities and the nations in which they live. The successful introduction of durable, scalable, sustainable ARV therapy holds the key. Successfully implemented ARV therapy has enormous potential to acutely put an end to the suffering and death of people living with HIV/AIDS worldwide. Long term, it can allow parents to raise their children and teachers to teach generations of children. Successful ARV treatment programs will reverse the trends of economic and geopolitical instability occurring in regions plagued by AIDS. Finally, a successful program, fueled by the resources of the wealthiest nations in the world, can make global health and equity of HIV care a reality, and may change the hearts and minds of many who may have pursued a path of terror to embrace civilization and peace. Yet in order for these outcomes to be realized, ARV treatment programs must be successful.

Antiretroviral therapy has major limitations that have appreciated over the last 15 years and caused HIV therapy to become more complex and costly in the developed world. It is our responsibility now, to build on the past 15 years of experience with ARV treatment and create durable treatment programs for those most in need. Successful strategies to bring HIV therapies for resource-limited settings need to be developed in the context of the complexities of using ARV in societies with minimal health care infrastructures, limited monitoring capabilities, different opportunistic infections and nutritional deficiencies, and different levels of HIV education and stigmatizations. Local solutions need to be developed, implemented and embraced. What works well in the US may not work well in Vietnam. What works well in China may not work well in Nigeria. Available data from African and Caribbean populations strongly suggest that the time needed to develop a clinical outcome, after HIV infection, is significantly compressed compared to the US and European populations, and that differences in the health care delivery systems account for only a part of this accelerated disease process. These therapeutic programs and approaches must also be carefully considered and anchored in what is known about the pathogenesis of HIV/AIDS in such populations and not simply the blanket application of known US and European therapeutic strategies (Kanki *et al.*, 1999; De Wit *et al.*, 2002; Morgan *et al.*, 2002; Constantine *et al.*, 2003).

This is not to suggest that large scale therapeutic interventions should not begin now, but that as treatment goes forward, systematic monitoring and evaluation of treatment outcomes should be central to the implementation of these programs. This will allow programs that work to be expanded, and programs with high failure rates to be eliminated. "Successful" ARV therapy should not merely count the number of patients treated, but rather programs must be measured by treatment outcomes and their consequences for society. This will be important to ensure that the programs that are ultimately recognized as failures within 5–10 years, do not get exponentially expanded prematurely. If they do, and ARV programs fail to meet goals of key donor countries, both the billions of dollars required to maintain these programs, and future opportunities to implement sustainable ARV treatment worldwide, could be severely compromised. However, if demonstrated success is linked to additional resources, and these programs are brought to scale as rapidly as possible, the integration of science, medicine, industry and public policy to deliver ARV treatment globally will successfully confront AIDS as we await the global deployment of an highly efficacious HIV vaccine.

REFERENCES

Boehringer Ingelheim Pharmaceuticals, Inc. (2003). Viramune package insert. Ridgefield, CT: revised Sept. 4, 2003.

Brindeiro R.M., Diaz R.S., Sabino E.C., Morgado M.G., Pires I.L., Brigido L., Dantas M.C., Barreira D., Teixeira P.R., Tanuri A. and the Brazilian Network for Drug Resistance Surveillance. (2003). Brazilian Network for HIV Drug Resistance Surveillance (HIV-BResNET): a survey of chronically infected individuals. *AIDS* 17:1063–1069.

Brinkman K., ter Hofstede H.J.M, Burger D.M., Smeitink J.A.M., and Koopmans P.P. (1998). Adverse effects of reverse transcriptase inhibitors: mitochondrial toxicity as common pathway. *AIDS* 12: 1735–1744.

British HIV Association (BHIVA) guidelines for the treatment of HIV-infected adults with antiretroviral therapy. (2001). *HIV Med.* 2:276–313.

Carr A., Samaras K., Burton S., Law M., Freund J., Chisholm D.J., Cooper D.A. (1998). A syndrome of peripheral lipodystrophy, hyperlipidemia and insulin resistance in patients receiving HIV protease inhibitors. *AIDS* 12:F51–F58.

Casado J.L., Perez-Elias M.J., Antela A., Sabido R., Marti-Belda P., Dronda F., Blazquez J., Quereda C. (1998). Predictors of long-term response to protease inhibitor therapy in a cohort of HIV infected patient. *AIDS* 12:F131–F151.

Chaisson, R.E., Keruly, J.C., and Moore, R.D. (2000). Association of initial CD4 cell count and viral load with response to highly active antiretroviral therapy. *JAMA* 284:3128–3129.

Chen, R.Y., Westfall A.O., Mugavero M.J., Cloud, G.A., Raper, J.L., Chatham, A.G., Acosta, E.P., Taylor, K.H., Carter, J., Saag, M.S. (2003). Duration of highly active antiretroviral therapy regimens. *Clin Infect Dis.* 37:714–722.

Chun T.W., Carruth, L., Finzi, D., Shen, X., DiGiuseppe, J.A., Taylor, H., Hermankova, M., Chadwick, K., Margolick, J., Quinn, T.C., Kuo, Y.H., Brookmeyer, R., Zeiger, M.A., Barditch-Crovo, P., Siliciano, R.F. (1997a). Quantification of latent tissue reservoirs and total body viral load in HIV-1 infection. *Nature* 387:183–188.

Chun, T.W., Stuyver, L., Mizell, S.B., Ehler, L.A., Mican, J.A., Baseler, M., Lloyd, A.L., Nowak, M.A., Fauci, A.S. (1997b). Presence of an inducible HIV-1 latent reservoir during highly active antiretroviral therapy. *PNAS* 94:13193–13197.

Chun, T.W., and Fauci, A.S. (1999). Latent reservoirs of HIV: Obstacles to the eradication of virus. *PNAS* 96:10958–10961.

Cochrane, J. (2000). Narrowing the gap; access to HIV treatment in developing countries. A pharmaceutical company's perspective. *J of Med Ethics* 26:47–50.

Constantine, N.T., Sill, A.M., Jack, N., Kreisel, K., Edwards, J., Cafarella, T., Smith, H., Bartholomew, C., Cleghorn, F.R., Blattner, W.A. (2003). Improved classification of recent HIV-1 infection by employing a two-stage sensitive/less-sensitive test strategy. *J Acquir Immune Defic Syndr.* 32:94–103.

Copeland, W.C., Chen, M.S., and Wang, T.S.F. (1992). Human DNA polymerases alpha and beta are able to incorporate anti-HIV deoxynucleotides into DNA. *J Biol Chem.* 267:21459–21464.

Deeks, S.G., Hecht, F.M., Swanson, M., Elbeik, T., Loftus, R., Cohen, P.T., Grant, R.M. (1999). HIV RNA and CD4 cell count response to protease inhibitor therapy in an urban AIDS clinic: Response to both initial and salvage therapy. *AIDS* 13:F35–F43.

de Truchis, P., Force, G., Welker, Y., Mechali, D., Pulik, M., Chemlal, K., Rouveix, E., Devidas, A., Praindhui, D., Mamet, J-P. (2001). An open-label study to evaluate safety and efficacy of a quadruple combination therapy without protease inhibitor (Combivir + abacavir + efavirenz) in antiretroviral therapy naïve adults (CNAF3008). XIII International AIDS Conference; July 9–14. Durban, South Africa. (abstract 3208).

DeWit, S., Boulme, R., Poll, B., Schmit, J.C., and Clumeck, N. (2002). Viral load and CD4 response to PI containing regimen in B versus non-B treatment-naïve HIV-1 patients. 2nd International AIDS Society Conference on HIV Pathogenesis and Treatment; July 13–16, 2002. Paris, France. (abstract 25).

Eshleman, S.H., Mracna, M., Guay G., Deseyve M., Cunningham, S., Musoke P., Mmiro, F. Jackson, J.B. (2001). Selection of nevirapine resistance (NVP^R) mutations in Ugandan women and infants receiving NVP prophylaxis to prevent HIV-1 vertical transmission (HIVNET-012). 8th Conference on Retroviruses and Opportunistic Infections; Feb 4–8. Chicago, IL. (abstract 516).

Farmer, P., Leandre, F., Mukherjee, J.S., Claude, M., Nevil, P., Smith-Fawzi, M.C., Koenig, S.P., Castro, A., Becerra, M.C., Sachs, J., Attaran, A., Kim, J.Y. (2001). Community-based approaches to HIV treatment in resource-poor settings. *Lancet* 358:404–409.

Farthing, C., Khanlou, H., and Yeh,V. (2003). Early virologic failure in a pilot study evaluating the efficacy of once daily abacavir, lamivudine, and tenofovir DF in treatment naïve HIV patients. Program and abstracts of the 2nd International AIDS Society Conference on Pathogenesis and Treatment; July 13–16. Paris, France. (abstract 43).

Finzi, D., Hermankova, M., Pierson, T., Carruth, L.M., Buck, C., Chaisson, R.E., Quinn, T.C., Chadwick, K., Margolick, J., Brookmeyer, R., Gallant, J., Markowitz, M., Ho, D.D., Richman, D.D., Siliciano, R.F. (1997). Identification of a Reservoir for HIV-1 in Patients on highly active antiretroviral therapy. *Science* 278:1295–1300.

Fortgang, I.S., Belitsos, P.C., Chaisson, R.E., and Moore, R.D. (1995). Hepatomegaly and steatosis in HIV-infected patients receiving nucleoside analog antiretroviral therapy. *Am J Gastroenterol.* 90:14336.

GlaxoSmithKline. (2003). Dear Health Care Provider Warning. Early virologic non-response in patients with HIV infection treated with lamivudine, abacavir, and tenofovir. (July 2003).

Hogg, R.S., Yip, B., Wood, E., Chan K., Craib, K.J.P., O'Shaughnessy, M.V., Montaner J.S.G. (2001). Diminished effectiveness of antiretroviral therapy among patients initiating therapy with CD4+ cell counts below $200/mm^3$. 8th Conference on Retroviruses and Opportunistic Infections; Feb 4–8. Chicago, IL. (abstract 342).

Joint United Nations Programme on HIV/AIDS. (2002). Accelerating access to care, Geneva.

Kanki P.J., Hamel D.J., Sankale J.L., Hsieh C., Thior I., Barin F., Woodcock S.A., Gueye-Ndiaye A., Zhang E., Montano M., Siby T., Marlink R., NDoye I., Essex M.E., MBoup S. (1999). Human immunodeficiency virus type 1 subtypes differ in disease progession. *J Infect Dis.* 179:68–73.

Kaplan, J., Hanson, D., Karon, J., Cohn, D., Thompson, M., Buskin, S., Fleming, P., Dworkin, M. (2001). Late initiation of antiretroviral therapy (at CD4+ lymphocyte count <200cells/ml) is associated with increased risk of death. 8th Conference on Retroviruses and Opportunistic Infections; Feb 4–8. Chicago, IL. (abstract 520).

Lalezari, J., Drucker, J., Demasi, R., Hopkins, S., and Salgo, M. (2001). A controlled phase II trial assessing three doses of T-20 in combination with abacavir, amprenavir, low dose ritonavir and efavirenz in non-nucleoside naïve protease inhibitor experienced HIV-1 infected adults. 8th Conference on Retrovirus and Opportunistic Infections; Feb 4–8. Chicago, IL. (abstract LB5).

Ledergerber, B., Egger, M., Opravil, M., Telenti, A., Hirschel, B., Battegay, M., Vernazza, P., Sudre, P., Flepp, M., Furrer, H., Francioli, P., Weber, R. (1999). Clinical progression and virological failure on highly active antiretroviral therapy in HIV-1 patients: A prospective cohort study. Swiss HIV Cohort Study. *Lancet* 353:863–868.

Little, S.J., Holte, S., Routy, J.P., Daar, E.S., Markowitz, M., Collier, A.C., Koup, R.A., Mellors, J.W.,

Connick, E., Conway, B., Kilby, M., Wang, L., Whitcomb, J.M., Hellmann, N.S., Richman, D.D. (2002). Antiretroviral-drug resistance among patients recently infected with HIV. *N Engl J Med.* 347:385–394.

Lucas, G.M., Chaisson, R.E., and Moore, R.D. (1999). Highly active antiretroviral therapy in a large urban clinic: Risk factors for virologic failure and adverse drug reactions. *Ann Intern Med.* 131:81–87.

Lucas, G.M., Chaisson, R.E., and Moore, R.D. (2003). Survival in an urban HIV-1 clinic in the era of highly active antiretroviral therapy: A 5-year cohort study. *J Acquir Immune Defic Syndr.* 33:321–328.

Medina, D.J., Tsai, C.H., Hsiung, G.D., and Cheng, Y.C. (1994). Comparison of mitochondrial morphology, mitochondrial DNA content, and cell viability in cultured cells treated with three anti-human immunodeficiency virus dideoxynucleosides. *Antimicrob Agents Chemother.* 38:18248.

Morgan, D., Mahe, C., Mayanja, B., and Whitworth, J. (2002). Progression to symptomatic disease in people infected with HIV-1 in rural Uganda: prospective cohort study. *BMJ* 324:193–196.

Office of the Press Secretary. (2003). Fact Sheet: The President's Emergency Plan for AIDS Relief. Vol. 2003.

Opravil, M., Ledergerber, B., Furrer, H., Gallant, S., Hirschel, B., Meienberg, F., Wagels, T., Bernasconi, E., Rickenbach, M., Weber, R. and the Swiss HIV Cohort Study. (2001). Clinical benefit of early initiation of HAART in patients with asymptomatic HIV infection and CD4 counts >350/mm^3. 8th Conference on Retroviruses and Opportunistic Infections; Feb 4–8. Chicago, IL. (abstract LB6)

Palella, F.J., Delaney, K.M., Moorman, A.C., Loveless, M.O., Fuhrer, J., Satten, G.A., Aschman, D.J., and Holmberg, S.D. (1998). Declining morbidity and mortality among patients with advanced human immunodeficiency virus infection. The HIV Outpatient Study Investigators. *N Engl J Med.* 338:853–860.

Paterson, D.L., Swindells, S., Mohr, J., Brester, M., Vergis, E.N., Squier, C., Wagener, M.M., Singh, N. (2000). Adherence to protease inhibitor therapy and outcomes in patients with HIV infection. *Ann Intern Med.* 133:21–30.

Robbins, G.K., De Gruttola, V., Shafer, R.W., Smeaton, L.M., Snyder, S.W., Pettinelli, C., Dube, M.P., Fischl, M.A., Pollard, R.B., Delapenha, R., Gedeon, L., van der Horst, C., Murphy, R.L., Becker, M.I., D'Aquila, R.T., Vella, S., Merigan, T.C., Hirsch, M.S., and the AIDS Clinical Trials Group 384 Team. (2003). Comparison of sequential three-drug regimens as initial therapy for HIV-1 infection. *N Engl J Med.* 349:2293–2303.

Staszewski, S., Gallant, J.E., Pozniak A.L., Suleiman, J.M.A.H., DeJesus, E., Lu, B., Sayre, J., Cheng, A. (2003). Efficacy and safety of tenofovir DF (TDF) versus stavudine (d4T) when used in combination with lamivudine and efavirenz in antiretroviral naive patients: 96 week preliminary interim results. 10th Conference on Retroviruses and Opportunistic Infections; Feb. 10–14. Boston, MA. (abstract 564b)

Sterling, T.R., Chaisson, R.E., Bartlett, J.G., Moore, R.D. (2001). CD4+ lymphocyte level is better than HIV-1 plasma viral load in determining when to initiate HAART. 8th Conference on Retrovirus and Opportunistic Infections; Feb 4–8. Chicago, IL. (abstract 519).

Sundar, K., Suarez, M., Banogon, P.E., and Shapiro, J.M. (1997). Zidovudine-induced fatal lactic acidosis and hepatic failure in patients with acquired immunodeficiency syndrome: Report of two patients and review of the literature. *Crit Care Med.* 25:1425–1430.

Tanuri, A. (2003). Brazilian Network of HIV Drug Resistance Surveillance (HIV-BResNet): Results from the National survey done in 2001. Presented at Global HIV/AIDS Program of the World Bank Group. Provision of ARV Therapy in Resource Limited Settings: The Challenges of Drug Resistance and Adherence; June 17–18. Washington D.C.

Tavel, J.A., Miller, K.D., and Masur H. (1999). Guide to major clinical trials of antiretroviral therapy in human immunodeficiency virus-infected patients: Protease inhibitors, non-nucleoside reverse transcriptase inhibitors, and nucleotide reverse transcriptase inhibitors. *Clin Infect Dis.* 28:643–676.

Van Der Horst, C., Sanne, I., Wakeford C., Quinn, J. and Rousseau, F. (2001). Two Randomized, Controlled, Equivalence Trials of Emtricitibine (FTC) to Lamivudine (3TC). 8th Conference on Retroviruses and Opportunistic Infections; Feb 4–8. Chicago, IL. (abstract 18).

Wong, J.K., Hezareh, M., Gunthard, H.F., Havlir, D.V., Ignacio, C.C., Spina, C.A., Richman, D.D. (1997) Recovery of replication-competent HIV despite prolonged suppression of plasma viremia. *Science* 278:1291–1294.

World Health Organization. (2002). Scaling-up antiretroviral therapy in resource-limited settings. Geneva.

30

Pediatric AIDS in Asia

Prevention, Treatment, and Government Intervention

Kenneth McIntosh

Harvard Medical School, Harvard School of Public Health, Division of Infectious Diseases, Children's Hospital Boston, Boston, Massachusetts, USA

INTRODUCTION

Pediatric HIV infection is generally of two types; that which is acquired from the mother before, during, or shortly after birth (perinatal infection), and that which is acquired later during childhood. In the latter category are infections transmitted through blood transfusions or other introductions of contaminated material through the skin (e.g., injection drug use, ritual scarification), sexual abuse, and early risky sexual behavior. The last category belongs in the field of "pediatrics" when local definitions of the pediatric age group include sexually active teenagers. In most societies, adolescents, particularly girls in their teens, are one of the most vulnerable groups for sexual transmission of HIV. Whether or not they are considered "children," it is important to highlight this problem in an effort to find ways to prevent it.

Perinatal HIV infection, which is the leading cause of HIV infection in young children, occurs during maternal gestation, at the time of delivery, or through breastfeeding. In the absence of intervention, the rate of transmission in an unselected group of HIV-positive pregnant women is 30–40%, and it is widely accepted that about one quarter of this occurs *in utero* (mostly in the last trimester), one half in the process of birth, and one quarter during breast feeding (Dabis and Ekpini, 2002). The latter depends very much on the length of breastfeeding, since the monthly risk of transmission appears to be about equivalent throughout this time (Fawzi *et al.*, 2002a; Miotti *et al.*, 1999).

Perinatally acquired HIV infection has several features that are physiologically and clinically different from HIV infection in adults. The effects of HIV on the developing immune system, the developing nervous system, and developing systems in general is different from those on mature physiologic systems, with the result that clinical presentations may be different, and the natural history of the disease is different. Response to antiretroviral therapy, while similar, is also different, and there are important considerations of developmental pharmacology that impact on the response of children and adolescents to treatment.

The other important pediatric aspect of the world HIV epidemic is the larger effect of HIV infection in families on the health and welfare of children in general. This includes, most notably, the widespread problem of "AIDS-orphans," children who have lost one or both parents to AIDS, and who therefore depend for their care and education on their extended family, or on society in general. Other important issues are the effects of family AIDS stigma on children during their growth and development, and the economic impact of this chronic, gradually fatal illness on children.

All aspects of pediatric AIDS in Asia vary in relation to the society of the particular country where a child is born and raised. As will become clear in this short review of a large subject, the impact of the HIV/AIDS epidemic on children is not usually the first subject that comes to mind in the early stages of any country's epidemic. As a consequence, the amount of information about the incidence, epidemiology, clinical presentation, and response to treatment of pediatric HIV infection is highly variable, and often severely limited.

HIV PREVALENCE IN PREGNANT WOMEN IN ASIAN COUNTRIES

It can be expected, *a priori*, that as soon as any society's HIV epidemic moves into women of child-bearing age, perinatally infected children will appear. The most important determinant of the size of the perinatal epidemic is, therefore, the prevalence of HIV infection in pregnant women. Many countries have found that carefully planned, periodic sampling of women in antenatal clinics, either conducted anonymously or, with voluntary counseling, carried out to inform women of their HIV status, is one of the most useful indices of HIV infection in the population in general.

Data on the prevalence of HIV infection in pregnant women in Asia are not universally available. Figures 1–5 show regional prevalence in the most recent maps available on the web, in India, Myanmar, Thailand, Cambodia, and Vietnam.

There are several observations one can make from these data. First, there are certain important Asian countries that are not represented. Since the maps were made by the United States Bureau of the Census, this may reflect either the interest of the Bureau in certain countries, or simply the unavailability of data in certain countries. In some cases it is likely a reflection of the low population prevalence of HIV infection in countries such as Japan and Korea.

Also shown is a graph of HIV antibody prevalence over the past 12 years in pregnant women and military male conscripts in Thailand (Figure 6). It is of interest that the epidemic in young men reached a peak of about 3.5% in 1992 and 1993, and, with aggressive promotion of condom use, began to abate, reaching a plateau around 2% in 1995. The prevalence in pregnant women rose more slowly, but in about the same year, 1995, it reached a level very close to that in male conscripts. Since then, it has held steady in a narrow range, and is now the same as, or higher than, that in young men. It is widely thought that the epidemic in young men in the military was driven in its earlier stages by unprotected sexual contact with sex workers who, in turn, had a high prevalence secondary to spread from the injection drug-using population. The young men then spread infection to their wives. This pattern, played out in the late 1980s and early 1990s in Thailand, was subsequently seen in Cambodia and Myanmar, and is likely also to unfold in Vietnam and China if steps are not taken to stop it, since the essential elements are present in both countries [a population of injecting drug users (IDU) with, at least locally, a very high prevalence of HIV infection, a commercial sex trade that is largely underground and uncontrolled, and only partial compliance with

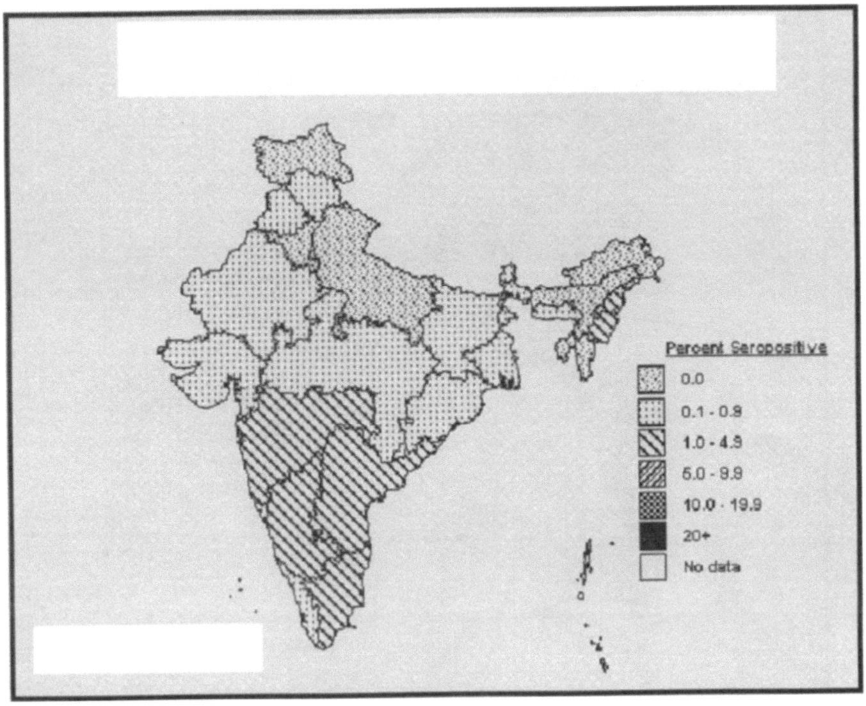

FIGURE 1. Seroprevalence of HIV-1 in pregnant women in India, 1999.
Source: United States Bureau of the Census, http://www.census.gov/ipc/aidsdb/.

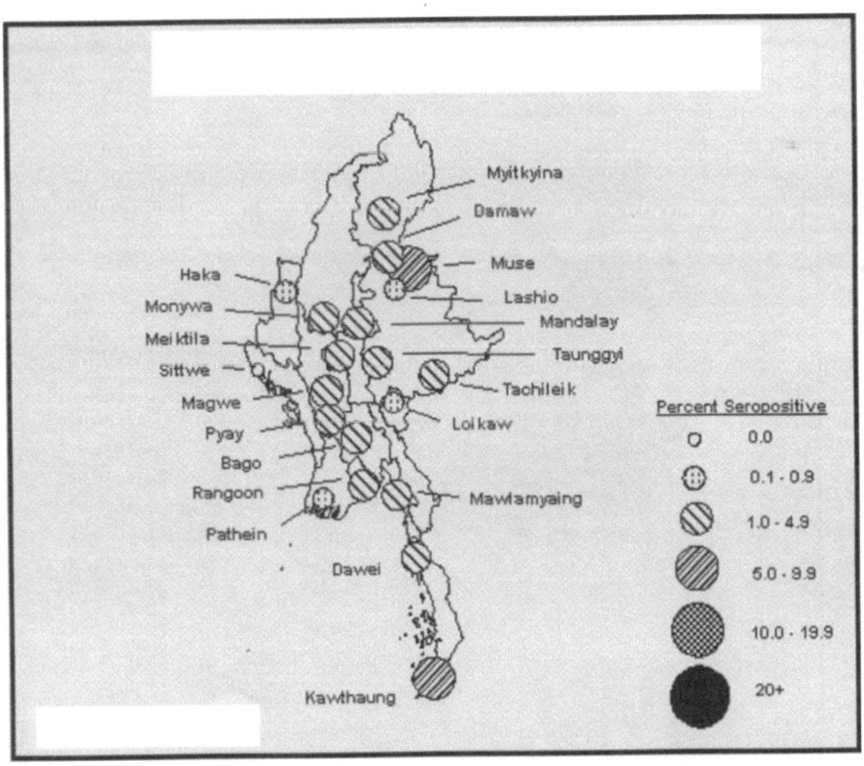

FIGURE 2. Seroprevalence of HIV-1 in pregnant women in Burma (Myanmar), 1999.
Source: United States Bureau of the Census, http://www.census.gov/ipc/aidsdb/.

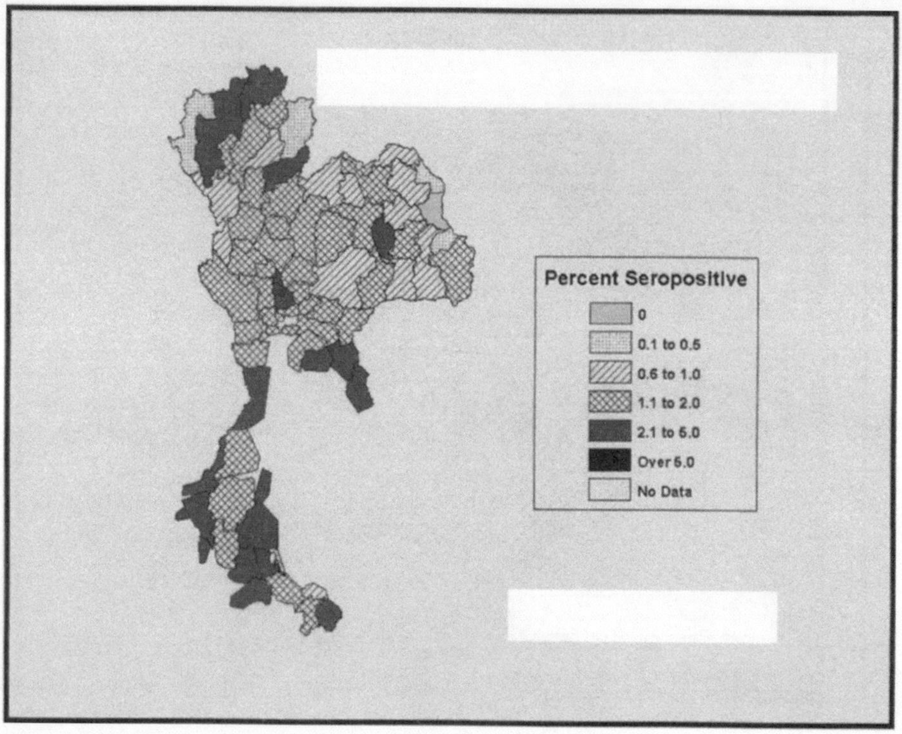

FIGURE 3. Seroprevalence of HIV-1 in pregnant women in Thailand, 2002.
Source: United States Bureau of the Census, http://www.census.gov/ipc/aidsdb/.

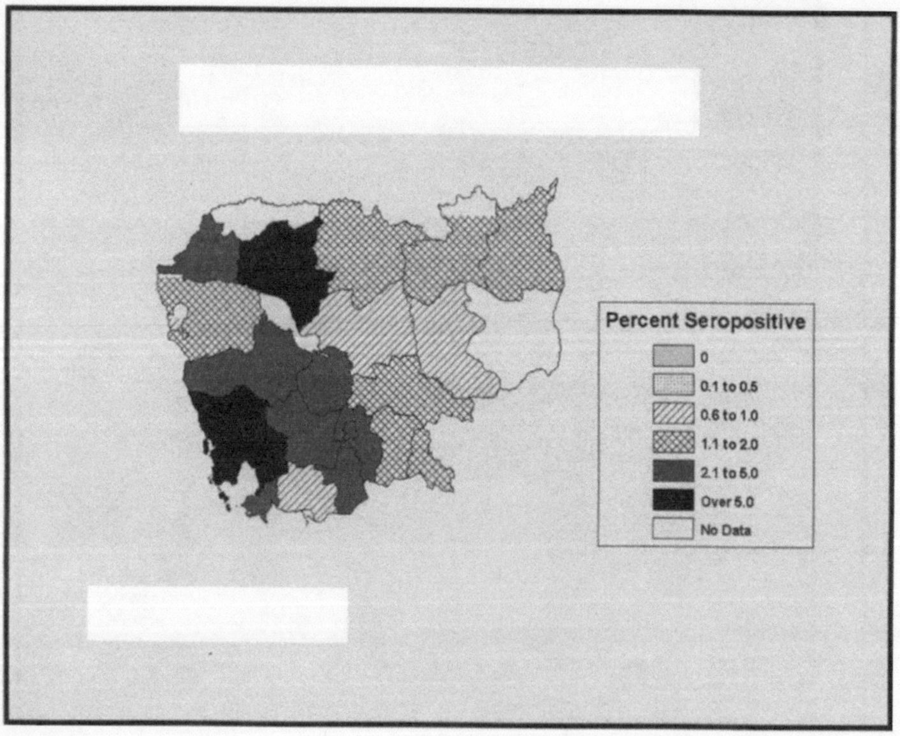

FIGURE 4. Seroprevalence of HIV-1 in pregnant women in Cambodia, 2000.
Source: United States Bureau of the Census, http://www.census.gov/ipc/aidsdb/.

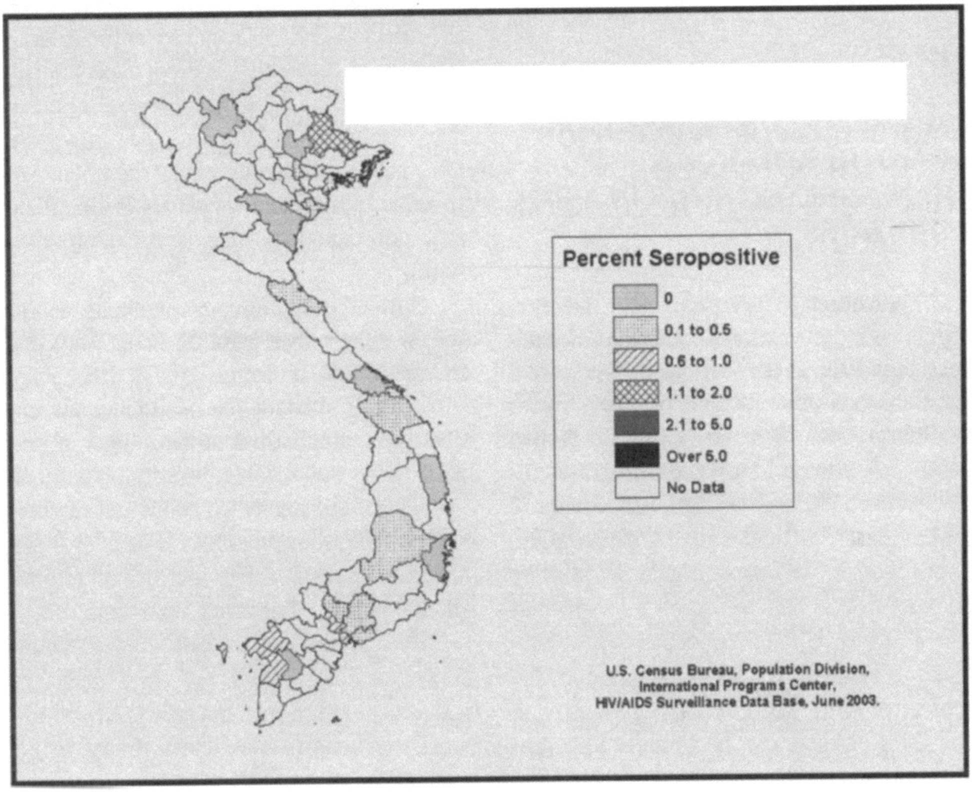

FIGURE 5. Seroprevalence of HIV-1 in pregnant women in Vietnam, 2001.

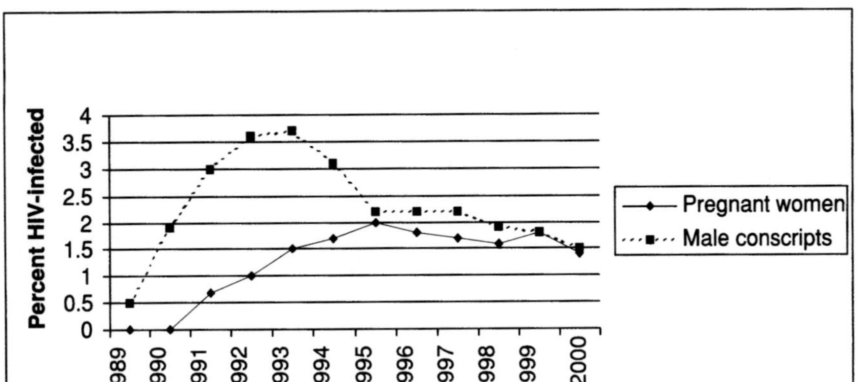

FIGURE 6. Seroprevalence of HIV-1 in sentinel populations of male military conscripts and pregnant women.

government programs urging universal condom use].

PROGRAMS FOR PREVENTION OF MOTHER-TO-INFANT TRANSMISSION OF HIV IN ASIAN COUNTRIES

Prevention of perinatal HIV infection begins with prevention of infection of child-bearing women in the first place. The second critical step is the institution of programs for voluntary counseling and testing of women during pregnancy. Many such programs include both men and women, and there are logical reasons to do this in a single program. Those women (or couples) who prove to be HIV-uninfected can be targeted for preventive messages. Uninfected women whose husbands or partners are HIV-infected can be the subject of particularly intensive counseling, and their partners can be brought into programs for care. Finally, women who are HIV-infected can be offered information and advice about their pregnancy, about breast feeding, and also about any programs available for prevention of vertical transmission.

A number of Asian countries have begun the complex process of counseling, serologic screening, and administration of antiretrovirals during pregnancy, at delivery, and in the newborn. In Thailand the process began in the mid 1990s, not long after the results of the PACTG 076 (Connor *et al.*, 1994) trial were published. Formula had been made available to the offspring of HIV-infected mothers even before this, as soon as it was becoming clear that breast-feeding was a significant route of transmission. Through funding from the Thai government, the Thai Red Cross, and a number of other sources, these programs were put in place so that, in a publication appearing in 2002 that covered one year in 2000–1, it was reported that 96.7% of more than half a million women received antenatal care, with 92.5% being counseled and tested. Of those found to be HIV-infected, 70.1% received antiretroviral treatment (zidovudine), using a short course regimen that emerged from several clinical trials conducted in Thailand (Amornwichet *et al.*, 2002). While this survey did not cover all births in Thailand (hospitals in Bangkok were not included), this is an impressive record.

Similar programs are regionally available in many other parts of Asia. With the emergence of data from HIVNET 012 (Guay *et al.*, 1999) to show that nevirapine administered as a single dose in the mother at onset of labor and a single dose in the baby at 2–3 days of age prevented about half of non-breastfeeding transmissions, in parts of India this drug has, as in Africa, become an important component of perinatal regimens.

Even in the areas where antiretrovirals are not available, there are ways that vertical transmission can be prevented. Nutritional deficiencies have been shown to be associated with HIV transmission from mother-to-infant, although this relationship is complex, and simple intervention, such as vitamin A supplementation, has not been successful in preventing transmission (Fawzi *et al.*, 2002b). General principles of antenatal health are particularly important in the presence of HIV infection, including treatment of any sexually transmitted diseases and optimization of nutrition (Dreyfuss and Fawzi, 2002). Finally, the process of delivery can be optimized to lessen transmission, with minimization of trauma to the mother or infant and avoidance of prolonged rupture of membranes.

It is clear that breastfeeding imposes a risk of HIV transmission, and equally clear that breastfeeding, particularly in areas where the water supply is unsafe, carries certain well accepted health benefits for the infant. These issues, as well as the availability or lack of availability of adequate formula, need to be discussed with the mother so she can make an informed choice about early feeding.

DIAGNOSIS OF PERINATAL HIV INFECTION IN CHILDREN

Because of the universal presence of transplacental antibody to HIV, the diagnosis of perinatally acquired HIV infection cannot be reliably made by serologic means until 18 months of age. Before that, tests that will detect the presence of virus in the blood are required. In reality this means either DNA or RNA polymerase chain reaction, or PCR (DNA being the preferred method for diagnosis), although it is likely that either acid- or heat-dissociated p24 antigen detection in serum or plasma would be a cheaper method that is marginally less sensitive (Schupbach, 2002). Diagnosis by clinical criteria is notoriously inaccurate, having both low sensitivity and low specificity (Chintu *et al.*, 1993).

Accurate and early diagnosis has many benefits both to the child and society. A reliable negative diagnosis (that is, a diagnosis of absence of HIV infection) relieves parental anxiety or, in orphanage situations, allows placement with the knowledge that the child should grow and develop normally. A reliable positive diagnosis (that is, a diagnosis of HIV infection) allows early institution of trimethoprim/sulfamethoxazole prophylaxis, preventing one of the most common serious or fatal infections in the first year of life. In societies where laboratories are equipped to enumerate CD4 cells, and where antiretroviral drugs are available, early diagnosis permits early institution of specific antiviral therapy, changing the entire natural history of pediatric HIV infection and converting the infection into a chronic disease with an unknown long term prognosis (Gortmaker *et al.*, 2001).

Thus, the availability of reliable, quality-assured, laboratory-based diagnosis, and, in particular, PCR is an important local consideration for pediatric HIV infection. Such diagnostic facilities are, in fact, available in certain areas of Asia—certain urban parts of Thailand, Phnom Penh, and larger academic facilities in many Asian countries, including India and China.

NATURAL HISTORY, MANAGEMENT, AND TREATMENT OF PERINATALLY ACQUIRED PEDIATRIC HIV INFECTION IN ASIA

Studies in the United States and Europe have shown that, in the absence of any intervention, the natural history of vertically transmitted HIV infection is most easily described by delineating two groups of infants, those with rapid progression of disease and those with slower progression (European Collaborative Study, 1994; Diaz *et al.*, 1998). The rapid progressors, about 20% of the whole, are more likely to be those infected *in utero*, but this is by no means exclusively the case. Rapid progressors have a rapid loss of immune competence, a drop in CD4 cells, and a series of clinical events, including poor growth, frequent infections, pneumonia due to *Pneumocystis jiroveci* (formerly *Pneumocystis carinii*), frequent and prolonged diarrhea, encephalopathy, and early death. The slower progressing group is heterogeneous, and resembles more closely a group of adults who acquire HIV infection horizontally. It includes children with lymphadenopathy and frequent infections, and children who do not progress until much later, coming to medical attention at the age of 9 or 10 years, or even later. Certain conditions are much more common in children than in adults: refractory thrush; recurrent, severe otitis media; recurrent or prolonged diarrhea; pneumococcal and other bacterial sepsis, including pneumonia; subacute parotitis; and a chronic, progressive, steroid-responsive pneumonia termed lymphocytic interstitial pneumonitis (LIP) that may be associated with infection by Epstein-Barr virus and that is seen only in children, usually between 18 months and 6 years of age.

In Asia there has been only one prospective, long-term study of perinatally infected infants and children followed from birth (Chearskul *et al.*, 2002). In this study, of 68 HIV-infected infants, 47 could be followed for clinical progression; 12 had what was described as rapid progression, approximately half of the rest had "intermediate" progression, and the remainder "slow" progression. Mortality was 31 of the total of 68 children, and many of those deaths were in the first year (12 of the total), and ascribed to "pneumonia" which may have been Pneumocystis pneumonia (PCP), undiagnosed, since PCP prophylaxis was not routinely administered. The most common AIDS-defining illness was recurrent serious bacterial infections (13 children), with wasting syndrome seen in eight children, encephalopathy in five, and PCP in four. Both wasting syndrome and encephalopathy had a particularly bad prognosis, as has been the case in the rest of the world. Interestingly, in this small, prospectively-followed cohort, tuberculosis was not seen, even though it is clear that tuberculosis in HIV-infected children is a growing problem in Thailand (Siriarayapon *et al.*, 2002). The authors felt that the study described a natural history with survival times shorter than those in the United States and Europe but longer than those in Africa. The clinical events described, although more frequent, were very similar to those described from Western cohorts.

Another study of the clinical manifestations of pediatric HIV infection emerges from a tertiary pediatric care center in Mumbai, India. This study, in contrast to the study from Bangkok, enumerates the findings in a referral population rather than in a cohort of infected children followed from birth (Merchant *et al.*, 2001). Thus, it is not a study of the "natural history" of perinatally acquired HIV infection, but rather a description of 285 children in whom the diagnosis was made, either serologically or (if less than 18 months of age) using serology plus WHO clinical criteria, after they were referred to an academic center. Nevertheless, this study presents very useful data. Most (87%) of the children were considered perinatally infected, whereas 12% had infection from blood or blood-product transfusion. The most frequently presenting finding was wasting syndrome (termed "protein energy malnutrition"), seen in 45%, and this was followed by tuberculosis, both pulmonary and extrapulmonary, seen in 29%.

Tuberculosis is difficult to diagnose in children under any circumstances. In the presence of HIV infection, it may be even more difficult, since infections of all types are so common, prolonged fevers are a frequent symptom, pneumonias of many types occur, and LIP, one of the most common syndromes, may be difficult to distinguish on clinical grounds from pulmonary tuberculosis. Moreover, children with advanced HIV infection, like adults, may be infected with non-tuberculous mycobacteria, and the overlap between these infections and systemic tuberculosis in HIV-infected children has not been well described. The management of tuberculosis in HIV-infected infants and children clearly represents one of the greatest challenges to both public health and the individual physician in Asia.

In both Thailand and India, dermatitis is very common in HIV-infected children. The etiologies are many, including candida, herpes simplex, herpes zoster, and an entity termed "pruritic papular eruption" which responds to topical steroids (Figure 7) (Wananukul and Thisyakorn, 1999). An opportunistic pathogen that is much more common in Southeast Asia than elsewhere in the world is *Penicillium marneffei* . This most commonly causes a generalized skin eruption with discrete, dome-shaped papules that are sometimes umbilicated (Figure 8) (Wananukul and Thisyakorn, 1999). As a generalized infection it can also cause localized or generalized lymphadenopathy, pneumonia, and other syndromes, including hemophagocytic syndrome (Chokephaibulkit *et al.*, 2001; Ukarapol *et al.*, 1998). The geographic distribution of this fungus extends from Thailand, to eastern India, Taiwan, Hong Kong, and southern China.

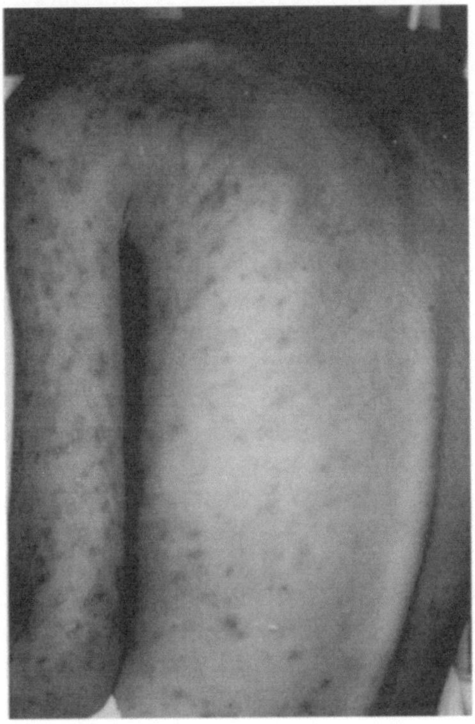

FIGURE 7. Pruritic papular eruption in a child in Thailand.
Source: Wananukul, S., and Thisyakorn, U. (1999). (Used with permission.)

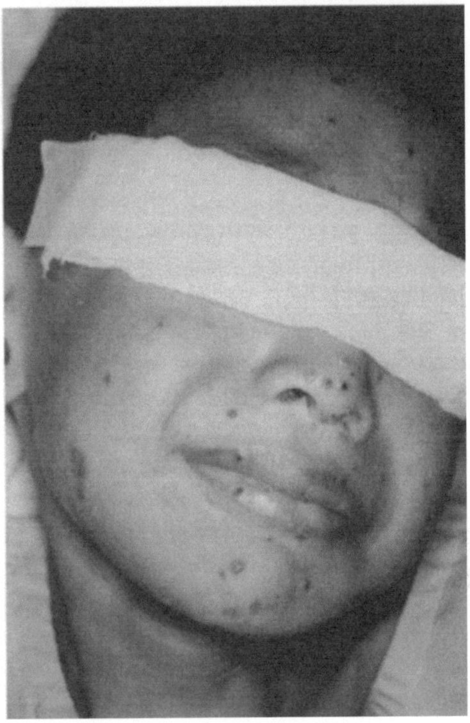

FIGURE 8. The rash of systemic *Penicillium marneffei* in a child in Thailand.
Source: Wananukul, S., and Thisyakorn, U. (1999). (Used with permission.)

Widespread use of trimethoprim/sulfamethoxazole (T/S) in HIV-positive infants is likely to change dramatically the natural history of pediatric HIV infection in Asia just as it did in the United States and Europe. While in present descriptions of the clinical findings in perinatally HIV-infected children PCP is not a common diagnosis, this was also the case early in the epidemic in Africa, and closer examination of the problem revealed that it was, in fact, extremely common (Ruffini and Madhi, 2002). The one study which examined the effect of T/S prophylaxis in infants in sub-Saharan Africa concluded that, while it did not appear to prevent *Pneumocystis jiroveci* infection, its use was associated with a significantly lower incidence of severe pneumonia and death (Madhi *et al.*, 2002). It seems likely that it will also be effective in Asia. Infections with *Haemophilus influenzae* type B, which are uncommon in the United States and Britain because of the general use of vaccine and its effect on carriage of the organism in the population, can be expected to be common, along with pneumococcal sepsis, pneumonia, and meningitis, in HIV-infected children in Asia.

Management of children with HIV infection is complex and involves both general and specialized pediatric care. General care includes particular attention to nutrition, prevention of common infections by immunization, and treatment of such infections when they occur. More specialized care includes prophylaxis to prevent opportunistic infections (OI), particularly PCP, and treatment of OI. It also involves decisions related to administration of antiretroviral drugs. Guidelines for management of children with HIV infection have been developed in a number of Asian countries. The guidelines in Thailand are in their Sixth Edition at this writing, and are frequently reviewed and updated (Ministry of Public Health Thailand, 2000). Guidelines in India emerged from the First National Conference on Pediatric HIV/AIDS in Delhi in late 2001 and have appeared on the web (http://www.pediatricskerala.com/html/hivguide.htm) under the sponsorship of the Indian Academy of Pediatrics. At this time, comprehensive pediatric guidelines have not appeared in other Asian countries.

The Thai guidelines recognize that laboratory diagnosis (or exclusion) of HIV infection in infancy is not always available, and T/S prophylaxis for *Pneumocystis jiroveci* in all offspring of HIV-positive women may not be practical. They list two options for primary prophylaxis in the first year of life: prophylaxis of all offspring until HIV infection is ruled out (similar to North American and European guidelines), and prophylaxis starting when suggestive symptoms or signs of HIV infection occur. Guidelines for older children are similar to those in adults and are based on (age-related) CD4 counts. In the web-based guidelines from India, primary Pneumocystis prophylaxis recommendations are similar to those of Europe and North America.

Guidelines for prevention and treatment of tuberculosis in HIV-infected children also have appeared both in Thailand and in India. Primary prophylaxis (isoniazid daily for 9–12 months) is indicated in situations of exposure to an infected adult, particularly a family member, as well as for a positive (>5 mm) PPD skin test. Treatment is similar to that of HIV-negative children, but there are warnings that it might have to be prolonged if response is delayed. Many countries have national tuberculosis programs with directly-observed therapy (DOT), and these programs clearly intersect with the treatment of HIV-exposed or -infected children. An additional important complication of the treatment of tuberculosis is the frequent and intense interaction of many anti-mycobacterial drugs with antiretroviral drugs, and the potential for synergistic toxicity. The latter pertains to both neurologic and hepatic toxicity. These problems are addressed briefly in the guidelines from the Indian Academy of Pediatrics, but are not addressed in the Thai guidelines. In fact, at the present time few children are receiving antiretroviral treatment, so the issue is moot, and, in addition, there is little information on solutions to this drug interaction problem in children.

As national programs are developed for the treatment of HIV-positive adults with antiretroviral drugs, it is inevitable that questions will arise about the treatment of HIV-infected children. Such treatment involves a number of very specific issues. First, pediatric formulations of antiretroviral drugs must be made available. This is not a trivial issue, since acceptable, tested formulations for children are not available in many parts of the world for many important antiretrovirals. Second, there is abundant experience to show that some formulations are more acceptable than others, on the basis of taste, volume to be consumed, and toxicity. Third, the dosage, frequency and pharmacokinetics of many antiretrovirals have not been worked out for children of all ages, and, more specifically, for children in Asian countries. Finally, despite many advances in the use of these drugs in children, there are still major questions that United States and Western European investigators have not answered concerning such basic issues as what are the best guidelines for beginning therapy in infants and children, how best to optimize therapy, and how to get children to take medicines rigorously and regularly.

ADOLESCENTS

No chapter on pediatric HIV infection would be complete without a section that recognizes the importance of adolescent HIV infections. In North American and European females, adolescents have the highest age-incidence of sexually transmitted infections (STI) of any age group and are therefore equivalently at risk for sexual transmission of HIV. The prevalence of HIV infection is known for adolescent populations in parts of Africa: in Kisumu, Kenya it is 8.3% in 15-year-old girls, rising to 29% by age 17; in boys of the same age it is much lower, rising only to 9% at 19 years of age (WHO, 2002). Similar population-based data are not available in Asia. However, a study of STI in a cohort of female sex workers in northern Thailand showed that 21% of 280 brothel workers began their commercial sex work when they were less than 15 years old. Beginning prostitution at this age was, in multivariate analysis, significantly associated with probability of being HIV-positive (Limpakarnjanarat *et al.*, 1999). Moreover, in India pediatric STI cases clearly begin to increase among children in the 10–14 year age group, demonstrating that this group, particularly street-children, is acutely vulnerable (Pandhi *et al.*, 2003).

Clearly, the prevalence of horizontally-transmitted HIV infection in older children of a community will depend on the particular cultural and behavioral practices, as well as accepted sexual norms, the activity of IDU, and the extent of the commercial sex industry and child prostitution. Also of importance in this equation are the educational measures that the community has put in place to inform children and young adults of HIV, its spread, and methods of prevention. At this writing, surveys among students in many Asian countries do not show a high level of knowledge about HIV/AIDS (Chatterjee *et al.*, 2001; Davis *et al.*, 1998; Ganguli *et al.*, 2002; Zheng *et al.*, 2002). Given the potential consequences of ignorance in this area, and the clear efficacy of the aggressive, open educational campaign in Thailand during the early 1990s, filling this information gap should be a top priority throughout the region.

ORPHANS

Estimates of the number of AIDS orphans in Asia can be obtained from the electronically available publication "Children on the Brink," updated in 2002 (TvTAssociates, The Synergy Project, 2002). It is estimated that in 2005 there will be 3 million "AIDS orphans" in Asia, most of them in Thailand, China, Cambodia, and Myanmar. The following table summarizes these estimates for those

TABLE 1. Orphan Estimates by Country

Country	Total No. of Children 0–14 years (1,000s)	Total Orphans as a % of All Children	Total No. of Orphans (1,000s)	Total No. of AIDS Orphans	AIDS Orphans as a % of All Orphans
Cambodia	6,160	8.2	508	105,000	20.7
China	287,706	4.7	13,386	206,000	1.5
India	342,054	7.4	25,159	2,086,000[a]	8.3[a]
Indonesia	63,868	6.3	4,029	37,000	0.9
Malaysia	7,857	4.1	325	23,000	7.2
Myanmar	15,635	8.3	1,303	101,000	7.7
Pakistan	65,417	7.4	4,861	53,000	1.1
Papua New Guinea	2,124	8.1	171	9,000	5.5
Thailand	16,787	6.5	1,094	380,000	34.8
Vietnam	24,376	5.6	1,367	47,000	3.4
Other	161,156	5.2	8,360	52,000	1.2
Total	993,140	6.2	61,563	3,099,000	5.0

Source: 2005 TvT Associates/The Synergy Project, 2002.
[a] Extrapolated from total figures given in the table.

countries where AIDS orphans are likely to represent a major numeric or proportional problem.

The projected total number of AIDS orphans in 2010 in this same report is 4,320,000 in the countries of Asia, with more than a doubling of numbers in China and Myanmar. AIDS orphans, at that point, will comprise 7.5% of all orphans.

This is clearly a crisis of enormous proportions. Depending very much on local conditions, the strength of extended families, school structures and community resources, and the commitment of governments, such a crisis has the capacity to disrupt societies and to extend the burden of the AIDS epidemic far into the future.

CONCLUSIONS

Pediatric HIV infections and AIDS are an extremely important piece of the wordwide epidemic, and one that often receives less attention than it deserves. It comprises both the infection of infants from their infected mothers during gestation, birth, and breastfeeding, and infections that occur later, including infections of young adolescents.

Adolescents are one of the most vulnerable and neglected populations in the worldwide HIV epidemic. The steps that need to be taken to protect these future adults are very clear: open education directed at prepubescent children about risks and how to avoid them; and vigorous and effective programs to prevent childhood drug abuse and prostitution.

The death of parents will leave many children without their usual and needed family support. This problem, which promises to grow to enormous size over the next decade, will tax all of the governments' and the societies' resources and extend the reach of the epidemic far beyond the burden of the disease itself.

The pattern of the pediatric HIV epidemic differs widely in the many nations and cultures of Asia. Nevertheless, early attention to all aspects of prevention, natural history, treatment, and care are essential to the health and welfare of children throughout the region.

REFERENCES

Amornwichet, P., Teeraratkul, A., Simonds, R.J., Naiwatanakul, T., Chantharojwong, N., Culnane, M., Tappero, J.W., and Kanshana, S. (2002). Preventing mother-to-child HIV transmission: the first year of Thailand's national program. *JAMA* 288:245–248.

Chatterjee, C., Baur, B., Ram, R., Dhar, G., Sandhukhan, S., and Dan, A. (2001). A study on awareness of AIDS among school students and teachers of higher secondary schools in north Calcutta. *Indian J Public Health* 45:27–30.

Chearskul, S., Chotpitayasunondh, T., Simonds, R.J., Wanprapar, N., Waranawat, N., Punpanich, W., Chokephaibulkit, K., Mock, P.A., Neeyapun, K., Jetsawang, B., Teeraratkul, A., Supapol, W., Mastro, T.D., and Shaffer, N. (2002). Survival, disease manifestations, and early predictors of disease progression among children with perinatal human immunodeficiency virus infection in Thailand. *Pediatrics* 110:e25.

Chintu, C., Malek, A., Nyumbu, M., Luo, C., Masona, J., DuPont, H.L., and Zumla, A. (1993). Case definitions for paediatric AIDS: The Zambian experience. *Int J STD AIDS* 4:83–85.

Chokephaibulkit, K., Veerakul, G., Vanprapar, N., Chaiprasert, A., Tanphaichitr, V., and Chearskul, S. (2001). Penicilliosis-associated hemophagocytic syndrome in a human immunodeficiency virus-infected child: The first case report in children. *J Med Assoc Thai.* 84, 426–429.

Connor, E.M., Sperling, R.S., Gelber, R., Kiselev, P., Scott, G., O'Sullivan, M.J., VanDyke, R., Bey, M., Shearer, W., Jacobson, R.L., Jimenez, E., O'Neill, E., Bazin, B., Delfraissy, J.F., Culnane, M., Coombs, R., Elkins, M., Moye, J., Stratton, P., and Balsley, J. for The Pediatric AIDS Clinical Trials Group Protocol 076 Study Group. (1994). Reduction of maternal-infant transmission of human immunodeficiency virus type 1 with zidovudine treatment. *N Engl J Med.* 331:1173–1180.

Dabis, F., and Ekpini, E.R. (2002). HIV-1/AIDS and maternal and child health in Africa. *Lancet* 359:2097–2104.

Davis, C., Noel, M.B., Chan, S.F., and Wing, L.S. (1998). Knowledge, attitudes and behaviours related to HIV and AIDS among Chinese adolescents in Hong Kong. *J Adolesc.* 21: 657–665.

Diaz, C., Hanson, C., Cooper, E.R., Read, J.S., Watson, J., Mendez, H.A., Pitt, J., Rich, K., Smeriglio, V., and

Lew, J.F. (1998). Disease progression in a cohort of infants with vertically acquired HIV infection observed from birth: The Women and Infants Transmission Study (WITS). *J Acquir Immune Defic Syndr Hum Retrovirol.* 18:221–228.

Dreyfuss, M.L., and Fawzi, W.W. (2002). Micronutrients and vertical transmission of HIV-1. *Am J Clin Nutr.* 75:959–970.

European Collaborative Study. (1994). Natural history of vertically acquired human immunodeficiency virus-1 infection. *Pediatrics* 94:815–819.

Fawzi, W., Msamanga, G., Spiegelman, D., Renjifo, B., Bang, H., Kapiga, S., Coley, J., Hertzmark, E., Essex, M., and Hunter, D. (2002a). Transmission of HIV-1 through breastfeeding among women in Dar es Salaam, Tanzania. *J Acquir Immune Defic Syndr.* 31:331–338.

Fawzi, W.W., Msamanga, G.I., Hunter, D., Renjifo, B., Antelman, G., Bang, H., Manji, K., Kapiga, S., Mwakagile, D., Essex, M., and Spiegelman, D. (2002b). Randomized trial of vitamin supplements in relation to transmission of HIV-1 through breastfeeding and early child mortality. *AIDS* 16:1935–1944.

Ganguli, S.K., Rekha, P.P., Gupte, N., and Charan, U.A. (2002). AIDS awareness among undergraduate students, Maharashtra. *Indian J Public Health* 46:8–12.

Gortmaker, S.L., Hughes, M., Cervia, J., Brady, M., Johnson, G.M., Seage, G.R., 3rd, Song, L.Y., Dankner, W.M., and Oleske, J.M. (2001). Effect of combination therapy including protease inhibitors on mortality among children and adolescents infected with HIV-1. *N Engl J Med.* 345:1522–1528.

Guay, L.A., Musoke, P., Fleming, T., Bagenda, D., Allen, M., Nakabiito, C., Sherman, J., Bakaki, P., Ducar, C., Deseyve, M., Emel, L., Mirochnick, M., Fowler, M.G., Mofenson, L., Miotti, P., Dransfield, K., Bray, D., Mmiro, F., and Jackson, J.B. (1999). Intrapartun and neonatal single-dose nevirapine compared with zidovudine for prevention of mother-to-child transmission of HIV-1 in Kampala, Uganda: HIVNET 012 randomised trial. *Lancet* 354:795–802.

Limpakarnjanarat, K., Mastro, T.D., Saisorn, S., Uthaivoravit, W., Kaewkungwal, J., Korattana, S., Young, N.L., Morse, S.A., Schmid, D.S., Weniger, B.G., and Nieburg, P. (1999). HIV-1 and other sexually transmitted infections in a cohort of female sex workers in Chiang Rai, Thailand. *Sex Transm Infect.* 75:30–35.

Madhi, S.A., Cutland, C., Ismail, K., O'Reilly, C., Mancha, A., and Klugman, K.P. (2002). Ineffectiveness of trimethoprim-sulfamethoxazole prophylaxis and the importance of bacterial and viral coinfections in African children with Pneumocystis carinii pneumonia. *Clin Infect Dis.* 35:1120–1126.

Merchant, R.H., Oswal, J.S., Bhagwat, R.V., and Karkare, J. (2001). Clinical profile of HIV infection. *Indian Pediatr.* 38:239–246.

Ministry of Public Health Thailand. (2000). National Guidelines for the Clinical Management of HIV Infection in Children and Adults. Ministry of Public Health, Bangkok.

Miotti, P.G., Taha, T.E., Kumwenda, N.I., Broadhead, R., Mtimavalye, L.A., Van der Hoeven, L., Chiphangwi, J.D., Liomba, G., and Biggar, R.J. (1999). HIV transmission through breastfeeding: A study in Malawi. *JAMA* 282:744–749.

Pandhi, D., Kumar, S., and Reddy, B.S. (2003). Sexually transmitted diseases in children. *J Dermatol.* 30:314–320.

Ruffini, D.D., and Madhi, S.A. (2002). The high burden of Pneumocystis carinii pneumonia in African HIV-1-infected children hospitalized for severe pneumonia. *AIDS* 16:105–112.

Schupbach, J. (2002). Measurement of HIV-1 p24 antigen by signal-amplification-boosted ELISA of heat-denatured plasma is a simple and inexpensive alternative to tests for viral RNA. *AIDS Rev.* 4: 83–92.

Siriarayapon, P., Yanai, H., Glynn, J.R., Yanpaisarn, S., and Uthaivoravit, W. (2002). The evolving epidemiology of HIV infection and tuberculosis in northern Thailand. *J Acquir Immune Defic Syndr.* 31: 80–89.

TvT Associates/ The Synergy Project. (2002). *Children on the Brink: A Joint Report on Orphan Estimates and Program Strategies.* UNAIDS (January 25, 2004); http://www.usaid.gov/pop_health/aids/Publications/docs/childrenbrink.pdf.

Ukarapol, N., Sirisanthana, V., and Wongsawasdi, L. (1998). *Penicillium marneffei* mesenteric lymphadenitis in human immunodeficiency virus-infected children. *J Med Assoc Thai.* 81:637–640.

Wananukul, S., and Thisyakorn, U. (1999). Mucocutaneous manifestations of HIV infection in 91 children born to HIV-seropositive women. *Pediatr Dermatol.* 16:359–363.

World Health Organization (WHO). (2002). HIV/AIDS in Sub-Saharan Africa, July 2002 (January 26, 2004); http://www.who.int/hiv/facts/en/SubSaharanAfrica.ppt.

Zheng, Y.H., Yi, L.X., and Yang, X. (2002). [Short-term effect evaluation of health education on the prevention of AIDS among university students in Changsha]. *Hunan Yi Ke Da Xue Xue Bao* 27:515–518.

31

Needs and Responses

Children Orphaned and Made Vulnerable by HIV/AIDS in the Mekong Subregion

Prudence Borthwick

UNICEF East Asia Pacific Regional Office, Bangkok, Thailand

INTRODUCTION

The plight of orphans has long been a theme of myths and folk narratives but it is only recently that orphans have become the subject of global advocacy, as AIDS removes a generation of parents across the world. The UN General Assembly Special Session (UNGASS) on HIV/AIDS in 2001 included this among commitments made by participating countries:

> "By 2003, develop and, 2005, implement national policies and strategies to build and strengthen governmental, family and community capacities to provide a supportive environment for orphans and girls and boys infected and affected by HIV/AIDS, including by providing appropriate counselling and psychosocial support, ensuring their enrollment in school and access to shelter, good nutrition and health and social services on an equal basis with other children; and protect orphans and vulnerable children from all forms of abuse, violence, exploitation, discrimination, trafficking and loss of inheritance" (UNAIDS, 2002).

As we draw close to the half way mark in the time frame for realizing UNGASS goals, countries around the world are beginning to take stock of their responses. How successful are we at providing the essentials orphaned children need to survive and develop: health care, education, protection from abuse and exploitation, a family, friends, and neighbors?

This paper looks at needs of and responses to children orphaned and made vulnerable by AIDS in the Mekong sub region. ("Orphans" in this paper, unless otherwise stated, refers to children who have lost mother, father, or both parents.)

The countries of the Mekong sub region are, in a sense, representative of the range of HIV/AIDS scenarios for countries in East Asia and the Pacific: three are high prevalence: Thailand, Myanmar, and Cambodia; two have large populations: China and Vietnam; and one is small and highly vulnerable: Lao People's Democratic Republic (Lao PDR).

Thailand has the most mature HIV/AIDS epidemic in the region. This is often described in terms of 'waves' of transmission. Sex workers, homosexually active men, and injecting drug users are considered the first wave; then male clients of sex workers and fellow injectors, and finally their non sex-worker partners. This is a pattern common in varying degrees throughout the region. Children were the last 'wave' of infections to emerge in any number (The World Bank, 2000).

Epidemiologists talk of waves of transmission, but there have also been waves of care: the small numbers of young women, homosexual men, and injecting drug users that became ill in the first wave; the much larger numbers of male clients of sex workers who succeeded them and filled hospital beds in northern provinces in the mid to late 1990s; and the wave that is still breaking in antenatal clinics throughout the country—the women who settled down with these men and had their children.

In 2000, the percentage of HIV-positive women in urban areas who tested pregnant was estimated at 1.6% in Thailand, 2.8% in Cambodia (UNAIDS, 2002), and between 2% and 2.5% in Myanmar (Myanmar National AIDS Programme, 2000). By now a proportion of these women will have transmitted HIV to their infants, although as prevention of mother-to-child transmission programs expand, the number of new infections in children will drop. In 2001, 38,753 children in the Mekong sub region were estimated to be living with HIV. These figures were compiled before the full gravity of China's blood contamination disaster emerged. The estimates of HIV-positive and HIV-affected children are likely to soar once the number of adults infected in the five worst hit provinces can be ascertained.

As with transmission, the last care wave to emerge is that of children orphaned by AIDS. Thailand's first children's homes and services set up to care specifically for children orphaned and affected by AIDS were established in the early nineties. By 2001 an estimated 289,000 children had lost at least one parent to AIDS (UNICEF, 2002a). By the late nineties Cambodian children's services were seeing the trickle of children orphaned and affected by AIDS turn into a stream, with an estimated one tenth of the total number of orphans losing mothers or fathers or both to AIDS by 2001 (UNICEF, 2002a).

Advances in access to antiretroviral therapy are bringing hope to affected families across the sub region. Yet it seems clear that the time lag in establishing services to procure and deliver the drugs to people with AIDS means children will continue to be orphaned by AIDS for some time, adding to the numbers already orphaned by AIDS over the past decade.

IMPACT ON CHILDREN

The impact on a child of losing one or both parents to AIDS has been well documented in African studies: impoverishment, loss of educational opportunities, deprivation, poor access to health services, increased risk of abuse, neglect and exploitation, depression, anxiety, stress, low self esteem, loss of inheritance, and discrimination. In the Mekong region less research has been done in this area but studies and experience suggest that children orphaned by AIDS face similar problems.

Economic Impact

AIDS means families spend more—on care and treatment for the ill family member and on their funeral—and receive less, losing the income of those caring for the sick and of the sick person themselves. A recent study of impact on adult parents of AIDS patients in two provinces in Thailand found that the combined costs of care, treatment, and funerals averaged 2.3 times and 1.8 times the average per capita income respectively. Poorer families spent less as a result of the illness, but more of them found the costs a serious burden. The main way families raised money was by borrowing money (two-fifths of cases) and selling possessions or property (one fifth of cases). Poorer families were more likely to sell possessions than rich and more likely to borrow, but they borrowed smaller sums. Government health insurance helped cover costs of medical treatment in about three fifths of cases (Knodel, 2002). The situation for HIV-affected families is somewhat worse in neighboring countries with a much lower per capita income and far fewer government services. In Cambodia, government sector health services are used in a minority of the cases of serious illness and around a tenth of all cases go completely untreated (Royal Government of Cambodia, 1999). Where government health services are used, the cost of transport must be factored in, as fewer services mean people have to travel greater distances. In Cambodia and Lao PDR, families may borrow rice from neighbors and/or money from moneylenders (KHANA, 2000). In Vietnam, affected families reported that their greatest problems were economic (UNICEF, 2003a). In Lao PDR, affected families were concerned with loss of earning ability, children's education and well being, and lack of access to medicine for themselves and their children. Access to medical care was the greatest priority for people with HIV/AIDS (UNICEF, 2003b). In China, HIV-affected families felt their economic situation was poorer than other non-affected families, and that family income decreased as workers had to stay home 4–8 days a month to take care of patients. Some families had to sell their land illegally or rent it out at a reduced price. Disposable family incomes were found to decrease by the equivalent of two years annual average income (Ionita *et al.*, 2002).

Emotional Impact

AIDS starts to have an impact on families long before the person with AIDS dies. As the first telling symptoms appear, family stress levels rise all around. Parents who are sick and worried may begin to fight with spouses and children. A Cambodian appraisal noted an increase in domestic violence and marital problems in families affected by HIV/AIDS (KHANA, 2000). In Thailand, between one third and one quarter of divorced HIV-affected couples were said to have broken up due to the illness (Knodel *et al.*, 2002).

Some research is emerging to suggest that at least educationally, children do better in school after they become orphaned, and that going to school and doing well at school is linked to children's happiness (Gilborn *et al.*, 2001). This could mean that for many children, the period of the parent's final illness may be worse than the period afterwards, when the nerve-wracking progression of the disease is finally resolved. Home care is now widely recognized as an effective way of reaching and assisting children in this difficult period.

After parents die, loss and grief set in. Children of different ages respond to loss in different ways. In the West, research indicates that children as young as 4 months old experience distress and loss at being separated from their mothers. Indeed, children from 4–6 months to 2–3 years are said to suffer the greatest distress when separated from their mothers and to experience the worst long-term developmental effects (Tolfree, 1995). In Mekong societies where grandparents and siblings can play an important part in parenting, the effects of maternal deprivation may not be quite so great. It is likely, however, that even very young children experience loss and deprivation upon the death of a parent. This contrasts with a common and often voiced perception of adults in the region that children under about age ten or eleven are too young to understand what is going on (KHANA, 2000).

Caring for Sick Parents

Children are faced with seeing the people they love and depend on ground down by the illness emotionally and physically. Physical symptoms can be frightening for younger children and the chores of caring for the sick can be burdensome for older ones.

In the Mekong region, it is customary for hospital nursing care to be provided by relatives. Doctors and nurses perform clinical care, providing medications, injections, and dressings. Relatives provide all other physical care. Where the sick have access to hospitals, older children may be deputized to sleep under their parents' hospital bed and, feed, toilet, and wash them. In some cases, children sleep under the hospital bed at night and go to school in the morning. In other cases they skip school or leave school to care for the parent. If the patient is at home, children may also be involved in care and may have to do the household tasks that the sick person would have done as well as their own.

Schooling

Children's schooling is generally affected by the disruption that occurs during parental illness and death, as well as by the subsequent impoverishment many families face. A teacher in the worst hit areas in Thailand tells of primary school children being distracted and inattentive in class around the time of a parent's death, and withdrawn and depressed afterwards (Ratri Lamnuan, Teacher, Hua Rin School, personal communication, November 2003). In 2000, Cambodian home care teams found that of their patients' children, 21% had to start working since their parent's illness, 30% were providing care, 40% had to go without things they needed and formerly had, 40% had to leave school, and 28% had to leave home (KHANA, 2000).

Discrimination can also affect a child's performance at school. Both HIV-positive and negative children of HIV-positive parents report name-calling and teasing at school in Thailand. Some children at the Camillian Centre in Rayong refused to go to school because they felt schoolmates "hated" them (Lakhonphon and Frederix, 2003). In the education arena, HIV-positive children experience both discrimination, if their status is known or if they are symptomatic; and disadvantage, on the basis of the impact of illness on their schooling. In some cases, adult caregivers remove children from school because they are always getting sick. This then makes it hard for children to catch up after long spells away from school.

Where school attendance is already low for a variety of reasons, as in Cambodia, the non-attendance of children affected by HIV/AIDS may not be remarkable. Poor attendance and performance and high dropout rates may be caused by other traumatic events, and they affect other vulnerable children.

Exploitation and Deprivation

The "Cinderella" syndrome—a situation in which children living with relatives or step parents are treated differently than the family's biological children and given more chores and fewer opportunities—is prevalent in the folk tales of the region, such as "Pla-Bu-Thong," a tale of a girl mistreated by a step parent. However, research findings in this regard vary. In Lao PDR, children living with only their mothers (due to either divorce or to the death of their fathers) had the heaviest workload, while double orphans had the same workload as other children (UNICEF, 2003b). In Cambodia, 39.3% of vulnerable adolescents reported being treated differently (commonly neglect, avoidance, and verbal and physical abuse) with 12.5% saying they were made to do more chores, 12.9% being underfed, and 6.9% not allowed to go to school. Only 1.4% reported being sexually abused. The number of HIV-affected children reporting being treated differently was higher than other vulnerable children but not significant at 43.1% as compared to 31.7% (O'Connell, 2003).

Abuse

Orphans lack the social protection that a parent provides. Evidence that orphans are vulnerable to abuse comes from a number of sources. In North America, studies have shown that foster parents are more than twice as likely to abuse children as biological parents (Tolfree, 1995).

A qualitative study on sexually abused and sexually exploited children in the Mekong, found that half the girls in the study came from single-parent families or were orphaned. In the case of 34 sexually abused children, uncles and stepfathers were the most frequent abusers followed by biological fathers and cousins. Of community members, neighbors were the most frequent abusers. Family break down was found to be common, and most children were in single-parent households and not closely supervised. Poverty contributed to vulnerability as parents worked long hours and left children in the care of adults who neglected or abused them. Cramped living quarters where adults shared rooms with children were also a factor. In three cases an unsafe school environment was a factor in the abuse (United Nations Economic and Social Commission for Asia and the Pacific, 2000). The study also found that sexual abuse was a contributing factor to girls' entry into the sex industry. Of 11 sexually abused children, eight entered the sex industry of their own accord (United Nations Economic and Social Commission for Asia and the Pacific, 2000).

A study of young Lao PDR sex workers revealed that 47% of the girls had a problem with their families, and of these, 18% reported domestic violence. Five of the girls reported sexual abuse and three had been abused by their step-fathers. The report noted that as the question on sexual abuse was often not answered, and researchers had been instructed not to persist with questions that made the girls uncomfortable, the percentage of girls experiencing sexual abuse could be higher (Ministry of Labour and Social Welfare/UNICEF Laos, 2001). Discomfort with the question or interview format may have affected responses to the Cambodian study cited above where only 1.4% of children reported experiencing sexual abuse.

Of course, children orphaned from other causes and children who are vulnerable for other reasons also face many of the economic and psychosocial problems noted above. A recent study in Cambodia found that matched groups of children affected by HIV/AIDS, including single and double orphans; and children not affected by AIDS, including orphans from other causes and other neglected, abused, or abandoned children, had similarly high levels of stress and anxiety and a similarly poor quality of life. In northern Thailand, participatory research in three villages found common ground among elderly people caring for children and youth from "problem-plagued" families (those affected by drugs, HIV/AIDS, and labor migration) (Duangsa *et al.*, 2000).

Workers in the field generally agree that the needs of children affected by HIV/AIDS must be considered on a case-by-case basis, as not all children affected by HIV/AIDS are vulnerable, and there is no point in seeking to somehow privilege suffering caused by AIDS over suffering caused by domestic violence, incest or, other family problems. Still, the double disadvantage of personal loss and economic deprivation that AIDS commonly confers, tilts children affected by the virus towards the bottom-most tier of disadvantage in society.

Discrimination on the Basis of HIV and AIDS

Children orphaned by AIDS are often said to be additionally disadvantaged by discrimination. In Vietnam and Lao PDR, focus groups found discrimination was a major issue of concern for people caring for children orphaned by AIDS and for service providers (UNICEF, 2003a; UNICEF, 2003b). Intense discrimination is often manifest at the earlier stage of the epidemic when fear and ignorance influence people's behavior. Many communities experience "boycotts" of funerals of people who die of AIDS. Health workers are generally the first to have to deal with HIV as people come for treatment and testing. Hence, hospitals are often the first location in which HIV-positive people face discrimination. In an environment in which numbers of HIV-positive people are increasing, health workers and community members embark on a steep learning curve. There is evidence that the situation improves over time. In northern Thailand, by the late 1990s, only about a quarter to a fifth of HIV-affected families reported a perception of rejection by the community. Less than 10% of these families felt that attendance at the funeral of HIV-positive family members was affected, and over half reported heath workers had been helpful (Knodel *et al.*, 2002).

In settings where there has been less exposure to HIV-positive people, like schools and urban communities in central Thailand, ignorance and fear persists and must be overcome. In Rayong, in central Thailand, HIV-positive children at the Camillian Social Centre (a hospice and children's home) experienced a number of forms of discrimination. These included being expelled from a school on the basis of parental HIV status, being excluded from school when their own status was known, being asked to get treatment before coming back to school, being asked to stay home until sores healed, and being called names such as "AIDS kid" by schoolmates. One girl was regularly addressed as "Miss AIDS" by her teacher, and some parents would not allow their children to play with the HIV-positive children (Lakhonphon and Frederix, 2003). In Rayong, the situation has improved over time, assisted by the effect of antiretroviral medications on the children's dermatological problems. Fourteen of the 30 children in the Camillian Social Centre were attending government schools in 2003 (Giovanni Contarin, personal communication, 2003). The Centre for AIDS Rights has documented similar instances of discrimination in schools or daycare centers in all regions of Thailand (Centre for AIDS Rights, 2003).

A large participatory research project involving 440 affected families in the northeast part of Thailand presented a slightly more optimistic picture. Despite the fact that the majority of parents had disclosed their children's HIV status, children generally appeared to be discriminated against only because they were symptomatic or thought to be symptomatic (Committee of the NGO AIDS Esan, 2003). In northern Thailand, children orphaned by AIDS were found to have a high rate of school attendance. Discrimination appeared to be a problem in two cases out of over one hundred. In these two cases, the school did not allow children to attend classes (Knodel *et al.*, 2002).

In Vietnam and China, affected and HIV-positive children have experienced problems in school (UNICEF, 2003b; Ionita *et al.*, 2003). In Lao PDR, discrimination was not identified as a problem specifically in schools, although ridicule of children by their peers, and community discrimination against adult family members was an issue (UNICEF, 2003b). Generally, community members and service providers appear to discriminate less as they learn more about HIV/AIDS. Given the pain and sadness discrimination causes for individuals, action to accelerate community understanding and acceptance must continue to be a priority.

Discrimination against Orphans and the Poor

Discrimination was the greatest predictor for stress and anxiety in a recent Cambodian study (O'Connell, 2003). However, the study also found that non HIV-affected children also experienced discrimination on the basis of being orphaned or poor. This is not surprising when we consider the social hierarchies based on relative wealth and poverty present in most societies, hierarchies that are frequently mirrored on the school playground, in the village square, and even, in places of worship.

In some cultures, orphans are implicated in the death of their parent through traditional beliefs. For example, in Nepal, orphans are called "mother-eaters" and widows are called "husband-eaters" (UNICEF, 2002b). While

TABLE 1. AIDS Orphan Estimates in Mekong Subregion, 2001[a]

Country	Total number of orphans (1,000s)	Total number of orphans due to AIDS (Absolute #)	Orphans due to AIDS as a percentage of total orphans %
Cambodia	478	52,000	10.9
China	14,827	76,000	0.5
Lao People's Dem. Rep	85	700	0.8
Myanmar	1,349	40,000	3.0
Thailand	1,048	289,000	27.6
Vietnam	124	22,000	17.7
Total	17,911	479,700	2.7

[a] *Source:* Children on the Brink, UNICEF 2002, with the exception of Lao PDR where figures for total number of orphans were taken from UNICEF MICS Survey 2000 and Viet Nam, where the official government estimate of total numbers of orphans is used. Total number of orphans is made up of the sum of maternal orphans and paternal orphans minus double orphans who will already have been counted in the previous categories. Government estimates of numbers of orphans tend to be somewhat lower than the "Children on the Brink" estimates. This is the case in China.

there is no such belief in the Mekong region, the Buddhist doctrine of Karma can suggest that negative life events are karmic consequences of wrongs committed in a previous life. The belief that orphans are destined to be "unlucky" may influence community expectations of the child, or indeed, the child's own expectations. This is suggested by qualitative interviews with children orphaned by AIDS in Cambodia, which included fatalistic comments like: "I have a bad fortune," and "I am not angry or disappointed at this [bad treatment] because I think I am a poor orphaned child" (O'Connell, 2003).

Inheritance

In Cambodia, focus groups told of bitter disputes over inheritance that had resulted in orphans forfeiting their rights to property. Despite a tradition of family inheritance, it was not uncommon for uncles and other relatives to contest inheritances (KHANA, 2000). Many countries have legislation acknowledging children's right to inherit, but the laws are not always enforced.

EXISTING RESPONSES

Currently, the Mekong region is preparing for increasing numbers of children orphaned by AIDS or living with a parent who is HIV-positive. With the increase in access to antiretrovirals, hopefully the numbers of orphans in Thailand have peaked, but the numbers continue to build in neighboring countries.

Experience from other parts of the world, such as sub Saharan Africa and countries which have had to learn a great deal about orphans, indicates that existing responses fall mainly into two categories. First, there is the government response that is usually in the form of direct care for a tiny percentage of children who cannot support themselves, have no income, and have no one to care for them. Second, there is the much-touted "social safety net" of extended family and community that cares for the vast majority of orphaned children. Many governments are now looking anew at their provisions for destitute children and at ways to extend and strengthen the social safety net, lest it collapse under the steadily increasing weight of numbers of children orphaned due to AIDS.

Children with HIV and AIDS

About 40,000 children are estimated to be living with HIV/AIDS in the sub region (UNAIDS, 2002). However, over half are living in one country, Thailand. In the Mekong sub region, as elsewhere, children

TABLE 2. Estimated Numbers of HIV-positive Children by Country

Country	Estimated number of Children (01–14) living with HIV/AIDS, end 2001
Cambodia	12,000
China	2,000
Lao PDR	<100
Myanmar	5,000
Thailand	21,000
Viet Nam	3,753
Total	38,753

Source: UNAIDS 2002

with HIV are initially the locus of government attention in relation to children affected by HIV/AIDS.

HIV-Positive Children Abandoned in the Hospital

In an environment where little is known about HIV, babies born to HIV-positive parents are assumed to be invariably HIV-positive themselves. This widespread misunderstanding is fall out from the "three modes of transmission" message. People remember only that vertical transmission is one of the three modes of transmission. They do not remember that only a third of HIV-positive women will go on to have HIV-positive children. Mothers abandon children to hospitals thinking the hospitals will be better able to care for their infants. In Thailand, a study of large government hospitals over the early years of the epidemic (from 1990–92), found that children of HIV-positive mothers were 5.4 times more likely to be abandoned (*Kong Rok Ed*, 1999). In Cambodia, increasing numbers of HIV-positive children have been left in the care of governmental and non-governmental children's homes, and some have been abandoned in hospitals (KHANA, 2000). Fifty HIV-positive newborns were abandoned in Tu Du hospital in Ho Chi Minh City in 2000, and in Hai Phong city, 47 babies had been abandoned by HIV-positive mothers by 2001 (Chung, 2001).

Residential Care for HIV-Positive Children

In Vietnam and Thailand, one response to HIV-infected children has been the development of specialized orphanages that care for HIV-positive children and children with AIDS. In Thailand, four out of 20 government orphanages have been designated for the care of HIV-positive children. Additionally, a number of private orphanages have been established specifically for HIV-positive children throughout the country.

The *Tam Binh* Centre was established in Vietnam in November 2002 to care for HIV-positive children. By July 2003, there have been 76 HIV-positive children at the center, of whom 12 had died. Eight children sero-converted and were moved from the center. There are now 56 HIV-positive children (28 boys and 28 girls) resident at the center in the following age groups: 0–18 months: 33; 19 months–5 years: 12; and 6–7 years: 11. Since September 2003, the center has had its own school class, and six children are now attending grade one. The center is also supporting three children that are cared for in the community (Van Trung, 2003). Lao PDR is one of the few countries that does not provide institutional care for HIV-positive children, as the only children's homes are the SOS children's villages, and these do not accept HIV-positive children at present (UNICEF, 2003b). In China, the Ministry of Social Welfare has not reported any HIV-positive children in Welfare Institutions as yet, and there are no facilities especially for HIV-positive children.

In Cambodia, children with chronic diseases (including HIV/AIDS) are accepted by 39 government and non-government residential centers throughout the country. Twenty-three residential centers (including five government orphanages) have segregated facilities for children with chronic disease. Children are chosen for these segregated facilities based on their need for special care and fear of contamination (Dybdal *et al.*, 2001).

Alternative Care for HIV-Positive Children

National governments are at different stages in the process of developing alternative care options such as adoption, foster care, and group homes. However, these alternative forms of care are currently less likely to be available to HIV-infected children. Overseas adoption generally excludes HIV-positive children. To date, few HIV-positive children have been fostered or adopted locally in Mekong countries. In Thailand, the Holt Sahathai Foundation began to offer foster home care to children born to HIV-positive mothers in 1999. By 2002, 19 children had been fostered under this program. Of the 19 children, only two were confirmed to be HIV-positive; one died before his first birthday and the other remained in foster care. The remaining 17 children sero-converted and were then put up for adoption (Holt Sahathai Foundation, 2002).

Community Care for HIV-Positive Children

As with other categories of orphaned children, the great majority of HIV-positive children are cared for by their extended families in communities. There is little data available about how these children are faring in countries other than Thailand. Lao PDR caregivers reported concern with lack of treatment for opportunistic infections and antiretrovirals (UNICEF, 2003b). In Cambodia, non-governmental organization (NGO) workers and government staff working with HIV-positive children felt they were less likely to be loved or benefit from education because they would die young. Hospital workers advised that caregivers need training and support so that they don't abandon children in hospitals (KHANA, 2000). Respondents on this issue may have been biased by their work experience in which they are more likely to see cases in which children are neglected than those in which they are cared for and loved.

A study by the NGO network in northeastern Thailand of 440 affected families found that children were usually living with a surviving parent on their parcel of land. Parents generally earned between 600 and 10,000 baht (US $15–250) per month. Mothers worked as rice planters and wage laborers, and fathers worked as laborers, farmers, seafarers, and army rangers or had done so before their deaths. The majority of children in the study who were HIV-positive were between zero and seven years old and were not symptomatic. They were studying in primary grade one or two and had the usual relationship with their peers at school despite the fact that the majority of parents had disclosed their own HIV status in the community. The children who were forced to leave school due to teasing had noticeable physical symptoms of opportunistic infections such as frequent coughing, sores, or spots. A number of HIV-positive children were receiving antiretroviral treatment. Those who were symptomatic had *Pneumocystis carinii* pneumonia, oral thrush, and wasting (Committee of the NGO AIDS Esan, 2003).

The problems most children (HIV-positive and negative) experienced were difficulties in meeting educational expenses such as the cost of uniforms, books and notebooks, shoes, physical education clothes, uniforms, and daily expenses. Other problems appeared to be more specific to HIV-positive children, including being unable to attend a school, having no money for transportation to the doctor, contracting opportunistic infections, and having no appetite. The children's career expectations were similar to those of other children; most wanted a higher education to become a doctor, nurse, teacher, soldier, or police officer, and to earn income to support their families (Committee of the NGO AIDS Esan, 2003).

Sometimes HIV-positive children in communities are not given access to treatment, as relatives do not want them to suffer unnecessarily and are convinced the children will die anyway (KHANA, 2000). This has been identified as a problem in Thailand as well, particularly in relation to children experiencing side effects from antiretroviral drugs. Dr. David Wilson, of Medecins Sans Frontieres (MSF) in Thailand, has identified denial of treatment as one of two forms of discrimination faced by HIV-positive children. The other form is lack of opportunity to attend school. Wilson has characterized relatives' responses as "Why should the child be treated because they will die anyway?" and, "Why should the child go to school when they won't live to adulthood?" MSF has developed a program of activities, games, and resources designed to address these issues. They inform caregivers and get them to take responsibility for ensuring the child is treated and adheres to his/her treatment regime. They also involve the child, so that he/she too is motivated and supported to take the prescribed medicine (Wilson, 2003).

Children Affected by HIV/AIDS

This category of children is challenging to governments, as they are frequently invisible in the early stages of the epidemic. Also, programming for these children overlap (almost entirely) with services provided for other vulnerable children. Experience in Africa and Asia suggests that not only are the services that are provided for orphans from other causes and other vulnerable children appropriate for children affected by HIV, but it also suggests that providing special services can be stigmatizing and can add to their burden. This can be hard for policy makers and planners to grasp as they are often asked what they are doing to prepare for increasing numbers of HIV-affected children while at the same time they are advised not to provide dedicated services. Workers in the field learn quickly that activity camps for HIV-affected children create resentment among their peers, while banners proclaiming "scholarships for the AIDS orphans" sadden recipients. This field experience is validated by emerging research from Africa and Asia which shows that children orphaned by causes other than AIDS, children in poverty, and children vulnerable for other reasons experience common problems and benefit from common solutions (O'Connell, 2003; Gilborn, 2001).

Residential Care for Children Orphaned by AIDS

HIV/AIDS private orphanages for both HIV-infected and HIV-affected children are proliferating in many countries, and are funded by religious groups, charitable individuals, and non-government organizations. Societies and cultures in the region appear to have a ready acceptance of institutional care as an acceptable solution to the needs of orphaned children generally, and HIV-positive children in particular (KHANA, 2000). Donors, often from overseas, seem happy to fund institutions using an antiquated model of care no longer tolerated in developed countries. This is the "institutional" model of care, in which large numbers of children are segregated by age and gender, cared for, and sometimes even educated, in isolation from surrounding communities and often from any family members they may have. Critics of such care are almost entirely confined to a handful of welfare professionals. How can we ensure that these children will be able to develop the skills and relationships we all need to develop emotionally and socially?

Existing responses from governments in the region display a heavy reliance on a limited number of residential care institutions of varying quality to care for abandoned and destitute children and orphans. The UNGASS commitments are stimulating both donor and government interest in improving provisions for orphans. A new menu of possible responses is now emerging—measures to support faltering families and to prevent institutionalization, development of alternatives, and regulations to improve standards of care.

One international NGO widely represented in residential care in the Mekong region is SOS-Kinderdorf International, an organization that came to Vietnam and Thailand in the late 1960s. Currently there are SOS villages in all Mekong countries except Myanmar. SOS Children's Villages are part of a movement to reform institutional care. Children are accommodated in family-like groups with a housemother situated in a "village" of similar houses. At present, SOS villages in the region do not accept HIV-positive children and are funded independently of the government. Another international NGO with an impact in this area is Holt International, which is working with governments in China, Vietnam, and Thailand (where it is called Holt Sahathai Foundation) towards family preservation and reunification on the basis that an institution, no matter how good, cannot substitute for a family.

Cambodia. In Cambodia, there are currently three forms of institutional care for orphaned, abandoned, and vulnerable children. These are comprised of 20 government centers, 88 NGO centers (70% of which are registered with the Ministry of Social Affairs, Labour, Vocational Training, and Youth [MoSALVY]), and an unknown number of privately run centers, some of which are registered with the government (Dybdal *et al.*, 2001).

Alternatives to residential care supported by the government include: re-integration with families, adoption (both domestic and inter-country), group homes based in communities, and outreach and foster care, although so far only a small number of children are in foster care under the auspices of government or NGOs. NGO centers support re-integration, adoption, fostering, group homes, extended family care or kinship care, and child-headed households.

MoSALVY is preparing for a dramatic increase in orphans due to AIDS with policies aimed at alternatives to institutional care and guidelines and a regulatory framework for care providers. In addition, MoSALVY has developed specific strategies to strengthen communities in order to cope with caring for these children.

China. Children affected by the blood contamination disaster will test China's resources for orphaned children. Given the higher fertility in country areas and among ethnic minorities, and the fact that in some villages, adults of a range of ages all sold blood, huge numbers of children could be affected by AIDS and could require care. At the same time, the impact of national family planning programs means a greater pool of adults available in the less affected communities to care for children through fostering and other arrangements.

The Ministry of Civil Affairs is responsible for orphans and abandoned children. To date, most children abandoned have been disabled and female. There are 54,550 orphaned or abandoned children living in child welfare homes, social welfare institutions, and children's villages, an increase of 10,000 over the previous three years. In 2002, there were about 38,000 social welfare institutions throughout China. Of these, 600 cared for orphans and abandoned children. There are also nine SOS villages. Recently, government has been promoting alternative forms of care for these children including adoption, fostering, and group homes based in communities. Foster care was initiated comparatively recently in 1997, and the Ministry of Civil Affairs has developed policy, standards, and guidelines to expand this option. The Adoption Law was passed in 1993 and in 1998 it was amended to enable more domestic adoption. Adoption is now well established, with 45,000 children adopted (both domestically and internationally) in 2001. The government of China acknowledges an imminent increase in the number of children orphaned by AIDS and is developing policies on the care of these children.

Lao PDR. There are five SOS villages in Lao PDR and 13 ethnic minority boarding schools. The former house around 500 single and double orphans and the latter house 2,752 mainly older children, about half of whom are orphaned. There is a popular perception that

SOS villages offer status and advantages in terms of education and facilities, as they are usually better equipped and resourced than the average villager's home. The Ministry of Labour and Social Welfare also has a positive view of the SOS villages and are consulted on placements made. Although some caregivers mentioned SOS villages, the majority of villagers and all children consulted in a recent UNICEF study said that extended family was the best form of care for orphaned children. SOS also runs three kindergartens, a vocational training center, and a social center. In addition they have three half-way houses available to boys from the village when they turn 15 (UNICEF, 2003b).

The ethnic minority boarding schools are run by the Ministry of Education and are provided with 90,000 kip (US $5.70) per month per child and rice as well. Budgets for the schools are very low, and students grow a lot of their own food. Participants are expected to return home to their villages once they complete their education (UNICEF, 2003b).

The Ministry of Labor and Social Welfare is in the process of creating a policy on alternative care. As yet, there are no alternatives to residential care supported by government such as fostering programs or group homes. Foreign adoptions have been prohibited since 1994 (UNICEF, 2003b).

Myanmar. Services supplied by the government include institutional care for orphans, abandoned, destitute, and street children, and children in conflict with the law (Myanmar National AIDS Programme, 2000).

The Department of Social Welfare (DSW) runs six residential nurseries that provide care for orphans, abandoned, and destitute children of both sexes ranging from newborn up to the age of five. At five years of age, these children are transferred to single sex training schools where they live together with street children, destitute children, and children in conflict with the law (up to age sixteen). The Department of Social Welfare operates eight training schools (six for boys and two for girls).

Some church groups, Buddhist monks, nuns, and private community based organizations also run children's homes. Officially, institutions with a capacity of more than 50 children need to be registered with the DSW and are subsidized for the cost of rice and clothing and for salary of the warden. The subsidies vary according to the number of children, the resources available, and recommendations made by the respective State and Divisional Social Welfare Officer. According to DSW rules and regulations, a supervisory committee should be formed in each institution to provide effective care services.

There is currently no systematic registration system in Myanmar making the exact number of children living in institutions or orphanages difficult to estimate. According to official figures, as of December 2003, there were about 200 institutions run by voluntary organizations and registered with the DSW, which accommodate about 10,500 children. In addition, there are other institutions that are not registered with the DSW. Even though these institutions call themselves orphanages, many resident children are not double orphans but children from single parent families or poor families.

Institutions continue to be the first choice for authorities responsible for supporting destitute children. Alternatives to institutional care for orphans, including fostering programs, group homes and outreach/ community support are not yet common policy or practice. A few international NGOs (INGOs) have initiated fostering and outreach community support programs. However, officially, under the Registration of Kittima Adoption Act of 1941, the DSW offers adoption services for children under five who are under the protection and care of DSW residential nurseries with the aim of enabling these orphans to grow up in a family (UNICEF Yangon, 2003).

In Myanmar, The Child Law of 1993 contains provisions on "children in need of protection and care," including those with "no parent or guardian," those "in the custody of cruel parents or guardians," or those "afflicted with a contagious disease" (Article 32 a,d,f). Article 12 refers to the right to live with, and be brought up by, both parents or any one parent if they are alive. It also provides that "children shall not be separated forcibly from his or her parents except, in a case where in accordance with law, separation is necessary for the best interests of the child." The Child Law further invokes the right to maintain contact on a regular basis with parents lawfully separated, if it is not prejudicial to the best interests of the child. This Law and the Rules Related to the Child Law (Dec 2001) contain detailed provisions of the State's responsibilities to children in need of protection and care, as well as adoption. There is no legal provision specifically addressing HIV-positive or affected children in the Child Law (1993), or in the National AIDS Program adopted in 1992.

Thailand. Institutional care continues to be popular among religious bodies, charitable organizations, and society in general. Although the Royal Thai Government is slowly moving away from a reliance on large-scale institutional care, there are still 20 government residential institutions in 15 provinces, mostly gender and age-segregated. These catered to about 6000 orphaned, abandoned, or neglected children in the year 2000, or under 1% of the total of 1,048,000 orphans from all causes (UNICEF, 2002a).

The most striking example of an alternative approach to care is the Wiengping Children's Home in Chiengmai, which aims to reduce the number of children in the Children's Home through a range of measures including: a program of family preservation and family reunion with a caseload of about 350 a year (15% of family preservation cases are those affected by HIV/AIDS); a local foster care program; adoption—facilitating 3,570 adoptions in 2000 (largely overseas); a shared care arrangement with 12 privately run children's homes (five of which only accept children living with HIV/AIDS); and ten group homes in the community (caring for nearly 100 children). Wiengping Children's Home also aims to prevent children from coming into the Home by providing benefits and support to families caring for orphans. Seven government babies and children's homes now have foster care programs, six of which involve placing children with families in land resettlement communities. The Holt Sahathai Foundation, an NGO dedicated to keeping families together and avoiding institutionalization, supports the foster care and family preservation programs.

The Ministry of Social Development and Human Security (formerly the Department of Social Welfare) estimates that they provided care to around 200,000 children affected by AIDS in Thailand. In 2001, the Department also supported and regulated 78 community day care centers for children aged three to six, in hill tribe communities, land resettlement communities, and disadvantaged communities (Sunthonthada *et al.*, 2002).

Vietnam. Vietnam has a range of institutions that provide care to orphans and HIV/AIDS-affected children including: Social Protection Centers, run by the Ministry of Labour, Invalids, and Social Affairs (MoLISA); charitable institutions and compassionate homes, sometimes run by Buddhist monks and nuns or Church based groups; SOS villages and reformatory schools for children in conflict with the law, run by the Ministry of Public Security. 13,000 children including orphans, street children, disabled, and HIV-positive children, live in 95 social protection centers funded by the government, benefactors, and NGOs. Government institutions are provided with VND100,000–115,000 (US $6.44–7.40) per month per child for children in their care. The government is proposing to increase this sum to VND140,000 (UNICEF, 2003a). There are also over 100 charitable institutions which provide for 4000–5000 children and ten SOS villages.

Community Care for Children Affected by HIV/AIDS

In most countries, governments are beginning to review their provision for orphans and vulnerable children in the light of what is best for the child's development. The family is often known as the social safety net. Governments need to strengthen this social safety net lest it become strained under the pressure of increasing numbers.

The Pool of Caregivers. The great majority of orphaned and vulnerable children in the Mekong sub region are cared for by their extended families. Grandparents are reported to be common providers of care for orphans in Lao PDR, Vietnam, and Thailand, particularly maternal grandparents, followed by aunts and uncles. In Cambodia, grandparents were the most highly regarded providers of care, followed by maternal aunts (KHANA, 2000). One problem with the dependence on grandparents is the shortage of people of this generation in Cambodia due to the deaths in the Pol Pot period and low life expectancy. At the same time, high fertility rates—the total fertility rate was 4.9 in 2001—mean a greater number of children will be orphaned in each family. In Lao PDR, although there has been no loss of population on the scale of Cambodia, life expectancy in 2001 was a low 54 and the total fertility rate was five births per woman (UNICEF, 2001).

This contrasts with the situation in China, Vietnam, and Thailand where total fertility rates are low—1.8, 2.3, and 2 respectively—and life expectancy is high—71, 69, and, 70 respectively (UNICEF Statistics, 2001). Myanmar is somewhat in between with a low life expectancy of 60.6 (male) and 63.4 (Female) (UNFPA, Myanmar, 2003), and a lower total fertility rate of 2.4 births per woman (UNFPA, Myanmar, 2002). Clearly, in China, Vietnam, and Thailand a larger number of grandparents will be around to care for a smaller number of children. In Lao PDR and Cambodia, and to some extent in Myanmar, a small number of grandparents will be inundated with children. If orphans are passed on to aunts and uncles in countries with high fertility rates they will be adding to the dependency rate in already large families. Demographics will also have an impact on the generation gap—in Thailand and China where the trend has been for women to marry later, there will be a bigger age difference between grandparents and grandchildren. This may translate into more problems at adolescence, as there will be an even wider generation gap.

According to the demographics, there is a smaller gap between generations in countries like Cambodia and Lao PDR. It may be that the generation gap is either less of a problem in these countries, or a cultural construct that has not been widely adopted in less urbanized, less westernized societies. The generation gap did not appear to be a problem for grandparents and relatives caring for adolescents in Cambodia. Adolescents in Cambodia did not mention it as a problem either. Caregivers said their primary problems were finding food and money to educate the children. Children's greatest wish was to get a job and earn money (KHANA, 2000). This contrasts with the situation in Chiengmai, Thailand, where caregivers, children, and youth frequently mentioned the generation gap in terms of differing expectations and poor communication between grandparents/caregivers and children and youth (Duangsa *et al.,* 2000). However, in both countries most children and youth spoke positively about their relationships with relatives (Duangsa *et al.*, 2000; O'Connell, 2003).

Another source of care and mutual support that is often overlooked, is siblings. Children in Cambodia mentioned being separated from sisters and brothers as a cause of unhappiness (O'Connell, 2003). Adults mentioned sibling relationships as a source of support for the children (KHANA, 2000). Both traditional community care and institutions often break up families of orphaned siblings. Relatives split siblings to ease the load on individual households, while institutions are frequently gender and age-segregated.

Community Support Mechanisms. Traditional care for orphans across the Mekong region includes informal fostering or adoption

TABLE 3. Ratio of Monks and Temples to Total Population

Country	No of monks[a]	No of temples[a]	Ratio of temples to population	Ratio of monks to population
Cambodia	50,000	3,700	1 : 3,632	1 : 268
Xishuangbanna, China	6,000	530	1 : 1,547	1 : 136
Lao PDR	19,000	2,900	1 : 1,863	1 : 284
Myanmar	400,000	50,000	1 : 967	1 : 120
Thailand	300,000	35,000	1 : 1,816	1 : 211
Viet Nam	28,900	14,544	1 : 5,444	1 : 2,740

[a] Figures supplied by National Buddhist Associations, 2001
Source: UNICEF EAPRO, 2002

by neighbors and care of children in a pagoda (temple) setting by Buddhist monks, including ordination of orphaned or vulnerable boys as novices. It is mainly boys who ordain as novices to complete their education, but in Lao PDR some older girls in need of care and protection ordain as nuns from about the age of 13 or 14. In Myanmar quite young girls of seven or eight ordain as nuns. The number of orphans supported by temples is not known. Few studies have been conducted on care for children in a temple setting. However, there is a very high level of community support and acceptance for temple based care, which, according to anecdotal evidence, serves many children very well. The impact of Buddhist practices and philosophies in relation to loss and grief in children also deserves more attention. In addition to temples taking in children, monks and nuns also frequently run orphanages, particularly in Myanmar and Vietnam. While most countries focus on the positive side of religious community care—keeping children in their birth communities and providing them with food, shelter, spiritual support, and an education—there is a down side common to many religious orders. It is not just celibate orders in the Christian church who are known to abuse children in their care. There are also cases of sexual abuse of children by monks in Buddhist temples and these are reported in the newspapers from time to time (United Nations Economic and Social Commission for Asia and the Pacific, 2000).

Although Christians are in a minority in the region they have been disproportionately involved in providing AIDS care. In Thailand, there are twenty-five Catholic HIV/AIDS projects many of which involve care and support of children both through orphanages and community care support schemes. Temples have even greater potential as providers of care for orphans in terms of their presence in the region.

In Thailand and Cambodia, monks and nuns have also become involved with community-based programs, supporting children so that they may remain with their extended families. Monks and nuns are involved in counselling as well as hospital and home visiting schemes (UNICEF EAPRO, 2002).

Religious leaders have been found to play an important role in reducing stigma and discrimination through teaching and practicing Buddhist values of compassion and loving kindness (UNICEF EAPRO, 2002). These teachings are also valued in other faith traditions.

Government Support of Affected Children Living in Communities. In Vietnam, the government also supports community-based care and provides emergency relief and recurrent benefits to disadvantaged groups in communities. Children in community care are entitled to VND45,000 (US $2.90) a month. In 1999, the government provided food, benefits, and institutional care to 155,000 orphans and 19,000 street children. In 2002, MoLISA provided 55,000 orphans and vulnerable children in communities with support and social allowance benefits. About 1.7 million children received a reduction or exemption from school fees, and 431,458 children received free health care insurance and health services (UNICEF, 2003a).

In Lao PDR and Cambodia, the government does not provide pensions or benefits for orphans living with their extended family or in the community. A recent UNICEF study in Lao PDR noted that orphans who were not being helped by their extended families really had no place to turn for help. No government workers or mass organizations were cited as providing support, and charitable support from unrelated community members was said to be limited. Provincial and District Social Welfare officers confirmed that they could help very few people, as they had a small budget for material assistance to needy families (UNICEF, 2003b).

In Cambodia, MoSALVY strategies for child protection include community-based child protection networks, community awareness, universal education, health services, information mobilisation, rural development, and birth registration.

In China, the government has a "socialization of social welfare" policy to develop new welfare responses including a variety of funding mechanisms. The government has run a state lottery since 1987 to raise funds for poverty alleviation, welfare assistance and, support of the disabled and elderly. Local governments are responsible for financing and providing services to children who need special care. The Ministry of Civil Affairs is planning a process of contracting foster families to care for children and providing allowances for living costs.

In Myanmar, the extended family is generally seen as the best source of support for HIV-affected individuals and children. Children who are affected by HIV/AIDS and live in institutions may benefit from government-supported schemes. However, these are heavily under-funded. At the local level, parent/teacher associations and community-based structures such as School Boards of Trustees sometimes support needy children such as orphans with school fees, books, stationery, and school uniforms in order to prevent them from dropping out of school (UNICEF, Yangon, 2003).

Home Care. Globally, home care is now seen as an extremely important intervention in caring for HIV-affected families. The greatest contribution of home care teams is always going to be the ability to treat their patients effectively and prolong their life and health, thereby preventing or delaying orphaning. While in the past, the most HIV-affected families could hope for was to gain a couple of years through timely diagnosis and treatment of opportunistic infections, the recent introduction of antiretrovirals could mean a dramatic reduction in the numbers of children orphaned by AIDS.

Home care services also play an important role in supporting affected families through the tumultuous period of illness, death, and loss. Home care services can identify children in affected families and assist them in coping with their parent's illness and preparing for their parents' death. Home care teams can do "succession planning" with parents and children and can observe and assess likely or feasible placements for the children before they are orphaned. Many home care services like the NGO Siam Care in Thailand have evolved to provide follow-up services for orphaned children after their parents' death. Siam Care estimates that the process of establishing children in alternative family care takes about three years and includes: the time involved in making plans with the parents, performing trial visits with the nominated family, moving the family to a new home, following up with the family, and evaluating the family. NGOs like Siam Care and Medecins Sans Frontieres (MSF) have shown that the effectiveness of services like arranging family placements for orphans can mean a financial savings in comparison to the cost of long-term institutionalization of children.

Home care has been introduced in all Mekong countries to different degrees, and is usually conducted in partnership between both local and international NGOs and government health services. In Thailand, networks of people with HIV/AIDS and self-help groups have also played an important role in home care. With the introduction of antiretroviral therapies, the involvement of such networks in home care is paying off, as they are able to offer the constant support and counseling for adherence to prescribed therapies which hospital clinics are unable to deliver. Despite the effectiveness of home care services in relation to affected families, there has been little systematic assessment of coverage, gaps, or capacity in most countries.

In China, home care projects of various kinds are operating in a number of provinces including Henan, Guizhou, Jilin, Jiangxi, Chongqing, Hubei, Sichuan, Shanxi, and Yunnan. They are supported by United Nations agencies, bilateral aid agencies, and NGOs and include groups like the Chinese Red Cross, MSF, and the Chinese Government.

Home care in Cambodia, as in neighboring countries, is generally provided by NGOs working in some cases with government. In Cambodia, UNICEF's Seth Koma program has developed community-based care activities in five of the poorest provinces: Stung Treng, Kompong Speu, Kompong Thom, Prey Veng, and Svay Rieng. A number of international and local NGOs conduct home care. Buddhist monks in pagodas also participate in home care projects with support from a range of donors and the Ministry of Cults and Religions (Royal Government of Cambodia, 2001).

In Myanmar, national and international NGOs and the Department of Health provide home care activities through local volunteers. Since many people do not know their HIV status, caregivers include chronically ill patients in the community targeting poor segments of the population rather than targeting only HIV-infected people. This also reduces discrimination and stigmatization in the community. The Myanmar Nurses Association (MNA) is implementing community home-based care in 15 townships where the prevalence of HIV infection is relatively high. The Myanmar Maternal and Child Welfare Association (MMCWA) implements care and support in seven selected townships in border areas and trade junction areas in Tachileik, Kawthaung, Lashio, Muse, Dawei, Myitkyina, and Monywa. World Vision International provides care and support activities in seafarer communities in southern Myanmar (UNICEF Yangon, 2003).

In 2003, the Lao PDR Youth Union and Provincial Committee for the Control of AIDS and the NGOs, the Lao PDR Red Cross and MSF, were involved in providing home-based care and other forms of support to affected families in three provinces: Savannakhet, Champassak, and Bokeo (UNICEF Vientiane, 2003).

Protection from Abuse. Social welfare ministries are beginning to develop preventative systems for child protection to detect and intervene in cases of child abuse in communities. Child protection programs are extremely relevant for children orphaned by AIDS, as they can be vulnerable to abuse by male family or community members. NGOs involved in provision of services to children report that monitoring of extended family placements is essential to ensure potential cases of abuse are identified and averted. In Thailand, the NGO Siam Care found building trust with children and maintaining regular communication with them was a large part of this process so that children would feel comfortable to report "odd behavior" on the part of caregivers (Somsak Wiengyangkung, personal communication, 2003).

In most countries of the sub region, there are no accurate figures on the number of children who have been sexually abused. Of the six Mekong countries all have provisions relating to sexual abuse in their penal codes. Only Thailand has a well- developed and comprehensive policy, legislation, and procedures to address abuse. However, in all countries existing laws are often not enforced (United Nations Economic and Social Commission for Asia and the Pacific, 2000).

Child protection is also hampered by the lack of welfare services to assist abuse survivors or to prevent abuse. Social welfare has not been based in a developed social work practice in Lao PDR, China, Cambodia, or Vietnam. In addition, social welfare structures tend to become more sparse as they are applied from a national to a local level. At the district level, social work is often a matter of officials distributing a small amount of resources, such as food for emergency relief (UNICEF EAPRO, 2002) rather than the more complex processes involved in preventing, assessing, and counseling cases of sexual abuse. National child protection networks are planned for all countries and are being piloted in some; however, the problem of limited local capacity must be addressed before they can be established nationally.

Lao PDR, Vietnam, Myanmar, and Cambodia have few trained social workers. In the sub region, social work as a professional discipline tends to be under developed, although governments and donors are working to remedy this situation. Lao PDR and Cambodia are worst off for social workers, as there have been no university-level courses available locally. Over the current period of UNICEF's Country Program of Cooperation, MoSALVY in Cambodia has been developing training and certification processes in social work within the Ministry (Royal Government of Cambodia, 2001). MoLISA, in Lao PDR, has also begun a process of needs assessments in this area (Government of the Lao PDR, 2001), and in Vietnam the Government is establishing degree courses in Social Work (The Government of Socialist Republic of Vietnam, 2002). China has professional social workers but many welfare staff working with orphaned and abandoned children are not trained in social work (Stockholm University, 2003). While social work is not a universal panacea, trained social workers can perform a valuable role in supporting community-based protection programs. As it is, abused children in the sub region often come into the orbit of state welfare assistance only when they leave their homes for the streets, the sex industry or criminal activities.

In Myanmar, the 1993 Child Law provides for the establishment of national, State, Divisional, District, or Township Committees on the Rights of the Child, which are responsible for protecting and safeguarding the rights of the child (Article 5). According to the provisions of the Child Law, social welfare officers are responsible for investigating child abuse and determining whether children are in need of care from the state or a custodian. To date, the follow-up on these tasks is constrained by the limited number of social welfare officers (UNICEF Yangon, 2003).

In Thailand, Parliament has passed very comprehensive legislation, the Child Protection Law, effective as of February 2004. It clearly spells out the role of the State in child welfare and protection, and for the first time calls for decentralization of both management and resources to provinces and communities. The law requires that each province establish appropriate systems to ensure the protection and welfare of children. UNICEF Thailand has provided support to selected provinces to prepare for the implementation of the law. They have supported development of a directory and a map of existing welfare homes of all types nationwide, and have provided training to child protection staff at both central and provincial levels. All provinces are required to establish a Provincial Child Protection Committee chaired by the governor and the Provincial Child Protection Multi-Disciplinary Team (UNICEF Thailand, 2003).

Daycare Centers. Reviews of the needs of relatives and community members caring for orphans have identified community-based daycare centers for pre-schoolers as an important form of support. In Thailand, the Ministry of Social Development and Human Security runs 78 child care centres for disadvantaged children between the ages of three and six whom live in hill tribe areas and land resettlement villages. In rural areas, day care centers are also set up by religious groups in churches, temples, and in villages. Typically, these are locally constructed and run very cheaply with support provided by government in the form of regulation, training, and monitoring. A number of countries regulate and monitor the establishment and operation of day care centers, but their potential to strengthen the communites capacity to care for HIV-affected children is only just recently being acknowledged.

Homework Centers. In Chieng Mai province, in a district seriously affected by AIDS, a Christian pastor has set up a community homework center after consultations with children orphaned by AIDS and their caregivers identified children's need for help with homework. The Homework Centre operates on Saturday morning and uses older children (including some who have themselves been orphaned by AIDS) as volunteers to assist younger children (Apidech Chairacha, Pastor, personal communication, March 2003). In Australia, the Commonwealth Government funds over 800 homework centers in aboriginal communities. These are run by communities, have registered tutors, and have been credited with improving the academic performance of aboriginal students (Johnston, 1991).

Programs Addressing Discrimination. The Centre for AIDS Rights and other NGOs in Thailand have acquired a body of experience in conciliating cases of discrimination by communities or schools against HIV-positive children and adults. In a case where a child is refused admission to a school, they have a repertoire of activities. These include visiting the area, talking to parents and teachers, and meeting with the district AIDS committee and the local network of HIV-positive people (Center for AIDS Rights, 2003).

In northern Thailand, the support the government has given to self-help groups for people with HIV/AIDS has had a major impact. Over the last ten years over two hundred of these groups have formed in the North alone, initially helped along by a government incentive paid to every village. The Thai programs have not been closely evaluated, but as we have seen, there has been a reduction in discrimination in the region in which people with HIV/AIDS have been most active (Knodel *et al.*, 2002). In addition, the self-help programs that were used to educate communities and give advice to HIV-positive people about caring for their health are now proving an important part of the movement to provide greater access to antiretroviral drugs for adults and children.

CONCLUSION

Numbers of orphans and vulnerable children are growing throughout the region for a number of reasons, HIV/AIDS being only one among them. Estimates of vulnerable children show that millions of children throughout the region are vulnerable, sad, stigmatized, exploited, poor, and hungry.

Traditionally, the extended family and the community have provided care for over 90% of orphaned children. Buddhist temples, Christian churches, and other faith-based organizations have also cared for orphans and poor children in the past and remain active in this field today. For a minority of vulnerable (and visible) children, governments have provided care, usually in the form of large-scale residential institutions.

The extended family is still an effective safety net. However, rapidly changing societies and the growing gap between rich and poor place both young and old under enormous pressure. Families need extra help to support extra children in difficult times. The safety net needs to be stronger and the mesh finer. Grandparents, for instance, can be great caregivers, but their increasing physical frailty and limited earning capacity mean they need all kinds of assistance to help them bring up happy, healthy children. Unfortunately, not all families provide nurturing environments for children. Children can be exploited and abused by family and community members unless protection mechanisms are in place.

Governments need to deliver support to all families caring for vulnerable and orphaned children, and to assist and protect the children in their care. To do this they must build local resources and local capacity in social welfare, health, and education. This will enable governments to support a wider range of alternative care options, including: family preservation and reunification, foster care and group homes, and the extension of benefits and community development programs.

Families with HIV report that their main concerns are discrimination and treatment for HIV-positive family members. Discrimination against people with HIV and AIDS causes untold distress. It is a barrier that prevents families from accessing services and obscures communities' understanding of the epidemic, particularly in its early stages. Yet we need to address more than one form of discrimination. It's not just children orphaned by AIDS who experience discrimination, but other poor and disadvantaged children who suffer in the same way. Welfare, health, and education services that are accepting and non-judgmental help children and families cope with difficult circumstances. Community leaders who advocate compassion and acceptance can make a difference for people with HIV and others who are disadvantaged by poverty or other adverse circumstances.

In terms of treatment, moves to extend access to antiretrovirals may prove to be the single most effective measure in caring for children affected by HIV, simply by returning their parents to health and employment. If the countries of the region succeed in obtaining universal access to antiretrovirals for adults and children with AIDS, the major work for the next few years will be supporting families to obtain and maintain treatment and helping them pick up the pieces of lives shattered by the virus.

Current global strategies—strengthening families' and communities' capacity to care for and protect their children, ensuring governments care for the most vulnerable, and ensuring access to services—are emerging as effective measures to address the needs of HIV-affected children. For governments and the communities they serve, the task of taking these strategies, turning them into policies, legislation, and services, and making sure it all works in practice, has only just begun. By 2005, when we fulfill the UNGASS goals, it will not be just children with HIV who benefit, but all orphaned and vulnerable children.

REFERENCES

Center for AIDS Rights. (2003). Sample Cases of Children Affected by HIV/AIDS with No Access to their Right to Education in Thai Society, CEO workshop on Measures to promote and protect the education rights of children affected by AIDS: From policy to practice, 5 June 2003, Bangkok.

Chung, A. (2001). *Children Infected and Affected by HIV/AIDS, Reality and Solutions*, MoLISA and UNICEF Workshop on Policy, law and model on care for children infected and affected by HIV/AIDS, 19–20 July 2001, Hanoi.

Committee of the NGO AIDS Esan, (2003). Surveying the difficult conditions of children affected by AIDS in five northeastern provinces, CEO workshop on Measures to promote and protect the education right of children affected by AIDS: From policy to practice, 5 June 2003.

Duangsa, D., Duongsaa, U., Wannarat, S., Rojanawaranon, M., and Wannarat, S., (2000). *Linkages between Children/Youth and Older Persons in the Community in Northern Thailand*. Helpaged International and UNICEF. Chengmai.

Dybdal, A-S., Daigle, G. And, Sabonne, S. (2001). *Analytical Report: The National Survey of Providers of Alternative Care for Children in Cambodia*. MoSALVY. Phnom Penh.

Gilborn, L.Z., Nyonyintono, R., Kabumbuli, R., and Jagwe-Wadda, G. (2001). *Making a Difference for Children Affected by AIDS: Baseline Findings from Operations Research in Uganda*. Population Council, Inc.

Government of the Lao PDR/UNICEF. (2001). *Master Plan of Operations for the 2002–2006: Country Programme of Co-operation*. Vientiane.

Government of Socialist Republic of Vietnam/UNICEF Vietnam. (2002). *A Programme to Advance Child Rights in Vietnam*: Plan of Operations 2001–2005, UNICEF Vietnam.

Holt Sahathai Foundation. (2002). *Holt Sahathai Foundation (HSF) Programs in the Area of Children Affected by HIV & HIV-Positive Children*. Bangkok. (Unpublished report).

Ionita,G., Hereward, M., Stewart, W., Yuan, J., Li, J., Zhang, J., and Li, X. (2002). *The Long Term Social-Economic Impact of AIDS on Children and Policy Response in China's Yunnan Province* (Unpublished report).

Johnston, E. (1991). *Royal Commission into Aboriginal Deaths in Custody, National Report*, Volume 4, AGPS, Canberra, Aboriginal Tutorial Assistance Scheme 33.1.49.

Khmer HIV/AIDS NGO Alliance (KHANA). (2000). *Children Affected by HIV/AIDS: Appraisal of Needs and Resources in Cambodia. Summary Report*. KHANA.

Knodel, J., Im-em, W., Saengtienchai, C., Vanlandingham, M., and Kespichayawattana, J. (2002). *The Impact of an adult child's death due to AIDS on older-aged parents*: Results from a direct interview survey. Institute for Population and Social Research, Mahidol University, Bangkok.

Kong Rok Ed. (1999). Kong khuap khum rok tid tor, Krasuang Satharanasu. (Mesayan 2542). Kan dulae dek thi dai rap phon krathop chak rok ed, Kan sammana radap chat ruang rok ed khrang thi 7 (translation: AIDS Division, Department of Communicable Diseases Control, Ministry of Health. (1999). The Care of Children Affected by AIDS, 7th National AIDS Conference).

Lakhonphon, S. and Frederix, K. (2003). *Children at the Camillian Social Centre (CSC) & Their Experience of Discrimination at School* (unpublished paper).

Ministry of Labour and Social Welfare, UNICEF Laos. (2001). *How I got here: Commercial Sexual Exploitation of Children in Lao PDR*.

Myanmar National AIDS Programme (2000). Sentinel Surveillance Data.

O'Connell, K. (2003). The Psychological Well Being of AIDS Affected and Vulnerable Children: A Cambodian Perspective. NYEMO, Phnom Penh. (unpublished draft report).

Royal Government of Cambodia (1999). *National Health Survey: Cambodia 1998*, Phnom Penh.

Royal Government of Cambodia/UNICEF Cambodia. (2001). *Investing in Children: Master Plan of Operations of the Royal Government of Cambodia/UNICEF*, Country Programme of Cooperation 2001–2005. UNICEF Cambodia, Phnom Penh.

Stockholm University. (2003). Country Reports 2003. New Strategies for a New Millenium, 2nd International Conference, Stockholm, May 12–15, 2003. Department of Social Work, Stockholm University, Stockholm.

Sunthonthada, K., Worasiri-amon, Y., Ondam, B. (2002). Rai ngan "Kan suksa klum paw mai dek lae tua chi wad kan damnoen ngan dan kan krum krong thang sangkhom khang krom pracha songkhro", (translation: Report from a Study of a Target Group of Children and Social Protection Implementation Indicators of the Social Welfare Division) Population and Society Research Institute, Mahidol University, Bangkok.

Tolfree, David. (1995). *Roofs and Roots: The care of separated children in the developing world*. Arena Publishing. Hants, England.

Joint United Nations Program on HIV/AIDS (UNAIDS). (2002). *Report on the Global HIV/AIDS Epidemic 2002*, UNAIDS, Geneva.

United Nations Population Fund (UNFPA). (2002). *Myanmar Fertility and Reproductive Health Survey, 2001*, Department of Population, UNFPA. Yangon.

United Nations Population Fund (UNFPA). (2003). *Human Resource Development Indicators, Myanmar, 2002*. Department of Labour, UNFPA. Yangon.

United Nations Children's Fund (UNICEF). (2001). UNICEF Statistics, End Decade Assessment, Multiple Indicator Cluster Survey MICS2—National reports http://www.childinfo.org/MICS2/ natlMICSrepz/MICSnatrep.htm. (accessed December 13, 2003).

United Nations Children's Fund (UNICEF). (2002a). *Children on the Brink 2002: A Joint Report on Orphan Estimates and Program Strategies*, UNICEF, New York.

United Nations Children's Fund (UNICEF). (2002b). *The Increasing Vulnerability of Children in Nepal*: Report of an Assessment of Children and Families Affected by HIV/AIDS in Nepal and the Response at Family, Community, District and National Level.

United Nations Children's Fund (UNICEF). (2003a). *The Situation of Families and Children Affected by HIV/AIDS in Vietnam: A National Overview*, Final Report, 30 August 2003 (In press).

United Nations Children's Fund (UNICEF). (2003b). *A National Study of Orphans and Children Affected by HIV/AIDS in Lao PDR: Preliminary Findings* (Unpublished).

United Nations Children's Fund East Asia and the Pacific Regional Office (UNICEF EAPRO). (2002). *Securing a Future: Mekong Children and HIV/AIDS*, Bangkok.

United Nations Children's Fund (UNICEF) Thailand (2003). *Report on Child Protection Law*. (Unpublished report).

United Nations Children's Fund (UNICEF) Yangon. (2003). Update to Securing A Future. UNICEF Yangon. (Unpublished report).

United Nations Children's Fund (UNICEF) Vientiane. (2003). Internal Report on Lao PDR HIV/AIDS Programme. UNICEF Vientiane. (Unpublished report).

United Nations Economic and Social Commission for Asia and the Pacific (2000). *Sexually Abused and Sexually Exploited Children and Youth in the Greater Mekong Sub region: A Qualitative Assessment of Their Health Needs and Available Services,* United Nations, New York.

Van Trung, N. (2003). Tam Binh Orphanage Presentation, Consultation on the situation of HIV+ abandoned children whose parents are HIV+ drug users, HCMC 4 December 2003, Ho Chi Minh City.

The World Bank. (2000). Thailand's Response to AIDS. Thailand Social Monitor V. Bangkok.

Wilson, D. (2003). Accessing the issue of discrimination against children with AIDS, Pre-Congress Workshop on Pediatric AIDS, The 11th Asian Congress of Pediatrics and the 1st Asian Congress on Pediatric Nursing. *From prevention to care and anti-stigmatization*, 2–3 November 2003, Bangkok.

32

Prevention of Mother-to-Child Transmission of HIV in Thailand

Striding towards Access to HAART for the Family

Sophie Le Coeur[1], Gonzague Jourdain[2], Intira Collins[2], Nicole Ngo-Giang-Huong[2], Vallop Thaineua[3], and Marc Lallemant[4]

[1]*Institut National d'Etudes Démographiques/Harvard AIDS Institute*
[2]*Harvard School of Public Health, Department of Immunology and Infectious Diseases, Boston, Massachusets USA; Perinatal HIV Prevention Trial, Chiang Mai, Thailand*
[3]*Ministry of Public Health, Bangkok Thailand*
[4]*Institut de Recherche pour le Développement/Perinatal HIV Prevention Trial, Chiang Mai, Thailand*

INTRODUCTION

The AIDS epidemic became visible in North America, Europe, and Africa at the beginning of the 1980s, but did not emerge in Asia until ten years later; some countries have only been experiencing the epidemic very recently. However, the lessons learned in countries which faced the epidemic 10 to 20 years ago seem to have had limited impact on the response to recent epidemics in Asia. In countries such as India, Myanmar, Cambodia, and Vietnam, the sad story of the HIV epidemic seems to be repeating itself. Thailand remains the exception.

To date, UNAIDS estimates that, among the 40 million persons living with HIV/AIDS at the end of the year 2003, 7.4 million live in Asia (UNAIDS, WHO, 2003). In the year 2003 alone, one million new HIV infections and 500,000 deaths occurred as a result of AIDS in Asia.

While HIV has spread in Africa mainly through casual heterosexual relationships in the population at large, in Asia the epidemic has consisted of multiple interrelated epidemics, affecting members of high risk groups and their immediate sexual partners first. (Brown *et al.*, 1994). This silent epidemic gradually spread into the general heterosexual population, most of whom are of reproductive age, increasing the chances of transmitting the virus to their offspring, with major consequences on child mortality.

Ironically, over the past three decades, maternal and child health programs such as immunization, oral rehydration, growth monitoring programs, and breast-feeding promotion were heavily emphasized to combat infant morbidity and mortality in developing countries and have been largely successful in lowering infant mortality, particularly in Asia. Yet today the HIV/AIDS epidemic has reversed this trend. Indeed, in 2003 alone, 2.5 million children under 15 years of age were infected with HIV/AIDS, and about 500,000 died of AIDS worldwide (UNAIDS, WHO, 2003). Most of these pediatric infections were due to mother-to-child transmission (MCT). Unfortunately in many developing countries, despite the major breakthrough of the PACTG 076/ANRS 024 trial in 1994 demonstrating the remarkable efficacy of zidovudine (AZT) in reducing perinatal transmission of HIV by 66% in non-breastfeeding women, perinatal infections continue to occur (Connor *et al.*, 1994). The number of pediatric AIDS cases in Asia is relatively low compared to Africa, reflecting lower HIV prevalence and the generally lower fertility level in Asia. However, when women are having fewer children, as is the case in some countries such as China and Thailand, families place a great emphasis on the child's well being. Therefore, the importance of MCT HIV prevention programs within these contexts should not be underestimated.

In this chapter, we will first describe the characteristics of the Thai epidemic, and outline the national response against it. We will then assess the different steps, which led to the implementation of the MCT prevention program, and how the interplay between research and policy was essential to its success. Finally, we will review the challenges of extending MCT HIV prevention into wider antiretroviral (ARV) access programs, providing long-term treatments to parents and infected children.

THAILAND'S EPIDEMIC

Of all Asian countries, Thailand was the first and one of the hardest hit by the HIV pandemic (Weniger *et al.*, 1991). Almost one million of its 60 million population are thought to have been infected (World Bank, 2000). The first wave of the epidemic, beginning in 1989, developed very rapidly through intravenous drug use and was essentially caused by HIV-1 subtype B, the virus found in the US and in Europe (Weniger *et al.*, 1991). The second wave of the epidemic was caused by HIV-1 subtype CRF01_AE and spread among female sex workers (FSW) (Sittitrai *et al.*, 1994). This virus then spread into the general heterosexual population, firstly from FSW to their clients, and then from the clients to their regular partners (Nelson *et al.*, 1996; Bunnell *et al.*, 1999). To date, more than 80% of women infected in Thailand have contracted HIV in what they thought was a "monogamous" relationship with their husbands (World Bank, 2000). In June 2002, the prevalence rate of HIV in pregnant women was 1.4% at the national level with the highest rates found in northern Thailand, according to sentinel surveillance (Ministry of Public Health, 2002).

THAI RESPONSE TO THE EPIDEMIC

The Royal Thai Government responded quickly to the HIV/AIDS epidemic and implemented a multi-sector AIDS program as early as 1987 (Phoolcharoen *et al.*, 1998). At its onset, this program involved all government ministries, non-governmental organizations, multilateral donors, and private businesses. Cooperation at the national level among ministries was carried out through the National AIDS Prevention and Control Committee chaired by the Prime Minister (Berman, 1999).

The National AIDS Program particularly focused on four areas of interventions against HIV/AIDS.

Public Information, Education, and Prevention

As early as 1989, bi-annual sentinel surveillance surveys were conducted in each province among intravenous drug users (IDU), direct and indirect FSW, military recruits, blood donors, and women receiving antenatal care. The data collected highlighted the most affected provinces and documented the dynamic of the epidemic spreading from one group of high-risk behaviors such as FSW to other sectors of the general population such as the military recruits (Nelson *et al.*, 1996). The publication of these survey results in the national newspapers, illustrating the visible progression of the epidemic, was instrumental in raising public/government awareness towards the spread of the HIV/AIDS.

The government responded with several national campaigns, bombarding the public with information on HIV/AIDS using all forms of mass media as well as innovative and powerful methods of communication. For example, a nationwide network of volunteers was mobilized to distribute cards, audiocassettes, and videos containing information about HIV/AIDS (World Bank, 2000). Condom use was heavily promoted through the 100% condom use campaign in which the active involvement of the charismatic public figure Mechai Viravaidya was critical to its success. Finally, HIV testing was rapidly made available in all government hospitals and in many private facilities.

The comprehensive monitoring and surveillance system in place since 1989 enabled the documentation of the success of these prevention programs in curtailing the spread of the epidemic (Bunnell *et al.*, 1999). Indeed, the impact of these preventive measures was particularly visible in the North. For example, prevalence rates in pregnant women dropped from more than 10% to less than 5% between 1994 and 1997 in the Phayao province (Ministry of Public Health, 2000). The surveillance system also allowed observers to follow the epidemic, demonstrating the overall prevalence of HIV decline in FSW and in the general population, while pointing out the relative failure of the campaign among IDU (Celentano *et al.*, 1998; Nelson *et al.*, 2002; World Bank, 2000; UNAIDS/WHO, 2003). We will see later in this chapter that a similar monitoring strategy also allowed the documentation of the successful Prevention of Mother-to-Child Transmission (PMTCT) program.

Human Rights and Social Support

A national counseling plan was launched in 1990 that included training of counselors, and promotion of voluntary anonymous HIV counseling and testing at the national level. This plan was expanded in 1993 to provide training for nurses in the antenatal care setting (Kanshana and Kullerk, 1998). In addition, the government took a clear stand against the discrimination of HIV-positive individuals and advocated for protection of their rights (Ainsworth *et al.*, 2000). For example, calls for mandatory blood testing and disclosure of results were strongly opposed. The government also supported many non-governmental organizations (NGOs) involved in various aspects of HIV/AIDS prevention and care including home care, building AIDS patients' networks, income generating activities, and family support groups. For example, the Thai Business Initiative in Rural Development is a project aimed at diverting young rural women away from prostitution by providing them with training and employment.

Promotion of Research

Important epidemiological, clinical, virological, and socio-behavioral research programs conducted in Thailand were encouraged and supported by the Ministry of Public Health (MOPH). The research allowed a better understanding of the dynamic of the epidemic and documented the unique success of the Thai prevention campaigns (Nelson *et al.*, 1996). These research programs also helped instigate pilot projects, which were launched at the regional level, and proved to be crucial in guiding interventions and policies at the national level (Thaineua *et al.*, 1998; Kanshana *et al.*, 2000). The close collaboration between policy makers at the MOPH and researchers was particularly effective in the field of mother-to-child prevention. Finally, Thailand was and continues to be actively involved at the forefront of the global research effort towards an HIV/AIDS vaccine, coordinated by a National HIV vaccine committee of knowledgeable experts (Natpratan *et al.*, 1996).

Medical Treatment and Care

The use of AZT was approved in 1987, and until the mid 1990s it was provided by the MOPH to HIV-positive Thais. The Thai Food and Drug Administration (FDA) then rapidly allowed the importation of many other antiretrovirals. Later, an agreement between the Thai government and the manufacturer of AZT allowed the Government Pharmaceutical Organization (GPO) to purchase the drug in bulk at a competitive price. The GPO is now producing several generic ARVs including GPOvir, a pill taken twice a day combining d4T, 3TC, and nevirapine. In 2003, the MOPH announced its collaboration with the Global Fund for AIDS, TB, and Malaria, to provide 70,000 HIV-positive individuals access to ARV treatment.

PREVENTION OF MOTHER-TO-CHILD TRANSMISSION PROGRAM: A SUCCESS STORY

The First Steps

Within the national HIV/AIDS prevention program, Thailand specifically targeted MCT of HIV. Beginning as early as 1990, even before any measures to reduce MCT were discovered, some hospitals were conducting HIV testing for pregnant women. At that time, this practice reflected general fears among health care workers who felt the need to know the HIV status of their patients in order to protect themselves. However, when discovered to be HIV-positive, most women were informed of their HIV status. Theoretically, the women could then make a decision with regard to the continuation of their pregnancy, about safe infant feeding practices, postpartum contraception, and prevention of sexual transmission to their partners. At this time, most women who were confirmed to be HIV-positive had their pregnancy terminated, while many of those who continued with their pregnancy were sterilized thereafter (Intaraprasert *et al.*, 1996; Paisarntantiwong *et al.*, 1995; Rugpao *et al.*, 1997). This trend reflected the fact that most health care workers felt they had nothing to offer these women, who were often perceived as unable to handle the crisis of HIV infection. This attitude amongst the health care workers changed significantly after 1993, when the intense training on HIV counseling provided by the MOPH was extended to nurses within antenatal care settings.

In the same year, while continuing to support the UNICEF Baby-Friendly Initiative and promoting breastfeeding, the MOPH recommended formula feeding to HIV-positive women in response to the clear evidence that HIV could be transmitted through breastfeeding (Le Coeur *et al.*, 1996; Dunn *et al.*, 1992). The MOPH ensured that this recommendation was only targeted towards HIV-positive women who could then decide on the safest mode of feeding for their infants. In the public hospitals, formula was provided for free to the poorest of HIV-positive women until the child reached 18 months of age (Kanshana and Kullerk., 1998). In response to concerns over a potential 'spill over' effect, a study performed in northern Thailand showed that formula feeding programs targeted towards women with HIV/AIDS did not negatively impact efforts to promote breastfeeding among the non-infected population (Talawat *et al.*, 2002).

As soon as the results of PACTG 076 were released in 1994, demonstrating the remarkable efficacy of AZT in reducing perinatal transmission of HIV, the MOPH reevaluated its HIV treatment program. In mid-1995, with the assistance of the World Bank and the World Health Organization, the MOPH analyzed the economics of antiretroviral therapy in Thailand (Prescott, 1997). They concluded that, given Thailand's budget for antiretrovirals and the quality of its health care infrastructure, AZT prophylaxis for HIV-positive pregnant women and their newborns was feasible, affordable, and by far the most cost-effective way to use the budget for antiretrovirals compared to the use of AZT monotherapy for patients. At about this time, the Thai FDA approved the use of AZT for the prevention of perinatal HIV.

In 1996–1997, after completing preliminary research studies, the Thai Red Cross, through its 79 nationwide affiliated hospitals, began providing AZT to HIV-positive pregnant women following the PACTG 076 regimen. Knowing that most MCT occurs close to delivery, the MOPH quickly initiated a pilot perinatal HIV prevention program in northern Thailand using a short course AZT treatment. At the same time, a large clinical trial was launched in parallel to the MOPH pilot program. The Perinatal HIV Prevention Trial (PHPT-1) was conducted by Harvard University, the Institut de Recherche pour le Dévelopement (IRD), and 27 hospitals of the Ministry of Public Health (Lallemant *et al.*, 2000). The main objective of this research trial was to compare the efficacy of abbreviated AZT treatments in mothers and/or children with the standard PACTG 076 regimen. PHPT-1 demonstrated that a long course of AZT prophylaxis (from 28 weeks' gestation, and 6 weeks in the newborn) was more effective than a short one (delayed until 35 weeks' gestation, and for 3 days in the newborn) with transmission rates of 4.1% versus 10.5%, respectively. Both programs, the MOPH program in the North and the PHPT-1 research project, complemented each other greatly and both benefited from the other in terms of training, coverage, and capacity building (Thaineua *et al.*, 1998). The economic analysis of the MOPH pilot program in the North proved it was highly cost-effective, and showed that the cost of drugs was relatively low compared to the cost of training for counseling, HIV testing, and provision of formula (Borand, 2000).

During the same period, the US-CDC, with the Bangkok Collaborative Perinatal HIV Transmission Study Group, was conducting a placebo-controlled trial in Bangkok which demonstrated that a short course AZT regimen starting at 36 weeks of pregnancy could reduce perinatal transmission of HIV by half in non-breastfeeding women (Shaffer *et al.*, 1999). Together with the MOPH, they carried out a pilot program in 1998 for the prevention of HIV perinatal transmission in the Northeast of Thailand (Kanshana *et al.*, 2000).

In December 1999, the MOPH convened a meeting to issue national guidelines on perinatal HIV transmission prevention, based on evidence from the clinical trials described above, along with the pilot programs in the North and Northeast. The MOPH decided to launch its first nationwide perinatal transmission prevention program.

The Evolving National Program for the Prevention of Perinatal Transmission of HIV

As part of the national program for the prevention of HIV perinatal transmission, voluntary counseling and testing were provided during the first antenatal visit. In all public hospitals (community, district, or provincial hospitals) nurses have been trained to provide HIV pre- and post-test counseling through a 5-day training curriculum. The hospital laboratories were equipped to perform HIV tests according to the MOPH algorithm. Antenatal women attending health care centers where HIV counseling and testing were not available were referred to higher-level health units. Pre-test counseling was generally provided in groups together with a video prepared by a group of counseling experts. Women who wanted to discuss further issues regarding HIV testing could speak privately

TABLE 1. Efficacy of the National PMTCT Program in 822 Public Hospitals in Thailand, October 2000 to September 2001

	Numbers	%
Births	573,655	100%
Women with antenatal care	554,912	96.7%
Women tested for HIV during pregnancy	517,488	93.3%
Women with no antenatal care	18,743	3.3%
Women tested for HIV at the time of delivery	13,314	71.0%
HIV-positive women	6,646	1.2%
HIV-positive women who received AZT during pregnancy	4,659	70.1%
Newborns from HIV-positive mothers	6,475	—
Newborns from HIV-positive mothers who received AZT	5,741	88.7%
Newborns from HIV-positive mothers who received formula feeding	5,386	83.2%

Source: Amornwichet *et al.*, 2002

with the counselor. HIV results were then provided individually during confidential post-test counseling sessions. Prevention methods were stressed for HIV-negative women. For HIV-positive women, the counselors discussed the issue of diagnosis disclosure to the partner and other family members. In some hospitals, couple counseling and testing was also promoted. AZT prophylaxis for women during pregnancy and labor, and for newborns was promoted, along with formula feeding of newborns to reduce MCT. For women who did not attend antenatal care, HIV counseling and testing was provided at the maternity ward.

According to the national program implemented in 2000, prophylactic treatment includes AZT, 300 mg twice a day from the 34th week of gestation, oral AZT, 300 mg every 3 hours as a loading dose from the onset of labor; and for the newborns, AZT oral suspension, 2 mg/kg every 6 hours, for 1 week or for 6 weeks if the mother had been treated for less than 4 weeks. Additionally, formula feeding was recommended and provided for free to the poorest of HIV-positive women for 12 months. HIV diagnosis of children was performed by serology at 12 months of age, HIV-positive children being re-tested at 18 months. Finally, the guidelines recommended 'appropriate' medical care for mothers and children. This ranges from child immunization, surveillance of growth and development, to the systematic provision of prophylaxis of opportunistic infections to all children before knowing their HIV status or/and to the identification and treatment of immunocompromised women and children.

This national PMTCT program was monitored and evaluated using the computerized database compiled over the first year of its implementation. The results are summarized in Table 1. Among all pregnant women who had antenatal care (97%), 93% were tested for HIV, while this percentage was only 71% among women who did not have antenatal care. Seventy percent of the HIV-positive women received AZT during pregnancy, 89% of the infants were treated with AZT and 83% of the children were formula fed. Assuming a 30% transmission rate in the absence of any intervention, and 8% with AZT, it is estimated that 2457 pediatric HIV infections were avoided this year through the PMTCT program (Kanshana *et al.*, 2000; Kanshana and Simonds, 2002; Amornwichet *et al.*, 2002).

These great achievements were made possible due to a variety of important factors, including effective and strong leadership by the MOPH, as it initiated and implemented programs in response to emerging domestic needs. Public health decision-makers did not wait for international calls for action or international endorsement or support; the actions of the ministry were independent and highly self-reliant. The effectiveness of

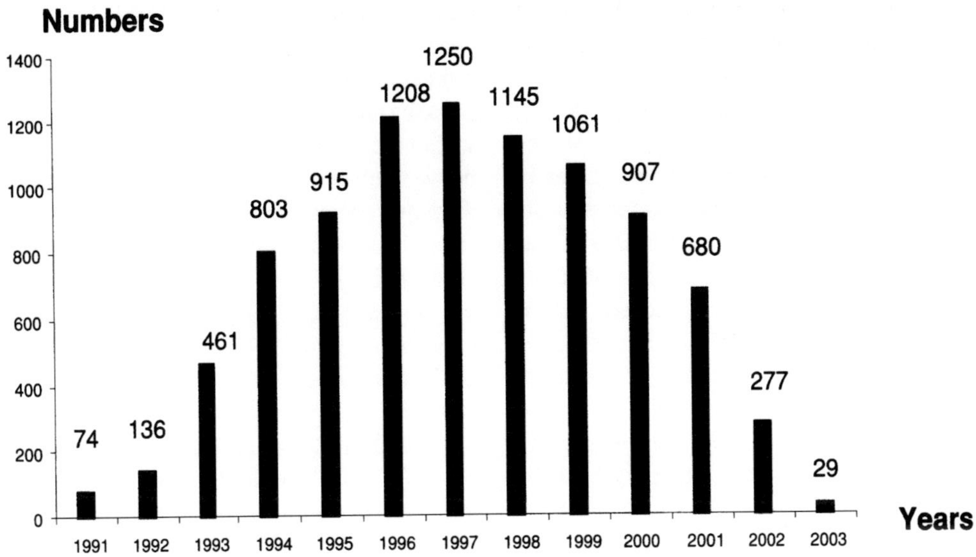

FIGURE 1. Number of Pediatric AIDS Cases (0 to 4 years old) Reported to the MOPH in Thailand from 1991 to May 2003. Source: Kanshana, 2003.

the PMTCT program reflects the pragmatic approach of the MOPH, using the latest scientific knowledge from clinical research, testing strategies through pilot projects before scaling up to the national level, and emphasizing training, particularly in HIV counseling. The high quality of HIV testing and health care system delivery were also extremely significant. It is clear that counseling played a crucial role in the success of this program not only for the patients but also in changing the attitudes of the health workers toward HIV-positive patients. Due to the high turnover of counseling personnel, and constant scientific developments, there has been a clear need for repeated training and refresher courses. Finally, the well-organized mother–child health system helped ensure the successful implementation of the program. This perinatal prevention program in turn contributed to the improvement of the mother-child health system beyond the HIV field, by creating a referral system from peripheral health centers to larger hospitals, facilitating communication and interaction within the different departments of the hospitals, and sensitizing the staff towards issues of confidentiality.

The success of the PMTCT program is uniquely illustrated by the dramatic drop in the number of pediatric HIV/AIDS cases reported to the MOPH, although this also reflects the impact of public campaigns on the prevention of sexual transmission (Figure 1).

To ensure the continued success of this program, the MOPH systematically reviews and updates its guidelines for the prevention of mother-to-child transmission of HIV in response to the latest scientific developments nationally and internationally.

Improving PMTCT Efficacy

Following the results of HIVNET 012, a trial in Uganda demonstrating the efficacy of a single dose of nevirapine (NVP) at onset of labor and 3 days after birth in the newborns, the Thai Red Cross decided to propose to all its network hospitals the addition of nevirapine to AZT for mothers at onset of labor and in neonates 48–72 hours after birth (Guay *et al.*, 1999).

New clinical trials have been conducted to improve the efficacy of the existing prophylactic programs using AZT monotherapy. The

Perinatal HIV Prevention Trial 2 (PHPT-2) in particular tested the addition of a single oral 200 mg dose of nevirapine at onset of labor, and one 6 mg dose for the newborn 48 to 72 hours after birth, to AZT starting at 28 weeks' gestation or as soon as possible thereafter (Lallemant *et al.*, 2002). The transmission rate in women who received AZT plus NVP was 2.0%, significantly lower than the 6.3% transmission rate experienced by women who received AZT alone. This simple regimen of AZT during the last trimester of pregnancy combined with a single dose of NVP at onset of labor is able to achieve a transmission rate as low as those obtained using highly active antiretroviral therapy (HAART) during pregnancy.

Following the remarkable results of this trial, the MOPH has again responded in a pragmatic manner, convening a meeting of experts and reviewing its national guidelines for the prevention of mother-to-child transmission of HIV in order to advance the initiation of zidovudine from 28 weeks gestation and incorporate NVP into the treatment package.

MOVING TOWARD ACCESS TO HAART

PMTCT Plus Programs

The extension of PMTCT to include long term provision of HAART to immunocompromised mothers and to the few HIV-positive children is referred to as PMTCT Plus. For example, all immuno-compromised HIV-positive mothers and infected children who had participated in the PHPT trials have received ARV drugs since 1999, and continue to be closely monitored. The follow-up of these cohorts has demonstrated that PMTCT Plus was feasible, well accepted, and highly beneficial to the patients involved. PMTCT Plus was also identified as a unique opportunity to reach out and treat HIV-positive fathers/partners so that both parents can care for their children. PMTCT Plus highlighted the need for further training of health workers, reorganization of the care system, patient networking, as well as improved communication within the health care network; as the linkage between obstetricians, pediatricians, internal medicine specialists, pharmacists, and counselors is critical to the successful implementation of HAART.

In May 2001, during the Third International Symposium on Pediatric AIDS in Thailand, in a public declaration, clinicians, researchers, and public health officers requested from the Ministry of Health the provision of HAART to HIV-positive mothers, children, and families within the Thai national PMTCT program. PMTCT Plus has since been prioritized in the program for access to care by the Ministry of Public Health. In 2002, the Department of Health at MOPH launched in four provinces a pilot PMTCT Plus program to provide HIV-positive mothers, fathers, and children with HIV care, including ARV treatment. The plan is to extend this "Care for HIV-infected mothers and families" program to the 76 provinces of Thailand by 2004.

Access to Care Pilot Programs

With the increasing production of generic drugs worldwide, the price of ARV drugs has dropped dramatically, and the possibility of providing long term ARV treatment to HIV-positive patients has become more realistic. In Thailand, the Government Pharmaceutical Organization (GPO) started producing GPOvir, a combination of d4T, 3TC, and nevirapine in a single pill to be administered twice a day, which costs approximately US$30 a month (Medecins Sans Frontiers, 2003).

To evaluate the feasibility of providing HAART to HIV-positive Thais, in addition to the PMTCT Plus cohort mentioned above, the AIDS division at the MOPH launched a pilot program, Access To Care (ATC) at the end of 2000. The goal of this program was to provide triple therapy (8 different combinations) to 2000 patients (CD4 <200 or viral load

>30,000 copies) mostly in the northern region of Thailand. This program demonstrated the feasibility of providing HAART at various levels of the health care system, through provincial, district, and community hospitals.

During this time, several research groups, in particular HIV-NAT, a consortium of Thai, Australian and Dutch researchers, were conducting important clinical trials providing crucial information on different combinations of ARV treatments, reduced dosages, and simplified intake schedules specific to the needs of the Thai population (Ruxrungtham *et al.*, 2000; Cardiello *et al.*, 2002; Cardiello *et al.*, 2003; Burger *et al.*, 2003). Researchers also tested the use of interleukin 2 in HIV-positive Thais, and investigated alternatives for cheaper techniques for monitoring treatment (CD4 enumeration, viral load measurements, and detection of resistance mutations) (Ruxrungtham *et al.*, 2000; Ruxrungtham *et al.*, 2002).

Using the same strategies of building upon the success of small pilot programs, and using the results of the clinical trials performed in Thailand, in 2003 the MOPH organized the revision of the national guidelines for the use of ARV. In the same year, the MOPH also launched, in collaboration with the Global Fund, a national program to provide access to HAART to 70,000 patients over the next five years.

CHALLENGES OF ACCESS TO CARE PROGRAMS

With the use of ARV combination therapies, HIV/AIDS has shifted from a deadly to a chronic disease. Physicians are eager to learn about HIV infection and various aspects of HAART, including baseline check-up before treatment initiation, adherence, potential side-effects/toxicity, monitoring of efficacy, management of resistance, and co-infections. Major issues related to the management of HIV-positive patients on treatment still need to be addressed in the specific context of Thailand: cancers such as cervical cancers in women, tuberculosis, immune reconstitution syndrome, management of co-infections in particular Hepatitis B and Hepatitis C, mitochondrial toxicity, lipodystrophy, pharmacokinetics of antiretroviral drugs, and monitoring strategies to decide when to switch from first line to further regimens.

As the field of HIV/AIDS medicine is a fast evolving discipline, there is a need for continuous training. Although the HIV medical training is much more complex, lessons can be learned from the successful nationwide training program on counseling organized by the MOPH.

The MOPH will need to set up necessary laboratory facilities at the local level to monitor treatment efficacy by performing CD4 count and possibly viral load. These techniques require expensive equipment and reagents, and extensive training for the laboratory workers. Although it is expected that the availability of "open system" machines and generic production of reagents will increase, innovative monitoring strategies and tremendous training will still be required. The MOPH is currently working in collaboration with the Harvard PHPT clinical research group in Chiang Mai to initiate a trial to compare two monitoring strategies- one based on the evolution of the CD4 count and the other on the viral load measure- for their efficiency in limiting the emergence of viral resistance in the hope of maintaining the maximum of regimen options. Combining this research project into Thailand's Global Fund program is a strategic and efficient use of the scientific resources within the country. It may, once again, prove instrumental for the future of the Thai public health policy for HIV medicine.

In contrast to the PMTCT model, which provides short term, simple ARV treatments in a standardized manner, access to care programs are much more difficult to implement. They require long term ARV treatments, good compliance, and protocols for tolerance and resistance issues, all of which need to be handled with a great deal of flexibility.

In order to assess the effectiveness of the access to care program, a comprehensive surveillance system at the national level is required to monitor both drug management and also treatment efficacy, safety, and resistance. This will help ensure the best use of expensive therapies and laboratory tests such as viral load, sequencing, and therapeutic drug monitoring.

As more and more patients receive ARV treatments over time, viruses with resistant mutations will emerge. In order to maintain clinical efficacy, patients will need to be switched to other ARV regimens. Since the priority was given to include the cheapest drugs into the first line combinations, as time passes, the number of complex cases requiring newer, more expensive drugs will add to the number of new patients needing ARV, resulting in increased costs. Generic versions of the newest ARV drugs have not been produced domestically due to Thailand's compliance with the TRIPS Agreement and intellectual property rights (IPR commission, 2002). Thailand would need to make use of the provisions laid out in the Doha Declaration for Public Health 2001, such as compulsory license or parallel import, to secure access to, or the production of generic versions of the drugs required to treat complex cases (WHO, 2002). Additionally, research into new generic combinations, formulations specific for children, and dosages adapted for Thai patients could help ensure the affordability and long term efficacy of the access to care program.

In the year 2001, the Thai government passed an historic Health Care System reform resulting in the "30 Baht policy." This new policy, highly progressive in its aim to provide universal health care, also reflects how health issues have, perhaps for the first time, risen to the forefront of the national political agenda. This policy was implemented with great speed, resulting in initial problems in areas of financial management and large influxes of patients awaiting complex and costly treatment. In response the MOPH is re-evaluating and redesigning the universal health care system to ensure that the 30 Baht system is sustainable, assessing for example, the effectiveness of decentralized financial management. Within this context, the provision of long-term ARV treatments will require significant political and financial commitment. Furthermore, the acceptability of public funding for such programs by the population at large may be challenged by conflicting demands for the use of limited financial resources in public health.

In addition to the need for a strong health care system, the involvement of patients' networks and NGOs in the provision of HIV/AIDS care is another important component to support patients receiving therapy, and could help them deal with issues of adherence, toxicity, and tolerance. The numerous organizations currently supporting people living with HIV/AIDS (PLWHA), by providing home care, income-generating activities, peer counseling, etc. will need to incorporate the ARV care component into their agenda.

To secure the successful implementation of PMTCT Plus, a prioritized aspect of Access to Care in Thailand, specific issues will have to be addressed, including the emergence of resistance to antiretrovirals provided for the prevention of mother-to-child transmission, especially nevirapine. Several studies (HIVNET 012, PACTG 316, SAINT) have reported a significant incidence of nevirapine-resistance-associated viral mutations within days to weeks after exposure (Guay *et al.*, 1999; Dorenbaum *et al.*, 2002; Moodley *et al.*, 2003; Eshleman *et al.*, 2001; Cunningham *et al.*, 2002). These mutations, which tend to fade over time, are likely associated with a subsequent decrease in efficacy of HAART regimens containing non-nucleoside reverse transcriptase inhibitors (NNRTI). Though for uninfected children the benefit associated with nevirapine is clear and permanent, solutions need to be found to overcome this issue.

CONCLUSION

Thailand has made great strides in the area of perinatal HIV prevention, and this experience offers many important lessons for both developed and developing countries. With strong political leadership through key individuals and the ministry of public health, Thailand showed how a pragmatic approach towards HIV/AIDS and public health was possible. The perinatal HIV prevention programs demonstrated the effectiveness of learning from international and domestic clinical research, experimenting with the results in small-scale pilot projects, and upon its success, scaling-up to the national level. Thailand's initiative to experiment, learn, and implement the national programs were done independently, in response to its unique needs as they emerged, and without external demands to act.

Thailand could retain its leadership in this field of PMTCT and extend it further to include PMTCT Plus and access to HAART by pursuing those strategies which have proved so effective in the past. These include informing the public, securing the human rights of patients, encouraging scientific research, using proven clinical research results for the definition of public health interventions, initiating and scaling up successful pilot programs to the national level as quickly as possible, and monitoring the effectiveness of the interventions. However, given the nature of HIV/AIDS, many challenges remain with regard to effective therapy.

REFERENCES

Ainsworth, M., Teokul, W. (2000). Breaking the silence: Setting realistic priorities for AIDS control in less-developed countries. *Lancet* 356:55–60.

Amornwichet, P., Teeraratkul, A., Simonds, R.J., Naiwatanakul, T., Chantharojwong, N., Culnane, M., Tappero, J., and Kanshana, S. (2002). Preventing mother-to-child HIV transmission. The first year of Thailand's national program. *JAMA* 288:245–248.

Berman, J. (1999). Thailand attacks AIDS with two-pronged approach. *Lancet* 353:1600.

Borand, L. (2000). Côut-efficacité de la prévention de la transmission mère-enfant du VIH dans le cadre du projet pilote du nord de la Thailande (zone 10). Master of Public Health Dissertation, Paris VI University. (Unpublished).

Brown, T., Sittitrai, W., Vanichseni, S., and Thisyakorn, U. (1994). The recent epidemiology of HIV and AIDS in Thailand. *AIDS* 8 Suppl 2:S131–S141.

Bunnell, R.E., Yanpaisarn, S., Kilmarx, P.H., Rhodes, P.H., Limpakarnjanarat, K., Srismith, R., Mastro, T., and St. Louis, M. (1999). HIV-1 seroprevalence among childbearing women in northern Thailand: monitoring a rapidly evolving epidemic. *AIDS* 13(4):509–515.

Burger, D., Boyd, M., Duncombe, C., Felderhof, M., Mahanontharit, A., Ruxrungtham, K., Ubolyam, S., Stek, M., Cooper, D., Lange, J., Phanupak, P., and Reiss, P. (2003). Pharmacokinetics and pharmacodynamics of indinavir with or without low-dose ritonavir in HIV-infected Thai patients. *J Antimicrob Chemother* 51:1231–1238.

Cardiello, P.G., Monhaphol, T., Mahanontharit, A., van Heeswijk, R.P., Burger, D., Hill, A., Ruxrungtham, K., Lange, J.M., Cooper, D.A., and Phanuphak, P. (2003). Pharmacokinetics of once-daily saquinavir hard-gelatin capsules and saquinavir soft-gelatin capsules boosted with ritonavir in HIV-1-infected subjects. *J AIDS* 32:375–379.

Cardiello, P.G., van Heeswijk, R.P., Hassink, E.A., Srasuebkul, P., Mahanontharit, A., Samor, T.M., Worarien, W., Beijnen, J.H., Hoetelmans, R.M., Ruxrungtham, K., Cooper, D.A., Lange, J.M., and Phanuphak, P. (2002). Simplifying protease inhibitor therapy with once-daily dosing of saquinavir soft-gelatin capsules/ritonavir (1600/100 mg): HIV-NAT 001.3 study. *J AIDS* 29:464–470.

Celentano, D.D., Nelson, K.E., Lyles, C.M., Beyrer, C., Eiumtrakul, S., Go, V.F., Kuntolbutra, S., and Khamboonruang, C. (1998). Decreasing incidence of HIV and sexually transmitted diseases in young Thai men: Evidence for success of the HIV/AIDS control and prevention program. *AIDS* 12:F29–F36.

Connor, E.M., Sperling, R.S., Gelber, R., Kiselev, P., Scott, G., O'Sullivan, M.J., VanDyke, R., Bey, M., Shearer, W., Jacobson, R.L., Jimenez, E., O'Neill, E., Bazin, B., Delfraissy, J.F., Culnane, M., Coombs, R., Elkins, M., Moye, J., Stratton, P., and Balsley, J. The Pediatric AIDS Clinical Trials Group Protocol 076 Study Group. (1994). Reduction of maternal-infant transmission of human immunodeficiency type I with Zidovudine treatment. *N Engl J Med* 331:1173–1180.

Cunningham, C.K., Chaix, M.L., Rekacewicz, C., Britto, P., Rouzioux, C., Gelber, R.D., Dorenbaum, A.,

Delfraissy, J.F., Bazin, B., Mofenson, L., and Sullivan, J.L. (2002). Development of resistance mutations in women receiving standard antiretroviral therapy who received intrapartum nevirapine to prevent perinatal human immunodeficiency virus type 1 transmission: A substudy of pediatric AIDS clinical trials group protocol 316. *J Infect Dis*186:181–188.

Dorenbaum, A., Cunningham, C.K., Gelber, R.D., Culnane, M., Mofenson, L., Britto, P., Rekacewicz, C., Newell, M.L., Delfraissy, J.F., Cunningham-Schrader, B., Mirochnick, M., and Sullivan, J.L. International PACTG 316 Team. (2002). Two-dose intrapartum/newborn nevirapine and standard antiretroviral therapy to reduce perinatal HIV transmission: A randomized trial. *JAMA* 288:189–198.

Dunn, D.T., Newell, M.L., Ades, A.E., and Peckham, C.S. (1992). Risk of human immunodeficiency virus type 1 transmission through breastfeeding. *Lancet* 340:585–588.

Eshleman, S.H., Mracna, M., Guay, L.A., Deseyve, M., Cunningham, S., Mirochnick, M., Musoke, P., Fleming, T., Fowler, M., Mofenson, L., Mmiro, F., and Jackson, J. (2001). Selection and fading of resistance mutations in women and infants receiving nevirapine to prevent HIV-1 vertical transmission (HIVNET 012). *AIDS* 15:1951–1957.

Guay, L.A., Musoke, P., Fleming, T., Bagenda, D., Allen, M., Nakabiito, C., Sherman, J., Bakaki, P., Ducar, C., Deseyve, M., Emel, L., Mirochnick, M., Fowler, M.G., Mofenson, L., Miotti, P., Dransfield, K., Bray, D., Mmiro, F., and Jackson, J.B. (1999). Intrapartum and neonatal single-dose nevirapine compared with zidovudine for prevention of mother-to-child transmission of HIV-1 in Kampala, Uganda: HIVNET 012 randomised trial. *Lancet* 354:795–802.

Intaraprasert, S., Taneepanichskul, S., and Chaturachinda, K. (1996). Laparoscopic sterilisation in HIV-1 positive women. *Contraception* 56:305–307.

Intellectual Property Rights Commission. (2002). Integrating Intellectual Property Rights and Development Policy: Report of the Commission of IPR. London, (September 12, 2002); www.iprcommission.org/papers/text/final_report/reportfinal.htm

Kanshana, S. (2003). A Stepwise Approach to PMTCT of HIV: Overcoming the Barrier for Implementation and Experience from the Field. 11th Asian Congress of Pediatrics, Bangkok, November 2–5, 2003. (Unpublished).

Kanshana, S. and Kullerk, N. (1998). Situation analysis: Current interventions to reduce vertical transmission of HIV in Thailand. UNICEF office for Thailand, July. p. 37.

Kanshana, S., Thewanda, D., Teeraratkul, A., Limpakarnjanarat, K., Amornwichet, P., Kullert, N., Akksilp, S., Sereesittipitak, V., Mastro, T., and Simonds, R.J. (2000). Implementing short-course zidovudine to reduce mother-infant HIV transmission in a large pilot program in Thailand. *AIDS* 14:1617–1623.

Kanshana, S. and Simonds, R.J. (2002). National program for preventing mother-child HIV transmission in Thailand: Successful implementation and lessons learned. *AIDS* 16:953–959.

Lallemant, M., Jourdain, G., Le Cœur, S., Kim, S., Koetsawang, S., Comeau, A.M., Phoolcharoen, W., Essex, M., McIntosh, K., and Vithayasai, V., for the Perinatal HIV Prevention Trial (Thailand) Investigators. (2000). A trial of shortened zidovudine regimens to prevent mother-to-child transmission of Human Immunodeficiency Virus 1. *N Engl J Med* 343:982–991.

Lallemant, M., Jourdain, G., Le Cœur, S., Mary, JY., Koetsawang, S., McIntosh, K., Ngo-Giang-Huong, N., Kanshana, S., and Thaineua, V. (2002). Nevirapine (NVP) during labor and in the neonate significantly improves zidovudine (ZDV) prophylaxis for the prevention of perinatal HIV transmission: results of PHPT-2 first interim analysis. XIV International AIDS. Conference, Barcelona, July 7–12, 2002. [Abstract Lb0r22]. (Unpublished).

Le Coeur, S. and Lallemant, M. (1996). Breastfeeding and HIV/AIDS. In: Mann, J. and Tarantola, D. (eds.), *AIDS in the World II*, Oxford University Press, Cambridge, pp. 273–278.

Medecins San Frontieres. (2003). Drugs under the Spotlight: Sharing practical knowledge about pharmaceutical patents. www.accessmed_msf.org_documents/patents_2003.pdf

Ministry of Public Health, Division of epidemiology. (2002). http://www.aidsthai.org/aidsenglish/situation_03.html

Ministry of Public Health, Provincial Health Office, Phayao Province. (2000). Annual report. pp. 141. (in Thai).

Moodley, D., Moodley, J., Coovadia, H., Gray, G., McIntyre, J., Hofmyer, J., Nikodem, C., Hall, D., Gigliotti, M., Robinson, P., Boshoff, L., and Sullivan, J., for the South African Intrapartum Nevirapine Trial (SAINT) Investigators. (2003). A multicenter randomized controlled trial of nevirapine versus a combination of zidovudine and lamivudine to reduce intrapartum and early postpartum mother-to-child transmission of human immunodeficiency virus type 1. *J Infect Dis* 187:725–735.

Natpratan, C., Nantakwang, D., Beyrer, C., Kunawararak, P., Gunhom, C., Celentano, D.D., Nelson, K.E., and Khamboonruang, C. (1996). Feasibility of northern Thai factory workers as participants in HIV vaccine trials. *Southeast Asian J Trop Med Public Health* 27:457–462.

Nelson, K.E., Celentano, D.D., Eiumtrakol, S., Hoover, D.R., Beyrer, C., Suprasert, S., Kuntolbutra, S., and Khamboonruang, C. (1996). Changes in sexual behavior and a decline in HIV infection among young men in Thailand. *N Engl J Med* 335:297–303.

Nelson, K.E., Eiumtrakul, S., Celentano, D.D., Beyrer, C., Galai, N., Kawichai, S., and Khamboonruang, C. (2002). HIV infection in young men in northern Thailand, 1991–1998: Increasing role of injection drug use. *J AIDS* 29:62–68.

Paisarntantiwong, R., Sathapornpong, G., and Kongsin, P. (1995). Female Sterilisation Following Pregnancy among HIV-Infected Women in Vajira Hospital, 3d International Conference on AIDS in Asia and the Pacific, Chiang Mai, September 17–21, 1995, Abstract PB2102. (Unpublished).

Phoolcharoen, W., Ungchusak, K., Sittitrai, W., Brown, T. (1998). Thailand: Lessons from a strong national response to HIV/AIDS. *AIDS* 12 Suppl B: S123–S135.

Prescott, N.M. Setting priorities for government involvement with antiretrovirals. (1997). In: Van Praag, E., Fernyak, S., Katz, A. (eds.), *The implications of antiretroviral treatments.* World Health Organization, Geneva, Switzerland, pp. 57–62.

Rugpao, S., Wongpun, P., de Boer, M., Tovanabutra, S., Celentano, D., Robinson, V., Duerr, A., Nagachinta, T., Nelson, K. E., and Suriyanon, V. (1997). Factors affecting reproductive and contraceptive decision making among HIV infected partners in Northern Thailand. Fourth International Conference on AIDS in Asia and the Pacific, Manila, The Philippines, October 25–29, 1997. (Unpublished).

Ruxrungtham, K., Kroon, E.D., Ungsedhapand, C., Teeratakulpisarn, S., Ubolyam, S., Buranapraditkun, S., van Leeuwen, R., Weverling, G.J., Kunanusont, C., Lange, J.M., Cooper, D.A., and Phanuphak, P. (2000). A randomized, dose-finding study with didanosine plus stavudine versus didanosine alone in antiviral-naive, HIV-infected Thai patients. *AIDS* 14:1375–1382.

Ruxrungtham, K., Suwanagool, S., Tavel, J.A., Chuenyam, M., Kroon, E., Ubolyam, S., Buranapraditkun, S., Techasathit, W., Li, Y., Emery, S., Davey, R.T., Fosdick, L., Kunanusont, C., Lane, H.C., and Phanuphak, P., Vanguard Study Group. (2000). A randomized, controlled 24-week study of intermittent subcutaneous interleukin-2 in HIV-1 infected patients in Thailand. *AIDS* 14:2509–2513.

Ruxrungtham, K., Ubolyam, S., Hassink, E.A., Ungsedhapand, C., Kroon, E., Duncombe, C., Weverling, G.J., Nookai, S., Lange, J., Cooper, D., and Phanuphak, P. (2002). Significant differences between plasma HIV-1 RNA assays in HIV-1 subtype E infected patients treated with antiretroviral therapy. *Asian Pac J Allergy Immunol* 20:105–111.

Shaffer, N., Chuachoowong, R., Mock, P.A., Bhadrakom, C., Siriwasin, W., Young, N.L., Chotpitayasunondh, T., Chearskul, S., Roongpisuthipong, A., Chinayon, P., Karon, J., Mastro, T., and Simonds, R.J., Bangkok Collaborative Perinatal HIV Transmission Study Group. (1999). Short-course zidovudine for perinatal HIV-1 transmission in Bangkok, Thailand: A randomised controlled trial. *Lancet* 353:773–780.

Sittitrai, W., Phanuphak, P., Barry, J., and Brown, T. (1994). A survey of Thai sexual behaviour and risk of HIV infection. *Int J STD AIDS* 5(5):377–378.

Talawat, S., Dore, G.J., Le Cœur, S., and Lallemant, M. (2002). Infant feeding practices and attitudes among women with HIV infection in northern Thailand. *AIDS Care* 14:625–631.

Thaineua, V., Petchsree, S., Aree, T., Lallemant, M., Soucat, A., and Lamboray, J.L. (1998). From efficacy to effectiveness: Routine prevention of mother-to-child HIV transmission by a short course of zidovudine in northern Thailand. *South East Asian J Trop Med Publ Health* 29:429–442.

UNAIDS, WHO. (2003). AIDS epidemic update, December 2003.

Weniger, B.G., Limpakarnjanarat, K., Ungchusak, K., Thanprasertsuk, S., Choopanya, K., Vanchseni, S., Uneklabh, T., Thongcharoen, P., and Wasi, C. (1991). The epidemiology of HIV infection and AIDS in Thailand. *AIDS* 5 Suppl 2:S71–S85.

World Bank. (2000). Thailand response to AIDS. Building on Success, Confronting the future. http://www.worldbank.or.th/social/pdf/Thailand's%20Response%20to%20AIDS.pdf

World Health Organization. (2002). TRIPS, Intellectual Property Rights and Access to Medicines. WHO HIV/AIDS Antiretroviral Newsletter:8.

33

Prevention of Sexual STI/HIV Transmission in Jiangsu Province, China

Yang Haitao[1], Ding Jian-ping[1], Du Yaping[2]

[1] *Jiangsu Provincial Center for Disease Prevention and Control, Nanjing, China*
[2] *Jingjiang Epidemic Prevention and Health Station, Jingjiang, China*

INTRODUCTION

The primary transmission route for HIV in China is injecting drug use. However, the proportion of new infections transmitted sexually is increasing rapidly. Chinese government officials are responding with prevention interventions, including the 100% Condom Use Program, which has been piloted in several sites in China, including Jingjiang, in Jiangsu province. A summary of this pilot program will be presented here. This intervention shows great promise and is being scaled up in China. However, sexual transmission between high risk groups like sex workers and the general population is not being adequately targeted by current interventions. Further, the current surveillance system is not equipped to accurately detect the movement of HIV in the general population.

SEXUAL TRANSMISSION OF HIV IN CHINA

Female Sex Workers (FSW)

Although sharing injection equipment among injecting drug users (IDU) has always been the main transmission route for HIV in China, the proportion of sexually transmitted HIV infections has increased from 5.5% in 1997 to 10.9% at the end of 2002 (MoH/UNAIDS, 2003). Data from sentinel surveillance show that the HIV prevalence among sex workers is increasing, and Mother to Child Transmission (MTCT) has continued to increase since the first reported case of MTCT in 1995 (MoH/UNAIDS, 2003).

There could be as many as six million female sex workers in China, among whom, HIV prevalence could be as high as 10.3%

in some areas (Bai, 2003). Sentinal surveillance data shows that about 10% of sex workers reported always using condoms, while about 49% reported never using condoms (UNAIDS, 2003).

Men Who Have Sex with Men (MSM)

The National Center for AIDS Prevention and Control (NCAIDS) estimates that there are 8–10 million men who have sex with men (MSM) in China, among whom HIV prevalence could be as high as 2–5% in some areas (Bai, 2003). Qiu Renzhong of the Chinese Academy of Social Sciences (CASS) estimates that men who have sex with men comprise 1–3% of the total Chinese population (which at 1% is 13 million men) (Qiu, 2002). In the mid-1990s in Beijing, over 50% of reported HIV cases were MSM (Zhang, 2001).

Migrant Workers

Approximately 80–120 million people are migrant workers, or members of the "floating population". Long distance truck drivers, a subpopulation of migrant workers, are identified nationally as a high-risk group and included in national and provincial sentinel surveillance. In a survey on long-distance truck drivers in Shandong, 7% were found to have an STI. However, there are no education or prevention interventions targeted towards this group, or to the larger group of migrant workers (MoH/UNAIDS, 1997).

Young People

The National Center for AIDS Prevention and Control estimates that about 364 million Chinese are young, unmarried, sexually active, and lacking in proper knowledge about safe sexual practices (Bai, 2003).

Former Plasma Donors

Other routes of sexually transmitted HIV-infection include secondary infections from HIV-infected former plasma donors, which have contributed to extremely high HIV prevalence rates in some villages in Henan and other provinces. In these villages, many poor farmers were infected by selling their plasma. Their blood was pooled with others' blood of the same type as the plasma was extracted, then a portion of this pooled blood was transfused back into the donors, a practice intended to prevent anemia, ensuring HIV infection of all donors in the pool if even one was previously infected (SCMP, 2002).

STI Patients

Through HIV testing among STI patients, NCAIDS estimates that prevalence in this group ranges somewhere between 2–8% (Bai, 2003). The sexual risk behaviors of this group, as evidenced by the spread of STI, provide another route for the sexual transmission of HIV in China.

PREVENTION OF SEXUAL TRANSMISSION: JIANGSU PROVINCE

This section presents a case study of Jiangsu Province. Unless otherwise noted, statistics on STIs and demographics in Jiangsu province in the following sections are unpublished statistics from the Jiangsu Provincial CDC.

There is evidence that risky sexual behavior is increasing in Jiangsu: it has the highest reported STI rates in the country (although this is probably due in part to the design of the reporting system). Rates of STI have been increasing steadily since 1990.

Jiangsu, like many other provinces in China, is investing heavily in transportation infrastructure. Several expressways and ports are under construction or have recently been completed. Typically such projects are built by a male migrant labor force, housed in single-sex dormitories near the construction site. A survey of construction workers in Jiangsu's floating population found that 4% had an STI (MoH/UNAIDS, 1997). It is common for FSW to establish themselves near such sites. There are an estimated 4.5 million migrant workers in Jiangsu, about half natives of the province and the other half having come from other provinces to work in Jiangsu. 88% of FSW in Jiangsu report never using a condom, while 0.4% report always using a condom.

100% Condom Use Program in Jingjiang, Jiangsu

Data from the 100% Condom Use Program in Jingjiang comes from the summary report of the project, an unpublished report compiled by staff members from the Jiangsu Provincial CDC and the Jingjiang Health and Anti-epidemic Station (Yang *et al.*, 2003).

The 100% Condom Use Program (100% CUP) among establishment-based sex workers was initiated in Ratchaburi Province, Thailand in 1989. Since then, such programs have been expanded nationally in Thailand in 1991, piloted in Cambodia in 1998, expanded nationally there in 2000, and piloted in China beginning in 2001 (Bai, 2003).

In China, 100% CUP is being rolled out in phases. It was first piloted in Jiangsu and Hubei provinces, next in Hunan and Hainan. The next provinces to launch pilot sites will be Sichuan, Shanxi, Yunnan, and Guangxi (Bai, 2003).

In March of 2001, Jingjiang, a city in Jiangsu, was selected as a pilot site for 100% CUP, a WHO supported program which had been successful in Thailand and Cambodia. Situated at the crossroads between the northern and southern parts of the province, near the Yangtze River, two and half hours drive from the capital city of Nanjing, Jingjiang is a common stopping point for travelers. The total population is 666,000, 250,000 of which live in the city. Of these, 150,000 are residents and approximately 100,000 are migrant workers. The incidence of STIs in Jingjiang is about average for Jiangsu province.

Nearly 100 Entertainment Establishments (EEs) where commercial sex work takes place were identified in Jingjiang for the purposes of the pilot program. Sex work is mainly concentrated in bathhouses and sauna centers, usually in small single rooms designated for massages. The total number of women who self-identified as sex workers in the EEs varies, from over 1000 in the peak season (winter) to 500 in the slower season (summer).

The overall objectives of the pilot 100% CUP program were as follows: 1) Determine the extent of HIV/AIDS awareness, risk behavioral characteristics, and STI infections among FSW, 2) establish an effective intervention model including all establishments which provide sex services, and 3) explore the potential for the effectiveness of the 100% CUP program in the context of China's culture, laws, and policies while collecting information helpful to the formulation of HIV/AIDS policy and interventions.

To achieve these objectives, 100% CUP employs the following strategies: provide education about STI/HIV transmission and prevention and condom use, persuade FSW to use condoms consistently and teach them how to persuade clients to use condoms, distribute IEC (Information, Education, and Communication) materials as teaching aids, provide education about where to obtain condoms and how to determine condom quality, refer clients and others with STIs to the project clinics, trace sexual contacts of STI infected patients, provide disincentives for EEs failing to comply with 100% CUP policies.

Phase I: Preparation, Training, and Baseline Survey

In March 2001, a steering committee composed of the Vice Mayor of Jingjiang government, officials of health department, public security, culture department, industrial and commercial administrative management department was formed. The project office was established, employing people from the county, municipal and provincial levels.

Six local STI clinics were evaluated by the National Center for STD Control (located in Nanjing, Jiangsu). The local health department and the 100% CUP office worked with these clinics to correct problems identified during this evaluation. Counseling rooms and additional testing equipment were added to STI clinics. The local STI surveillance system was expanded.

IEC materials were designed and produced for 100% CUP and distributed to EEs. Large scale HIV/AIDS awareness efforts were focused on Jingjiang around World AIDS Days 2001 and 2002.

Since November of 2001, 52 condom vending machines have been installed around the EEs. The quality of condoms available on the local market was evaluated and a system put in place for monitoring the distribution and quality of local condoms.

Workshops on STI/HIV counseling skills, STI comprehensive services, outreach skills, development of effective IEC materials, and the fundamentals of 100% CUP were given for local health professionals and program staff. A series of seminars and meetings on STI/HIV awareness and 100% CUP was organized for the owners of local EEs.

During the baseline study, in late 2001, 355 FSW were interviewed, and 303 samples were collected for testing. The majority of the FSW, at the age of 17–39 years old, migrated from rural areas within Jiangsu and from other provinces. 70.98% had junior high school level education, 54.08% were unmarried, and 41.41% were married. Many were highly mobile and usually stayed at an establishment for less than three months (50.90%).

The mean number of sexual partners in the last week (preceding the day of the interview) was 6.54. 52.61% of the respondents had regular boyfriends or sexual partners outside of providing commercial sex services.

In the three months preceding the interview, 31% of the respondents reported consistent condom use, 35% frequent use, 11% occasional use, and 23% no use; 56% reported condom use during their last sexual encounter. 55% of respondents bought condoms at private healthcare shops, 39% at pharmacies. 96% of the respondents would ask the clients to use a condom; however, if the clients didn't want to, 9% would still provide sex services, and 28% of the respondents may still provide sex services, depending on the price and on whether the client's genitals appeared healthy. 97% of respondents found it convenient to obtain condoms in Jingjiang.

Though 95% of the FSW had heard of STI and 97% heard of AIDS, 21% did not know the common STIs or how they are transmitted; 17% did not know how HIV was transmitted. They had obtained their STI/HIV/AIDS knowledge from doctors, health education, television, and print media.

Based on laboratory tests and clinical examinations, 25% of the FSW were diagnosed with an STI (gonorrhea: 3%, chlamydia: 21%, syphilis: 0.33%, condyloma acurinatum: 2.31%), none were found to be HIV-positive.

The results of baseline survey demonstrated that unprotected sexual practices, lack of knowledge, and high prevalence of STI have put the FSW at risk of HIV infection. Comprehensive measures (including an IEC campaign, provision of affordable STI services, and supply of good quality condoms) are necessary to mitigate this risk. The local 100% CUP pilot was approved as a means by which to do this.

From June of 2002 to May of 2003, program staff traced the sexual contacts of 164 male STI cases treated in the project clinic; of them, 75 cases were linked with the EEs. 150 STI cases have been diagnosed in the project surveillance clinic, of them 22 cases were FSWs. All the cases were given services such as counseling, sex partner tracing and condom use education. Owners of EEs linked to these infections were warned.

Phase 2: Implementation

Beginning in January of 2002, program staff visited EEs regularly to provide behavior change education, disseminate IEC materials, and establish good relationships with owners and FSW. STI cases among FSW discovered during the baseline survey exams were followed up with treatment. EEs linked with male STI through contact tracing were given warnings. In 2002 and 2003, 5,000 FSW were reached with 18 different variations of education interventions. Because of the mobility and turnover of FSW, program staff tried to visit EEs often, and employ many different modes of communication and education.

Phase 3: Monitoring and Evaluation

A rapid assessment was done in May 2002, followed by Stage 1 Evaluation in November 2002 and Stage 2 Evaluation in April 2003:

After the project was initiated, the rates of reported condom use went up steadily, with both commercial and non-commercial sex partners.

Based on laboratory tests and clinical examinations, the total STI prevalence rates in the first and second stage evaluation were 24.7% and 14.10%, respectively.

The quarterly distribution of condoms was monitored: it grew steadily over the course of the pilot program, from 50,000 during the second quarter of 2001 to 1,230,000 during the second quarter of 2003.

Awareness about STI/HIV transmission and prevention among FSW increased in some key areas, but the results were not consistent. For example, only 35% knew how HIV was transmitted at the time of the baseline survey; at the time of the Stage 1 evaluation, this number had increased to nearly 75%. However, the percentage of respondents correctly answering that question actually decreased between the Stage 1 and Stage 2 evaluations, with the final result being about 62%.

Challenges and Lessons Learned

According to NCAIDS, the biggest challenges for 100% CUP in China have been: mobility of sex workers, condom quality and distribution, police crackdowns on prostitution, sustainability, and scale-up (Bai, 2003). Challenges to the implementation and success of 100% CUP in Jingjiang included (Yang *et al.*, 2003):

- non-standard or sub-standard care in STI clinics;

TABLE 1. Consistent Use of Condoms among FSW in Entertainment Establishments in Jingjiang (%)

			At last sexual encounter	
	In the last three months	In the last week	With commercial sex partner	With non-commercial sex partner
Baseline Survey (2001.11)	31.1	38.1	74.9	27.2
Rapid Assessment (2002.6)	46.00	62.0	84.4	33.3
Stage Evaluation 1 (2002.11)	57.69	75.1	89.1	55.3
Stage Evaluation 2[a] (2003.4)	74.2	87.6	92.3	68.5

Source: (Yang, *et al.*, 2003)
[a] The increase in consistent condom use from the Baseline Survey to the Stage 2 evaluation was statistically significant ($P < 0.01$) in each case.

TABLE 2. Prevalence of STI/HIV Among FSW in Entertainment Establishments in Jingjiang (%)

	Gonorrhea	Chlamydia	Condyloma acurinatum	Syphilis	HIV	Total
Method	Culture	"Clearview"	Clinical Symptoms	Clinical Symptoms	ELISA	
Baseline Survey (2001.11)	3.3	21.12	2.31	0.33	0	25.08
Stage Evaluation 1 (2002.11)	7.57	17.93	2.39	0	0	24.70
Stage Evaluation 2 (2003.4)	—	13.68	0.85	0	0	14.10

Source: Yang, *et al.*, 2003

TABLE 3. STI/HIV Transmission and Prevention Awareness Among FSW in Entertainment Establishments in Jingjiang

Knowledge		Baseline survey	Rapid assessment	Stage evaluation 1	Stage evaluation 2
6 common STDs	Correct	3.81	15.38		
	Partially correct	70.84	61.54		
	Didn't know	20.95	23.08		
Modes of HIV transmission	Correct	35.06	61.54	74.62	61.76
	Partially correct	46.26	15.38	20.08	27.94
	Didn't know	18.68	23.08	5.30	10.29
How to avoid HIV transmission	Correct	7.53	30.77	51.31	45.59
	Partially correct	65.22	61.54	43.82	43.38
	Didn't know	27.25	7.69	4.87	11.03

Source: Yang, *et al.*, 2003

- failure to track information on sexual contacts of male STI patients;
- unwillingness of STI clinics to distribute information about condom use;
- lack of/difficulty of enforcement of relevant public health laws and regulations for entertainment establishments;
- difficulty of evaluating project's effect given the constant mobility of the target population; and
- irregular quality of condoms available on the local market.

The Jingjiang pilot project staff found that the keys to successfully implementing 100% CUP were: government commitment; multisectoral collaboration between health, public security, family planning, and information/propaganda; policies issued jointly by different government sectors (particularly a cooperative agreement on strengthening the prevention and control of STI/HIV issued by the health and public security bureaus of Jingjiang); identification and training of a capable and experienced team; up to date knowledge on outreach work, counseling, and development of effective IEC materials; and education targeted not only towards FSW, but to the general population, in order to raise awareness about prevention and about the program's merit (Yang *et al.*, 2003).

Prevention Efforts Targeted towards the General Population

In Jiangsu, middle and high school students are taught nationally standardized content on health and sexually transmitted infections. The Jiangsu CDC's HIV/AIDS section provides educational materials for distribution at universities and in public places around World AIDS Day. They also try to utilize media outlets (newspapers, radio, television) to distribute information to the public. The provincial Health Education Institute holds educational events and distributes materials at business centers and universities. Some hospitals provide pamphlets and counseling to pregnant women, engaged couples, and in some workplaces (Meyers and Stiefvater, 2002).

No measures are in place, with the exception of the 100% CUP pilot in which sexual contacts of FSW are being tracked, to target any of the bridges into the general population.

Thc current surveillance system in Jiangsu is not equipped to detect an emerging HIV epidemic in the general population, since little testing is done outside of high risk groups. This is a common problem in many countries. However, there are examples in which testing of certain groups of the general population has been initiated and has served as an important indicator. For example, after preliminary data showed that about 450 members of its force of 38,000 tested positive for HIV, the Mumbai, India police department plans to build a database of the HIV status of its employees, and to implement an AIDS awareness program in which over 800 police officers have already been trained to participate. In addition, all police officers will undergo mandatory HIV testing every six months. The department is also trying to identify how the police were infected: it is well-known that some Mumbai police officers are customers of sex workers (Kaisernetwork.org, 2004) Currently, there are no programs like this in China, in which large numbers of "upstanding citizens" are being tested for HIV.

RISKS FOR A GENERALIZED EPIDEMIC: JIANGSU AS A CASE STUDY

Located on the eastern coast of China, Jiangsu is one of China's strongest provincial economies. Average per capita income ranges from RMB 10,000 (US$1200) in Kunshan (near Shanghai) to RMB 4000 (US$480) in Xuzhou (near the border with Henan in the northern part of the province). Jiangsu's HIV/AIDS budget has significantly increased over the last few years. It increased from RMB 1.2 million (US$145,000) in 2001 to RMB 3.5 million (US$423,000) in 2002.

HIV/AIDS classifies as a low-level epidemic in Jiangsu, according to UNAIDS/WHO guidelines; HIV prevalence has not consistently exceeded 5% in any defined subpopulation, although HIV infection has existed for many years.

Bridges from High-Risk Groups to the General Population

Sex between female sex workers and their clients is an obvious bridge between a "high-risk" group and the general population. One study found that "rich men" are ten times as likely to visit a FSW than physical laborers in a city, and 22 times as likely as a man from a rural area (Pan, 2001).

It is generally known that it is not uncommon for businessmen and government employees (often married) to be clients of sex workers (Meyers and Stiefvater, 2002). However, no surveillance measures are currently in place to identify HIV-infection in these specific groups. HIV-infection in these men would only be detected if they submitted to an HIV test prior to giving blood or having surgery, during a pre-marital check up, at an STI clinic, or at a voluntary testing site (Meyers and Stiefvater, 2002).

Other high risk groups also provide bridges for HIV to move into the general population. As 10% of China's population continues to "float", many of them maintain sexual contacts in their hometowns, as well as in the cities in which they are working. Most MSM in China have wives or girlfriends, and many also have children. Former plasma donors—mostly farmers—have unknowingly spread HIV to their wives and children, causing prevalence rates in many villages to reach crisis proportions.

HIV Surveillance in the General Population: Jiangsu Province

Jiangsu's HIV/AIDS surveillance (like China's national surveillance system) is focused on the following high-risk groups: STI patients, FSW, IDU, blood donors, and long distance truck drivers. Surveillance activities are focused on these groups via testing at national as well as provincial sentinel surveillance sites.

Members of the general population currently being tested for HIV may not be a representative sample. There are 202 screening labs in Jiangsu that carry out routine HIV/AIDS testing; these include comprehensive hospitals, mother-child hospitals, STI clinics, blood collection stations, and the HIV/AIDS section of the CDC. The test cost 90RMB in 2002 (13% of the average monthly income of a Nanjing resident, and 27% of the average monthly income in a poorer rural area) at most clinics and is more expensive in some hospitals (Meyers and Stiefvater, 2002). The number of people who test positive through routine surveillance is very low, and HIV/AIDS section staff suspect that those who do test positive are actually members of high risk groups.

Members of the general population tested through routine surveillance include surgery patients, pregnant women (but not all pregnant women), blood donors, and voluntary testers (Meyers and Stiefvater, 2002). In China's rapidly reforming health system, patients pay most medical costs out of pocket, so it is possible that surgery patients represent a higher-than-average income group.

Prenatal care is not routine for all pregnant women; it is much more common in urban than rural areas and is more common for higher income women. It may be that the pregnant women tested are more urban and higher-income, and therefore have better access to education and health care, than a random sample of pregnant women.

The government's campaign to encourage blood donations through government work units and university campuses uses a quota system that requires certain employees and students to donate blood twice per year. These "model citizens" may not represent the average citizen.

So far, relatively few HIV cases have been discovered through voluntary testing in China. In Jiangsu province, this number is zero (Meyers and Stiefvater, 2002). However, the number of voluntary testers remains very low. CDC staff report that most voluntary testers believe they have engaged in risky behavior, so they would expect a positive correlation between voluntary testing and likelihood of HIV infection. However, voluntary testing is likely also correlated with a higher than average level of HIV/AIDS awareness, which may lessen an individual's overall likelihood of HIV infection. Since rates of voluntary testing still remain so low, the statistical characteristics of the voluntary testing population are not yet well-known (Meyers and Stiefvater, 2002).

CONCLUSION

Interventions to prevent sexual transmission of HIV are increasing in number and scale in China. 100% CUP is an example of one such program that is currently being scaled up. Results of pilot programs show that this program can be used to increase condom usage, foster multisectoral cooperation, improve STI and HIV surveillance data, collect data on FSW and STI patient sexual contacts, and curb sexual risk behaviors.

However, the focus of most promising interventions is only on high risk groups. They indirectly protect the general population by preventing further infection in these high risk groups. 100% CUP sets a good example by building in a component of the intervention that traces sexual contacts of FSW. However, few efforts target the general population or these bridge groups into the general population specifically.

Because of the presence of HIV in high-risk groups, evidence of sexual risk behaviors in the general population resulting in STIs, the many bridges connecting high risk groups to the general population, and the lack of accurate HIV prevalence data on the general population, there is potential in China for a hidden epidemic. The current surveillance system may not detect such an epidemic in the general population until many more people become symptomatic, potentially years after they were infected.

Continued and expanded emphasis on behavioral surveillance is needed to find out more about the sexual contacts of high risk groups. Some of this data is already being collected, as part of 100% CUP and as part of MSM interventions in Heilongjiang and other places. The next step is deciding what to do with such data. Will HIV-positive people be counseled to share their status with their sexual contacts? Can more information about these sexual contacts lead to the design of better educational materials, media campaigns, and more targeted behavioral interventions? Results of another 100% CUP pilot suggest that peer education should accompany 100% condom use programs and recommend that new HIV interventions target the partners of sex workers. (Kim *et al.*, 2002)

Finally, national and provincial surveillance efforts must continue efforts to increase voluntary counseling and testing in the general population and to improve surveillance data on prevalence in the general population.

REFERENCES

Bai, Y. (2003). 100% Condom Use Program in China. Presentation available online at http://www.chain.net.cn/PDF/P7.pdf. National Center for AIDS Prevention and Control, Beijing, China (July 23, 2003).

Kaisernetwork.org. (2004). Mumbai, India, Police Dept. Mandates HIV Testing, Creates AIDS Awareness Program After 450 Officers Test HIV-Positive. (report summarized from a *Times of India* report, 1/8/04) (January 9, 2004) http://www.kaisernetwork.org/daily_reports/rep_index.cfm?hint=1&DR_ID=21587.

Kim, A., Samnang, P., BunLeng, H., Van Griensven, G.J.P., Mandel, J., Page-Shafer, K. (2002). HIV and correlates of consistent condom use among fishermen who have sex with sex workers, SihanoukVille, Cambodia, 2000. AIDS Research Institute, University of California San Francisco, poster presented at the International AIDS Conference, Barcelona, July 2002.

Meyers, K. and Stiefvater, E. (2002) Preparing for Crisis: Jiangsu, China's AIDS Response. Paper submitted in fulfillment of the Master in Public Policy thesis requirement at the John F. Kennedy School of Government at Harvard University. (April 2002) (unpublished paper).

Ministry of Health, China (MoH)/Joint United Nations Program on HIV/AIDS (UNAIDS). (1997). China Responds to AIDS: HIV/AIDS Situation and Needs Assessment Report. Jointly prepared by MoH and the UN Theme Group on HIV/AIDS in China. (November, 1997).

Ministry of Health, China (MoH)/Joint United Nations Program on HIV/AIDS (UNAIDS). (2003). A Joint Assessment of HIV/AIDS Prevention, Care, and Treatment in China. UN Theme Group on HIV/AIDS in China. (December 1, 2003).

Pan, S. (2001). Draft paper presented at the 1st Annual National AIDS Conference in Beijing, China. (November, 2001).

Qiu, R. (2002). Draft Proposal to the Legislation and Law Reform in Relation to AIDS in the People's Republic of China. (January 2002) (unpublished document).

South China Morning Post. (2002). Taskforce supervises Aids relief efforts. October 28, 2002.

United Nations Joint Program on AIDS (UNAIDS). (2003) www.unaids.com, accessed November 15, 2003.

Yang, H., Du, Y., Ding, J., Qian, W., Li, L., Zhou, Z. (2003) China/Jiangsu 100% Condom Use Programme Summary Report. China/Jiangsu 100% CUP Office (September 14, 2003) (unpublished).

Zhang, B. (2001). Consensus and Suggestions on Homosexuality and related AIDS Issues. The Group of Friends Exchange. Qingdao, China.

V

The Decisive Battleground

Collaborations, Impacts, and Potential Forces

34

AIDS in Asia

What Can We Learn from the Rest of the World?

Alan Whiteside

Health Economics and HIV/AIDS Research Division, University of KwaZulu-Natal Durban, South Africa; School of Tropical Medicine, University of Liverpool

INTRODUCTION

In many parts of Asia, HIV/AIDS is a relatively recent phenomenon; not many Asians (outside of the HIV/AIDS community) honestly believe that it is or will be an issue for the continent. But there is no room for complacency. Indeed, there is a growing fear that parts of Asia may experience an explosive epidemic. In Bangkok in September 2003, Dr. Nafis Sadik (2003), Special Envoy of the Secretary-General for HIV/AIDS in Asia and the Pacific, warned Asian leaders of the impending epidemic. He noted that although adult HIV prevalence rates exceed 1% in only three countries, there are severe localized outbreaks in several countries, including India and China.

One of the earliest lessons learned from the HIV/AIDS epidemic was that it leads to denial and stigmatization. This, in turn, made dealing with the disease more difficult. During the early identification of the disease in the USA, it was linked with homosexuals, Haitians and hemophiliacs, and in the case of the first two was thought to be linked to lifestyle (Shilts, 1987). These communities suffered blame and stigmatization. The idea that HIV was associated with particular groups also led to denial that it was a problem for those outside of those groups. This was extended to nationalities and indeed continents.

The same pattern of stigmatization was seen in Africa. AIDS was regarded as someone else's problem. The Ugandans (who were among the first to be open about the disease and discuss it) believed that the initial impetus for the spread of HIV was the invasion of the Tanzanian army in 1979. In South Africa, it was regarded as a central African problem.

Globally, for the past 15 years, AIDS has been indelibly associated with Africa. The image on CNN is of skeletal adults dying miserably in the corner of some mud and thatch hut, and of wide-eyed, ragged and malnourished but photogenic orphans. When the global community thinks of AIDS, it is generally an African picture that springs to mind. This is misplaced.

The most rapidly rising epidemic curves are among some drug using populations in Eastern Europe. This has been mirrored in Indonesia, where HIV has been seen in 26 of the 30 provinces and HIV prevalence rose from zero to 50% between 1998 and 2001 in a Jakarta clinic (UNAIDS, 2002b). The country with the second largest number of AIDS cases in the world is India. At the end of 2001, the last year for which there is data, it was estimated that there were about four million people living with HIV in India. This was exceeded only by the 5 million infected South Africans. The next closest was Nigeria with 3.5 million infections (UNAIDS, 2002b). Soon China and India will have the bulk of the world's HIV/AIDS cases; UNAIDS estimates that there will be 10 million cases in China by 2010 (UNAIDS, 2003) while at a 2002 Centre for Strategic and International Studies conference, Mrs. Ghosh, the project director of the Indian National AIDS Control Organization warned that if the country achieved its epidemic control objectives there would be nine million HIV infections by 2006 and if there was a 50% slippage the number of infections would rise to 14.7 million (Center for Strategic and International Studies, 2002).

Despite this there is a general unwillingness to learn from Africa or indeed even to engage with the African experience. Between 1996 and 2002, I co-directed training workshops on "Planning for HIV/AIDS in Developing Countries" in India, Nepal, Malaysia and the Philippines, and as a result, interacted with participants from every Asian country apart from the Central Asian Republics of the former Soviet Union. The one message we were constantly given by senior officials and sponsors was: "Don't mention Africa—Asia is not like Africa, and people will be offended by the comparison." This apparent racism was also evident when we worked in Eastern Europe, only here the message was: "Don't mention Africa or Asia—we are not like those people". (In fairness to the participants in the workshops, they were almost all open-minded and willing to learn from the African experience; the problem lay at the donor and senior government level.)

It is against this background that this chapter is being written. The reality is that we all have much to learn from each other. Most of Asia is fortunate, in that the epidemic has not taken hold and the successes and failures of prevention in the rest of the world can still be applied. Equally, where there is an epidemic, we need to look at the impact in places that are further ahead, and work out strategies for mitigation. As treatment options expand, lessons can be applied from one resource-poor environment to another.

In this chapter, I will explore what Asia can learn from the rest of the world. The chapter will look at the drivers of the epidemic and the responses to it, warning that the western biomedical response is inadequate. In the second part of the chapter, I build on the drivers to look at a paradigm for understanding why the epidemic has spread in some parts of the world and not in others. We will see how this might be applied in Asia. The third part of the chapter looks at denial and division and identifies this as the main area where Asia needs to learn from the rest of the world. Finally, I bring together the discussion in a conclusion that seeks to draw out the main lessons.

THE DRIVERS OF THE EPIDEMIC

In some sub-Saharan African countries, over 30% of adults are infected, while in others, HIV is relatively under control. Haiti has an adult HIV prevalence of 6.1% while the contiguous Dominican Republic has one of 2.5%. In Asia, adult prevalence in Cambodia is 2.7%, in neighboring Vietnam it is 0.3%, while in Laos it is estimated to be less than 0.1%. Why is there this difference across and within continents?

The first lesson is that AIDS is not globally an homogenous epidemic. But it also

TABLE 1. Understanding the Determinants of HIV/AIDS

	Distal determinants		Proximal determinants	
Determinants	Macro-environment	Micro-environment	Behaviour	Biology
	Wealth	Mobility	Rate of partner change	Virus sub-types
	Income distribution	Urbanisation	Prevalence of concurrent partners	Stage of infection
	Culture	Access to health care	Sexual mixing patterns	Presence of other STDs
	Religion	Levels of violence	Sexual practices and condom use	Gender
	Governance	Women's rights and status	Breast feeding	Circumcision
		Health resources	Drug use patterns	Drug use Blood and medical safety
Interventions	Social policy—redistribution Legal Reform— Human Rights Taxation Debt relief Terms of Trade	Social Policy Economic Policy Legal Reform Employment legislation	Behaviour change communication Condom promotion and marketing	STD treatment Blood safety Anti-retroviral therapy during pregnancy

Source: Barnett *et al.*, 2000

varies within countries. What is unique about Asia is the size of the populations and the countries. The epidemiology of the epidemic in Asia is discussed elsewhere in this volume and here we will only draw examples to illustrate specific cases.

Understanding the differences in epidemics means understanding the drivers of HIV/AIDS. A methodology for this is illustrated in Table 1.

The first set of drivers are medical-clinical factors that help in explaining why people become infected if they are exposed to HIV. This is shown in the column 'biology' of Table 1. This is also the 'modern', western interpretation: the view that HIV/AIDS is a problem of the body alone. If that view is accepted, then HIV/AIDS will be seen as a problem to be solved by medical science, clinical practices, epidemiological knowledge and behavioral interventions.

Thus far, the history of interventions in the HIV/AIDS epidemic shows the dominance of the clinical-medical approach in dealing with an epidemic of infectious, sexually-transmitted disease. This trend is continuing with the Global Fund and the recent World Health Organization (WHO) initiatives and their current emphasis on the idea of anti-retroviral therapy. There has been consistent opposition to the medicalization of the disease and oversimplification of the response. This was epitomized by the late Jonathan Mann and his associates at the WHO/GPA and at the Francois-Xavier Bagnoud Center for Health and Human Rights at Harvard University. They saw HIV/AIDS as more than a medical-clinical problem, one that required a broader perspective. The link they developed was between HIV/AIDS, health and human rights. We need to go further than this.

The third column of Table 1 adds behavior to the drivers. In order for a person to be exposed to HIV and have a chance of being infected they need to have certain behaviors. (The exception to this is mother to child transmission, where the risk for the infant is determined by the mother's HIV status and the access to drugs.)

Adding behavior to the diagram moved the focus of concern away from the body to the mind. This was an improved conceptual approach, and indicated further possible interventions and areas of engagement with the disease. The biological goal of any program aimed at tackling an epidemic disease is to reduce the rate of transmission by intervening in the process of disease communication from one individual to another. In the case of sexually transmitted disease, this meant a focus on the "core transmitters". In the drug-driven epidemics, it meant trying to identify the drug users and intervene with them (needle exchanges were very successful in some settings—but in others the more draconian method of identifying and arresting people has been tried).

In order for people to have behaviors which result in them being exposed to HIV, we need to understand that they operate in a micro- and a macro- environment. The whole story of how epidemics come into existence, who has the highest likelihood of being infected and therefore who is most exposed, is indicated by the first two columns in Table 1. Epidemic disease, and HIV/AIDS in particular, is indeed a disease of the body—but that is only the presenting symptom. The epidemic is more deeply seated. An HIV/AIDS epidemic reveals many of the fractures, stresses and strains in a society. Concern with medical-clinical issues and with individual behavior change, to the almost total exclusion of the structural and distributional factors which result in those behaviors, has had serious implications. In particular, the links between poverty and disease have been obscured (for example, Wilkinson, 1986; Fox, 1989; Blaxter, 1990; Backlund *et al.*, 1996). These are the areas where policy is likely to require a long term perspective and is most likely to run into the problem where people throw up their hands, saying that it is all too complicated or impossible. Their reaction is to stick to the easier, more familiar and pragmatic interventions that can be undertaken with individuals: the biomedical and behavioral responses.

Are there drivers that are peculiar to different part of the world? The vast majority of infections in Africa have been heterosexually transmitted and Table 1 was originally developed for the African setting. In Asia, the situation is complex but at present the epidemic is concentrated (and spreading) in specific population groups chiefly injecting drug users, sex workers, men who have sex with men, and people exposed through unsafe medical practices. Some of the Asian drivers have been added to the table and it can be developed further.

According to the UNAIDS December 2002 epidemic update: "Throughout the region, injecting drug use offers the epidemic huge scope for growth. Upwards of 50% of injecting drug users already have acquired the virus in parts of Malaysia, Myanmar, Nepal, Thailand and in Manipur in India, while HIV infections among Indonesia's growing population of injecting drug users is soaring" (UNAIDS, 2002a). This report also noted that high rates of needle-sharing have been documented among users in Bangladesh and Viet Nam and there was evidence that "a considerable proportion" of street-based sex workers in Viet Nam also inject drugs (a phenomenon detected in other countries, too). The 2003 epidemic update includes data from Guangxi province in China and Ho Chi Minh in Vietnam. In Guangxi HIV prevalence among IDU rose from zero to over 15% between 1996 and 2000, Ho Chi Minh it rose from zero in 1992 to over 80% in 2001. (UNAIDS, 2003).

Male-to-male sex occurs in all countries of the region and features significantly in the epidemic. Countries that have measured HIV prevalence among men who have sex with men have found it to be high—14% in Cambodia in 2000 and roughly the same level among male Thai sex workers. (UNAIDS, 2002a). The cultural norms mean that lots of men who have sex with men hide that aspect of their sexuality. Many might marry and have sexual relationships with women.

In Thailand, meanwhile, recent modeling suggests that the main modes of transmission have been changing. Whereas most HIV transmission in the 1990s occurred through commercial sex, half of the new HIV infections now appear to be occurring among the wives and sexual partners of men who were infected several years ago. There are also indications that unsafe sexual behavior is on the increase among young Thais (UNAIDS, 2002a).

In China and, to a lesser extent, India, there have been reports of significant transmission as a result of unsafe medical practices, in particular, the use of untested blood. We have no way of knowing how many people have sero-converted as a result of this—the data are simply not available, but there are some indications of the scale of the problem. In India, the National AIDS Control Organization listed risk/transmission categories and in 2001, of AIDS cases, 4.1% were infected through contaminated blood or blood products (Barnett and Whiteside, 2002). In China, it was estimated that 9.7% of HIV cases were transmitted through illegal blood plasma collection. (Center for Strategic and International Studies, 2002). In a number of Chinese villages, blood donations were taken from villagers for plasma extraction and pooled by blood type, then transfused back into the donors. A more efficient way of spreading HIV would be hard to find. In many other Asian countries, the practice of paying donors resulted in contaminated blood being collected.

There is a need for actions to be taken in terms of the biological and behavioral columns in Table 1. Indeed, the point about the interventions in the table is that these responses remain valid, but have more chance of success if they are supported by the other responses. Blood safety, for example, is crucial. (Indeed this was an early response in Uganda, Zimbabwe and South Africa). Condoms are effective but problematic, in part because they require male compliance. Treating other sexually transmitted infections reduces rates of HIV transmission, but there are questions as to the sustainability and cost of such programs. Behavior change interventions do work as long as they are maintained. This has been seen in the US and Western gay male communities, Thai brothels, and among intravenous drug users with needle exchange programs in the UK and the Netherlands. But these interventions are aimed at core transmitters. In epidemics that spread beyond core transmitters, such strategies will not be adequate.

THE JAIPUR PARADIGM: AN APPROACH TO EXPLAINING AND PREDICTING THE HIV EPIDEMIC

What was lacking in epidemiological analysis developed to respond to the epidemic was a way of predicting if HIV might move beyond core transmitters. Here we turn to the "Jaipur Paradigm" (named the Jaipur Paradigm because the initial ideas were developed with participants at a Policy Research Workshop at the Indian Institute of Health Management Research in Jaipur, India in 1996). The paradigm evolved because attempts to explain the different profiles of HIV epidemics by developing indices or measures of correlation had not been successful (Fransen and Whiteside, 1995; Filmer, 1996). Some African countries with high scores on income and development indexes, for instance, have very serious HIV epidemics, while in others the epidemic seemed to have stabilised despite poor economic performance and slow development.

We developed an hypothesis that the susceptibility of a society to HIV spread, and thereby the profile of its epidemic, are determined by two variables:

- the degree of social cohesion;
- the overall level of wealth.

This paradigm has been presented and published in a number of fora (Barnett *et al*, 2000a; Barnett and Whiteside, 2002), and judging by the way it has been taken up is regarded as a useful framework for analysis (UNAIDS and International Institute of Migration, 2003; Fourie and Schönteich, 2001).

Social cohesion is an analytical concept used without value judgement. It may be the expression of cultural homogeneity of a society, the product of good governance and a strong civil society, related to a prescriptive religious culture, or the result of a controlling authoritarian political system or military dictatorship. While cohesion may be a deciding factor in determining a society's susceptibility to HIV infection, the analysis can not be turned into a justification for oppression and social homogenisation.

Wealth and income are relatively unproblematic concepts. In addition to overall wealth, the degree of inequality in distribution is an important factor. The relationship between health, economic inequality, and social support is important and has been explored by other authors (Wilkinson, 1996). It should be noted that wealth is, in this analysis, relative. South Africa may not be wealthy by comparison to Japan but in relation to Mozambique it is. Teachers in Mozambique are paid a pittance by most international standards but compared to the peasant farmers they are extremely well off.

Combining the two variables allows the categorisation of groups and societies along two axes into four broad "types" each with a distinct epidemic pattern of HIV prevalence.

Pattern 1: High social cohesion and high wealth. This is characterised by slow growth followed by a low peak and slow decline with low endemic prevalence.

Pattern 2: Low social cohesion and high wealth. These societies exhibit a sharp increase in prevalence followed by a relatively rapid decline as the society mobilises the means for an appropriate response.

Pattern 3: Low social cohesion and low wealth. A society with low levels of social cohesion and low income would show an epidemic which may take some time to gain momentum, but once it does, rises rapidly and the prevalence of infection remains high.

Pattern 4: High social cohesion and low wealth. The fourth epidemic pattern is characterised by slow epidemic growth to a plateau of low HIV prevalence.

The four hypothetical HIV prevalence curves corresponding to each one of the patterns are presented in Figure 1.

The classification of societies and the four epidemic profiles were developed on the basis of case studies of the UK, the Philippines, Botswana, South Africa, Uganda, Ukraine and India (Barnett and Whiteside, 2002). In the detailed discussion of the case studies, the UK was held up as an example of a country with high income and high social cohesion—a Pattern 1 country.

Examples of high income, low social cohesion countries (Pattern 2) were provided by Botswana and South Africa. Botswana's Gross National Income per capita in 2001 was \$3630, while in South Africa it was \$2900. This is three or more times higher than every other sub-Saharan African country, with the exception of Gabon (\$3160) and Namibia (\$1960) (African Development Bank, 2003). The lack of social cohesion in South Africa with its traumatic past is clear—Botswana does not have this, but has a very mobile population.

Pattern 3 countries—low wealth and low social cohesion—were more difficult to find (at least ones where there were good data). In the end, the examples we used were both experiencing transition. Ukraine had had relatively high income, and under the old regime high and enforced social cohesion, but it provides

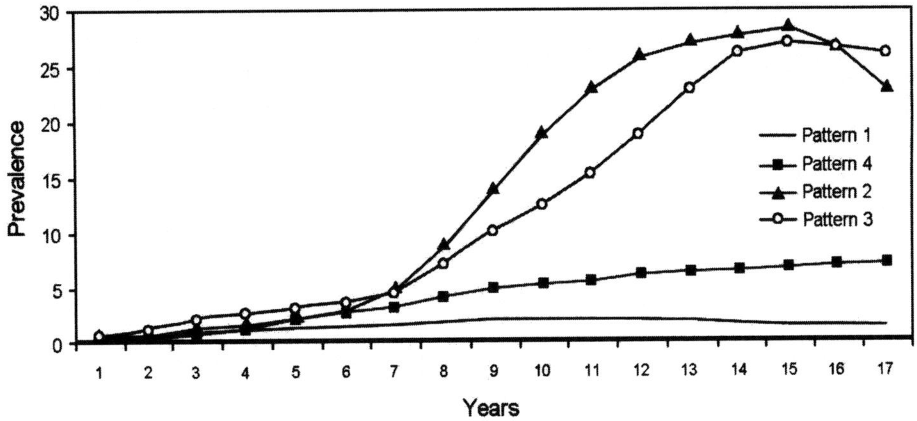

FIGURE 1. Hypothetical epidemic patterns of HIV. (Barnett and Whiteside, 2002)

an example of where this has broken down, and so the country may be in transit to a Pattern 3 country. Uganda under Amin and Obote was a country with low wealth and low social cohesion, and experienced a Pattern 3 epidemic. When Musevini came to power, the emphasis was on building the economy and society, and it can be argued that Uganda is transitioning to a Pattern 4 epidemic. The Philippines has low income but high levels of social cohesion and so is a Pattern 4 country. India provided a second example of a Pattern 4 country, but this was put forward some four years ago and there was a degree of ambivalence in our analysis.

Revisiting this paradigm for this chapter, in early 2004, I would argue it remains applicable to Asia. We did not have an Asian example of Pattern 1 or Pattern 2 countries in the original analysis. However, Pattern 1 (high income and high social cohesion) countries are not hard to find on the continent: Singapore and Japan are two examples. Pattern 2 (high income and low social cohesion) countries are harder to identify. Revisiting the paradigm and looking at the data it is possible that Thailand might have proved an example of high income and, at the time the epidemic began to spread, and among certain groups, low social cohesion. HIV came at a moment when there had been sustained economic growth, increased mobility and urbanization and some political unease. Equally, it could be argued that the underlying strength of the society allowed a rapid response.

Cambodia or Vietnam might provide examples of Pattern 3 (low income and low social cohesion) countries. What is interesting is the way that these countries have responded to the epidemic. It appears that in part the responses and their success have centred around building social cohesion. In both these countries there is evidence to show that condom use among female sex workers is significant and increasing (UNAIDS, 2002a; UNAIDS, 2003). UNAIDS wrote in 2002, "Cambodia's epidemic appears to be stabilizing, thanks to sustained prevention programs that link government and civil society and that span various sectors of society" (UNAIDS, 2002a). There is a degree of openness in both countries which, along with leadership, I would argue, is building social cohesion—something that is happening in the broader political arena anyway.

The Philippines, in the original discussion provided an example of a Pattern 4 (low income high, social cohesion) country. The Jaipur Paradigm was applied by Filipino colleagues, who concluded that the paradigm was of value in the "diagnosis" in their country. The high social cohesion in Philippines may seem contrary to some outside perceptions of easy sexuality, a flourishing commercial sex trade, and a mobile and poor population. However the evidence is of a low, slow epidemic: the first AIDS cases were reported in 1984 but the annual number of cases has never exceeded 60 cases per year (UNAIDS, 2000a). The authors of the National Economic Development Authorities Report (2000) suggest that factors slowing the epidemic are:

- The country is an archipelago detached from the Asian mainland. The lack of land borders has helped to reduce the spread of the disease.
- Most Filipino men are circumcised.
- The society is sexually conservative which includes late sexual debut and low rates of extra marital sex and resort to sex workers.
- Low rates of injecting drug use.
- The church is a powerful moral force in Filipino society.
- Literacy rates are high, over 90%.
- There have been multi-sectoral awareness and information campaigns involving government, NGOs, academics, the wider community as well as people living with HIV/AIDS.
- The NGO sector is strong and vocal, and an important part of a political system where popular mobilization and street protest has shown itself able to change governments relatively peacefully.

In addition, HIV/AIDS interventions in the Philippines have taken place in a supportive environment. In 1998, the legislature passed the AIDS Prevention and Control Act (RA 8504). This prohibited compulsory testing for HIV, emphasised human rights, provided that individuals with HIV should have basic health and social services, that there should be accredited HIV testing centres, and finally, that HIV/AIDS education should be integrated into schools at all levels. Filipino informants said that the moral authority of the church, the vibrancy of the NGO community and strength of family discipline all contribute to social cohesion in the face of large scale public corruption and political uncertainty (Barnett and Whiteside, 2002).

Adding Transition to the Paradigm

Since this paradigm was first developed, it has undergone many iterations and refinements through workshops, presentations and application. In this chapter, I want to add one further variable which is particularly important in Asia—that of transition. This was underestimated in the earlier work. Transition—economic, social, or political—is a powerful driver. But, as important, transition can be from "good" to "bad" or from "bad" to "good".

The rapid economic transition in China might be argued to be economically good but socially disruptive. The economic growth may create the environment in which HIV spreads. Susceptible groups include migrants—it is estimated that China has a migrant population of 120 million people, "huge populations of poor people are moving from rural areas to more developed cities" (Center for Strategic and International Studies, 2002). Both commercial sex and homosexual behavior are illegal, pushing them underground and creating problems for openly addressing these behaviors. The political and economic changes are also leading to a "fraying health care system (which) lacks sufficient capacity at this point to deal with HIV/AIDS". (Center for Strategic and International Studies, 2003). All this is also implicated in the epidemic HIV transmitted via plasma donation.

The Cambodian transition from genocide and the brutal Pol Pot regime was, in almost every sense, good. However, the arrival of UN troops as peacekeepers and the subsequent peace which resulted in new mobility and economic growth all assisted the spread of HIV. Indonesia's economic and political upheavals may be implicated in the spread of HIV there. Thailand is hailed as the first country to bring the HIV epidemic under control. The evidence for this was a decline in prevalence in pregnant women—in urban areas the median prevalence rose to a peak of 1.93% in 1995, falling to 1.28% in 1997 (UNAIDS, 1998); among army conscripts the peak was

4% in May 1993, falling to under 2% by 1996 (World Bank, 1997); and a massive decline in recorded sexually transmitted diseases among men—from 225,000 in 1988 to fewer than 50,000 by 1995 (World Bank, 1997). However, soon after these achievements were recorded, Thailand saw a severe economic slowdown. GDP growth from 1980 to 1990 was 7.6%; from 1990 to 1998 it was 7.4%, but in 1997/98 fell to −7.7% and only recovered to 1% in 2000/01 (World Bank, 2000a; World Bank, 2000b). This has meant fewer resources to fight the disease, in addition to the increased poverty and social stress. Data from 2000 shows that HIV infections stabilized and in many cases there has been a slight increase. For example the data on urban pregnant women shows slight increases in every region apart from the Southern Region, although this was just a few tenths of a percent (US Bureau of the Census, 2004).

The argument is simple. Transition—any transition—creates stresses and inequalities. However, transition is part of the human condition and is how we develop, evolve, and move forward as societies, nations and communities. The problem is that it also creates the space for HIV transmission.

Applying the Paradigm to Sub-Regions and Sub-Groups

National HIV epidemics are rarely homogenous. Each country has distinct social pockets of susceptibility and vulnerability, as well as regions and groups with discrete epidemic profiles. In the original work, we included India as a case study of a Pattern 4 country, but noted that there are many distinct epidemics in India. In Maharashtra, it is concentrated in urban centers among female sex workers and their clients and is now spreading into the general population. In Manipur and the northeast of the country, the epidemic is centered in IDU, but is also, according to recent reports, spreading beyond this group. We used Rajasthan and Manipur as case studies.

Rajasthan has a population of over 44 million people. It is one of the driest areas of India, with frequent droughts. Twelve percent of the population are "tribal" peoples, nearly double the national average. They are among the very poorest in India and their livelihood strategy exposes them to potential infection. Poor peoples' income potential in this part of India is probably constrained less by access to land itself—although this can be a problem—than by access to irrigation. Unable to provide for themselves and their households from their land (a situation often exacerbated by drought), both men and women enter various forms of laboring work. This may be daily, involve travel to nearby towns, or more distant migration to other states. Rajasthani people travel to neighbouring Gujarat to work on the commercial cotton plantations for months at a time. They also travel to other countries, including the Gulf states.

Raised levels of sexually transmitted infection prevalence, close urban/rural relations, marked income and wealth inequalities, complex inter-ethnic relations and identities, gender inequality, heavy dependence upon long-distance lorry transport, and labor migration all contribute to the creation of a risk environment. In such circumstances, social and economic conditions facilitate rapid transmission of infection once bridging has occurred between high prevalence urban subpopulations and the general population. At present there are no data to show that this has occurred in Rajasthan; but the potential is there.

The same dearth of data applies in Manipur, but here the dynamic of the epidemic is different. The state has only 0.2% of India's population (about 2 million people), but over 7% of the total number of reported HIV infections in the country (National AIDS Control Organization, 1998). Manipur's first AIDS case was identified in 1990 in an IDU. There are few time series data, but the HIV epidemic has been tracked among drug users in Imphal, Manipur's capital. In 1994, 85.6% of IDU tested in Imphal were infected. This had fallen slightly to 69.8% in 1998 (National AIDS Control Organization, 1998). In 1999, Imphal also recorded 2.3% of pregnant women infected at one site (UNAIDS 2000b).

Manipur is currently experiencing an epidemic among young urban men. There are factors peculiar to this state that increase susceptibility. It is geographically isolated and culturally distinct from much of the rest of India. It became part of the Indian union only in 1949, after a brief period of independence following the departure of the British. The relationship between Manipur and India is "colonial". The area was starved of investment until it achieved statehood in 1972. However, since then it has seen little in the way of development. This lack of economic activity, combined with disrupted livelihoods and central government neglect, creates high levels of youth unemployment. This, in turn, drives injecting drug use.

Proximity to Myanmar (with which it shares a long border) and the Golden Triangle are additional factors. Indeed, drug-smuggling routes pass through Manipur. Activists suggest that, ironically, it was sometimes the relatively wealthy sons of Indian officials who were among the first IDU. With increasing urbanization, the decay of the extended family and household system, few significant local industries, and little sign of development, the situation is not going to change—except that the disease is now spreading from the IDU community to the general population of the state. In 1990, 95% of those who were HIV-positive were IDU; by 1997, this had dropped to 75%, indicating the spread into the wider population (Barnett and Whiteside, 2002).

The paradigm can also be applied to groups in a country. For example, long distance truck-drivers in Asia may enjoy high income, but because of the nature of their work, escape much of the control which ensures social cohesion in their culture. Relative to their community of origin, which may have a Pattern 3 or Pattern 4 epidemic, the epidemic curve among truck drivers would be expected to tend towards Pattern 2. Migrant workers, as alluded to in the case of Rajasthan, may be separated from families in poor working conditions for periods of time, greatly increasing the risk of unsafe sex. In an extreme example of this, entire cohorts of young women have been forced into sex work from impoverished Nepali communities (Hannum, 1997).

DENIAL AND DIVISION

The discussion of the drivers of the epidemic and the Jaipur Paradigm provide analytical tools for understanding what is driving the epidemic and where it may be located. The case studies are mostly taken from parts of the world other than Asia, but I have updated the original analysis and applied it to Asia. The question is what other lessons can we learn from the rest of the world that can advise the response.

HIV/AIDS has the potential to be divisive, and denial of the problem will exacerbate this. In most of the world, denial of the epidemic was the first response. For example, in Kenya, between 1984 and 1987, the existence of the epidemic was questioned, and even when it was recognized there was a sense that it was not a serious problem. "AIDS was described in the press and by policymakers as a 'disease of Westerners' " (Family Health International, 1996). Furthermore, there was a real concern in the government that HIV/AIDS would be bad for business, especially tourism. This came to a head when, in 1987, the British army banned soldiers from taking leave in Mombasa because of high levels of HIV infection among prostitutes. The Minister of Health responded swiftly and "blamed the foreign press for distorting the issue and 'creating panic' " (Family Health International, 1996).

There was a similar response in the former Soviet Union. Here, the data distinguished between foreigners and locals. For example, in Ukraine during the initial period of the epidemic (from 1987 to 1994), there was mass HIV testing. Over 39 million (39,226,986) tests were carried out. These were performed on all blood donors, pregnant women, sexual partners of HIV-positive persons, social and professional contacts of HIV-positive people, hospitalized patients, military personnel, people who were abroad for more than three months, "promiscuous persons"(sic), patients with sexually transmitted diseases, prisoners, men who had sex with men, and drug addicts. Of the 39 million tests only 398 were positive, and the majority of these (215) were foreigners. AIDS was seen as a foreigner's problem. However, in 1995, of the 1489 HIV-positive people identified, only nine were foreigners, and this trend has continued (Barnett *et al.*, 2000b).

In Asia, an analogous pattern of denial was widespread during the early years of the epidemic. In some instances, foreigners were required to prove that they were HIV negative before being allowed to enter countries. There were stories of HIV-positive sex workers being dumped across the border from Thailand to Myanmar. The estimated 100,000 to 200,000 Nepali female sex workers in India were identified with the spread of HIV and subjected to discrimination (Hannum, 1997).

While denial continues to be an issue in parts of Africa and Eastern Europe, in some other areas there is a new openness and acceptance of the epidemic as a problem. For example, in Botswana, the President has acknowledged the epidemic as the primary challenge for the state, and has suggested that Botswana might not survive as a nation. "We stand at the crossroads of a threat of annihilation of our nation," he said (Mogae, 2000). In Ukraine, HIV/AIDS has been taken seriously by the government. In 2000, there was a presidential decree "On Urgent Measures on Prevention of HIV/AIDS", describing the state policy on the issue. A governmental commission for HIV/AIDS prevention was established within the Cabinet of Ministers. The Vice Prime Minister heads the commission. At the national level, there was a National Plan for Responding the HIV/AIDS epidemic for 2001–2003, and 2002 was declared "the year of HIV/AIDS"(Balakireva *et al.*, 2001).

What, then, is the situation in Asia? As would be expected, it is mixed. Dr. Nafis Sadik, the Special Envoy for HIV/AIDS in Asia and the Pacific commented in 2003:

> "In my one year as the Secretary-General's Special Envoy for HIV/AIDS in Asia and the Pacific, I have met and talked with many government and civil society leaders and I have addressed meetings at global, regional and national levels. Despite all that has been written and said about HIV/AIDS, despite international conferences and national meetings; despite unremitting advocacy by UNAIDS; despite many, many expressions of commitment to urgent action against HIV/AIDS, it has become clear to me that national and local authorities are not yet convinced. We have simply not seen the extraordinary responses that ESCAP members need to turn back the infection in the Asia-Pacific region.
>
> Leaders have certainly changed their attitudes. They now recognize that HIV/AIDS is present among their various constituencies. But then again, many of them have said nothing, because the issues are too sensitive and broaching them always invites controversy. Too few leaders are willing to stand up to say what must be said, that however unpleasant the reality may be, ESCAP countries have to face it.
>
> Some leaders have also buried themselves in the illusion that HIV/AIDS is not really an Asian problem: that the infection will somehow restrict itself to the high-risk groups-sex workers, drug injectors and men who have sex with men. These groups have little sympathy and support. The wider community sees their behavior as "deviant", if not actually illegal—as indeed they are in many countries. People extend this disapproval and stigma to all HIV/AIDS patients, and even to those living with HIV/AIDS." (Sadik 2003)

On the other hand, the experience of openness in Thailand and the Philippines is instructive. In Thailand, there was early acknowledgement of the potential problem. In the late 1980s, HIV spread among IDU and FSW. In 1991, the government of Prime Minister Anand Panyarachun mounted a massive national prevention effort. One of the key components was the 100% condom use program, which sought to ensure that condoms were used in all commercial sex establishments. The result was a dramatic decline in the number of new sexually transmitted infections and, over time, a decline in HIV prevalence was been tracked (World Bank, 1997).

One of the main lessons to be learned in stopping the spread of HIV is about openness and leadership. Thus, we have to conclude that much of Asia has far to go in this.

It may be that particular features of Asian life in some countries have prevented the issue from being addressed. The politics of AIDS policy is tightly tied to the political and cultural processes whereby complex nations are constructed. The Indian state has to come to grips with an epidemic that is bound up with areas of taboo such as gender, caste, ethnicity, masculinity, and money. In Malaysia and Indonesia, religion plays an important role in the response, and this, along with drug use, create problems for the state and state apparatus.

Sadik (2003) can have the final word: "... African countries have seen the full, appalling impact. Two of the most advanced countries in that region, Botswana and South Africa, are looking at the possibility of economic disaster and social disintegration as the result of HIV/AIDS. It could happen here. I believe that if all of us unite and act together—and only if we unite and act together—can we prevent the same fate overtaking the ESCAP region".

CONCLUSION

Testing and Learning from the Paradigm

The argument in this chapter is that we need to understand the drivers of the epidemic in order to prevent it. One tool, which may help us do this, is the Jaipur Paradigm, which, through an assessment of susceptibility, allows the prediction of an HIV epidemic in a specific society or group. This is based on a mixture of qualitative and quantitative variables. This paradigm needs to be refined to take into account the transition that so many countries are going through.

It is a practical and valuable tool and has been applied in the Philippines where the National Department of Health used it to ask if the epidemic would remain "low and slow". It carried out "Risk analysis... to look at how our susceptibilities and vulnerabilities might change, for the worse" (National Economic and Development Authority, 2000). Issues they identified were: increased population mobility, including militarization, especially in Mindanao; sexual conservatism which can result in unwillingness to discuss sex and promote condom use; low and incorrect condom use; lacerating sexual practices such as insertion of bolitas (small metal balls) into the penis; gender inequity; and invisibility of the epidemic.

In huge and populous societies, such as India and China, it is helpful to consider the enormous diversity of the country. We have the example of our Indian case studies. The situation in Rajasthan suggests a high level of susceptibility associated with population movement between rural and urban areas, especially medium- and long-term labor migration. Levels of rural and urban poverty and marked income and wealth inequality indicate that many population sub-groups are likely to pursue livelihood strategies which expose them to infection. Poor households will be vulnerable to the impact of excessive death and illness, and health systems will certainly be affected. Manipur's isolation suggests its epidemic is unlikely to contribute markedly to generalization of the Indian epidemic. However, considered regionally, in relation to adjoining areas of Myanmar and China, the Manipur epidemic may generalize.

Societies can, and do, change. Social cohesion may break down or build up; countries may experience economic growth or decline. Social cohesion is particularly fragile if it is maintained by authoritarian social control. Analysis has to be performed with a historical perspective. The interpretation of the profile of the HIV epidemic in Uganda, for instance, has to take account of the transition from social chaos and economic decline in the 1970s and 1980s to economic stability and greater order in the 1990s. It will be particularly important to follow and try to anticipate the epidemics in the countries of Eastern Europe and Asia, which are undergoing profound political, social, and economic transitions.

Implications for Social Interventions

The analysis provided in the Jaipur paradigm and as developed above also provides justification for interventions at the socio-economic level and adds weight to the view that governments have a substantial responsibility in this area (World Bank, 1997). It also shows that economic growth alone is not the panacea, but has to be accompanied by social development. This means addressing issues of equality, human rights and the construction of "civil society". HIV/AIDS interventions that ignore these issues may not be effective or sustainable in the long term.

One of the barriers to conceptualizing social policy interventions in response to AIDS is the difficulty of moving from understanding individual infection to seeing this as mediated by the social, economic and cultural context. Small changes in social norms may have a major impact on HIV incidence.

We suggest four areas of social policy for the strengthening of social cohesion, acting on a society's susceptibility to HIV and also on its vulnerability to the impacts of HIV:

- Altering social norms and standards: for example, increasing pressure to raise the age of first intercourse by a series of measures which might include extending compulsory schooling.
- Improving the status of women: for example, by increasing their access to capital through legislative and other positive action programs such as micro-finance initiatives.
- Improving the performance of social institutions through health and education sector reforms.
- Improving the quality of controlled social environments. This means looking at situations where people are forced to live together, in army barracks, on ships or in labor camps and either trying to avoid this happening or targeting interventions towards these people.

These areas were identified as being particularly applicable to Africa, but they are equally relevant for Asia.

Africa's epidemic is, in some parts, horrific, in terms of the proportion of sexually active adults who are infected (Botswana, Swaziland and Zimbabwe). In other areas, the actual numbers are startling (South Africa and Nigeria). With the exception of Thailand, where the epidemic took off and thus far has been brought under control, most of Asia is poised on a knife edge. Proportionately, the rates of infection may be lower; but even low rates will result in a human tragedy.

Asia can learn from Africa, Eastern Europe and the Caribbean. The question is, will it?

REFERENCES

African Development Bank. (2003). African Development Bank Report Globalisation and Africa's Development. Oxford University Press, Oxford.

Backlund, E., Sorlie, P.D., and Johnson, N.J. (1996). The shape of the relationship between income and mortality in the United States: Evidence from the National Longitudinal Mortality Study. *Annals of Epidemiology* 6:12–20.

Balakireva, O., Galustian, Y., Yaramenko, O., Scherbyns'ka, A., Kruglov, Y., Levchuk, N., Onikienko, V., and Andruschak, L. (2001). HIV/AIDS social and economic impacts in Ukraine: Report by the Ukrainian Institute of Social Research. British Council and Ukrainian Institute of Social Research, Kyiv City.

Barnett, T., and Whiteside, A. (2002). *Aids in the Twenty-first Century: Disease and Globalization.* Palgrave Macmillan, Basingstoke.

Barnett, T., Whiteside, A. and Decosas, J. (2000a). The Jaipur paradigm: A conceptual framework for understanding social susceptibility and vulnerability to HIV. *Journal of the South African Medical Association* 90:1098–1101.

Barnett, T., Whiteside, A., Khodakevich, L., Kruglov, Y., and Steshenko, V. (2000b). The social and economic impact of HIV/AIDS in Ukraine. *Soc Sci Med* 51(9):1387–1403.

Blaxter, M. (1990). *Health and Lifestyles.* Routledge, London.

Center for Strategic and International Studies. (2002). The second wave of the HIV/AIDS pandemic: Conference report. CSIS Press, Washington, DC.

Center for Strategic and International Studies. (2003). Averting a full-blown HIV/AIDS epidemic in China: A report of the CSIS HIV/AIDS delegation to China, January 13–17, 2003. Centre for Strategic and International Studies, Washington, DC.

Family Health International. (1996). AIDS in Kenya: Socioeconomic impact and policy implications. Family Health International and AIDS Control and Prevention Project, Washington, DC.

Filmer, D. (1996). The socio-economic correlates of 'risky' sexual behavior: Results from an analysis of DHS surveys. World Bank, UNAIDS and EU AIDS Task Force Seminar, Chateau Limelette, Belguim.

Fourie, P., and Schönteich, M. (2001). Africa's new security threat: HIV/AIDS and human security in Southern Africa. *Afr Security Rev* 10(4):29–42.

Fox, A. J. (ed). (1989). *Health Inequalities in European Countries.* Gower, Aldershot.

Fransen, L., and Whiteside, A. (1995). Assessing national and regional risk of HIV/AIDS. Economic Research Unit, University of Natal, Durban. (Unpublished paper).

Hannum, J. (1997). AIDS in Nepal: Communities confronting an emerging epidemic. American Foundation for AIDS Research in association with Seven Stories Press, New York.

Mogae, F. quoted in a BBC Report headed AIDS Kills 50% in Botswana and dated 7th November 2000, http://news.bbc.co.uk/2/hi/africa/1011639.stm, accessed October 1, 2003.

National AIDS Control Organization. (1998). http://www.naco.nic.in/1998, accessed January 11, 2003.

National Economic and Development Authority. (2000). Living with HIV/AIDS: Case study on Filipinos living with HIV/AIDS. Health Action Information Network for NEDA, Manila.

Sadik, N. (2003). Speech to the United Nations Economic and Social Commission for Asia and the Pacific Ministerial Round Table. (September 11, 2003); http://www.unaids.org/en/about+unaids/speeches.asp

Shilts, R. (1987). *And the Band Played on: Politics, People and the AIDS Epidemic.* St Martin's Press, New York.

UNAIDS. (1998). Thailand Epidemiological Fact Sheet on HIV/AIDS and Sexually Transmitted Diseases. UNAIDS and WHO, Geneva.

UNAIDS. (2000a). Phillipines epidemiological fact sheet on HIV/Aids: update. UNAIDS, Geneva.

UNAIDS. (2000b). India epidemiological fact sheet on HIV/AIDS. UNAIDS, Geneva.

UNAIDS. (2002a). Epidemic update. UNAIDS, Geneva.

UNAIDS. (2002b). Report on the global HIV/AIDS epidemic. UNAIDS, Geneva.

UNAIDS. (2003). Epidemic update. UNAIDS, Geneva.

UNAIDS and International Institute of Migration. (2003). Mobile populations and HIV/AIDS in the Southern African region: recommendations for action. Desk review and bibliography on HIV/AIDS and mobile populations. UNAIDS, Geneva.

US Bureau of the Census. (2004). HIV/AIDS Profile: Thailand. http://www.census.gov/ipc/hiv/thailand.pdf., accessed January 12, 2003.

Wilkinson, R.G. (1986). *Class and Health: Research and Longitudinal Data.* Tavistock, London.

Wilkinson, R. G. (1996). *Unhealthy Societies: the Afflictions of Inequality.* Routledge and Kegan Paul, London.

World Bank. (1997). Confronting AIDS: Public priorities in a global epidemic: A World Bank policy research report. Oxford University Press for the World Bank, New York and Oxford.

World Bank. (2000a). *World Development indicators.* World Bank, Washington.

World Bank. (2000b). *World Development Report 1999/2000.* Oxford University Press, New York.

35

Preventive HIV-1 Vaccines

Prelicensure Development

Karen L. Goldenthal[1], Rebecca L. Sheets[2], Therese Cvetkovich[1], Donna K. F. Chandler[1], Julienne M. Vaillancourt[1], and Antonia Geber[1]

[1]*Division of Vaccines and Related Products Applications, Office of Vaccines Research and Review, Center for Biologics Evaluation and Research, Food and Drug Administration, Rockville, Maryland, USA*
[2]*Vaccine Research Center and Division of AIDS, National Institutes of Health Bethesda, Maryland, USA*

INTRODUCTION

Overview of HIV-1

The World Health Organization (WHO) has estimated that 40 million individuals are living with HIV-1 as of 2003 (UNAIDS/WHO, 2003). In addition, approximately 14,000 people are newly infected with HIV-1 each day, worldwide (UNAIDS/WHO, 2003). Thus, there is tremendous public health interest in developing safe and effective preventive HIV-1 vaccines. Vaccines have proven to be one of the most effective means of preventing serious infectious diseases. The contribution of vaccines toward markedly decreasing the incidence of many of the once-common childhood infectious diseases has been particularly notable (CDC, 1999). Thus, the public health goal is to develop an effective HIV-1 vaccine that will achieve a similar success in controlling the AIDS epidemic. However, the development of an HIV-1 vaccine has a unique and complex set of scientific, clinical, social, ethical, and economic challenges (Amara and Robinson, 2002; Esparza and Osmanov, 2003; Fast *et al.*, 1995; Goldenthal *et al.*, 1998; Klausner *et al.*, 2003; Nathanson and Mathieson, 2000). Collaborative efforts in the development of an effective HIV-1 vaccine are ongoing among government agencies, academic investigators, and pharmaceutical and biotechnology companies. Even more organization on a global scale has been strongly encouraged (Klausner *et al.*, 2003).

More than 45 HIV-1 vaccine candidates have been studied in U.S. clinical trials to date (Amara and Robinson, 2002; NIH, 2002; McMichael and Hanke, 2003). These candidates have included recombinant proteins, synthetic peptides, DNA vaccines, and live viral and bacterial vectors expressing HIV-1 antigens. Some recombinant protein vaccine formulations have included adjuvants not previously used in licensed vaccines. Also, the "prime-boost" approach (which uses more than one vaccine in the same regimen) is common in HIV-1 vaccine development studies (Amara and Robinson, 2002; McMichael and Hanke, 2003).

Overview of Vaccine Regulation

The focus of this chapter is the prelicensure development of preventive HIV-1 vaccines. In the U.S., vaccines to prevent infectious diseases are regulated by the Office of Vaccines Research and Review (OVRR) located within the Center for Biologics Evaluation and Research (CBER), U.S. Food and Drug Administration (FDA). Vaccine development occurs in several stages. Usually, an immunogen(s) is identified based on the pathogenesis of the disease to be prevented by the vaccine. The manufacturing process for the vaccine is developed, and appropriate preclinical studies are performed to support initiation of human clinical trials. In the U.S., clinical studies in humans to assess the safety, immunogenicity and efficacy of the candidate vaccine are performed under an Investigational New Drug application (IND). The phases of clinical development are described below. Nonclinical studies as well as product and manufacturing refinements continue during the IND stage. Following the completion of Phase 3 clinical development, a Biologics License Application (BLA) may then be submitted to CBER/FDA for approval to market the vaccine. FDA will perform a facility inspection during the BLA phase. Often, sponsors make commitments at the time of approval to perform specific post-marketing clinical studies. Following licensure, FDA usually approves the release of each vaccine lot prior to commercial use (unless a different plan is approved), and FDA conducts periodic inspections of the manufacturing facility. Also, following licensure, a supplement to an approved BLA may be submitted to support a clinical change (e.g., expanded age indication) or certain product/manufacturing/facility changes.

FDA Documents and Other Resources

A wide variety of FDA and related resources are available to sponsors of vaccines under development. U.S. FDA regulations [from Title 21 of the Code of Federal Regulations (CFR)] relevant to the manufacture, product quality and clinical testing of vaccines are provided in Table 1. In addition, FDA provides advice and guidance to vaccine developers in a variety of ways, e.g., FDA guidance documents, FDA letters to sponsors regarding specific regulatory submissions such as INDs, and regulatory meetings.

Regarding guidance document development, the FDA continues to play an active role in the International Conference on Harmonisation (ICH) by participating in various working groups. ICH was organized to harmonize the technical requirements for drug approval among three regions: the European Union, Japan, and the United States. These activities have resulted in the issuance of ICH documents that have official FDA concurrence.

Tables 2 and 3 provide some of the relevant documents available from the FDA and the ICH, respectively. Some of these FDA and ICH documents have a particular focus on clinical trial-related topics and statistics. A major goal of the clinical documents is facilitating "Good Clinical Practice" (GCP) in addition to providing specific technical direction. GCP is an internationally recognized ethical and scientific quality standard for the design, conduct, documentation, and reporting of clinical trials that enroll human subjects. Compliance with this standard provides assurance that the rights, safety and well being of trial participants are protected and that the trial results are credible (ICH, 1997a).

TABLE 1. U.S. FDA Regulations Relevant to the Manufacture, Product Quality and Clinical Testing of Vaccines[a]

21 CFR 25	Environmental impact considerations
21 CFR 50	Protection of human subjects
21 CFR 56	Institutional Review Boards
21 CFR 58	Good laboratory practice for nonclinical laboratory studies
21 CFR 201	Labeling
21 CFR 202	Prescription drug advertising (promotional labeling)
21 CFR 210	Current good manufacturing practice in manufacturing, processing, packing, or holding of drugs; general
21 CFR 211	Current good manufacturing practice for finished pharmaceuticals
21 CFR 312	Investigational new drug application (IND)
21 CFR 314, 126	Adequate and well-controlled studies
21 CFR 600	Biological products: general
21 CFR 601	Licensing
21 CFR 610	General biological products standards

[a] Regulations covering the U.S. Food and Drug Administration (FDA) are located in Title 21 of the Code of Federation Regulations (CFR). These may be obtained as provided in Table 2 or directly from the Government Printing Office, Washington, D.C. 20402-9328. Also, the CFR can be accessed and searched on line directly from http://www.gpoaccess.gov/cfr/index.html.

TABLE 2. Examples of FDA Documents Relevant to the Manufacture, Product Quality and Clinical Testing of HIV Vaccines[a]

Points to Consider (PTC)

- Draft PTC in the production and testing of new drugs and biologicals produced by recombinant DNA technology (1985)
- Supplement to the PTC in the production and testing of new drugs and biologicals produced by recombinant DNA technology: Nucleic acid characterization and genetic stability (1992)
- Draft PTC in the characterization of cell lines used to produce biologicals (1993)
- PTC on plasmid DNA vaccines for preventive infectious disease indications (1996)
- PTC in the manufacture and testing of monoclonal antibody products for human use (1997)

Guidelines

- Guideline for submitting documentation for the stability of human drugs and biologics (1987)
- Guideline for submitting documentation for packaging for human drugs and biologics (1987)
- Guideline on general principles of process validation (1987)
- Guideline for the format and content of the clinical and statistical sections of an application (CDER) (1988)
- Test for residual moisture for biological products (1990)

Guidances and Related Documents

- Guidance on alternatives to lot release for licensed biological products (1994)
- Guidance for industry—Changes to an approved application: Biological products (1997)
- Guidance for industry—The sourcing and processing of gelatin to reduce the potential risk posed by Bovine Spongiform Encephalopathy (BSE) in FDA-regulated products for human use (1997)
- Guidance for industry for the evaluation of combination vaccines for preventable diseases: Production, testing and clinical studies (1997)
- Guidance for industry—Providing clinical evidence of effectiveness for human drug and biological products (1998)
- Guidance for industry—Content and format of chemistry, manufacturing and controls information and establishment description information for a vaccine or related product (1999)
- Refusal to file procedures for biologics license applications (SOPP 8404) (2002)
- Draft guidance for industry: Sterile drug products produced by aseptic processing—Current good manufacturing practice (2003)

[a] Other FDA documents may also be of interest to vaccine developers. FDA documents are available from the Office of Communication, Training and Manufacturers Assistance, HFM-40, CBER, 1401 Rockville Pike, Rockville, MD 20852-1448. Also, documents may be obtained by calling 1-800-835-4709 or 301-827-1800. Also, many documents can be downloaded from CBER's internet site at http://www.fda.gov/cber/publications.htm.

TABLE 3. Examples of International Conference on Harmonisation (ICH) Documents Relevant to the Manufacture, Product Quality and Clinical Testing of Vaccines[a]

Clinical

- E3: Structure and content of clinical study reports (1996)
- E6: Good clinical practice: Consolidated guideline (1997)
- E8: General considerations for clinical trials (1997)
- E5: Ethnic factors in the acceptability of foreign clinical data (1998)
- E9: Statistical principles for clinical trials (1998)
- E11: Clinical investigation of medicinal products in the pediatric population (2000)

Manufacture and Product Quality

- Q2A: Validation of analytical procedures (definitions and terminology) (1995)
- Q2B: Validation of analytical procedures: Methodology (1997)
- Q5B: Analysis of the expression construct in cells used for production of r-DNA derived protein products (1996)
- Q5D: Quality of biotechnological/biological products: Derivation and characterization of cell substrates used for production of biotechnological/biological products (draft) (1998)
- Q5A: Viral safety evaluation of biotechnology products derived from cell lines of human or animal origin (1998)

[a] Other ICH documents may also be of interest to vaccine developers. ICH documents can be obtained by telephone or accessing the FDA web site (see Table 2) and are also available from http://www.ich.org/.
Note: year in parenthesis refers to year of publication in the Federal Register.

Additionally, FDA and ICH documents pertaining to cell substrates, viral safety evaluation, manufacturing, product characterization, stability testing, and nonclinical toxicology are also available.

Regulatory meetings with the Agency play a critical role in vaccine development. Minutes of these meetings are prepared by FDA and shared with the sponsor. At a minimum, sponsors are strongly encouraged to have official meetings with FDA at critical times in the drug development process, e.g., prior to the submission of an IND (pre-IND meeting), before initiation of a Phase 3 efficacy study (end-of-Phase 2 meeting), and prior to submission of a BLA (pre-BLA meeting) (U.S. FDA, 2000a; 2002). Also, CBER staff may be contacted for assistance with scientific and regulatory matters at any time during development.

Sponsors should remain attentive to the availability of new FDA and ICH documents, etc., during drug development, through Federal Register notices and several internet sites (see Tables 2 and 3). Also, CBER/FDA has co-sponsored a variety of vaccine-related workshops, especially with other U.S. Public Health Service Agencies, WHO, and foreign regulatory authorities on important and/or emerging issues of relevance to vaccine developers. Additional information regarding vaccine development is available from a number of publications (Baylor and Midthun, 2004; Goldenthal and McVittie, 1997; Goldenthal *et al.*, 2001).

PRODUCT AND QUALITY CONTROL

FDA-regulated biological products, including vaccines, must be safe (relative freedom from harmful effect when prudently administered) [21 CFR 600.3(p)], pure (relative freedom from extraneous matter) [21 CFR 600.3(r)], potent (defined as the specific ability of product... to effect a given result) [21 CFR 600.3(s)], and manufactured consistently according to current good manufacturing practice [21 CFR 210–211]. In order to meet regulatory requirements, common principles of vaccine production and quality control include the following: detailed and documented manufacturing procedures to ensure consistency of production; defined compatible components; product characterization and specifications; testing to identify any adventitious agents; examination for extraneous materials (purity); and stability, including genetic stability.

There are many product issues for sponsors to address in vaccine development. The source and quality of all starting materials should be documented. For the cell substrate used to produce the vaccine, the history and identity of the cells, cell banking system, characterization of any endogenous viruses, and adventitious agent testing for the cell substrate should be described. For example, tests will be needed to rule out specific viral contaminants that could potentially be present in the cell substrates used for vaccine production. Well-documented banks should be prepared for bacterial seeds, viral seeds, and cell substrates according to current good manufacturing practice (cGMP). The history and characterization of the viral or bacterial seeds should be documented. If relevant, validation of the manufacturing process for the removal and/or inactivation of viruses or bacteria is required. In-process testing to determine the acceptability of product intermediates for further manufacturing, as well as tests for the release of bulk and final products, must be developed (including the appropriate specifications). The sponsor will also need to generate real-time stability data to justify expiry for the final container product as well as holding times for the bulk product(s) and critical intermediates.

A critical component of vaccine development is the establishment and refinement of lot release criteria. Even vaccine lots used for Phase 1 clinical studies will have lot release testing, although the testing and acceptance criteria may be modified during drug development. By the initiation of Phase 3 clinical studies, product specifications and formulation should be established. Lot release criteria typically include sterility (most situations), the general safety test in guinea pigs and mice to detect extraneous toxic contaminants, and an identity test (e.g., SDS-PAGE, Western blot, amino acid analysis, or immunologic assay). Purity tests may include the percent moisture for a lyophilized product, endotoxin content, and SDS-PAGE or HPLC analyses. Tests may be required to document removal of certain process contaminants. A potency test (*in vivo* or *in vitro*, depending on the parameter) may include assessment of immunogenicity or protection, antigen content, or chemical composition.

PRECLINICAL AND NONCLINICAL STUDIES

A safety study compliant with good laboratory practice (GLP) (21 CFR 58) is often needed to support the initiation of a Phase 1 clinical trial with a novel product. (See also next paragraph regarding GLP safety studies.) In addition, other nonclinical data may be needed to fulfill the requirement that adequate information be provided "to conclude that it is reasonably safe to conduct the proposed clinical investigations" [21 CFR 312.23(a)(8)]. Such data could include product characterization information, demonstration of adequate attenuation (for live organisms), completeness of inactivation and lack of reversion for inactivated organisms or toxoids, the absence of adventitious agents, and assessment of pyrogenicity. Specific testing recommendations exist for plasmid DNA vaccines (U.S. FDA, 1996b). Also, guidance is available regarding developmental toxicology studies for vaccines (U.S. FDA, 2000b). Animal studies may be used to evaluate potency or to demonstrate immunogenicity. Often, challenge/protection studies are carried out in animals to demonstrate proof of concept for vaccine activity, but these are not usually required to initiate Phase 1 studies.

If a preclinical GLP safety study is conducted, the following principles should be considered: The study design should be based on the intended clinical use, including route and device of administration, formulation and dose (to include the highest dose). An extra dose (N + 1) should be given compared to that proposed in the clinical trial(s). A somewhat compressed immunization schedule (which will ordinarily still be at least several weeks between doses) compared to the proposed clinical use may be employed as long as it permits time for an immune response to develop. A relevant animal model should be used, i.e., the vaccine should be immunogenic in the animal species selected for the safety study. Chemistry, hematology, necropsy, histopathology and other appropriate assessments at pre-specified times are expected. Safety data in non-human primates are usually not necessary to support a Phase 1 study. The GLP safety study protocol(s) should be submitted to FDA for review and concurrence prior to implementation.

Adjuvants are often included in the vaccine formulation. An adjuvant is defined as an agent that enhances specific immune responses to antigens. Aluminum compounds are the only adjuvants included in currently licensed U.S. vaccines. The specific vaccine/adjuvant formulation is licensed, rather than an adjuvant alone (Goldenthal *et al.*, 1993). The need for an adjuvant should be justified.

ASSAYS

Early and adequate attention should be given to assay development and validation (Schofield, 2000; ICH, 1995; 1997b). Validation involves detailed assessment and acceptance of performance characteristics (e.g., precision, accuracy, specificity, limits of detection and quantitation, linearity, range and systems suitability) of the assay.

The potency assay(s) used to qualify the product is critical to vaccine development. Information on the validation of the vaccine potency assay(s) used to qualify products is available (Taffs, 2001). During the course of vaccine development, a suitable quantitative assay measuring a biologically relevant effect will need to be fully developed and validated. However, a provisional potency assay may be used for lots to be tested in early, non-pivotal trials.

Validation of immune response and virologic assays used in HIV vaccine clinical trials is another critical area. The performance characteristics of assays intended to evaluate the subjects' vaccine-induced immune responses and HIV-1 virologic status should be submitted to the IND prior to using the assays in a clinical trial, even for early studies. For example, this may include the description of immunological assays intended to distinguish the vaccine-induced immune response from that elicited by wild-type infection. Clade specific assays may be needed in order to evaluate vaccine-induced immune responses and document new infections. Also, the performance of viral load assays based on DNA or RNA signal amplification may be affected by the clade of the virus. Thus, considerable research and development may be necessary to provide adequate assay validation, especially when multiple endemic subtypes (clades) are present in the proposed trial population. While assays may undergo refinement during early clinical studies, the development, testing and validation of definitive laboratory assays to be used for the efficacy trial case definition should be implemented early enough to avoid delays in starting such trials.

CLINICAL DEVELOPMENT

Phase 1

Phase 1 vaccine trials are primarily designed to evaluate safety and immunogenicity in a limited number, e.g., 20–80 per study, of closely monitored subjects. Clinical evaluation of new vaccines usually starts with Phase 1 testing in healthy adult volunteers 18 to 40 years of age who are at low risk of contracting HIV-1 infection. The primary objective will be safety assessment of the experimental vaccine.

More than one vaccine dose level may be evaluated in a Phase 1 study, usually in a step-wise manner of increasing dose by group, called dose-escalation. Details of any dose-escalation plan should be clearly described in the protocol. The acceptability of any plans to proceed with dose-escalation before completion of the vaccination regimen in each lower dose group will depend on factors such as the characteristics of the investigational vaccine, as well as reactogenicity detected in preclinical models or clinical data for the same or similar products.

Clinical evaluations of safety in Phase 1 studies should include both local injection site and systemic reactions. At predefined intervals, periodic assessments of the local injection site and systemic signs and symptoms will be recorded. Pre and post-vaccination evaluation of serum chemistry and hematology values of volunteers (at least for the first Phase 1 study) may be appropriate in addition to product-specific safety evaluations. The prototype case report form (CRF) or subject diary should list each item to be assessed and the predefined times of assessment (e.g., baseline, 24 hours post-vaccination, etc.).

The appropriate timeframe for active monitoring of adverse events will depend on the vaccine. For HIV-1 vaccines, active monitoring for at least one week post-vaccination for recombinant protein and peptide vaccines, and at least 14 days post-vaccination for novel live, vectored vaccines is recommended. Solicited events should include symptoms appropriate for the type of vaccine and study population, e.g., detailed solicitation of gastrointestinal symptoms when evaluating live, oral vaccines. Subjects should also be questioned about adverse events when they return for immunogenicity studies, usually within one month post-immunization. An additional follow-up at 6 months after the last dose, focused on serious adverse events (SAEs), new onset of chronic illness, and (if applicable) worsening of chronic illness, is also recommended.

Specific adverse event (AE) criteria for discontinuing further vaccinations for both an individual subject as well as for the overall study (i.e., stopping rules) should be clearly described in the protocol. In this regard, a grading scale for solicited adverse events, e.g., fever, should be included in the protocol and should be appropriate for assessing toxicity in healthy volunteers. The criteria for discontinuing further vaccinations should be linked to the AE grading scale(s). Investigators should explicitly attempt to anticipate situations that may lead to safety problems for the vaccinees and provide mechanisms to address these situations in the protocol.

For studies of products using non-HIV live, replicating organisms (e.g., vaccinia-vectored HIV-1 vaccines), sponsors should describe their proposed procedures for containment of the live biological material during their clinical studies and should provide data on the expected survival of the organism in the environment (if applicable). To date, this issue has been addressed for live viral-vectored and bacterial-vectored HIV-1 vaccines studied under IND. At a minimum, shedding of live vaccine organisms should be evaluated in the first Phase 1 study. The physical isolation of volunteers early in clinical development may be necessary to assess shedding of attenuated and revertant organisms and the potential for spread to contacts. The FDA reviews the sponsor's summary of containment procedures to determine whether such procedures are adequate. If appropriate, the protocol should include a procedure for eradication of the vector organisms (e.g., antibiotics) in the event that shedding persists beyond a pre-specified number of days.

Phase 2

In general, Phase 2 vaccine studies enroll more subjects than Phase 1 studies, i.e., Phase 2 studies enroll up to several hundred per trial. Phase 2 studies are often randomized and controlled. During Phase 2 development, a preferred vaccine formulation, dose, and regimen are identified for further evaluation in an efficacy trial. Phase 2 studies also provide more precise estimates of the rates of common local and systemic reactions. In addition, Phase 2 studies provide feasibility information relevant to the conduct of Phase 3 studies, e.g., subject accrual, acceptance of vaccine regimens, compliance with study protocols, etc. At this stage, some subjects at high risk for acquiring HIV-1 infection may be enrolled.

The evaluation of vaccinees who become infected during the trial is a critical component of Phase 1 and 2 vaccine studies. Information gathered from these subjects may lead to a better understanding of humoral and cell-mediated immunity (CMI) against HIV-1 (McElrath *et al.*, 1996; Kahn *et al.*, 1995; O'Toole *et al.*, 1996; Belshe *et al.*, 1994). For example, the analysis of genotypes and phenotypes of the breakthrough viruses could be very informative (Graham *et al.*, 1998; Connor *et al.*, 1998; Berman *et al.*, 1997).

Advantages and disadvantages of large-scale Phase 2 intermediate-size trials for screening candidate HIV-1 vaccines have been discussed (Rida *et al.*, 1997).

Phase 3

Phase 3 studies are large trials that will, in most cases, include the principal efficacy and safety data needed for licensure. Phase 3 studies should be discussed with CBER well in advance of study implementation to ensure that such studies are appropriately designed (including an adequate sample size) to meet intended goals, especially support of product licensure. Important potential populations for preventive HIV-1 vaccine efficacy trials include adolescents and adults, as well as infants born to HIV-1 infected mothers (Safrit, 2003). With regard to design of efficacy trials for the latter population (to evaluate mother to infant transmission), the experiences with the PACTG 076 (zidovudine) and PACTG 185 (HIV immune globulin) clinical trials may be instructive (Connor *et al.*, 1994; Stiehm *et al.*, 1999).

In preparation for Phase 3 efficacy studies, background epidemiological data (including recent seroincidence and endemic HIV clade data, and if applicable, serology to the vaccine vector) should be obtained in the intended efficacy trial population to support the rationale for selecting that specific population and the specific vaccine antigens. In this regard, useful information may be available through the Los Alamos HIV sequence database in New Mexico and from the Centers for Disease Control and Prevention (CDC). Preliminary safety and immunogenicity data obtained from the efficacy trial target population should also be available (see below). Logistical issues such as data collection systems and vaccine distribution (e.g., maintaining cold chain) should be addressed during the Phase 1 and 2 studies that precede the Phase 3 efficacy trial.

Prior to starting an efficacy trial, sponsors should provide their scientific rationale (i.e., the basis for expecting the product to be effective) along with supporting safety and immunogenicity data from Phase 1 and 2 to CBER, and will likely be asked to present such information to an FDA advisory committee. However, the FDA does not have pre-specified rationale requirements for a sponsor to advance to a Phase 3 efficacy study of a preventive HIV-1 vaccine, e.g., a certain type and level of immune response that must be attained, a requirement for specific successful animal protection studies, etc. The sponsor's entire data set and rationale will be evaluated to determine whether initiating Phase 3 studies is appropriate.

Elements of efficacy protocols are presented in Table 4 (Goldenthal and McVittie, 1997; ICH, 1996, 1997c, 1998a; Friedman *et al.*, 1996; Dixon *et al.*, 1993). Selection of the vaccine dose and schedule for the efficacy trial should be based on the results of Phase 1 and 2 studies. The study should be carefully designed to allow a valid estimate of efficacy; precision in the 95% confidence limits on the efficacy estimate should be considered in the calculation of sample size (O'Neill, 1988). Most prelicensure vaccine efficacy trials are well-controlled studies that have a double-blind, randomized design. Ideally, information would be obtained concerning the duration of efficacy and immunity over a period of at least several years.

A vaccine efficacy trial will usually have a single primary endpoint. In most

TABLE 4. Basic Elements of an HIV Vaccine Efficacy Trial Protocol

A. Study hypothesis

B. Study population
- Inclusion/exclusion criteria, e.g., age, sex, health status, occupation, laboratory values, allowed concurrent medications
- Basis for determining risk status
- Background data on disease incidence in target population (see below)

C. Vaccine (and placebo) composition (clades, strains, adjuvants, etc.), dose, schedule, route, and anatomic site of administration

D. Study design
- Control group
- Randomization scheme/implementation plan
- Study masking
- Items to be assessed/time schedule: clinical and laboratory parameters for safety, immunogenicity, virology and efficacy
- Case (endpoint) definition(s)
- Clearly stated primary and secondary endpoints to define efficacy [Include or provide reference to details of methodology (immune assays, viral load, etc.)]
- Plan for individuals who become HIV-1 infected during the study

E. Surveillance plans
- Frequency
- Methods of assessment
- Personnel

F. Statistical section
- Background data to support assumptions for sample size estimation
- Prospective statistical methods for obtaining point estimate of vaccine efficacy and 95% Confidence Intervals (CIs) for the primary endpoint
- Level of vaccine efficacy anticipated; lower CI obtainable with sufficient power for the primary endpoint
- Prospective statistical analysis plan for other endpoints
- Method of covariate adjustment and list of covariates, if applicable
- How adverse event rates will be compared statistically and at what significance level
- Estimated number of drop-outs and losses-to-follow-up, and their handling in analyses
- Interim analyses, including early stopping guidelines
- Method of adjustment for multiplicity, if needed
- Justification for trial sample size based on the preceding items in this section

G. Plan for an independent DMC (including membership)

H. Prototype case report forms (CRFs)[a], subject diaries[a], and informed consent forms (CFs)[a]

I. Model scripted interviews[a] for any protocol-specified telephone follow-up

[a] These model forms and documents should be submitted to the IND at the same time as the protocol.

circumstances, this endpoint is a laboratory test result(s), a clinical finding(s) or outcome(s), or a specifically defined combination. There should be a well-defined and validated case definition of the disease or infection(s) under study (Ad hoc group, 1988; Blackwelder *et al.*, 1991; Storsaeter *et al.*, 1990). The CRF and subject diary, as applicable, should be submitted with the protocol; these should be designed to systematically assess information pertinent to the primary and secondary efficacy endpoints, and safety parameters including quantification of severity (e.g., grading scale for toxicities). The potential for vaccinee self-unblinding to alter risk behavior, and thus trial endpoints and outcomes, has been discussed (Fast *et al.*, 1995; Schaper *et al.*, 1995).

A variety of potential clinical trial endpoints for preventive HIV-1 vaccine trials have been discussed in the literature (Schaper *et al.*, 1995; Hoff and Barker, 1995). Among these endpoints have been the following: (a) acute HIV-1 infection ("sterilizing immunity"); (b) chronic HIV-1 infection; and (c) clinical disease progression of HIV-1 disease in vaccinees who become infected during the study. Also, there is interest in examining viral load and CD4 cell counts in vaccinees who become infected. Evaluation of virologic failure or treatment initiation with antiretroviral drugs in vaccinees who become infected has also been discussed (Gilbert *et al.*, 2003). Additionally, the effect on horizontal transmission from an infected vaccinee has been discussed as a possible endpoint in the literature. This proposal is based on the postulate that a vaccine might decrease virus transmission by decreasing the infectiousness of the vaccinee, without necessarily conferring benefit to the vaccinee (Schaper *et al.*, 1995). Assessment of these endpoints could be affected by the limits of detection of viral load/viral detection assays, as well as confounded by the use of anti-retroviral drugs (Bloom, 1998; CDC, 2002), especially soon after infection, or by the use of postexposure prophylaxis (CDC, 1998).

It is not clear whether an HIV-1 vaccine derived from one clade will confer protection against infection with HIV-1 of a different clade, or even against a divergent strain within the same clade (Rowe, 1996; Nathanson and Mathieson, 2000). Consensus or ancestor sequences have been proposed in vaccine design to minimize the genetic differences between vaccine strains and contemporary isolates (Gaschen *et al.*, 2002). Also, targeting a single gene product may not be sufficient. Readers are referred to a publication (Goldenthal *et al.*, 2001) and an FDA guidance document (U.S. FDA, 1997) for further information on the development of combination vaccines.

In general, a correlate of protection for vaccine efficacy may be identified by analysis of results from a successful clinical efficacy trial, or may be suggested from sources such as population-based studies of immunized persons. Ideally, the correlation of clinical protection with the post-vaccination immune response at selected time points (e.g., one month post-vaccination and at other specified time points) should be evaluated. The critical time points may differ for serological and cell-mediated immune (CMI) response parameters. Searching for an immunological correlate(s) of protection in a vaccine efficacy trial is particularly relevant if one has not been identified previously.

Insights into the immunologic correlates of protection from HIV-1 infection may be obtained from sources such as (i) animal challenge protection trials, (ii) long-term survivors, and (iii) multiply exposed and uninfected persons (Haynes *et al.*, 1996; Kaul *et al.*, 2001; Zhu *et al.*, 2003). Aspects of both the humoral and cell-mediated immune responses have been implicated in the host's partial control of viral replication (Fauci, 2003). The host's genetic background can play an important role in protection, e.g., individuals who are homozygous for a deletion mutant of the CCR5 receptor appear to be less susceptible to HIV-1 infection (Samson *et al.*, 1996; Dean *et al.*, 1996; Paxton *et al.*, 1998).

Identification of an HIV-1 vaccine-induced immune correlate of protection may improve the scientific rationale for extrapolating clinical efficacy data across clades by use of comparative immune responses, as well as for evaluating data from other clinical "bridging" studies (see below). Such information may also help with the design of future vaccines. However, identifying a correlate of protection is not a requirement for licensure. There are licensed vaccines for which an immunological correlate of protection has not been identified, e.g., acellular pertussis and typhoid vaccines.

Special mention should be made of vaccine efficacy studies conducted outside of the United States. In many instances, foreign efficacy trials are performed for epidemiological reasons, e.g., because the disease of interest has a low incidence in the United States. Vaccines for indications such as the prevention of typhoid fever, Japanese encephalitis, pertussis and hepatitis A have been licensed in the U.S. using foreign efficacy data. However, immunogenicity (and efficacy) differences between populations may result from differences in factors such as genetics, nutritional status, and background infections; therefore, safety and immunogenicity data should be obtained in the specific population in which the efficacy trial will be performed (ICH, 1998b; Katz, 1983; Patriarca *et al.*, 1991). Additionally, if efficacy is based on data from a foreign trial(s), then safety and immunogenicity data with the vaccine in U.S. populations will likely be expected to support licensure in the United States (See section on Clinical Bridging Studies).

Sponsors may decide to conduct foreign studies under U.S. FDA IND even when they are not required to do so, i.e., when the vaccine is manufactured in a foreign country. This practice is encouraged in order to receive FDA recommendations prospectively for trials that may be used to support licensure in the U.S. Any foreign study not performed under an IND must comply with 21 CFR 312.120 in order to use the data to support U.S. licensure.

A vaccine efficacy trial should have a formally established independent Data Monitoring Committee (DMC) [formerly referred to as a Data and Safety Monitoring Board (DSMB)] with relevant multidisciplinary membership (e.g., biostatisticians, clinicians, and bioethicists). If the DMC will conduct an interim analysis of the data, the following information should be provided prospectively as part of a detailed statistical plan in the protocol: (a) The conditions (e.g., specific schedule, number of events, etc.) which must be met before performing the interim analysis; (b) The criteria for early study termination; and (c) A list of the individuals who will have access to the interim data. Any unmasked review of the data, including any review of the data by treatment group (regardless of whether or not the group identities are revealed), would be considered an interim analysis. Excellent discussions of DMCs and interim analysis concepts are available (Ellenberg *et al.*, 1993; Ellenberg *et al.*, 2002; Emerson and Fleming, 1990; Geller and Pocock, 1987; O'Brien and Fleming, 1979; U.S. FDA, 2001).

The first preventive HIV-1 vaccine efficacy trial, the AIDSVAX B/B trial, was started in 1998 in the USA, Canada, Puerto Rico and the Netherlands (Francis *et al.*, 2003). Results from this trial were announced in the first quarter 2003. Analysis of this trial data failed to show vaccine efficacy for the primary endpoint, prevention of HIV-1 infection in the overall trial population. The second efficacy trial, the AIDSVAX B/E trial, was started in Bangkok, Thailand, in 1999 (Francis *et al.*, 2003). Preliminary results from this second trial, announced in late 2003, indicate that the respective candidate vaccine did not show efficacy. Yet, much can be learned from examination of the protocol designs, and issues encountered during the conduct of these trials.

Additional Considerations for Safety Data

Large numbers of healthy individuals will typically receive a new vaccine, and safety data are critically important. Licensure decisions are definitely affected by the quality and quantity of available safety data. High quality case report forms (CRFs) and, when applicable, scripted telephone interviews are necessary to obtain interpretable data. In addition, vaccine-specific safety questions should be carefully addressed during clinical development.

Safety data are most interpretable when obtained from *randomized, controlled* studies. In most clinical development schemes, the majority of prelicensure safety data is obtained from the efficacy trial(s). For large Phase 3 trials (e.g., thousands of subjects), it may be appropriate to evaluate only a subset of the trial population for common local and systemic events. In this case, all trial subjects would be monitored for SAEs by pre-specified methods (Goldenthal *et al.*, 2001).

Consent Forms, Institutional Review Boards (IRBs), and Related Topics

The elements of informed consent forms (CFs) are stated in 21 CFR 50. Discussions of issues for CFs for preventive HIV-1 vaccine trials are available (Fast *et al.*, 1995; Bloom, 1998). There is an appropriate emphasis on informing the subjects of potential medical and social implications of trial participation as well as identifying and addressing issues for special populations, e.g., adolescents. Information contained in the CF should be consistent with the model CF submitted to the FDA, as well as with the protocol and investigator's brochure. Careful review of the site-specific CFs for consistency of important items across the study is critical. Integrated, repeated counseling of trial subjects about avoiding high risk behavior for acquisition of HIV-1 infection has been an important part of preventive HIV-1 vaccine trials.

The requirements for Institutional Review Boards (IRBs) are stated in 21 CFR 56. In ICH parlance, a committee in a foreign country serving a similar function may be referred to as an Independent Ethics Committee (IEC). 21 CFR 312.120 discusses the use of foreign clinical studies not conducted under an IND to support licensure in the U.S., including ethical principles, as noted earlier. Reviews of the complex and evolving ethical issues for HIV-1 vaccine trials are available (Fast *et al.*, 1995; Bloom, 1998; Guenter *et al.*, 2000).

Clinical "Bridging" Studies

A clinical bridging study is a trial in which a parameter (or parameters) of interest for a vaccine, e.g., study population, manufacturing scale, formulation, dosing schedule, is directly compared with a different version of that parameter with respect to the effect of the change on the product's clinical performance. For example, a bridging study may be needed to address the concern that certain changes (e.g., in procedures or production scale) might have resulted in a different vaccine that is no longer clinically equivalent to the previous version with proven efficacy (Goldenthal *et al.*, 1998; U.S. FDA, 1996a). Also, a clinical bridging study could be used to provide scientific support that efficacy data obtained with one population can be extrapolated to a different population (ICH, 1998b; WHO, 2003).

Bridging studies should have a prospective statistical plan. These studies should be adequately designed (including sample size) to address the relevant questions. The primary objective of a clinical vaccine bridging study is usually to determine whether or not the immune response(s) elicited in the new group (e.g., receiving new product) is "non-inferior" to that of the control group (e.g., receiving the earlier version) (Goldenthal *et al.*, 1998). Comparisons of immune response data are most interpretable when obtained from randomized, controlled studies (U.S. FDA, 1997; Goldenthal and McVittie, 1997). Safety comparisons are also an important component of these studies. Confidence limits on differences between comparison groups (as well as for each group separately) should be provided for immune response parameters, such as seroconversion rates and geometric mean concentration (GMC) of antibody (Horne *et al.*, 2001). CMI response parameters may also be of interest in this regard, although validation of such assays has been difficult in the past. When there is no clearly identified immune correlate of protection, the clinical relevance of a decreased immune response for the new product or formulation (or in a new population) may be unclear, and thus, it may not be possible to conclude that the two versions are clinically equivalent (Goldenthal *et al.*, 1998).

FDA ADVISORY COMMITTEES

Sponsors may be requested to present their data and clinical development plans to the U.S. FDA Vaccines and Related Biological Products Advisory Committee (VRBPAC) (or to other appropriate FDA advisory committees) at various times during development. The following are examples of stages of development where FDA may request advisory committee input: (a) Prior to the initiation of Phase 1 clinical studies, to consider safety issues pertaining to a novel vaccine strategy; (b) Prior to the initiation of a Phase 3 efficacy study, to review the trial design as well as supporting data; and (c) Prior to licensure, following FDA's review of the license application. The FDA staff prepares relevant questions for the VRBPAC and may also prepare briefing documents and make technical presentations at the meeting. A discussion of FDA advisory committees is available (Freas and Gertzog, 1997). Transcripts and other documents from open sessions of FDA advisory committee meetings are available at http://www.fda.gov/ohrms/dockets/ac/acmenu.htm.

CONCLUSION

Sponsors have the complex responsibility of coordinating the manufacturing, product testing, and nonclinical and clinical evaluation, so that vaccine development can advance in a timely manner. HIV-1 vaccines present a number of unique and evolving considerations with regard to clinical trial design, clinical development in general, and risk/benefit assessments for healthy populations. Clinical protocols should be designed to meet their stated objectives as well as to optimize the protection of trial participants. Careful overall planning includes anticipating needs of future trials (e.g., validation of critical assays). For example, such preparation will lessen the likelihood of delays in initiating large efficacy trials and other pivotal studies due to inadequately validated immunologic or virologic assays. The FDA offers specific regulatory guidance through communications with Agency staff as well as documents relevant to vaccine development. Sponsors and others considering HIV-1 vaccine development are encouraged to utilize these resources.

ACKNOWLEDGEMENTS. The authors would like to acknowledge the review and helpful suggestions provided by the following colleagues: Karen Midthun, M.D., Marion Gruber, Ph.D., and Theresa Finn, Ph.D.

This article reflects the authors' assessment of the approach to development for HIV-1 preventive vaccines and is not intended to represent the official position of the FDA.

REFERENCES

Ad Hoc Group for the Study of Pertussis Vaccines. (1988). Placebo-controlled trial of two acellular pertussis vaccines in Sweden—Protective efficacy and adverse events. *Lancet* 1:955–960.

Amara, R.R., and Robinson, H.L. (2002). A new generation of HIV vaccines. *Trends Mol Med.* 8:489–495.

Baylor, N.W., and Midthun, K. (2004). Regulation and testing of vaccines. In: Plotkin, S.A., and Orenstein, W.A. (eds.), *Vaccines*, 4th ed. W.B. Saunders, Philadelphia, pp. 1539–1556.

Belshe, R.B., Bolognesi, D.P., Clements, M.L., Corey, L., Dolin, R., Mestecky, J., Stablein, D., and Wright, P. (1994). HIV infection in vaccinated volunteers. *JAMA* 272:431. [Letter]

Berman, P.W., Gray, A.M., Wrin, T., Vennari, J.C., Eastman, D.J., Nakamura, G.R., Francis, D.P., Gorse, G., and Schwartz, D.H. (1997). Genetic and immunologic characterization of viruses infecting MN-rgp120-vaccinated volunteers. *J Infect Dis.* 176:384–397.

Blackwelder, W.C., Storsaeter, J., Olin P., and Hallander, H.O. (1991). Acellular pertussis vaccines. Efficacy and evaluation of clinical case definitions. *Am J Dis Child.* 145:1285–1289.

Bloom, B.R. (1998). The highest attainable standard: Ethical issues in AIDS vaccines. *Science* 279:186–188.

CDC. (1998). Management of possible sexual, injecting-drug use, or other nonoccupational exposure to HIV, including considerations related to antiretroviral therapy. Public Health Service Statement. *MMWR* 47 (No. RR-17):1–14.

CDC. (1999). Impact of vaccines universally recommended for children—United States, 1990–1998. *MMWR* 48:243–248.

CDC. (2002). Guidelines for using antiretroviral agents among HIV-infected adults and adolescents: recommendations of the Panel on Clinical Practices for Treatment of HIV. *MMWR* 51(No. RR-7):1–56.

Connor, E.M., Sperling, R.S., Gelber, R., Kiselev P., Scott G., O'Sullivan, M.J., VanDyke, R., Bey, M., Shearer, W., Jacobson R.L., Jimenez E., O'Neill, E., Bazin, B., Delfraissy, J.F., Culnane, M., Coombs, R., Elkins, M., Moye, J., Stratton, P., and Balsley, J. (1994). Reduction of maternal-infant transmission of human immunodeficiency virus type 1 with zidovudine treatment. Pediatric AIDS Clinical Trials Group Protocol 076 Study Group. *N Engl J Med.* 331:1173–1180.

Connor, R.I., Korber, B.T., Graham, B.S., Hahn, B.H., Ho, D.D., Walker, B.D., Neumann, A.U., Vermund, S.H., Mestecky, J., Jackson, S., Fenamore, E., Cao, Y., Gao, F., Kalams, S., Kunstman, K.J., McDonald, D., McWilliams, N., Trkola, A., Moore, J.P., and Wolinsky, S.M. (1998). Immunological and virological analyses of persons infected by human immunodeficiency virus type 1 while participating in trials of recombinant gp120 subunit vaccines. *J Virol.* 72:1552–1576.

Dean, M., Carrington, M., Winkler, C., Huttley, G.A., Smith, M.W., Allikmets, R., Goedert, J.J., Buchbinder, S.P., Vittinghoff, E., Gomperts, E., Donfield, S., Vlahov, D., Kaslow, R., Saah, A., Rinaldo, C., Detels, R., and O'Brien, S.J. (1996). Genetic restriction of HIV-1 infection and progression to AIDS by a deletion allele of the CKR5 structural gene. Hemophilia Growth and Development Study, Multicenter AIDS Cohort Study, Multicenter Hemophilia Cohort Study, San Francisco City Cohort, ALIVE Study. *Science* 273:1856–1862.

Dixon, D.O., Rida, W.N., Fast, P.E., and Hoth, D.F. (1993). HIV vaccine trials: Some design issues including sample size calculation. *J AIDS* 6: 485–496.

Ellenberg, S., Geller, N., Simon, R., and Yusuf, S. (eds.) (1993). Practical issues in data monitoring of clinical trials. *Statistics in Medicine* 12:419–616. [Proceedings of a meeting, Bethesda, MD, USA, January 27–28, 1992]

Ellenberg, S.S., Demets, D.L., and Fleming, T.R. (eds.). (2002). *Data Monitoring Committees in Clinical Trials: A Practical Perspective*, John Wiley & Sons, Ltd; Chichester, England.

Emerson, S.S., and Fleming, T.R. (1990). Interim analyses in clinical trials. *Oncology* 4:126–133.

Esparza, J., and Osmanov, S. (2003). HIV vaccines: a global perspective. *Curr Mol Med.* 3:183–193.

Fast, P.E., Sawyer, L.A., and Wescott, S.L. (1995). Clinical considerations in vaccine trials with special reference to candidate HIV vaccines. *Pharm Biotech.* 6:97–134.

Fauci, A.S. (2003). HIV and AIDS: 20 years of science. *Nat Med.* 9:839–43.

Francis, D.P., Heyward, W.L., Popovic, V., Orozco–Cronin, P., Orelind, K., Gee, C., Hirsch, A., Ippolito, T., Luck, A., Longhi, M., Gulati, V., Winslow, N., Gurwith, M., Sinangil, F., and Berman, P.W. (2003). Candidate HIV/AIDS vaccines: lessons learned from the World's first phase III efficacy trials. *AIDS* 17:147–156.

Freas, W., and Gertzog, J. (1997). The FDA's biological products advisory committees. In: Mathieu, M., (ed.), *Biologics Development: A Regulatory Overview*, 2nd ed. Parexel, Waltham, Mass., pp. 253–268.

Friedman, L.M., Furberg, C.D., and DeMets, D.L. (1996). *Fundamentals of Clinical Trials*, 3rd ed. Mosby, New York.

Gaschen, B., Taylor, J., Yusim, K., Foley, B., Gao, F., Lang, D., Novitsky, V., Haynes, B., Hahn, B.H., Bhattacharya, T., and Korber, B. (2002). Diversity considerations in HIV-1 vaccine selection. *Science* 296:2354–2360.

Geller, N.L., and Pocock, S.J. (1987). Interim analyses in randomized clinical trials: Ramifications and guidelines for practitioners. *Biometrics* 43:213–223.

Gilbert, P.B., DeGruttola, V.G., Hudgens, M.G., Self, S.G., Hammer, S.M., and Corey, L. (2003). What constitutes efficacy for a human immunodeficiency virus vaccine that ameliorates viremia: Issues involving surrogate end points in phase 3 trials. *J Infect Dis.* 188:179–193.

Goldenthal, K.L., and McVittie L.D. (1997). The clinical testing of preventive vaccines for infectious disease indications. In: Mathieu, M. (ed.), *Biologics Development: A Regulatory Overview,* 2nd Ed. Parexel, Waltham, Mass., pp. 123–139.

Goldenthal, K.L., Cavagnaro, J.A., Alving, C.R., and Vogel, F.R. (1993). Safety evaluation of vaccine adjuvants. *AIDS Res. Hum. Retroviruses* 9:S47–S51.

Goldenthal, K.L., Vaillancourt, J.M., Geber, A., and Lucey, D.R. (1998). Preventive HIV-1 vaccine clinical trials: A regulatory perspective. *AIDS Res Hum Retroviruses* 14:S333–S340.

Goldenthal, K.L., Falk, L.A., Ball, L., and Geber, A. (2001). Prelicensure evaluation of combination vaccines. *Clin. Inf. Dis.* 33:S267–S273.

Graham, B.S., McElrath, M.J., Connor, R.I., Schwartz, D.H., Gorse, G.J., Keefer, M.C., Mulligan, M.J., Matthews, T.J., Wolinsky, S.M., Montefiori, D.C., Vermund, S.H., Lambert, J.S., Corey, L., Belshe, R.B., Dolin, R., Wright, P.F., Korber, B.T., Wolff, M.C., and Fast, P.E. (1998). Analysis of intercurrent human immunodeficiency virus type 1 infections in phase I and II trials of candidate AIDS vaccines. AIDS Vaccine Evaluation Group, and the

Correlates of HIV Immune Protection Group. *J Infect Dis.* 177:310–319.

Guenter, D., Esparza, J., and Macklin, R. (2000). Ethical considerations in international HIV vaccine trials: Summary of a consultative process conducted by the Joint United Nations Programme on HIV/AIDS (UNAIDS). *J Med Ethics* 26:37–43.

Haynes, B.F., Pantaleo, G., and Fauci, A.S. (1996). Toward an understanding of the correlates of protective immunity to HIV infection. *Science* 271;324–328.

Hoff, R., and Barker, L.F. (1995). Trial objectives and end points for measuring the efficacy of HIV vaccines. *Infect Agents Dis.* 4:95–101.

Horne, A.D., Lachenbruch, P.A., Getson, P.R., and Hsu, H.S. (2001). Analysis of studies to evaluate immune response to combination vaccines.*Clin Infect Dis.* 33:S306–S311.

ICH. (1995). Q2A: Validation of analytical procedures (definitions and terminology). *Federal Reg.* 60:11259–11262.

ICH. (1996). Structure and content of clinical study reports. *Federal Reg.* 61:37319–37343.

ICH. (1997a). Good clinical practice: Consolidated guideline. *Federal Reg.* 62:25691–25709.

ICH. (1997b). Q2B: Validation of analytical procedures: Methodology. *Federal Reg.* 62:27463–27467.

ICH. (1997c). General considerations for clinical trials. *Federal Reg.* 62:66113–66119.

ICH. (1998a). Statistical principles for clinical trials. *Federal Reg.* 63:49583–49598.

ICH. (1998b). Ethnic factors in the acceptability of foreign clinical data. *Federal Reg.* 63:31790–31796.

Kahn, J.O., Steimer, K.S., Baenziger, J., Duliege, A.M., Feinberg, M, Elbeik, T, Chesney, M., Murcar, N., Chernoff, D., and Sinangil, F. (1995). Clinical, immunologic, and virologic observations related to human immunodeficiency virus (HIV) type 1 infection in a volunteer in an HIV-1 vaccine clinical trial. *J Infect Dis.* 171:1343–1347.

Katz, S.P. (1983). Effects of malnutrition and parasitic infections on the immune response to vaccines: Evaluation of the risks associated with administering vaccines to malnourished children. In: Halsey, N.A., and de Quadros, C.A. (eds.), *Recent Advances in Immunization. Scientific Publication #451.* Pan American Health Organization, Washington, D.C., pp. 81–89.

Kaul, R., Dong, T., Plummer, F.A., Kimani, J., Rostron, T., Kiama, P., Njagi, E., Irungu, E., Farah, B., Oyugi, J., Chakraborty, R., MacDonald, K.S., Bwayo, J.J., McMichael, A., and Rowland-Jones, S.L. (2001). CD8(+) lymphocytes respond to different HIV epitopes in seronegative and infected subjects. *J Clin Invest.* 107:1303–1310.

Klausner, R.D., Fauci, A.S., Corey, L., Nabel, G.J., Gayle, H., Berkley, S., Haynes, B.F., Baltimore, D., Collins, C., Douglas, R.G., Esparza, J., Francis, D.P., Ganguly, N.K., Gerberding, J.L., Johnston, M.I., Kazatchkine, M.D., McMichael, A.J., Makgoba, M.W., Pantaleo, G., Piot, P., Shao, Y., Tramont, E., Varmus, H., and Wasserheit, J.N. (2003). The need for a global HIV vaccine enterprise. *Science* 300:2036–2039.

McElrath, M.J., Corey, L., Greenberg, P.D., Matthews, T.J., Montefiori, D.C., Rowen, L., Hood, L., and Mullins, J.I. (1996). Human immunodeficiency virus type 1 infection despite prior immunization with a recombinant envelope vaccine regimen. *Proc Natl Acad Sci.* USA 93:3972–3977.

McMichael, A.J., and Hanke, T. (2003). HIV vaccines 1983-2003. *Nat Med.* 9:874–880.

Nathanson, N., and Mathieson, B.J. (2000). Biological considerations in the development of a human immunodeficiency virus vaccine. *J Infect Dis.* 182:579–589.

NIH, NIAID. (2002). *The Jordan Report 20th Anniversary: Accelerated Development of Vaccines.* [To obtain this document, connect to http://www.niaid.nih.gov/dmid/vaccines/jordan20/.]

O'Brien, P.C., and Fleming, T.R. (1979). A multiple testing procedure for clinical trials. *Biometrics* 35:549–556.

O'Neill, R.T. (1988). On sample sizes to estimate the protective efficacy of a vaccine. *Statistics in Medicine* 7:1279–1288.

O'Toole, C., Muller, S., Nara, P., and Kohler, H. (1996). Immunologic mechanism for human immunodeficiency virus type 1 gp120 vaccine failure. *J Infect Dis.* 173:512–513.

Patriarca, P.A., Wright, P.F., and John, T.J. (1991). Factors affecting the immunogenicity of oral poliovirus vaccine in developing countries: Review. *Reviews of Infectious Diseases* 13:926–939.

Paxton, W.A., Kang, S., and Koup, R.A. (1998). The HIV type 1 coreceptor CCR5 and its role in viral transmission and disease progression. *AIDS Res Hum Retroviruses* 14 Suppl 1:S89–S92.

Rida, W., Fast, P., Hoff, R., and Fleming, T. (1997). Intermediate-size trials for the evaluation of HIV vaccine candidates: A workshop summary. *J AIDS* 16:195–203.

Rowe, P.M. (1996). HIV subtypes raise vaccine anxieties [news]. *Lancet* 347:603.

Safrit, J.T. (2003). HIV vaccines in infants and children: Past trials, present plans and future perspectives. *Curr Mol Med.* 3:303–312.

Samson, M., Libert, F., Doranz, B.J., Rucker, J., Liesnard, C., Farber, C.M., Saragosti, S., Lapoumeroulie, C., Cognaux, J., Forceille, C., Muyldermans, G., Verhofstede, C., Burtonboy, G., Georges, M., Imai, T., Rana, S., Yi, Y., Smyth, R.J., Collman, R.G., Doms, R.W., Vassart, G., and Parmentier, M. (1996). Resistance to HIV-1 infections in caucasian individuals bearing mutant alleles of the CCR-5 chemokine receptor gene. *Nature* 382:722–725.

Schaper, C., Fleming, T.R., Self, S.G., and Rida, W.N. (1995). Statistical issues in the design of HIV vaccine trials. *Ann Rev Public Health* 16:1–22.

Schofield, T.L. (2000). Assay development: Assay validation. In: Chow S. C. (ed.), *Encyclopedia of Biopharmaceutical Statistics.* Marcel Dekker, New York, pp. 13–30.

Stiehm, E.R., Lambert, J.S., Mofenson, L.M., Bethel, J., Whitehouse, J., Nugent, R., Moye, J. Jr., Glenn Fowler, M., Mathieson, B.J., Reichelderfer, P., Nemo, G.J., Korelitz, J., Meyer, W.A. 3rd, Sapan, C.V., Jimenez, E., Gandia, J., Scott, G., O'Sullivan, M.J., Kovacs, A., Stek, A., Shearer, W.T., and Hammill, H. (1999). Efficacy of zidovudine and human immunodeficiency virus (HIV) hyperimmune immunoglobulin for reducing perinatal HIV transmission from HIV-infected women with advanced disease: results of Pediatric AIDS Clinical Trials Group protocol 185. *J Infect Dis.* 179:567–575.

Storsaeter, J., Hallander, H., Farrington, C.P., Olin, P., Mollby, R., and Miller, E. (1990). Secondary analyses of the efficacy of two acellular pertussis vaccines evaluated in a Swedish phase III trial. *Vaccine* 8:457–461.

Taffs, R.E. (2001). Potency tests of combination vaccines. *Clin Infect Dis.* 33 Suppl 4:S362–S366.

UNAIDS/WHO (2003). AIDS Epidemic Update. December 2003. Geneva, Switzerland.

U.S. FDA, Center for Biologics Evaluation and Research (CBER), Center for Drug Evaluation and Research (CDER). (1996a). FDA guidance concerning demonstration of comparability of human biological products, including therapeutic biotechnology-derived products. [To obtain this document, connect to http://www.fda.gov/cber/guidelines.htm.

U.S. FDA, Center for Biologics Evaluation and Research, Office of Vaccines Research and Review. (1996b).Points To Consider on Plasmid DNA Vaccines for Preventive Infectious Disease Indications. [To obtain this document, connect to http://www.fda.gov/cber/gdlns/plasmid.pdf.]

U.S. FDA, Center For Biologics Evaluation and Research. (1997). Guidance for Industry for the Evaluation of Combination Vaccines for Preventable Diseases: Production, Testing and Clinical Studies. [To obtain this document, connect to http://www.fda.gov/cber/guidelines.htm.]

U.S. FDA. (2000a). Guidance for Industry: Formal Meetings With Sponsors and Applicants for PDUFA Products. [To obtain this document, connect to http://www.fda.gov/cber/guidelines.htm.]

U.S. FDA. (2000b). Draft Guidance for Industry: Considerations for Reproductive Toxicity Studies for Preventive Vaccines for Infectious Disease Indications. [To obtain this document, connect to http://www.fda.gov/cber/guidelines.htm.]

U.S. FDA. (2001). Draft Guidance for Clinical Trial Sponsors On the Establishment and Operation of Clinical Trial Data Monitoring Committees. [To obtain this document, connect to http://www.fda.gov/cber/guidelines.htm.]

U.S. FDA, Center for Biologics Evaluation and Research. (2002). Standard Operating Procedures and Policies (SOPP 8101.1): Scheduling and Conduct of Regulatory Meetings with Sponsors and Applicants. [To obtain this document, connect to http://www.fda.gov/cber/regsopp/81011.htm.]

WHO. (2003). Guidelines on Clinical Evaluation of Vaccines: Regulatory Considerations. (http://www.who.int/.)

Zhu, T., Corey, L., Hwangbo, Y., Lee, J.M., Learn, G.H., Mullins, J.I., and McElrath, M.J. (2003). Persistence of extraordinarily low levels of genetically homogeneous human immunodeficiency virus type 1 in exposed seronegative individuals. *J Virol.* 77:6108–6016.

36

United States Department of Defense HIV-1 Vaccine Development in Thailand

Deborah L. Birx[1], Arthur E. Brown[2], Philip O. Renzullo[1], Mark S. de Souza[2], and John G. McNeil[1,3]

[1] *U.S. Military HIV Research Program, Rockville, Maryland, USA*
[2] *Armed Forces Research Institute of Medical Sciences, Bangkok, Thailand*
[3] *Vaccine Research Center, National Institute of Allergy and Infectious Diseases, National Institutes of Health, Bethesda, Maryland*

INTRODUCTION AND HISTORY

History of the Armed Forces Research Institute of Medical Sciences (AFRIMS)

For nearly 40 years, the AFRIMS, located in Bangkok, Thailand, has been the cornerstone of many research efforts essential for the Royal Thai Army (RTA), Thailand and the U.S. Department of Defense (DoD). The primary focus of this joint activity has been research into the prevention of endemic infectious diseases affecting both the RTA and the U.S. deployed forces in Southeast Asia.

The AFRIMS traces its origin to the year 1958 when a group of scientists from the United States and Thailand undertook a joint study of a cholera epidemic in Thailand. The Southeast Asia Treaty Organization (SEATO) recognized the significance of the cholera problem and established the SEATO Cholera Research Laboratory, Bangkok, in 1959. Although initially tasked to conduct scientific research on various aspects of the cholera epidemic, the laboratory's mission was expanded in 1961 to include research on other tropical diseases and renamed the SEATO Medical Research Laboratory. The laboratory became the AFRIMS upon dissolution of SEATO in 1977 and today operates as a joint Thai–American military medical research venture. It is comprised of both Royal Thai and U.S. Army Research Components. Overall command rests with a RTA officer. The U.S. Component functions as a Special Foreign Activity of the Walter Reed Army Institute of Research (WRAIR) in Washington, D.C., and of the U.S. Army Medical Research and Materiel Command (USAMRMC). The Thai Component of AFRIMS is a subordinate command of the RTA Medical Department.

The mission of the AFRIMS is medical research, disease surveillance, and development and evaluation of medical products for militarily relevant infectious and tropical infectious diseases. The primary objectives of the U.S. Component of AFRIMS include: i) monitor and assess potential disease threats, especially emerging infectious diseases; ii) evaluate new drugs and vaccines for prophylaxis and treatment of militarily important infectious diseases; iii) develop and test new forward-deployable rapid diagnostic methods; iv) investigate and test new control measures against infectious disease vectors to interrupt disease transmission; v) define the epidemiology of militarily important diseases endemic to tropical regions; vi) advise the Commander-in-Chief, Pacific Command, and the U.S. Ambassador, Thailand, on tropical disease threats; and vii) develop infrastructure and continue proactive training, development, and technology transfer to Thai medical research for Thai control and responsibility.

Research programs within AFRIMS include enteric diseases (infectious causes of diarrhea), malaria vaccine and drug research, viral diseases, especially dengue fever and hepatitis. In addition, the Departments of Entomology, dedicated to the study of disease vectors, and Retrovirology, focused on HIV vaccine development and evaluation, exist at AFRIMS. AFRIMS also supports emerging disease threats as a part of a Global Emerging Infections Surveillance program.

The USAMRMC conducts the majority of its research and development activities at military medical research institutes, and a minority through contracts and cooperative research and development agreements with universities and other institutions. AFRIMS has a long and outstanding reputation as the military's premier biomedical research institution in Thailand, focusing primarily on research in the field of military preventive medicine. It is the largest overseas U.S. Army biomedical research laboratory and plays a vital role in the study of tropical infectious diseases, conducting cutting-edge research and development projects which address the medical threats facing U.S. forces deployed in over 75 countries worldwide.

The United States Army Medical Component—AFRIMS conducts collaborative research with government, academic, and industrial partners to develop and evaluate diagnostic tests, vaccines, and drugs against tropical infectious diseases of military importance.

Personnel assigned to AFRIMS have contributed to medical policy on troop deployment and troop readiness by providing expert medical advice to combatant commanders. For example, AFRIMS has supported joint U.S.–Thai military exercises in Thailand for the last decade (Cobra Gold and Balance Torch). This support included surveying diarrheal diseases to define antibiotic susceptibility patterns and recommend prevention and treatment, presenting lectures to medical units, and providing current epidemiological data to personnel responsible for preventive medicine. AFRIMS also provided laboratory support for Operations Desert Storm and Restore Hope.

AFRIMS directly employs over 250 people, including 20 U.S. officers and enlisted personnel, and 120 Thai scientific, technical, and administrative personnel. In addition, numerous contractors and visiting scientists work at AFRIMS. AFRIMS undertakes collaborative projects not only with other U.S. military research units, but also with the Thai government and with scientists in universities in Thailand and in other countries worldwide.

USAMRMC, the senior military medical research command, unlike private pharmaceutical companies, is concerned with medical threats during military deployment, and thus is not limited to only drug or vaccine development which has viable commercial potential. Pharmaceutical companies are often willing to enter into cooperative agreements with AFRIMS to develop and test new drugs and vaccines, enabling them to leverage their research dollars. Nearly one-half of the budget of AFRIMS now comes from such partnerships with the private sector.

The capacity of AFRIMS to conduct field studies outside of its laboratories in Bangkok is extensive. Currently, several dozen field sites are in operation, staffed by personnel from Bangkok, as well as local paid and volunteer staff. Infectious disease investigations can be initiated on short notice and at any location in the country once proper approvals are obtained. Some of AFRIMS' field sites have been in operation for more than a decade, bringing sophisticated equipment to focal points of study. Good working relationships within the Thai Ministry of Public Health (MoPH), the RTA, and individual hospitals and clinics all over Thailand allow for mutually productive collaborations in studying diseases and medical products. AFRIMS' personnel also travel regionally to study diseases of interest in Nepal, Laos, Cambodia, and Vietnam.

For more than four decades, AFRIMS has conducted ground breaking research and conducted clinical trials on experimental therapeutics and vaccines for malaria (Brown *et al.*, 1994), scrub typhus (Watt *et al.*, 2000), dengue (Endy *et al.*, 2002), enteric diseases (Hoge *et al.*, 1998), Japanese encephalitis (Hoke *et al.*, 1988), Hepatitis A, B, C, E (Innis *et al.*, 1991; Maneerat *et al.*, 1996; Kozik *et al.*, 2000), and, since 1991, HIV-1. Two pivotal vaccine efficacy trials have been performed collaboratively between AFRIMS and the MoPH, leading to product licensure. The HIV-1 vaccine development effort in Thailand builds on this longstanding bilateral partnership. AFRIMS partnered with the MoPH to carry out phase III trials of Japanese encephalitis and hepatitis A vaccines, and provides the administrative foundation supporting the personnel and services required for the ongoing Phase III HIV vaccine trial. USAMRMC is supporting the involvement of an additional 400 individuals in the conduct of the trial through expanded contractual relationships with the Thai Ministry of Health, Mahidol University, and the RTA.

History of the U.S. Military HIV Research Program

In the mid 1980s, the U.S. military recognized the emerging HIV-1 epidemic as a new threat to U.S. forces. In response to this threat, a Congressionally-mandated research program was initiated in 1986 to monitor and to mitigate the impact of HIV/AIDS on the U.S. military's readiness. The U.S. Military HIV Research Program (USMHRP) was initiated as a result of the Congressional and military directive to develop effective preventive measures against HIV to include: education, testing both the blood supply and military members, vaccine development, and implementation of novel anti-viral therapies and clinical management tools. In 2003, HIV-1 continues to pose a significant and persistent threat to the U.S. military. The risk of infection with HIV-1 is similar to the well-documented risk of infection with hepatitis B. Consequently, the military requirement for an HIV-1 vaccine is as urgent as was the need for hepatitis B vaccine for the military in the 1980s.

The incidence of new HIV-1 infections in the active and reserve force has remained constant over the past decade at approximately 400–500 each year (Renzullo *et al.*, 2001). Infections have been documented as occurring in the United States and during international deployment as the global epidemic continues to expand unabated throughout Eastern and Central Europe, Asia, and Sub-Saharan Africa. The risk for exposure to the virus by DoD personnel increases during deployments, peacekeeping missions, and humanitarian aid missions as the epidemic spreads in local populations. There are more deployment-associated HIV-1 infections in DoD personnel annually than any other life-threatening infectious disease, including malaria and multi-drug resistant tuberculosis. These infections are occurring in highly trained senior enlisted personnel and junior officers. The primary risk for deployment-associated infection is local heterosexual exposure. Currently, 5–10% of recent HIV-1 infections in the U.S. military active duty force are non-B subtype. HIV-1 type E infections have been associated with Naval ports-of-call exposures while HIV-1 A, C, D type infections are associated with

African deployments and U.S. Embassy guard assignments (Brodine *et al.*, 1999; Brodine *et al.*, 2003). With the increasing deployment of U.S. forces to areas of the globe in which the HIV-1 epidemic is characterized by a non-B subtype, the focus of the military's HIV vaccine development strategy is to develop a globally effective HIV-1 vaccine with emphasis on non-B subtypes.

The Program has addressed blood exposure risk to active duty troops in the military's health care delivery system, as such troops are co-deployed with other foreign militaries that have high HIV-1 infection rates. The prevalence of the virus in African troop populations ranges from less than 1% to more than 50%. A potential for co-casualty exposure due to field contamination in co-joint military operations or from blood supplies obtained from foreign nationals (the U.S. Embassy bombings) is another area of concern to the U.S. military. In addition, exposure of active duty troops on humanitarian missions, where the local population as well as the co-deployed troops may have a substantial but undocumented of HIV-1 prevalence, must be considered.

The Program builds on the strength of the greater research initiatives within the U.S. military medical research command and continues to address specific HIV requirements essential to meet its mission: prevention of HIV-1 disease in the active force. These requirements include: defining the HIV epidemic on a global level; developing diagnostics and immunologic assays critical for vaccine development; designing, evaluating, and testing of vaccine immunogens from pre-clinical through Phase III efficacy trials; and translating this research to the care and treatment of HIV-infected personnel. The need to develop a globally effective vaccine is critical and the USMHRP is working toward that goal. Recently, the Program's efforts have been further augmented and focused following a ground breaking agreement between the DoD and the Department of Health and Human Services through USAMRMC and the National Institute of Allergy and Infectious Diseases (NIAID). This 2003 agreement brings together the broad comprehensive talent and global strategic planning of the Division of AIDS (DAIDS), NIAID, for HIV prevention, vaccines, and treatment research to the USMHRP. Through the execution of this agreement there is an unprecedented alignment of U.S. government activities to enhance efficacy and ensure non-duplicative complementary initiatives in both programs. All strategic and long term planning of the USMHRP is done jointly with DAIDS and this planning process is further facilitated through the Partnership for AIDS Vaccine Evaluation, which includes the U.S. Centers for Disease Control and Prevention (CDC). For the first time all U.S. government HIV-1 research agencies are united in their mission to control this global epidemic. Although the USAMRMC-NIAID agreement is less than 15 months old, tremendous benefits to the USMHRP have already been seen. DAIDS has brought to the USMHRP expertise in protocol development; statistics; comprehensive aspects of adverse event reporting; preclinical research knowledge; and novel therapeutic initiatives essential to the integrated approach to global HIV prevention through education, vaccine development, and disease prevention through treatment. USMHRP brings to the U.S. government collaboration a strong knowledge of international site development inclusive of all aspects of HIV vaccine development, vaccine production capacity, and a well-defined racially diverse HIV-seropositive cohort without barriers to care and treatment.

KEYS TO INTERNATIONAL VACCINE DEVELOPMENT: ROLE OF PARTNERSHIPS AND HOST GOVERNMENT COMMITMENT

A significant element of Thailand's success in HIV research can be attributed to an excellent public health network, broad access to health care, superb universities, and highly accomplished clinical researchers. In the late 1980s, there was an alarming increase in the prevalence of HIV in Thailand, most notably in the northern region. This dramatic increase continued, peaking in 1992–1993. Since that time there has been an equally dramatic decline, as Figure 1 shows (Torugsa *et al.*, 2003).

There is little doubt that this dramatic decline in HIV prevalence mirrors the development and implementation of Thailand's extensive nation-wide HIV intervention program. Thailand's successful response to the HIV epidemic is a model of what can be accomplished by a government, public health infrastructure, and a population willing to face and address the difficult issues surrounding HIV intervention and control in a concerted, national effort. This same spirit of cooperation and willingness to address HIV control issues, in addition to a highly developed public health infrastructure, are among the reasons that the World Health Organization (WHO) selected Thailand as one of four countries to lead the assessment of HIV vaccines (Esparza, 1993).

Another important component of the success is the ongoing cooperation and linkages between the major sponsors. More than a decade ago, UNAIDS and the United States National Institutes of Health/National Institute of Allergy and Infectious Diseases (NIH/NIAID) recognized the critical role of HIV vaccine development in confronting the global epidemic and began investing early in the characterization of potential vaccine cohorts (Mann and Kay, 1991; Esparza *et al.*, 1991; Nelson *et al.*, 1994; Gao *et al.*, 1994; Pau *et al.*, 1994). Through various collaborative programs, Thailand, Uganda, and Brazil were among the first countries to move forward on their respective continents, leading global HIV vaccine development both politically and scientifically. Dissecting the successes of these early initiatives leads to several insights. Early investment in country-specific, scientific leadership directly impacted government awareness of the HIV/AIDS epidemic, provided critical leadership to HIV/AIDS control programs, and ultimately, helped form the design and implementation of national HIV/AIDS plans (Ungphakorn and Sittitrai, 1994; Phoolcharoen *et al.*, 1998) and the Thai National HIV Vaccine Development Plan (Division of AIDS/MoPH, 1993). The national plans in turn provided the framework for the review, and implementation and execution of

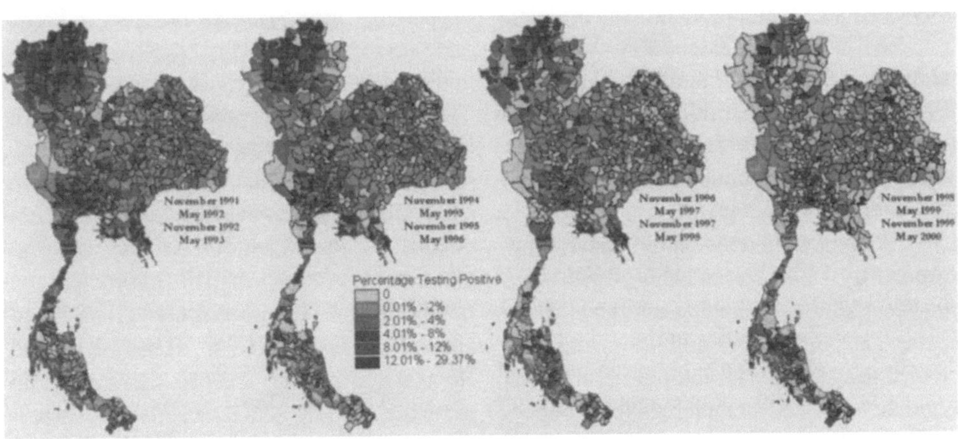

FIGURE 1. Choropleth maps of HIV prevalence in four classes of young men at time of entry into the Royal Thai Army, Thailand, 1991–2000. Location determined by residence during the previous 2 years. Prevalence is stratified by color and localized to district or group of districts so that calculations are based on >20 men.

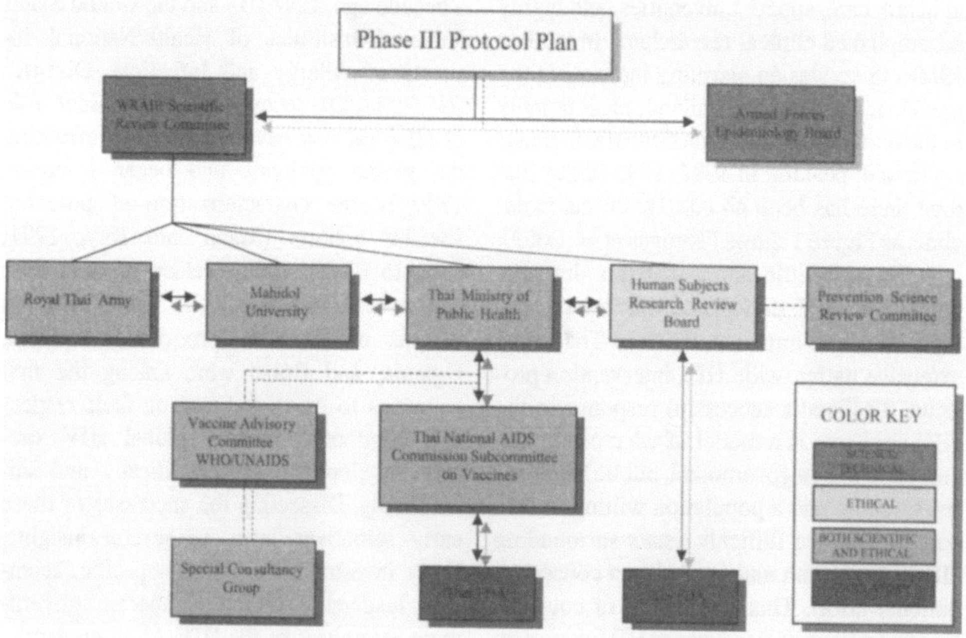

FIGURE 2. Thailand HIV Vaccine Review Process.

HIV protocols. These plans also created objective national standards and requirements that sponsors were expected to meet, and provided a framework for country-specific infrastructure development. All necessary scientific and human subject use review/approval processes were defined, thus permitting sponsors to accurately predict a pathway and timeline for evaluation of their products (see Figure 2).

The Thailand National HIV/AIDS Plan and its companion the Thai National Plan for HIV/AIDS Vaccine Development and Evaluation, continues to evolve as the needs of the country evolve and continues to provide a critical framework for sponsors.

The momentum created by the early investment by UNAIDS and the NIH/NIAID attracted additional collaborations and investments. The U.S. CDC and the DoD followed these efforts with the development of comprehensive and complementary country programs (MacQueen *et al.*, 1999). The CDC efforts centered at the MoPH, while the DoD effort was based at AFRIMS, the site of long term collaborative efforts on regional infectious diseases (Carr *et al.*, 1994; Mason *et al.*, 1995).

The United States government and academic institutions, as well as many international research and policy organizations, have supported Thailand's vaccine development strategy. Millions of dollars have been directed to Thailand over the past decade, expanding infrastructure, funding training, and providing technology transfer. The Thai government has worked in partnership with Thai universities to promote the investment in human resources and to expand training. Additionally, the Thai vaccine development effort has moved forward because of the fundamental commitment to ongoing and aggressive prevention activities promoted and funded by the Thai government (Tanasugarn and Wienrawee, 1994; Hanenberg and Rojanapithayakorn, 1996; Kanshana and Simonds, 2002). Most recently, a comprehensive HIV care and treatment plan has been developed and implemented through the Thai MoPH with support from the Global Fund.

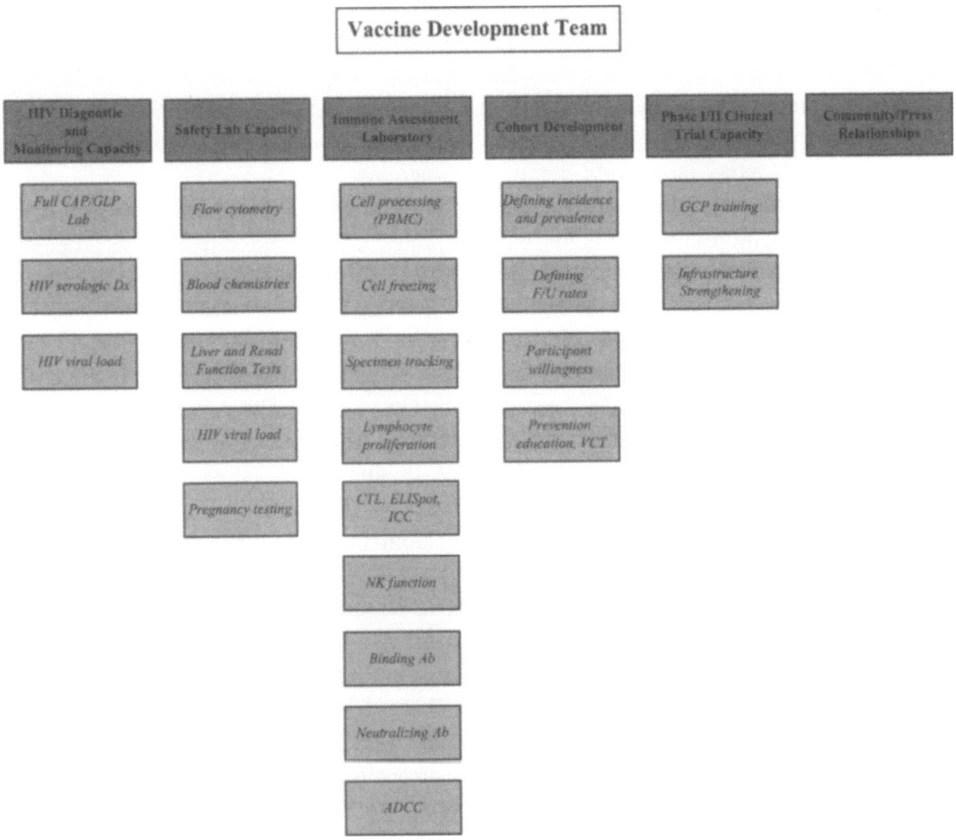

FIGURE 3. Vaccine Development Elements Proceeding in Parallel.

Establishing the Team and Vision

The Program's strategy for the design and development of an HIV vaccine is directed by the DoD's mandate to provide a product for prevention of HIV-1 disease that is globally effective. The primary opportunity to initiate this process existed in the research collaborations and long term investments in laboratory facilities in Thailand established by the RTA and the U.S. military. Thailand was confronted with an expanding HIV-1 epidemic as evidenced among young Thai army recruits. The initial international response of the U.S. DoD to the global HIV threat was the establishment of the Department of Retrovirology at AFRIMS in 1993. A strategic plan was developed linking the mandate for the development of an effective global HIV-1 vaccine development with the opportunity of combating the expanding HIV-1 epidemic in Thailand. The mission of this newly-formed department at AFRIMS linked to the USMHRP focused on the evaluation of vaccines for prevention of infection and the establishment of all the necessary elements for full U.S. Food and Drug Administration and ICH (International Conference on Harmonisation)-compliant phase III efficacy trials.

An in-country collaborative team was developed, through extensive training of RTA officers and cooperation with leading Thai Universities (Figure 3).

Emphasis on the single mission of vaccine development for the global prevention of HIV-1 disease kept the team focused and generated incremental progress toward a Phase III efficacy trial. Members of the U.S.–Thai team focused on specific issues including: core prevention activities focused on providing voluntary counseling and testing and accurate GLP (Good Laboratory Practice) HIV-1 diagnosis; establishing an immune assessment laboratory and a safety assay laboratory; defining the depth, breadth, and subtype of the epidemic; defining appropriate cohorts for large vaccine trials; establishing sophisticated clinical research networks for Phase I/II testing; defining the HIV-1 subtype of the epidemic; and convincing vaccine companies to design and manufacture the vaccines. All of these activities, including the development of a world-class laboratory in Thailand, began in parallel, rather than in series, with team leaders in the U.S. and Thailand.

The key element of the progress was the commitment to in-country support staff. As HIV-1 vaccine development moved from an envelope vaccine based on laboratory strains to complex immunogens derived from primary isolates, the DoD program began a comprehensive vaccine development initiative bringing together clinical researchers and immunologists from the premier Thai universities. Infrastructure development for the complex process of immunogenicity assessment, diagnostic, and safety laboratory assessment meeting Good Laboratory Practices and College of American Pathology (CAP) standards moved forward alongside prevention education and cohort development, all in an integrated and simultaneous effort.

Building Laboratory Capacity

Since 1994, the Program has developed a clinical trials support laboratory in Thailand. These facilities include a CAP-approved diagnostic laboratory and full immune assessment laboratories with the capacity to perform Cytotoxic T Lymphocyte (CTL) assays. The Program has trained and built the infrastructure through multilateral, binational agreements, necessary for effective collaborations in international vaccine development research. The Program has been instrumental in implementing and supporting flow cytometric quality assessment/quality control (QA/QC), 3 CTL laboratories, data management, Good Clinical Practices, and local monitoring of trial conduct and in-country preventive educational programs.

The DoD focused infrastructure development on the critical specimen processing aspects of vaccine research, creating Standard Operating Procedures (SOPs) and QA/QC parameters to maximize lymphocyte viability and functional integrity after freezing and thawing cycles. The program invested substantial time and resources into specimen processing and cell preservation. As cellular function assays were a key to the vaccine development efforts, maintaining cell function in addition to general cell viability was critical. To facilitate and maximize QA/QC and to allow rapid (4–6 hour) processing of cells, local processing units were set-up in the north (Chiang Mai), southeast (Chon Buri) and centrally (Bangkok) to support the vaccine research efforts. Routine HIV-1 diagnosis was being performed and was augmented to include the extensive QA/QC procedures required for full CAP approval. Training in all aspects of diagnostic and safety lab assay performance in compliance with CAP standards was performed and permanent staff were hired to oversee this long-term process. Flow cytometric and immunoassessment workshops and working groups were established to facilitate assay optimization and manage the institution of regular proficiency panel assessments.

Establishing Accurate HIV-1 Diagnostic and Monitoring Capability

In the early 1990s, a standardized program of HIV testing of all recruits was established in collaboration with the WRAIR, which had established a similar program for the U.S. Army (Brown *et al.*, 1996). Centralized testing at the Army Institute of Pathology utilized a diagnostic algorithm consisting of two sequential HIV enzyme immunoassays (EIAs) followed by confirmation with an HIV-1 Western blot. More than 50,000 sera per year were tested from this low prevalence (1–4% HIV-positive) population. The RTA confirmed the very low frequency of false positivity (0.11%) associated with the WHO's recommendations (1997) for use of sequential EIA assays alone (Chanbancherd *et al.*, 1999). Substudies have shown that false reactivity of some HIV rapid tests may occur with malaria and dengue infections and that HIV-2 continues to be absent in Thailand (Chanbancherd *et al.*, 2000).

Using the Capacity to Define the Natural History of HIV-1 Subtype E (CRF01-AE) HIV Infection in Thai adults

While the ideal HIV vaccine would prevent infection, it may also ameliorate or delay onset of disease. Thus, it is essential to characterize the course of disease in Thais infected with the prevalent strain of HIV (CRF01_AE). To fully assess HIV disease progression and immune responses, accurate quantitation of viral load is required. AFRIMS and collaborators have shown that methods based on both template (nucleic acid) and signal amplification are reliable, with the latter giving approximately 0.3-fold lower values of RNA log copies/ml (Elbeik *et al.*, 2002). Among recruits, 80% or more of HIV infections are caused by subtype E HIV (Chanbancherd *et al.*, 2003). In a study of the natural history of HIV infection and disease, the viral load of 255 adult subjects with HIV genotype E infections was detectable in 93% with a mean of 4.09 log RNA copies/ml prior to the start of therapy (Trichavaroj *et al.*, 2001). The concentration of plasma RNA was directly related to the presence of AIDS-defining illnesses, inversely related to CD4 count, and independent of gender after adjustment for CD4 count.

Techniques were developed to evaluate immune responses and viral load at mucosal surfaces. HIV-infected volunteers and seronegative vaccine recipients were enrolled to assess virus at mucosal surfaces, key to heterosexual transmission of HIV (de Souza *et al.*, 2001). In about one third of these subjects, HIV nucleic acid was detectable in the naso-pharynx, with RNA concentrations lower than, but correlated with, those in matched plasma. Since the virus was not successfully isolated in culture, it is believed that these nasopharyngeal findings do not suggest the infectiousness of these secretions yet may provide an accessible site reflecting the virologic findings of vaginal and urethral mucosa. This information will be applied to breakthrough infections in the efficacy study.

Delayed-type hypersensitivity (DTH) skin tests allow *in vivo* assessment of cellular immune responses and provide independent prognostic information of HIV-infected patients (Birx *et al.*, 1993). This immune response was assessed using a panel of four recall antigens (tetanus toxoid, Candida, mumps, and Trichophyton) in 221 adult Thai subjects from across the HIV disease spectrum (Brown *et al.*, 2000). Frequency of anergy was found to be inversely related to CD4 cell count; 38% of patients with CD4 counts of 0-200 cells/mm^3 were completely anergic. The study confirmed that DTH skin testing provided a low-tech method of assessing the integrity of cellular immune function in HIV-infected adults, and thus stage of disease and susceptibility to opportunistic infections.

Establishing Comprehensive Safety Labs

Safety labs were crucial in preparation for the execution of phase I/II vaccine trials. The Thai Component of AFRIMS and RIHES (Research Institute for Health Sciences) in Chiang Mai had established biochemistry laboratories with highly experienced personnel. However, difficulties were faced with differing assay methodologies, the continuity of reagent supplies, normal values based on the Thai population, and a lack of external proficiency panels and documentation

TABLE 1. Summary of Laboratory Capacity Building Successes to Date

- Built laboratory infrastructure for HIV-1 diagnosis, safety labs, and immune assessment in Bangkok and Chiang Mai Thailand with establishment of Standard Operating Procedures (SOPs), Quality Assurance/Quality Control (QA/QC), and proficiency panels.
- Established centralized specimen processing facilities in Bangkok, Chon Buri and Chiang Mai with on-going QA/QC for viability and function
- Established clinical trials network TAVEG—Thai AIDS Vaccine Evaluation Group
- Five phase I/II clinical trials involving approximately 800 volunteers
- Developed College of American Pathology (CAP)-approved laboratory in Bangkok
- Developed Phase III trial protocol and implementation of infrastructure

that would satisfy most laboratory accrediting bodies. A unified working group comprised of members of the two laboratories was established. Samples were shared between the two laboratories to determine whether different testing methodologies were comparable (they were). Discussions with reagent suppliers resulted in improved supply of reagents and equipment maintenance documentation. Normal value was rapidly established by collaborations between the laboratories and regional blood banks, thus resulting in considerable cost-savings compared to implementing a protocol. External proficiency panel testing was more problematic to obtain due to the problems of international shipment of biological materials. It was decided to use two sources of external proficiency panels to circumvent the problem of panels being delayed or lost in shipment/customs. Documentation was achieved by interactive dialogue as well as a commendable commitment on the part of the laboratory supervisors to provide SOPs and corrective action reports in a foreign language and work towards international laboratory accreditation (see Table 1).

Establishing Immune Assessment Laboratory

In preparation for this trial, the program supported the development of classic chromium release CTL assays throughout Thailand, training scientists from the north and the capital, and equipping laboratories at major universities. Each piece of infrastructure and each training opportunity focused on the requirements for HIV-1 vaccine development. But the equipment, laboratories, and techniques were applicable to all aspects of clinical trials and were utilized by the universities to support other non-HIV-1 projects that enhanced the long term stability and sustainability of the investment. HIV-specific CTLs are part of the acquired immune response to HIV infection and are a goal of vaccine-induced immune responses. WRAIR/AFRIMS scientists compared the CTL responses of 12 subtype E-infected Thai patients with 10 B-infected American patients (Lynch *et al.*, 1998). Responses in both groups were most frequent against the *gag* protein, which was also the most frequent target of cross-reactivity. This reactivity was also confirmed using CD8 gamma-interferon production as endpoint in an Elispot assay (Currier *et al.*, 2002).

Induction of antibodies which neutralize HIV is a goal of vaccine design. Assays for neutralization of subtype E viruses were developed at WRAIR, (Mascola *et al.*, 1996), transferred to AFRIMS, and further modified to include a flow cytometric endpoint (Darden *et al.*, 2000). Neutralizing antibodies from subjects with subtype E infection tend to be subtype specific (Polonis *et al.*, 2001). Dual reactivity in the B/E serotyping assay (anti-V3 loop) was associated with increased cross-neutralizing antibodies. The well-characterized viruses and polyclonal antibodies form a valuable set of reagents for study of pathogenesis and design of future candidate vaccines. Among patients with subtype E infections, it was found that rising neutralizing antibody titers were associated with slower disease progression (Chuenchitra *et al.*, 2003). Also, similar to subtype B infections, p24 antibody titers fell in patients with more rapid progression.

Prior to adaptive cellular immune responses, innate immune mechanisms in the form of natural killer (NK) cells may provide a first line of defense against infection. NK cell number and function were assessed (Cox and de Souza, 2000), comparing Thais and Americans with and without HIV infection (de Souza *et al.*, 2000). While having similar numbers (and percentages) of NK cells, the lytic function of NK cells was greater in Thais than Americans. This greater NK cell function of Thais persisted despite HIV infection. Thus, if a vaccine modifies and delays the course of HIV disease, the mechanisms involved may be population-specific and will require direct assessment.

Defining the Epidemic and Risk Factors for Transmission

Beginning in 1989, the RTA began HIV-1 screening of new recruits. HIV prevalence data generated from this screening program provides an unparalleled window on the HIV epidemic in Thailand. It provided the first strong data that the HIV epidemic in the Thai general population had peaked in the early 1990s and then declined (Mason *et al.*, 1995). This followed the start of intensive education and behavioral interventions by the military medicine and public health communities, as well as non-governmental organizations. The decline, although most clear in the north, has continued nationally (Mason *et al.*, 1998), with the characterization of these trends being further refined through the use of geographic information systems (Torugsa *et al.*, 2003).

Formal epidemiological studies were also carried out via multiple U.S.–Thai collaborations. RTA recruits were shown to be at greater risk of HIV infection if they lived in non-rural areas, were unmarried or less educated (Sirisopana *et al.*, 1996). A behavioral survey of 5474 recruits in 1996 suggested that past risk behavior among young northern men may have contributed to the intensity of the epidemic in that region (Kitsiripornchai *et al.*, 1998).

Although heterosexual transmission accounts for the large majority of infections in Thailand (UNAIDS/WHO, 2000) injecting drug users (IDU) form an important subgroup. Since hepatitis C (HCV) infection has been found in more than 95% of a Bangkok IDU cohort (Vanichseni *et al.*, 2001), HCV antibodies were utilized as a marker of exposure to injection drugs. In 2000, 57% of HIV-positive RTA recruits were found to be coinfected with HCV (Chanbancherd *et al.*, 2001). This information may refocus public health interventions. Importantly, the mode of HIV transmission may also influence the efficacy of an HIV vaccine.

The RTA recruit data and the government's sentinel surveillance together have produced the world's most complete characterization of a national HIV epidemic, and documented that the epidemic trend can be reversed. The molecular definition of the HIV-1 epidemic in Thailand occurred in parallel to all the above work ,demonstrating the CRF01-AE subtype. This information is not covered here as it appears in the Tovanabutra *et al.* chapter of this book.

Evaluation and Development of Cohorts for Vaccine Trial

The cohort of subjects for an HIV vaccine trial must be characterized in terms of HIV incidence, rate of follow up, willingness to participate, and migration patterns. The evaluation of potential cohorts has been a continuing process by AFRIMS investigators and their collaborators. Evaluations began with military medical and research staff and Army recruits (Jenkins *et al.*, 1995), then expanded to collaborations with the MoPH to assess sexually transmitted disease (STD) and family planning clinic attendees and members of the general community.

Recruits into the RTA were evaluated as potential vaccine trial subjects in two longitudinal cohort studies. The first study was carried out among 17,615 men recruited in 1991–92 (Carr *et al.*, 1994). HIV incidence ranged from 0.5 to 3.2/100 person-years (p–y) during the 2-year periods of military service. The follow-up rate was only 50% due to reassignments and other logistical problems, a level too low for a vaccine trial. Volunteers who became HIV-infected developed viral loads at set point which ranged more than 100-fold, with median values of 13,000–28,000 RNA copies/ml in the 6–18 months post-diagnosis . Interestingly, 21% of 29 subjects were found to have been in the "window period" of infection (RNA positive, antibody negative) during semiannual blood collections.

A more intensive cohort evaluation was then carried out in a large Army training base in the southern province of Prachuap Khiri Khan (Torugsa *et al.*, 1997). Among the nearly 4000 soldiers in this study, HIV prevalence was 1.8% and incidence was 0.38/100 p-y, less than the previous study situated largely in northern Thailand. Behavioral interventions for reduction of HIV risk were provided and assessed (Jenkins *et al.*, 1999; Jenkins *et al.*, 2000). Among the successful outcomes observed, visits to female sex workers (FSW) fell from 33% to 19% per 6-month interval. The HIV prevention interventions shown effective in this trial have been transitioned from research to operations and are now utilized throughout the RTA, providing a model for militaries of other countries.

Additional research associated with these studies of RTA recruits involved attempts to continue following recruits who left military service upon completion of their tours of duty (Renzullo *et al.*, 1999). Eighteen months after these young men left service, HIV-1 incidence rate in the cohort was sufficient to support a phase III HIV vaccine trial. However, follow-up was low (70%). Further, the rates of several sentinel risk factors for HIV infection in these men after leaving military service had declined compared to when the men were in the military. Taken together, these findings suggested that while ex-military service cohorts might contribute to a comprehensive vaccine cohort, they by themselves would be unable to sustain a phase III trial.

Attendees of STD clinics, considered a group at risk for HIV infection, were assessed as a potential vaccine trial cohort (Markowitz *et al.*, 1999). AFRIMS investigators collaborated with MoPH staff to enroll 371 male and 161 female attendees (FSW excluded). HIV incidence was 1.4/100 p–y in men and 0 in women; follow-up at 12 months was 78%. Total numbers of STD clinic attendees had already fallen in Thailand and this relatively low incidence showed that achieving an appropriate sample size for a phase III trial would be difficult.

Expanding the collaboration with the MoPH, women attending family planning clinics were evaluated (Sirisopana *et al.*, 2001). Women (n = 1115) aged 20 to 30 years old were enrolled; of note, 98% were married or in stable relationships. HIV prevalence was 4%, and incidence was 0.39/100 p–y. Follow-up was 86% and 82% at 6 and 12 months, respectively. More than 50% of volunteers said they would definitely, or very likely, join a future vaccine trial.

A second model utilizing the MoPH infrastructure assessed a potential community cohort in Chon Buri Province, with enrollment of 2500 adults (73% were 20–30 years) and an 18-month follow-up rate (Benenson *et al.*, 2001). HIV prevalence was 4.8%; incidence, in the presence of special counseling, was 0.55/100 p-y (0.70/100 p-y for those less than 30 years old). Mode of transmission among HIV-positive subjects was explored using HCV antibodies as a surrogate marker of injection drug exposure. Approximately 50% of the HIV-infected men were also HCV-positive, while rates of co-infection among women were similar to the 4% rates observed in HIV-uninfected women (Paris *et al.*, 2003). Overall follow-up rates were 84% and 81% at 6 and 12 months, respectively. This model,

TABLE 2. Summary of the U.S. Military HIV Research Program Trials Conducted in Thailand

Study Designation	Phase	Vaccine Antigen(s)	Manufacturer	Number of Volunteers	Year Initiated	Year Completed
RV-99	Phase I	gp120-SF2	Chiron Biocine	52	1995	1997
		gp120-SF2				
RV-114	Phase I/II	gp120-CM235	Chiron Vaccines	285	1997	1999
			Pasteur Merieux			
RV-132	Phase I/II	vCP1521	Connaught	130	1999	2001
			Pasteur Merieux			
		gp160-92TH023	Connaught			
		gp120-SF2				
		gp120-CM235	Chiron Vaccines			
RV-135	Phase I/II	vCP1521	Aventis Pasteur	125	1999	2001
		gp120-MN				
		gp120-A244	VaxGen			
RV-144	Phase III	vCP1521	Aventis Pasteur	16000	2003	2008*
		gp120-MN				
		gp120-A244	VaxGen			

utilizing MoPH staff to implement the study and enrolling through health centers and community hospitals, was assessed to be feasible for use in the recruitment and follow-up of volunteers for a phase III trial.

Through the 1990s, several collaborations assessed multiple potential cohorts for an efficacy trial of an HIV vaccine. With the exception of IDU attending Bangkok Metropolitan Authority clinics, HIV incidence and follow-up were inversely related. High-risk groups tended to be hard to identify and follow. Thus, after these studies throughout the 1990s, AFRIMS investigators approached the MoPH with a proposal to design and carry out a community-based trial based on the Chon Buri model described above (See Table 2).

Establishing Phase I/II Vaccine Testing Sites

In 1991, WHO selected Thailand and three other countries as potential HIV vaccine evaluation sites (Esparza, 1993). Since that time, Thailand has led the less-industrialized world in the clinical assessment of candidate HIV vaccines (Esparza and Bhamarapravati, 2000). In a manner unique outside the industrialized West, candidate HIV vaccines designed to match the locally-prevalent variant were produced by private sector partners. Recombinant DNA technology was used by Chiron Vaccines and VaxGen to produce monomeric glycoprotein (gp)120 antigens and by Aventis Pasteur to produce an oligomeric gp140 and a live canarypox vector with multiple HIV genes. These candidate vaccines were all based on envelope gene sequences from subtype E viruses isolated in Thailand (McCutchan *et al.*, 1992). The AFRIMS/Thai AIDS Vaccine Evaluation Group (TAVEG) collaboration assessed all four of these subtype E candidate vaccines for safety and immunogenicity. More TAVEG volunteers completed phase I/II clinical trials of preventive HIV vaccines in Thailand than the rest of the developing world combined (Esparza, 1993).

The initial phase I trial of a gp120 B vaccine in 1995 was followed by a focus on gp120 E primary isolates with the intent on moving forward into efficacy trials (Table I). If safety parameters were met during the Phase I trials, the product moved forward into Phase II testing, where clear immunogenicity (and safety) thresholds were set for moving forward into Phase III efficacy trials. The default was always to move forward unless the product did not meet predefined criteria.

AFRIMS' initial phase I/II HIV vaccine trial was carried out at the Pramongkutklao Army Medical Center (Bangkok) and at Chiang Mai University. This trial of 52 adult seronegative volunteers utilized a subtype B candidate vaccine (HIV SF2 gp120/MF59 from Chiron Vaccines) as a way to further develop: the in-country capacity for review, approval, oversight, and conduct of an HIV vaccine trial; the training of clinical and laboratory staff; the methods of volunteer recruitment; culture-specific educational materials and consent forms; and the knowledge base of the media and general public in relation to HIV vaccine trials. The vaccine was found to be safe and immunogenic in Thai adults (Nitayaphan *et al.*, 2000). The majority of volunteers described altruistic motivation for their interest in the trial (Jenkins *et al.*, 1998). Levels of risk behavior were reported as relatively low (Thapinta *et al.*, 1999) and no HIV infections occurred during the trial. About one fifth of volunteers reported negative reactions from family or friends, but none reported discrimination related to jobs, health care or insurance (Thapinta *et al.*, 1999).

Chiron Vaccines produced the first subtype E-specific, HIV candidate vaccine, a recombinant gp120 derived from CM235, a primary (C5, or CCR5 receptor usage virus) subtype E virus isolated at WRAIR. The AFRIMS collaboration expanded to become the TAVEG consisting of four academic clinical trial sites. A phase I/II trial of 380 volunteers evaluated the Thai E gp120 antigen in different doses and combinations with a subtype B gp120 antigen (Pitisuttithum *et al.*, 2003). The vaccine was found to be safe; subtype E-specific neutralizing antibodies (NAb) were detected in 85% of vaccinees, similar to the 84% of subtype B-specific NAb in subtype B vaccinees.

As an addendum to this protocol, 24 volunteers who had received the 100 ug dose of Thai E gp120 consented to receive two booster doses (200 ug) of this antigen after a rest interval of at least 12 months from their last vaccination. Both binding and neutralizing antibody titers were boosted more than 2-fold above the responses of the original immunization series but were not sustained at this level with the second booster dose (Chuenchitra and Polonis, unpublished data). Factors important in recruitment and the motivation of volunteers were again evaluated and found to be more complex than previously appreciated; but again altruism was found to be associated with volunteer retention (Thapinta *et al.*, 2002). The relationships which developed between the volunteers and members of the research team also appeared to be important in volunteer compliance and retention (Triampon, 2001).

The strategically defined goal of developing a vaccine which induces both humoral and cellular immunity was pursued through the evaluation of a "prime-boost" vaccine combination (Tartaglia *et al.*, 1998). Aventis Pasteur developed an attenuated canarypox virus which incorporated both subtype B and E (*env*) gene sequences (ALVAC-HIV vCP1521). This vectored vaccine, boosted by 1 of 3 Env protein vaccines, was evaluated in phase I/II clinical trials. As "boost," one combination utilized the bivalent B/E gp120 vaccine from Chiron Vaccines described above (Suriyanon *et al.*, 2002). The second combination assessed an oligomeric Thai E (TH023) gp140 as boost (Thongcharoen *et al.*, 2002). The third assessed the bivalent gp120 vaccine from VaxGen, AIDSVAX" B/E, as the boost (Nitayaphan *et al.*, 2002). All combinations were found to be well tolerated and safe; no volunteers became HIV-infected during the trials. As in previous trials, motivation and other factors were involved in recruitment and retention were assessed (Chinaworapong *et al.*, 2001; Khamboonruang *et al.*, 2001; Thapinta *et al.*, 2002).

The ability to move four products through Phase I and Phase II testing in Thailand within five years is a reflection of the commitment of the Thai investigators, the political will of the Thai government, and the team building between the laboratory and the clinic. Throughout the process, there was continued support from the U.S. State Department through the U.S. Embassy in Thailand, and the DoD through USAMRMC and WRAIR.

Building Community and Press Relationships

Vital to the success of any vaccine trial is willingness of members of the population targeted for enrollment to participate in the research. If substantial barriers or obstacles to participation exist, or if knowledge of scientific research or vaccines is lacking, vaccine trails will not succeed no matter how great the incidence rate is. Thus, community involvement in all aspects of planning for phase III trials is crucial. Research studies are well equipped to characterize knowledge about trials, as well as obstacles to participation. Research has found that despite awareness of vaccines and AIDS vaccine efforts being generally high in Thai populations, significant barriers to participation do exist (Jenkins *et al.*, 1995; Celentano *et al.*, 1995; Jenkins *et al.*, 1998; Thapinta *et al.*, 2002). These have included a fear of discrimination, fear of vaccine side effects, concern about disability or death, and concerns about adverse effects on personal relationships. However, characterizing the concerns is not enough. Once identified, obstacles to participation must be addressed. This can only be achieved through research marketing to the entire community.

In the case of the prime boost phase III, once the appropriate population was identified for phase III participation, research marketing was initiated through a well-defined community outreach plan. As a response to the need to maintain effective communication, a community outreach office (COO) was established and is located within the region from which the phase III population is being recruited. The COO facilitates activities to ensure maximum recruitment of volunteers using all the media at its disposal. Such media include not just standard print and broadcast (and other electronic) media, but also activities such as concerts, meetings, health fairs, and the like which community members might regularly attend. In addition, the COO has informed and continues to educate community leaders, as well as the media. It is through these avenues that the general public is most likely to be informed of the existence of the trial, which is expected of participants in order to enroll. Finally, the COO serves as the clearinghouse for all trial information and, most importantly, responds to all inquiries and requests for information from the media, community groups, and international organizations. The MoPH and all Thai and U.S. partners have worked to maintain positive community and press relationships since the onset of these efforts.

Phase III Trial: From Design to Implementation

The vaccine development strategy for Thailand during the 1990s focused on matching the vaccine to the circulating epidemic subtype (HIV-1 B and E) to minimize the question of cross-clade immunity and to directly address the question of protective immune responses (correlates of protection). Prior to 1996, prevalence data suggested an expanding epidemic in young males and sex workers and an implied incidence of 2–3%/year. A phase III trial was designed in 1996 to evaluate the specific immune effector arms of HIV-1 viral control using the projected incidence numbers. This specific strategy was developed in concert with Thai colleagues and was scrutinized by the Thai Ministry of Public Health. Pharmaceutical and biotech companies were contacted, Commercial Research and Development Agreements (CRADAs) and Material Transfer Agreements (MTAs) were established, and vaccines were designed and manufactured for evaluation in Thailand. Timelines were established for each of the critical elements and the work moved forward (Figure 4).

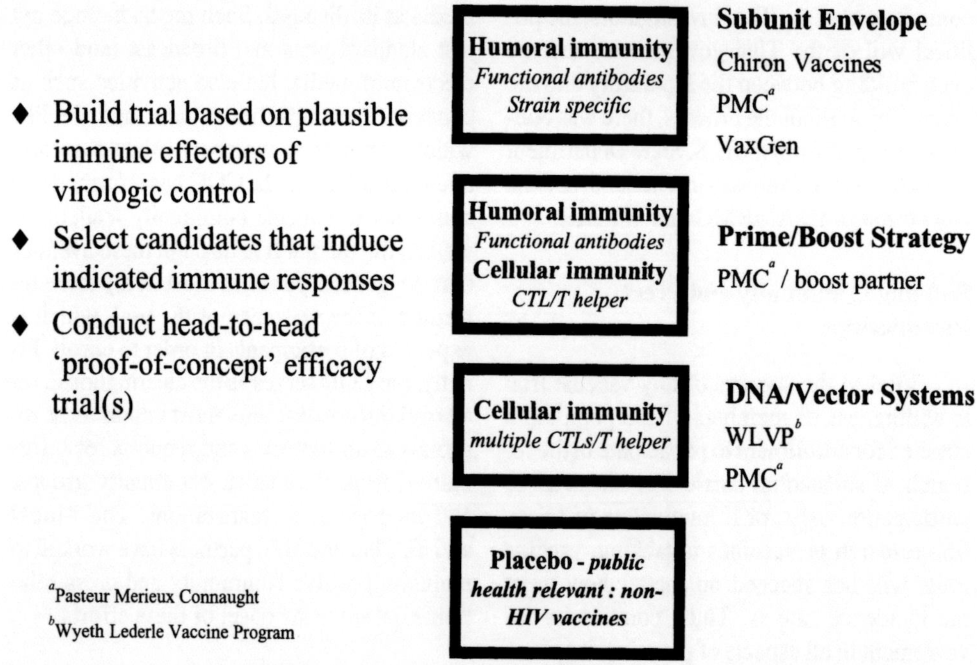

FIGURE 4. Correlates of Protection Trial Design circa 1995.

However, by 1998, data from incidence studies throughout the country demonstrated a significant diminution of the HIV-1 epidemic in Thailand. Six different cohort studies showed an incidence of sexually-acquired HIV-1 infection in the <1% range. The 100% condom use campaign, an inter-ministerial program of the Thai government, had resulted in a dramatic attenuation of the rising epidemic. The vaccine development strategy was thus redesigned to a two arm trial design: a placebo arm and an arm focusing on the induction of cellular and humoral effector immune responses. The best available vaccine candidates inducing these effector classes were evaluated for safety and immunogencity in Thai volunteers. Clear immunologic and safety milestones were defined in conjuction with Thai collaborators prior to beginning the critical Phase II trials of the proposed vaccine candidates. This was a critical decision as the intent at the end of the Phase II trials was to move forward with the pivotal Phase III trial with the best candidate.

Of the prime-boost vaccine combinations evaluated by the TAVEG in phase II trials, the combination of ALVAC-HIV and AIDSVAX®B/E was selected for advancement to phase III (efficacy) testing. The vaccine combination induced subtype E-specific NAb in 71% of vaccinees, lymphoproliferative responses in 58%, and CD8 cytotoxic T-lymphocyte responses in 23% of vaccinees. Safety profiles were based on extensive experience: more than 1800 people had received ALVAC-HIV constructs while more than 7500 people had received AIDSVAX® constructs (>2500 had received the B/E antigen combination in an ongoing phase III trial in Bangkok). The immunogenicity and safety milestones were met and in 2003 the Program launched the Phase III trial of a prime boost vaccine strategy demonstrated to induce both the humoral and cellular arms of the immune system. This complex trial is being executed through the Thai MOPH network, with additional fiscal and personnel support mechanisms. A senior member of the MoPH leads

TABLE 3. Summary of Immunogenicity Data From Phase II Prime/Boost Trial RV 132/RV135

CTL[a]	Percent response (%)		
N = 45 vaccine, 15 placebo	VAXGEN Boost 600 ug	Chiron Boost	Aventis Boost
PBMC CTL (vaccine)	28	25	16
PBMC CTL (placebo)	7	13	7
CD8 CTL (vaccine)	23	25	11
CD8 CTL (placebo)	0	13	7
LPA[b]			
N = 45 vaccine, 15 placebo	VAXGEN Boost 600 ug	Chiron Boost	Aventis Boost
vaccine	58	75	93
placebo	7	13	7
Neutralization[c]			
N = 45 vaccine, 15 placebo	VAXGEN Boost 600 ug	Chiron Boost	Aventis Boost
vaccine	71	100	96
placebo	0	0	0

[a] Cytotoxic T lymphocyte (CTL) (whole peripheral blood mononuclear cells (PBMC) and CD8 specific) in standard HIV Vaccine Trial Network definitions of positive response
[b] Lymphocyte Proliferation Assay (LPA) □ (positive response lymphocyte stimulation index (LSI)≥5)
[c] Neutralization: Tissue culture lab adapted (TC □ LA) or R5 expressing line E viruses screened at 1:10

the investigator team with collaboration from the Faculty of Tropical Medicine, Mahidol University, the RTA and U.S. Army Components of AFRIMS and the WRAIR. The vaccine manufacturers are Aventis Pasteur and VaxGen. Also contributing to the trial under cooperative agreement and contracts are the Henry M. Jackson Foundation for the Advancement of Military Medicine, EMMES Corporation, and Bangkok Pathology Laboratories.

The immunogenicity data, established prior to the onset of the Phase II trial, formed the basis for determining whether to go forward to the Phase III trial. These data are summarized in Table 3.

The 18 months prior to start of the phase III trial focused on expanded training and infrastructure development to allow execution of the first Phase III trial with a complex immunogen combining a cellular immunity inducing prime (ALVAC-HIV 1521) with a gp120 B/E boost of humoral immunity (VaxGen B/E). The Program has supported extensive Good Clinical Practice training of trial staff and expanded laboratory and data management facilities as required for the conduct of the trial. However, the capacity built will be available in the future to support other clinical research in Thailand.

The phase III trial is community-based among young adults in Chon Buri and Rayong Provinces using a double-blind, placebo-controlled, randomized study design (Rerks-Ngarm *et al.*, 2002). Immunization occurs over 6 months, followed by a 3-year follow-up period. While safety will continue to be assessed, the primary efficacy endpoint is HIV infection with secondary endpoints being viral load and CD4 count among those volunteers who develop intercurrent HIV infections. The laboratory measurements are performed centrally in the AFRIMS laboratories, accredited by the College of American Pathologists. The trial is powered to detect a reduction in HIV incidence of 50% or greater among the 16,000 volunteers, half of whom will receive vaccine. The size of this trial carries great logistical challenges and requires optimal engagement and education of the local and national communities. The efficacy of this prime boost strategy will be known in 2008 upon completion of the phase III trial.

TABLE 4. Lessons Learned from Vaccine Development Work in Thailand: Comprehensive Development Strategy Addressing all Requirements from Onset of Collaboration

- Long-term commitment of financial and human resources
  - ~60–70 million dollars in direct support of collaborative R&D to date
  - ~30 FTEs in Thailand, many more in direct support from US
- Epidemiological surveillance: collaborative study with RTA of recruits
  - Kinetics of Epidemic
  - Establish predominance / importance of CRF01_AE in Thailand
- Active vaccine cohort exploration and development
  - Chiang Mai, Phayao, Bangkok, Prachuap Kiri Khan, Rayong, Chon Buri
- Network established to conduct Phase I/II human trials—TAVEG (N ~ 700)
  - Gp120/160 (Chiron, VaxGen, Aventis)
  - vCP1521 (Aventis)
- Team building—long-term commitment
  - Training (GLP, GCP, QA/QC, immunology, data management, epidemiology & statistics)
  - Laboratories (diagnostics, immunology)
  - Agreement for provision of ARTs
  - Full participation in "Down stream" issues related to vaccine access/availability

The essential lessons learned and requirements from vaccine development in Thailand are summarized in Table 4. It was critical to the process to define in advance, through consensus of all stakeholders, the required parameters to move forward from one step in the pathway to the next. This brought clarity and transparency to the process of HIV-1 vaccine development.

Phase III Trial Approval: Science Bridges the Politics of HIV Vaccine Development

The United States and Royal Thai governments are both committed to prevention and control of, and ultimately to ending, the global HIV/AIDS pandemic. Towards that end, the development of a safe, effective, and deployable prophylactic vaccine is a priority. Scientists and public health experts from both governments, in collaboration with partners from academia, private industry, and affected communities—collectively referred to TAVEG—have been involved with joint development of HIV vaccines since 1991. This cooperative partnership has always been based on the active and equivalent participation of its members, and commitment to shared goals, sound science, highest ethics, and complete transparency.

Development of prophylactic vaccines is most effectively conducted when there is good evidence that a particular immune response is associated with a desirable clinical outcome, such as amelioration or complete abrogation of disease. Regarding HIV vaccine development, such evidence emanating from humans and HIV would be ideal; however evidence from animal models (such as from non-human primates with simian or chimeric simian-human immunodeficiency viruses) also informs rational vaccine design and development. Unfortunately, after nearly two decades of scientific exploration there are no such clear-cut immune response(s) defined to compel the development of a specific HIV vaccine candidate. Rather, there is evidence to support the putative importance of many different effector responses potentially inducible by vaccine candidates (Franchini *et al.*, 1995; Andersson *et al.*, 1996; Myagkikh *et al.*, 1996; Leno *et al.*, 1999; Hel *et al.*, 2001; Currier *et al.*, 2002; Hel *et al.*, 2002; Mothe *et al.*, 2002; Pal *et al.*, 2002; Santra *et al.*, 2002; Marthas, 2003). Contemporary convention hypothesizes that efficacious HIV vaccines may require the induction of both cell-mediated and antibody-mediated adaptive immunity. No single existing vaccine candidate adequately provides such a full constellation of immune responses. A prime boost regimen (PBR) which is used in phase III is comprised of two vaccine components—one primarily designed to stimulate cell-mediated immunity and the other antibody-mediated immunity—capable of inducing a broad-based, complex repertoire of anti-HIV responses.

In 1997, TAVEG initiated development of a PBR comprised of Aventis Pasteur's canarypox vector ALVAC-HIV (vCP1521) as a priming agent with recombinant envelope glycoproteins (gp120s or gp160) as boosting agents. All PBR components were specifically constructed for development in Thailand through the inclusion of *env* genes and proteins from prevalent endemic subtype E HIVs. Initially, three glycoprotein (gp) candidates were paired with ALVAC-HIV: gp160 from Pasteur Merieux Connaught (PMC); gp120 from Chiron Vaccines; and gp120 from VaxGen. PMC and Chiron subsequently withdrew their candidate glycoproteins secondary to technical and corporate business considerations. Between 1997 and 2002, a PBR development plan was collectively constructed and executed to assemble the data required for subsequent decision-making regarding efficacy testing of TAVEG's PBR. TAVEG advancement criteria required that the PBR be safe, well-tolerated, and induce cell-mediated and antibody-mediated responses. Immune response metrics were prospectively established for cytotoxic T-lymphocyte, lymphocyte proliferative, and neutralizing antibody responses. These immunological targets were established based on a hypothesized relevance for efficacy as well as what was deemed to be achievable within the state-of-the-art of HIV vaccinology at the beginning of the 21st century. Notably, the specific nature of vaccine-induced immunity (both type and degree) required to affect protection against HIV/AIDS is completely unknown. Moreover, our knowledge of immune responses induced *in vivo* by candidate vaccines is defined by the immunological tools available to us, which are more numerous and improving over time. Within this context, TAVEG's pivotal phase II data were deemed entirely supportive of further development and efficacy testing of the ALVAC-HIV + gp120 PBR.

In January 2002, as TAVEG's phase II PBR data were being considered, NIAID and its HIV Vaccine Trials Network (HVTN) were equally evaluating immune response data from a similar ALVAC-HIV + gp120 PBR that was nearing completion of phase I/II evaluation in the Americas. NIAID/HVTN's considerations and decision-making occurred simultaneously and in coordination with TAVEG's decision-making concerning efficacy testing of their PBR. A decision was made not to proceed with further investigation of their ALVAC-HIV + gp120 PBR because their phase II milestone for cell-mediated immunity (CD8 + ELISPOT), required for the design and implementation of a subsequent study to correlate this response with efficacy, was not achieved. It was collectively decided that the TAVEG development plan was better positioned to assess efficacy of the ALVAC-HIV + gp120 PBR. On February 25, 2002 the NIAID Office of Communications and Public Liaison announced that TAVEG's phase III trial would be supported through a combined NIAID-USAMRMC program. This did not represent a decision double standard, but rather an informed choice to assess efficacy under the most favorable circumstances available.

During 2002–2003, TAVEG (now including the critical support of NIAID) developed and initiated a phase III clinical protocol in Thailand. This trial is designed to assess the efficacy of vCP1521 + AIDSVAX gp120 B/E in both preventing and/or controlling HIV infection. The efficacy trial, initiated in October 2003, seeks to enroll 16,000 volunteers from the provincial communities of Rayong and Chon Buri in southeastern Thailand.

Throughout the 18 month period prior to its initiation, TAVEG's phase III plan and protocol was reviewed and approved by 11 different governmental and academic scientific, ethical, and regulatory review bodies in Thailand and the United States, and by WHO/UNAIDS. Additionally, the PBR development plan and protocol was widely presented publicly at national and international meetings. It is believed that this represents one of the most widely-vetted and transparent vaccine research and development initiatives ever conducted.

During 2003, results from two efficacy trials of AIDSVAX gp120s indicated that this component of the PBR, by itself, had no efficacy. Based on these findings, why should TAVEG continue to support an AIDSVAX component in the PBR? The PBR represents a significantly different vaccine. An analogy may be drawn with treatment of monotherapy vs. combination therapies, where a single agent may have poor or no efficacy vs. substantial efficacy in a combination. The addition of gp120 significantly augments the immune response profile of ALVAC-HIV alone by additive and interactive means. In addition to the additive impact of each PBR component on the other (eg. CTL and Nab), there is an interaction of ALVAC-HIV priming with gp120 boosting in that T helper responses are both broader and increased in frequency, cytokine expression profiles are broadened, and antibody-dependent cellular cytotoxicity is induced (Pialoux *et al.*, 1995; Excler and Plotkin, 1997; Clements-Mann *et al.*, 1998; Tartaglia *et al.*, 1998; Barnett *et al.*, 1998; Sabbaj *et al.*, 2000; Gorse *et al.*, 2001; Ratto-Kim *et al.*, 2003). This complex immune response profile forms the very basis of the vaccine hypothesis TAVEG is testing in the phase III trial in Thailand. It is the induced complexity and frequency of anti-HIV immune responses that is deemed worthy of efficacy evaluation, not any particular single (e.g., CD4 + T cell) immune response.

The development of drugs and vaccines is an inherently linear process that requires milestones and advancement criteria, consensus-building, and consistency. When milestones are achieved, forward progress ensues. From a development science perspective, development should cease only when milestones are not achieved, or an underlying hypothesis is debunked. Vaccine development is a generational and iterative process with successfully-conducted efficacy trials of pivotal importance, importantly informing subsequent development and efficacy testing.

Nearly 20 years after the discovery of HIV, the TAVEG prime boost phase III study is the first government-sponsored efficacy trial of a candidate prophylactic HIV vaccine. The efficacy of the PBR will be known in 2008 upon completion of the phase III trial. Unfortunately the prospect for advanced development of next-generation HIV candidates is only just now appearing on the horizon. Much remains to be done.

SUMMARY

Early lessons reinforce the need to start simply and build to greater complexity. Partnerships need to be formed at the earliest stages of immunogen development, and expanded and built upon during the process of preclinical development through all stages of human testing. The DoD joined forces with the RTA, building the HIV-1 diagnostic infrastructure to begin mass HIV-1 testing and counseling in young males. These early data clearly identified the foci of the highest HIV prevalence and identified initial educational interventions. The RTA, in coordination with a well-funded national campaign, pursued 100% condom use and aggressive prevention education research, with evaluative techniques to access educational effectiveness supported by the DoD (Rojanapithayakorn and Hanenberg, 1996). In concert, the group collaborated on mapping the epidemic with molecular techniques and the earliest characterized strains were made available to international HIV-1 vaccine developers (McCutchan *et al.*, 1996; McCutchan *et al.*, 2000). VaxGen and Chiron gp120 E vaccines that were developed specifically for testing in Thailand were derived from these strains. The early collaborations also focused on developing clinical vaccine testing infrastructure and recruiting capability to permit Phase I/II vaccine testing of these candidates (Nitayaphan *et al.*, 2000; Kim *et al.*, 2000).

Each piece of infrastructure and each training opportunity focused on the requirements for HIV-1 vaccine development. But the equipment, laboratories, and techniques were applicable to multiple aspects of clinical trials, and were utilized by the universities to support other non-HIV-1 projects that enhanced the long-term stability and sustainability of the investment.

AFRIMS research has contributed significantly to the characterization of the HIV epidemic in Thailand. One of the lessons recognized is that this very process of building collaborations and carrying out studies in accordance with international ethical and regulatory standards helps to develop the infrastructure required for an efficacy trial. 'Infrastructure' is used here in its widest sense: human, physical, scientific, behavioral, and ethical. Benefits are bidirectional; the Americans involved have become more knowledgeable regarding the disease and its control, and how goals are pursued with colleagues in a resource-constrained environment. The recipe for success here included a long-standing joint research institute which allowed the development of personal and institutional relationships and provided technical training and full emersion with the endemic disease, including its socioeconomic dimensions. This type of binational organization requires sustained political and personnel commitments from both partners, as well as funding stability. Such international collaborative efforts are crucial in building global capacity to control HIV/AIDS and other major diseases which threaten the less developed regions and, thus, the whole world.

CONCLUSION

International HIV vaccine development has taken impressive steps forward over the past decade through multilateral, multinational partnerships (Berkley, 1999; Schultz and Bradac, 2001; Esparza, 2001; Makgoba *et al.*, 2002; Esparza *et al.*, 2002). The worldwide HIV vaccine development effort has brought together countries, investigators, and pharmaceutical companies from the Northern and Southern Hemisphere to work towards a common goal—the development of a global HIV vaccine. The world can look to the vaccine development efforts in Thailand as a model for successful implementation of this process. A partnership, which includes Thai Universities, the Thai Government, pharmaceutical companies, and international sponsors, has been the basis for carrying out a series of highly regarded Phase I, II, and III trials. No other country in the world has moved forward with this momentum and singleness of purpose (UNAIDS/WHO, 1998; Brown and McNeil, 1998; Nitayaphan and Brown, 1998; Berman, 1999; Nitayaphan *et al.*, 2000).

As the HIV-1 epidemic wreaks havoc throughout the globe, Thailand has quietly and persistently moved forward toward the goal of an efficacious HIV-1 vaccine. The Thai investigators are now providing their experience to other countries in the early stages of developing HIV vaccine programs of their own. In addition to the practical information provided by Thai vaccine developers, obstacles encountered and remedies constructed are also being conveyed. The extensive work in Thailand is an example of the concerted effort required to move from Phase I to Phase III trials and is a benchmark and inspiration for the rest of the world.

Acknowledgements. The views and opinions expressed herein are those of the authors and do not purport to reflect the official policy or position of the United States Army or the Department of Defense. The U.S. Military HIV Research Program is a cooperative program with the National Institute of Allergy and Infectious Diseases, Division of AIDS.

REFERENCES

Andersson, S., Makitalo, B., Thorstensson, R., Franchini, G., Tartaglia, J., Limbach, K., Paoletti, E., Putkonen, P., and Biberfeld, G. (1996). Immunogenicity and protective efficacy of a human immunodeficiency virus type 2 recombinant canarypox (ALVAC) vaccine candidate in cynomolgus monkeys. *J Infect Dis.* 174:977–985.

Barnett, S.W., Klinger, J.M., Doe, B., Walker, C.M., Hansen, L., Duliege, A.M., and Sinangil, F.M. (1998). Prime-boost immunization strategies against HIV. *AIDS Res Hum Retroviruses* 14 Suppl 3:S299–S309.

Benenson, M.W., Sirisopana, N., Amphaipit, R., Tungsakul, V., Pumratana, K., Santativongchai, S., Nitayaphan, S., and Brown, A.E. (2001). Cohort development for future HIV-1 efficacy vaccine trials: a community cohort, Chon Buri Province, Thailand, In Sixth International Congress on AIDS in Asia and the Pacific, Melbourne, Australia.

Berkley, S. (1999). An AIDS vaccine for all the world. Interview by Matthew O'Rourke. *AIDS Clin Care* 11:55–57.

Berman, J. (1999). Thailand attacks AIDS with two-pronged approach. *Lancet* 353:1600.

Birx, D.L., Brundage, J., Larson, K., Engler, R., Smith, L., Squire, E., Carpenter, G., Sullivan, M., Rhoads, J., Oster, C., James, W., Lupton, G., Wierzba, T., Burke, D., Redfield, R., and the Military Medical Consortium for Applied Retroviral Research. (1993). The prognostic utility of delayed-type hypersensitivity skin testing in the evaluation of HIV-infected patients. *J Acquir Immune Defic Syndr Hum Retrovirol.* 6:1248–1257.

Brodine, S.K., Shaffer, R.A., Starkey, M.J., Tasker, S.A., Gilcrest, J.L., Louder, M.K., Barile, A.,VanCott, T.C., Vahey, M.T., McCutchan, F.E., Birx, D.L., Richman, D.D., and Mascola, J.R. (1999). Drug resistance patterns, genetic subtypes, clinical features, and risk factors in military personnel with HIV-1 seroconversion. *Ann Intern Med.* 131: 502–506.

Brodine, S.K., Starkey, M.J., Shaffer, R.A., Ito, S.I., Tasker, S.A., Barile, A.J., Tamminga, C.L., Stephan, K.T., Aronson, N.E., Fraser, S.L., Wallace, M.R.,Wegner, S.A., Mascola, J.R. , and McCutchan, F.E. (2003). Diverse HIV-1 subtypes and clinical, laboratory and behavioral factors in a recently infected US military cohort. *AIDS* 17:2521–2527.

Brown, A.E. and McNeil, J.G. (1998). HIV vaccine development: a subtype E-specific strategy. *Southeast Asian J Trop Med Public Health* 29:377–382.

Brown, A.E., Singharaj, P., Webster, H.K., Pipithkul, J., Gordon, D.M., Boslego, J.W., Krinchai, K., Suarchawaratana, P., Wongsrichanalai, C., W.R., Perpamich, B., Kain, K.C., Hollingdale, M.R., Wittes, J., Que, J.U., Gross, M., Cryz, S.J. and Sadoff, J.C. (1994). Safety, immunogenicity and limited efficacy study of a recombinant Plasmodium falciparum circumsporozoite vaccine in Thai soldiers. *Vaccine* 12:102–108.

Brown, A.E., Brundage, J.F., Tomlinson, J.P., and Burke, D.S. (1996). The U.S. Army HIV testing program: the first decade. *Mil Med* 161:117–122.

Brown, A.E., Markowitz, L., Nitayaphan, S., Morgan, P., Sukwit, S., Chinaworapong, S., Leelasupasri, S., and Birx, D. (2000). DTH responsiveness of HIV-infected Thai adults. *J Med Assoc Thai.* 83:633–639.

Carr, J.K., Sirisopana, N., Torugsa, K., Jugsudee, A., Supapongse, T., Chuenchitra, C., Nitayaphan, S., Singharaj, P., and McNeil, J.G. (1994). Incidence of HIV-1 infection among young men in Thailand. *J Acquir Immune Defic Syndr Hum Retrovirol.* 7:1270–1275.

Celentano, D.D., Beyrer, C., Natpratan, C., Eiumtrakul, S., Sussman, L., Renzullo, P.O., Khamboonruang, C., and Nelson, K.E. (1995). Willingness to participate in AIDS vaccine trials among high-risk populations in northern Thailand. *AIDS* 9:1079–1083.

Chanbancherd, P., Jugsudee, A., Thanomklom, S., Limpairojn, N., Julananto, P., Thienamporn, P., Markowitz, L.E., de Souza, M.S., and Brown, A.E. (1999). Frequency of HIV false positivity from two sequential enzyme immunoassays in 111 639 sera. *AIDS* 13:2182–2183.

Chanbancherd, P., Limpairojn, N., Benenson, M., Jugsudee, A., Julananto, P., Tienamporn, P., Luecha, W., and Tasaniyananda, C. (2000). HIV-2 infection in Thailand. *Asian Pac J Allergy Immunol.* 18:245–248.

Chanbancherd, P., Julananto, P., Tienamporn, P., Chitripong, A., Tasaniyananada, C., Torugsa, K., de Souza, M., and Brown, A.E. (2001). The epidemiology of the hepatitis C virus among HIV-infected young Thai men in the year 2000, In Sixth International Congress on AIDS in Asia and the Pacific, Melbourne, Australia.

Chanbancherd, P., Paris, R.M., Torugsa, K., de Souza M., Myint K.S.A., Chitpong A., and Brown, A.E. (2003). High frequency of HIV-1 and hepatitis C co-infection among young Thai men: evidence for a changing pattern of HIV transmission in Thailand. *Southeast Asian J Trop Med Public Health* 34:580–582.

Chinaworapong, S., Nitayaphan, S., Morgan, P.A., Wongkamheang, S., Naksrisuk, S., Pitisuttithum, P., Buapunth, P., and Triampon, A. (2001). Motivation and recruitment for phase I/II HIV-1 prime-boost vaccine, In Sixth International Congress on AIDS in Asia and the Pacific, Melbourne, Australia.

Chuenchitra, T., Wasi, C., Louisirirojchanakul, S., Nitayaphan, S., Sutthent, R., Cox, J.H., de Souza, M.S., Brown, A.E., Birx, D.L., and Polonis, V.R. (2003). Longitudinal study of humoral immune responses in HIV type 1 subtype CRF01-AE (E)-infected Thai patients with different rates of disease progression. *AIDS Res Hum Retroviruses* 19:293–305.

Clements-Mann, M.L., Weinhold, K., Matthews, T.J., Graham, B.S., Gorse, G.J., Keefer, M.C., McElrath, M.J., Hsieh, R.H., Mestecky, J., Zolla-Pazner, S., Mascola, J., Schwartz, D., Siliciano, R., Corey, L., Wright, P.F., Belshe, R., Dolin, R., Jackson, S., Xu, S., Fast, P., Walker, M.C., Stablein, D., Excler, J.L., Tartaglia, J., Paoletti, E., and the NIAID AIDS Vaccine Evaluation Group. (1998). Immune responses to human immunodeficiency virus (HIV) type 1 induced by canarypox expressing HIV-1MN gp120, HIV-1SF2 recombinant gp120, or both vaccines in seronegative adults. *J Infect Dis.* 177: 1230–1246.

Cox, J.H., and de Souza, M. (2000). Evaluation of natural killer cell activity. *Mol Biotechnol.* 15:147–154.

Currier, J.R., de Souza, M., Chanbancherd, P., Bernstein, W., Birx, D.L., and Cox, J.H. (2002). Comprehensive screening for human immunodeficiency virus type 1 subtype-specific CD8 cytotoxic T lymphocytes and definition of degenerate epitopes restricted by HLA-A0207 and -C(W)0304 alleles. *J Virol* 76:4971–4986.

Darden, J.M., Polonis, V.R., deSouza, M.S., Chantakulkij, S., Brown, A.E., Birx, D.L., and Pattanapanyasat, K. (2000). A flow cytometric method for measuring neutralization of HIV-1 subtype B and E primary isolates. *Cytometry* 40:141–150.

de Souza, M.S., Karnasuta, C., Brown, A.E., Markowitz, L.E., Nitayaphan, S., Garner, R.P., McNeil, J.G., Birx, D.L., and Cox, J.H. (2000). A comparative study of the impact of HIV infection on natural killer cell number and function in Thais and North Americans. *AIDS Res Hum Retroviruses* 16:1061–1066.

de Souza, M.S., Trichavaroj, R., Sripliencham, S., Buapunth, P., Renzullo, P.O., Chuenchitra, C., Birx, D.L., Robb, M.L., and Brown, A.E. (2001). Detection and quantification of HIV type 1 RNA in nasopharyngeal washes from HIV-infected subjects. *AIDS Res Hum Retroviruses* 17:229–232.

Division of AIDS, Department of Communicable Disease Control. (1993). Thai National HIV Vaccine Development Plan. Ministry of Public Health, Bangkok, Thailand.

Elbeik, T., Alvord, W.G., Trichavaroj, R., de Souza, M., Dewar, R., Brown, A., Chernoff, D., Michael, N.L., Nassos, P., Hadley, K., and Ng, V.L. (2002). Comparative analysis of HIV-1 viral load assays on subtype quantification: Bayer Versant HIV-1 RNA 3.0 versus Roche Amplicor HIV-1 Monitor version 1.5. *J Acquir Immune Defic Syndr Hum Retrovirol.* 29:330–339.

Endy, T.P., Chunsuttiwat, S., Nisalak, A., Libraty, D.H., Green, S., Rothman, A.L., Vaughn, D.W., and Ennis, F.A. (2002). Epidemiology of inapparent and symptomatic acute dengue virus infection: a prospective study of primary school children in Kamphaeng Phet, Thailand. *Am J Epidemiol.* 156:40–51.

Esparza, J. (1993). Development of WHO-sponsored sites for HIV vaccine evaluation. *AIDS Res Hum Retrovir.* 9:1333–1334.

Esparza, J. (2001). An HIV vaccine: how and when? *Bull World Health Organ.* 79:1133–1137.

Esparza, J., and Bhamarapravati, N. (2000). Accelerating the development and future availability of HIV-1 vaccines: why, when, where, and how? *Lancet* 355:2061–2066.

Esparza, J., Osmanov, S., Kallings, L.O., and Wigzell, H. (1991). Planning for HIV vaccine trials: the World Health Organization perspective. *AIDS* 5 Suppl 2:S159–S163.

Esparza, J., Osmanov, S., Pattou-Markovic, C., Toure, C., Chang, M.L., and Nixon, S. (2002). Past, present and future of HIV vaccine trials in developing countries. *Vaccine* 20:1897–1898.

Excler, J.L. and Plotkin, S. (1997). The prime-boost concept applied to HIV preventive vaccines. *AIDS* 11 Suppl A:S127–S137.

Franchini, G., Robert-Guroff, M., Tartaglia, J., Aggarwal, A., Abimiku, A., Benson, J., Markham, P., Limbach, K., Hurteau, G., Fullen, J., Aldrich, K., Miller, N., Sadoff, J., Paoletti, E., and Gallo, R.C. (1995). Highly attenuated HIV type 2 recombinant poxviruses, but not HIV-2 recombinant Salmonella vaccines, induce long-lasting protection in rhesus macaques. *AIDS Res Hum Retroviruses* 11:909–920.

Gao, F., Yue, L., Craig, S., Thornton, C.L., Robertson, D.L., McCutchan, F.E., Bradac, J.A., Sharp, P.M., and Hahn, B.H. (1994). Genetic variation of HIV type 1 in four World Health Organization-sponsored vaccine evaluation sites: generation of functional envelope (glycoprotein 160) clones representative of sequence subtypes A, B, C, and E. WHO Network for HIV Isolation and Characterization. *AIDS Res Hum Retroviruses* 10:1359–1368.

Gorse, G.J., Patel, G.B., Mandava, M.D., Arbuckle, J.A., Doyle, T.M., and Belshe, R.B. (2001). Cytokine responses to human immunodeficiency virus type 1 (HIV-1) induced by immunization with live recombinant canarypox virus vaccine expressing HIV-1 genes boosted by HIV-1(SF-2) recombinant GP120. *Vaccine* 19:1806–1819.

Hanenberg, R. and Rojanapithayakorn, W. (1996). Prevention as policy: How Thailand reduced STD and

HIV transmission. *Aidscaptions* 3:24–27.

Hel, Z., Tsai, W.P., Thornton, A., Nacsa, J., Giuliani, L., Tryniszewska, E., Poudyal, M., Venzon, D., Wang, X., Altman, J., Watkins, D.I., Lu, W., von Gegerfelt, A., Felber, B.K., Tartaglia, J.,Pavlakis, G.N., and Franchini, G. (2001). Potentiation of simian immunodeficiency virus (SIV)-specific CD4(+) and CD8(+) T cell responses by a DNA-SIV and NYVAC-SIV prime/boost regimen. *J Immunol.* 167:7180–7191.

Hel, Z., Nacsa, J., Tryniszewska, E., Tsai, W.P., Parks, R.W., Montefiori, D.C., Felber, B.K., Tartaglia, J., Pavlakis, G.N., and Franchini, G. (2002). Containment of simian immunodeficiency virus infection in vaccinated macaques: correlation with the magnitude of virus-specific pre- and postchallenge CD4 + and CD8 + T cell responses. *J Immunol.* 169:4778–4787.

Hoge, C.W., Gambel, J.M., Srijan, A., Pitarangsi, C., and Echeverria, P. (1998). Trends in antibiotic resistance among diarrheal pathogens isolated in Thailand over 15 years. *Clin Infect Dis.* 26:341–345.

Hoke, C.H., Nisalak, A., Sangawhipa, N., Jatanasen, S., Laorakapongse, T., Innis, B.L., Kotchasenee, S., Gingrich, J.B., Latendresse, J., Fukai, K., and Burke, D.S. (1988). Protection against Japanese encephalitis by inactivated vaccines. *N Engl J Med.* 319:608–614.

Innis, B.L., Snitbhan, R., Hoke, C.H., Munindhorn, W., and Laorakpongse, T. (1991). The declining transmission of hepatitis A in Thailand. *J Infect Dis.* 163:989–995.

Jenkins, R.A., Temoshok, L.R., and Virochsiri, K. (1995). Incentives and disincentives to participate in prophylactic HIV vaccine research. *J Acquir Immune Defic Syndr Hum Retrovirol.* 9:36–42.

Jenkins, R.A., Chinaworapong, S., Morgan, P.A., Ruangyuttikarn, C., Sontirat, A., Chiu, J., Michael, R.A., Nitayaphan, S., and Khamboonruang, C. (1998). Motivation, recruitment, and screening of volunteers for a phase I/II HIV preventive vaccine trial in Thailand. *J Acquir Immune Defic Syndr Hum Retrovirol.* 18:171–177.

Jenkins, R.A., Torugsa, K., Mason, C.J., Jamroenratana, V., Lalang, C., Nitayaphan, S., and Michael, R.A. (1999). HIV risk behavior patterns among young Thai men. *AIDS and Behavior.* 3:335–346.

Jenkins, R.A., Torugsa, K., Markowitz, L.E., Mason, C.J., Jamroentana, V., Brown, A.E., and Nitayaphan, S. (2000). Willingness to participate in HIV-1 vaccine trials among young Thai men. *Sex Transm Infect.* 76:386–392.

Kanshana, S. and Simonds, R.J. (2002). National program for preventing mother-child HIV transmission in Thailand: Successful implementation and lessons learned. *AIDS* 16:953–959.

Khamboonruang, C., Ruengyutthikarn, C., Taejaroenkul, S., Sornsathapornkul, P., Brown, A.E., and Thongcharoen, P. (2001). Demographic characteristics and motivation of Thai HIV-seronegative volunteers participating in a phase I/II prime-boost vaccine trial in Bangkok and Chiang Mai Province, Thailand, In Sixth International Congress on AIDS in Asia and the Pacific, Melbourne, Australia.

Kim, J., Mascola, J., Frankel, S., VanCott, T., de Souza, M., Polonis, V., McLinden, R., Louder, M., Sambor, A., Brown, A.E., Nitayaphan, S., Duliege, A.M., Robb, M., McNeil, J., and Birx, D. (2000). Specific antibody responses to vaccination with bivalent CM235/SF2 gp120: Detection of homologous and heterologous neutralizing antibody (NAb) to subtype E HIV-1, In 7th Conference on Retroviruses and Opportunistic Infections, San Francisco, California.

Kitsiripornchai, S., Markowitz, L.E., Ungchusak, K., Jenkins, R.A., Leucha, W., Limpitaks, T., and Sangkharomya, S. (1998). Sexual behavior of young men in Thailand: Regional differences and evidence of behavior change. *J Acquir Immune Defic Syndr Hum Retrovirol.* 18:282–288.

Kozik, C.A., Vaughn, D.W., Snitbhan, R., and Innis, B.L. (2000). Hepatitis B virus infection in Thai children. *Trop Med Int Health* 5:633–639.

Leno, M., Carter, L., Venzon, D.J., Romano, J., Markham, P.D., Limbach, K., Tartaglia, J., Paoletti, E., Benson, J., Franchini, G., and Robert-Guroff, M. (1999). CD8 + lymphocyte antiviral activity in monkeys immunized with SIV recombinant poxvirus vaccines: Potential role in vaccine efficacy. *AIDS Res Hum Retroviruses* 15:461–470.

Lynch, J.A., de Souza, M., Robb, M.D., Markowitz, L., Nitayaphan, S., Sapan, C.V., Mann, D.L., Birx, D.L., and Cox, J.H. (1998). Cross-clade cytotoxic T cell response to human immunodeficiency virus type 1 proteins among HLA disparate North Americans and Thais. *J Infect Dis.* 178:1040–1046.

MacQueen, K.M., Vanichseni, S., Kitayaporn, D., Lin, L.S., Buavirat, A., Naiwatanakul, T., Raktham, S., Mock, P., Heyward, W.L., Des Jarlais, D.C., Choopanya, K., and Mastro, T.D. (1999). Willingness of injection drug users to participate in an HIV vaccine efficacy trial in Bangkok, Thailand. *J Acquir Immune Defic Syndr Hum Retrovirol.* 21:243–251.

Makgoba, M.W., Solomon, N., and Tucker, T.J. (2002). The search for an HIV vaccine. *BMJ.* 324:211–213.

Maneerat, Y., Wilairatana, P., Pongponratn, E., Chaisri, U., Puthavatana, P., Snitbhan, R., Raengsakulrach, B., Clayson, E.T., Vaughn, D.W., Kurathong, S., Pramoolsinsup, S., and Juthaputhi, A. (1996). Etiology of acute non-A, B, C hepatitis in Thai patients: preliminary study. *Southeast Asian J Trop Med Public Health* 27:844–846.

Mann, J.M. and Kay, K. (1991). Confronting the pandemic: the World Health Organization's Global

Programme on AIDS, 1986–1989. *AIDS* 5 Suppl 2:S221–S229.

Markowitz, L.E., Sirisopana, N., Charonwatanachokchai, A., Julvanichpong, W., Siraprapasiri, T., Palanuvej, T., Siriwongrangsun, P., Tungsakul, V., Pumratana, K., Chitwarakorn, A., Michael, R.A., and Brown, A.E. (1999). Feasibility of a preventive HIV-1 vaccine cohort among persons attending sexually transmitted disease clinics in Thailand. *J Acquir Immune Defic Syndr Hum Retrovirol.* 20:488–494.

Marthas, M., Van Rompay, K., McChesney, M., Miller, C.J., Evans, T., Schmidt, K., Lawson, J., Singh, R., Pahar, B., Earl, P., Moss, J., Franchini, G., Tartaglia, J., and Montefiori, D.C. (2003). Recombinant Poxviruses expressing SIV proteins are immunogenic in newborn rhesus macaques and protect against multiple, low-dose oral SIV challenge, In AIDS Vaccines 2003, New York, New York.

Mascola, J.R., Louder, M.K., Surman, S.R., Vancott, T.C., Yu, X.F., Bradac, J., Porter, K.R., Nelson, K.E.,Girard, M., McNeil, J.G., McCutchan, F.E., Birx, D.L., and Burke, D.S. (1996). Human immunodeficiency virus type 1 neutralizing antibody serotyping using serum pools and an infectivity reduction assay. *AIDS Res Hum Retroviruses.* 12:1319–1328.

Mason, C.J., Markowitz, L.E., Kitsiripornchai, S., Jugsudee, A., Sirisopana, N., Torugsa, K., Carr, J.K., Michael, R.A., Nitayaphan, S., and McNeil, J.G. (1995). Declining prevalence of HIV-1 infection in young Thai men. *AIDS* 9:1061–1065.

Mason, C.J., Kitsiripornchai, S., Markowitz, L.E., Chanbancherd, P., Supapongse, T., Jugsdee, A., Sirisopana, N., Chuenchitra, C., Torugsa, K., VanCott, T., Michael, R.A., and Nitayaphan, S. (1998). Nationwide surveillance of HIV-1 prevalence and subtype in young Thai men. *J Acquir Immune Defic Syndr Hum Retrovirol.* 19:165–173.

McCutchan, F.E., Hegerich, P.A., Brennan, T.P., Phanuphak, P., Singharaj, P., Jugsudee, A., Berman, P.W., Gray, A.M., Fowler, A.K., and Burke, D.S. (1992). Genetic variants of HIV-1 in Thailand. *AIDS Res Hum Retroviruses* 8:1887–1895.

McCutchan, F.E., Artenstein, A.W., Sanders-Buell, E., Salminen, M.O., Carr, J.K., Mascola, J.R., Yu, X.F., Nelson, K.E., Khamboonruang, C., Schmitt, D., Kieny, M.P., McNeil, J.G., and Burke, D.S. (1996). Diversity of the envelope glycoprotein among human immunodeficiency virus type 1 isolates of clade E from Asia and Africa. *J Virol.* 70:3331–3338.

McCutchan, F.E., Viputtigul, K., de Souza, M.S., Carr, J.K., Markowitz, L.E., Buapunth, P., McNeil, J.G., Robb, M.L., Nitayaphan, S., Birx, D.L., and Brown, A.E. (2000). Diversity of envelope glycoprotein from human immunodeficiency virus type 1 of recent seroconverters in Thailand. *AIDS Res Hum Retroviruses* 16:801–805.

Mothe, B.R., Horton, H., Carter, D.K., Allen, T.M., Liebl, M.E., Skinner, P., Vogel, T.U., Fuenger, S., Vielhuber, K., Rehrauer, W., Wilson, N., Franchini, G., Altman, J.D., Haase, A., Picker, L.J., Allison, D.B., and Watkins, D.I. (2002). Dominance of CD8 responses specific for epitopes bound by a single major histocompatibility complex class I molecule during the acute phase of viral infection. *J Virol.* 76:875–884.

Myagkikh, M., Alipanah, S., Markham, P.D., Tartaglia, J., Paoletti, E., Gallo, R.C., Franchini, G., and Robert-Guroff, M. (1996). Multiple immunizations with attenuated poxvirus HIV type 2 recombinants and subunit boosts required for protection of rhesus macaques. *AIDS Res Hum Retroviruses* 12:985–992.

Nelson, K.E., Beyrer, C., Natpratan, C., Eiumtrakul, S., Celentano, D.D., and Khamboonruang, C. (1994). Preparatory studies for possible HIV vaccine trials in northern Thailand. *AIDS Res Hum Retroviruses* 10 Suppl 2:S243–S246.

Nitayaphan, S. and Brown, A.E. (1998). Preventive HIV vaccine development in Thailand. *AIDS* 12 Suppl B:S155–S161.

Nitayaphan, S., Khamboonruang, C., Sirisophana, N., Morgan, P., Chiu, J., Duliege, A.M., Chuenchitra, C., Supapongse, T., Rungruengthanakit, K., de Souza, M., Mascola, J.R., Boggio, K., Ratto-Kim, S., Markowitz, L.E., Birx, D., Suriyanon, V., McNeil, J.G., Brown, A.E., and Michael, R.A. (2000). A phase I/II trial of HIV SF2 gp120/MF59 vaccine in seronegative thais. AFRIMS-RIHES Vaccine Evaluation Group. Armed Forces Research Institute of Medical Sciences and the Research Institute for Health Sciences. *Vaccine* 18:1448–1455.

Nitayaphan, S., Pitisuttithum, P., de Souza, M.S., Kim, J., Polonis, V., Heyward, W.L., Gurunathan, S., Ratto-Kim, S., and Brown, A.E. (2002). Safety and immunogenicity of live recombinant ALVAC-HIV (vCP1521) priming with AIDSVAX B/E gp120 boosting in Thai HIV-negative adults, In XIV International AIDS Conference, Barcelona, Spain.

Pal, R., Venzon, D., Letvin, N.L., Santra, S., Montefiori, D.C., Miller, N.R., Tryniszewska, E., Lewis, M.G., VanCott, T.C., Hirsch, V., Woodward, R., Gibson, A., Grace, M., Dobratz, E., Markham, P.D., Hel, Z., Nacsa, J., Klein, M., Tartaglia, J., and Franchini, G. (2002). ALVAC-SIV-gag-pol-env-based vaccination and macaque major histocompatibility complex class I (A*01) delay simian immunodeficiency virus SIVmac-induced immunodeficiency. *J Virol.* 76:292–302.

Paris, R., Sirisopana, N., Benenson, M., Amphaiphis, R., Tuntichaivanich, C., Myint, K.S., and Brown, A.E. (2003). The association between hepatitis C virus and HIV-1 in preparatory cohorts for HIV vaccine trials in Thailand. *AIDS* 17:1363–1367.

Pau, C.P., Kai, M., Holloman-Candal, D.L., Luo, C.C., Kalish, M.L., Schochetman, G., Byers, B., and George, J.R. (1994). Antigenic variation and serotyping of HIV type 1 from four World Health Organization-sponsored HIV vaccine sites. WHO Network for HIV Isolation and Characterization. *AIDS Res Hum Retroviruses* 10:1369–1377.

Phoolcharoen, W., Ungchusak, K., Sittitrai, W., and Brown, T. (1998). Thailand: Lessons from a strong national response to HIV/AIDS. *AIDS* 12 Suppl B:S123–S135.

Pialoux, G., Excler, J.L., Riviere, Y., Gonzalez-Canali, G., Feuillie, V., Coulaud, P., Gluckman, J.C., Matthews, T.J., Meignier, B., Kieny, M.P., the AGIS Group, and l'Agence Nationale de Recherche sur le SIDA. (1995). A prime-boost approach to HIV preventive vaccine using a recombinant canarypox virus expressing glycoprotein 160 (MN) followed by a recombinant glycoprotein 160 (MN/LAI). *AIDS Res Hum Retroviruses* 11:373–381.

Pitisuttithum, P., Nitayaphan, S., Tongcharoen, T., Khamboonruang, C., Kim, J.,de Souza, M., Chuenchitra, T., Garner, R., Thapinta, D., Polonis, V., Ratto-Kim, S., Chanbancherd, P., Chiu, J., Birx, D.L., Duliege, A.M., McNeil, J.G., and Brown, A.E. (2003). Safety and immunogenicity of combinations of recombinant subtype E and B HIV-1 envelope gp120 vaccines in healthy Thai adults. *J Infect Dis.* 188:219–227.

Polonis, V.R., de Souza, M.S., Chanbancherd, P., Chantakulkij, S., Jugsudee, A., Loomis-Price, L.D., Vancott, T.C., Garner, R., Markowitz, L.E., Brown, A.E., and Birx, D.L. (2001). HIV type 1 subtype E-infected patients with broadened, dual (B/E) V3 loop serology have increased cross-neutralizing antibodies. *AIDS Res Hum Retroviruses* 17:69–79.

Ratto-Kim, S., Loomis-Price, L.D., Aronson, N., Grimes, J., Hill, C., Williams, C., El Habib, R., Birx, D.L., and Kim, J.H. (2003). Comparison between *env*-specific T-cell epitopic responses in HIV-1-uninfected adults immunized with combination of ALVAC-HIV(vCP205) plus or minus rgp160MN/LAI-2 and HIV-1-infected adults. *J Acquir Immune Defic Syndr Hum Retrovirol.* 32:9–17.

Renzullo, P.O., Celentano, D.D., Beyrer, C., Eiumtrakul, S., McNeil, J.G., Garner, R.P., Ruangyuttigarn, C., Khamboonruang, C., and Nelson, K.E. (1999). HIV infection and risk behaviors in Thai men after their service in the Royal Thai Army: Informing vaccine cohort development. *AIDS and Behavior* 3: 25–32.

Renzullo, P.O., Sateren, W.B., Garner, R.P., Milazzo, M.J., Birx, D.L., and McNeil, J.G. (2001). HIV-1 seroconversion in United States Army active duty personnel, 1985–1999. *AIDS.* 15(12):1569–1574.

Rerks-Ngarm, S., Pitisuttithum, P., Kitayaporn, D., Brown, A.E., and McNeil, J.G. (2002). Joint Thai-US phase III trial of HIV prime-boost vaccines, In XIV International AIDS Conference, Barcelona, Spain.

Rojanapithayakorn, W. and Hanenberg, R. (1996). The 100% condom program in Thailand. *AIDS* 10:1–7.

Sabbaj, S., Mulligan, M.J., Hsieh, R.H., Belshe, R.B., and McGhee, J.R. (2000). Cytokine profiles in seronegative volunteers immunized with a recombinant canarypox and gp120 prime-boost HIV-1 vaccine. NIAID AIDS Vaccine Evaluation Group. *AIDS* 14:1365–1374.

Santra, S., Schmitz, J.E., Kuroda, M.J., Lifton, M.A., Nickerson, C.E., Lord, C.I., Pal, R., Franchini, G., and Letvin, N.L. (2002). Recombinant canarypox vaccine-elicited CTL specific for dominant and subdominant simian immunodeficiency virus epitopes in rhesus monkeys. *J Immunol.* 168:1847–1853.

Schultz, A.M. and Bradac, J.A. (2001). The HIV vaccine pipeline, from preclinical to phase III. *AIDS* 15 Suppl 5:S147–S158.

Sirisopana, N., Torugsa, K., Mason, C.J., Markowitz, L.E., Jugsudee, A., Supapongse, T., Chuenchitra, C., Michael, R.A., Burke, D.S., Singharaj, P., Johnson, A.E., McNeil, J.G., McCutchan, F.E., and Carr, J.K. (1996). Correlates of HIV-1 seropositivity among young men in Thailand. *J Acquir Immune Defic Syndr Hum Retrovirol.* 11:492–498.

Sirisopana, N., Benenson, M.W., Tontichaivanich, C., Pumratana, K., Tungsakul, V., Santativongchai, S., Teppatiphat, P., and Brown, A.E. (2001). Cohort development for future HIV-1 efficacy vaccine trials: women attending family planning clinics in Rayong Province, Thailand, In Sixth International Congress on AIDS in Asia and the Pacific, Melbourne, Australia.

Suriyanon, V., Thongcharoen, P., Khamboonruang, C., de Souza, M., Gurunathan, S., Ratto-Kim, S., Kim, J.,Duliege, A.M., and Brown, A.E. (2002). Safety and immunogenicity of live recombinant ALVAC-HIV (vCP1521) priming with gp120 boosting in Thai HIV seronegative adults, In XIV International AIDS Conference, Barcelona, Spain.

Tanasugarn, C. and Wienrawee, P. (1994). Community mobilization for AIDS prevention in Bangkok. *Aidscaptions* 1:10–15.

Tartaglia, J., Excler, J.L., El Habib, R., Limbach, K., Meignier, B., Plotkin, S., and Klein, M. (1998). Canarypox virus-based vaccines: Prime-boost strategies to induce cell-mediated and humoral immunity against HIV. *AIDS Res Hum Retroviruses* 14 Suppl 3:S291–S298.

Thapinta, D., Jenkins, R.A., Celentano, D.D., Nitayaphan, S., Buapunth, P., Triampon, A., Morgan, P.A., Khamboonruang, C., Suwanarach, C., Yutabootr, Y., Ruckphaopunt, S., Suwankiti, S., Tubtong, V., Cheewawat, W., McNeil, J.G., and Michael, R.A. (1999). Evaluation of behavioral and social issues among Thai HIV vaccine trial volunteers. *J Acquir Immune Defic Syndr Hum Retrovirol.* 20:308–314.

Thapinta, D., Jenkins, R.A., Morgan, P.A., Chiu, J., Boenim, W., Bussaratid, V., Chaddic, C., Naksrisook, S., Phonrat, B., Sirijongdee, N., Sornsathapornkul, P., Sontirat, A., Srisaengchai, P., Suwanarach, C., Wongkamhaeng, S., Brown, A.E., Khamboonruang, C., Nitayaphan, S., Pitisuttithum, P., and Thongchareon, P. (2002). Recruiting volunteers for a multisite phase I/II HIV preventive vaccine trial in Thailand. *J Acquir Immune Defic Syndr Hum Retrovirol.* 30:503–513.

Thongcharoen, P.T., Suriyanon, V.S., Khamboonruang, C.K., Kim, J., Polonis, V., de Souza, M., Gurunathan, S., and Brown, A.E. (2002). Safety and immunogenicity of live recombinant ALVAC-HIV (vCP1521) priming with an oligomeric gp160 boost in Thai HIV-seronegative adults, In XIV International AIDS Conference, Barcelona, Spain.

Torugsa, K., Jenkins, R.A., Krinchai, K., Lalang, C., Jugsudee, A., Brown, A.E., and Mason, C.J. (1997). Trend of HIV-1 seroincidence among young Thai men, In 4th International Congress on AIDS in Asia and the Pacific, Manila, Philippines.

Torugsa, K., Anderson, S., Thongsen, N., Sirisopana, N., Jugsudee, A., Junlananto, P., Nitayaphan, S., Sangkharomya, S., and Brown, A.E. (2003). HIV epidemic among young Thai Men, 1991–2000. *Emerg Infect Dis.* 9:881–883.

Triampon, A. (2001). Experience from the successful conduct of a phase I/II trial of a gp120 vaccine in Bangkok, In Sixth International Congress on AIDS in Asia and the Pacific, Melbourne, Australia.

Trichavaroj, R., de Souza, M.S., Buapunth, P., Markowitz, L., Sukwit, S., Nitayaphan, S., and Brown, A.E. (2001). HIV viral load in Thai men and women with subtype E infections. *J Acquir Immune Defic Syndr Hum Retrovirol.* 26:345–347.

UNAIDS/WHO (1998). AIDS vaccine research in Asia: Needs and opportunities, In Report from UNAIDS/WHO/NID meeting, Tokyo, Japan.

UNAIDS/WHO (2000). Epidemiological fact sheet on HIV/AIDS and sexually transmitted infections: Thailand—2000 update.

Ungphakorn, J. and Sittitrai, W. (1994). The Thai response to the HIV/AIDS epidemic. *AIDS* 8:S155–S163.

Vanichseni, S., Kitayaporn, D., Mastro, T.D., Mock, P.A., Raktham, S., Des Jarlais, D.C., Sujarita, S., Srisuwanvilai, L.O., Young, N.L., Wasi, C., Subbarao, S., Heyward, W.L., Esparza, L., and Choopanya, K. (2001). Continued high HIV-1 incidence in a vaccine trial preparatory cohort of injection drug users in Bangkok, Thailand. AIDS 15:397–405.

Watt, G., Kantipong, P., Jongsakul, K., Watcharapichat, P., Phulsuksombati, D., and Strickman, D. (2000). Doxycycline and rifampicin for mild scrub-typhus infections in northern Thailand: a randomised trial. *Lancet* 356:1057–1061.

World Health Organization. (1997). Revised recommendations for the selection and use of HIV antibody tests, *In Wkly Epidemiol Rec*, Vol. 72, pp. 81–87.

37

The Thailand MoPH–U.S. CDC Collaboration in Asia

Jordan W. Tappero[1,2], Taweesap Siraprapasiri[1,3], William C. Levine[1,2], Sombat Thanprasertsuk[3], Scott Dowell[1,2], Khanchit Limpakarnjanarat[1], and Timothy D. Mastro[2]

[1] *Thailand Ministry of Public Health-U.S. Centers for Disease Control and Prevention Collaboration; Nonthaburi, Thailand*
[2] *U.S. Centers for Disease Control and Prevention; Atlanta, Georgia, USA*
[3] *Thailand Ministry of Public Health; Nonthaburi, Thailand*

INTRODUCTION

In 1990, a joint activity between the Thailand Ministry of Public Health (MoPH) and the U.S. Centers for Disease Control and Prevention (U.S. CDC) known as the "HIV/AIDS Collaboration" was born, its primary objective was to conduct HIV prevention research to contribute to HIV/AIDS control efforts in Thailand. The Collaboration maintained an office and a laboratory on the campus of the MoPH in Nonthaburi, a Bangkok suburb. U.S. CDC scientists and public health advisors were assigned to live and work in Thailand alongside Thai MoPH colleagues. Local staff were hired and supported by the U.S. Embassy in Bangkok and the MoPH. This research initiative built on the trust established between the Thai MoPH and the U.S. CDC through the Thai Field Epidemiology Training Program (FETP), which was inaugurated in 1980, becoming the first FETP program outside North America. The Thai FETP is modeled on U.S. CDC's Epidemic Intelligence Service (EIS) program, both striving to improve public health surveillance, prevention and disease control efforts.

In 2001, Thailand became one of 25 partner countries participating in U.S. CDC's Global AIDS Program (GAP), an effort of the U.S. Department of Health and Human Services to assist countries with a high burden of HIV/AIDS by providing support for HIV prevention programs, care for persons living with HIV/AIDS, and capacity building in training, laboratory testing, surveillance, and monitoring and evaluation. Also in late 2001, the Collaboration welcomed the U.S. CDC's first International Emerging Infections Program (IEIP) to Thailand. The IEIP aims to integrate disease surveillance, applied research, training and capacity development and support for outbreak investigations of emerging infections. The addition of GAP and IEIP to the joint activity between the MoPH and U.S. CDC prompted a name change to the "Thailand MoPH–U.S. CDC Collaboration," which more accurately reflects the Collaboration's research and programmatic activities in HIV/AIDS, sexually transmitted infections (STIs), tuberculosis (TB), and other emerging infections.

This chapter reviews some of the Collaboration's major contributions in HIV/AIDS research over its 13-year history, and its new activities through GAP and IEIP.

HIV/AIDS RESEARCH

Descriptive Epidemiology

In 1988–1991, Thailand experienced an explosive HIV epidemic among injection drug users (IDU) and persons with sexual risk behaviors (World Bank Thailand Office, Bangkok, 2000; Weniger *et al.*, 1991; Nopkesorn *et al.*, 1993). In 1991, an analysis of HIV strains collected among high risk transmission populations across Thailand identified two distinct HIV-1 subtypes that could be segregated by transmission group (IDU, subtype B; persons with heterosexual risk behaviors including female sex workers, subtype E [later known as CRF 01_AE]), suggesting that the HIV epidemics in these two populations were largely independent (Ou *et al.*, 1993; Wasi *et al.*, 1995; Kalish *et al.*, 1995). However, this relatively clear HIV-1 subtype segregation by risk category was not sustained; by the mid 1990s, HIV-1 subtype E accounted for an increasing proportion of infections among IDU, in addition to the great majority of infections among persons with heterosexual risk behaviors (Subbarao *et al.*, 1998; Kitayaporn *et al.*, 1998; Limpakarnjanarat *et al.*, 1998). Spread of HIV from high risk groups to the general population was rapid, as evidenced by HIV prevalence among pregnant women attending antenatal clinics where HIV climbed steadily from 0.6% in 1991, peaking at 2.3% in 1995 (Kanshana and Simonds, 2002), and dropping slowly, yet steadily, to 1.4% in 2002 (Thai MoPH, 2002). Through the year 2000, nearly one million Thais became infected with HIV, with an additional 29,000 new infections estimated to have occurred in 2001; roughly 650,000 Thais are living with HIV/AIDS (CDC/Thai MoPH, 2003).

In 1988, a severe HIV epidemic was recognized among Bangkok's IDU, with prevalence rising from less than 1% to greater than 40% by years end, and later spreading to all provinces of Thailand and to other IDU populations in the Southeast Asia region (World Bank Thailand Office, Bangkok, 2000; Weniger *et al.*, 1991). Although the MoPH is rightfully touted for its success in dampening the spread of new HIV infections among female sex workers, their male clients, military conscripts, and pregnant women (Rojanapithayakom and Hanenberg, 1996; Nelson *et al.*, 1996; Kilmarx *et al.*, 2000b; Mastro and Limpakarnjanarat, 1995; Weniger and Brown, 1996; Torgusa *et al.*, 2003), the median prevalence of HIV-infection among IDU in Thailand has climbed steadily, reaching a peak of 50% in 2002 (Thai MoPH, 2002). In the absence of an effective HIV intervention targeting IDU, such as an HIV-1 vaccine, the overall proportion of new HIV infections in Thailand due to injection drug use, including women infected by needle-sharing partners, is projected to increase to 41% by 2005 (World Bank Thailand Office, Bangkok, 2000).

HIV Transmission among IDU and HIV Vaccine Evaluation

In 1991, the World Health Organization (WHO) initiated an HIV vaccine development program, including support to establish preparatory cohorts for HIV-1 vaccine trials (Esparza *et al.*, 1991; Heyward *et al.*, 1996). Simultaneously, the Royal Thai Government developed a National Plan for HIV/AIDS Vaccine Development and

Evaluation (Phoolcharoen *et al.*, 1998). With the political will of the MoPH behind it, an HIV vaccine preparatory cohort study was initiated to assess the feasibility of conducting an HIV vaccine efficacy trial among IDU at high risk for acquiring HIV infection.

In Bangkok, an extensive network of 17 outpatient narcotic clinics operated by the Bangkok Metropolitan Administration (BMA) provides free methadone treatment services annually for 6000 to 8500 IUD (Mastro *et al.*, 1994a). To assess the feasibility of conducting a large-scale HIV-1 vaccine trial in this population, the BMA, in partnership with Mahidol University, WHO, the Joint United Nations Programme on HIV/AIDS (UNAIDS), and the Collaboration conducted an HIV vaccine preparatory cohort study among IDU who were 18 to 50 years of age and attending BMA drug treatment clinics and testing negative for HIV-1 antibodies. This 1995–1998 BMA cohort study of 1209 IDU (median age, 31 years; 93% male) revealed a follow-up time contribution of 88.2% at 12 months, an annual HIV-1 incidence rate of 5.8 per 100 person-years, an HIV-1 subtype distribution of 21% B and 79% E (Vanichseni *et al.*, 2001), the clinical course of HIV infection by subtype (Hu *et al.*, 2001), the presence of intersubtype superinfections (Ramos *et al.*, 2002), and the willingness of a majority of IDU to participate in an large-scale efficacy trial (MacQueen *et al.*, 1999). The subtype distribution validated early genetic characterization work from this cohort (Subbarao *et al.*, 2000; Phan *et al.*, 2000), prompting the formulation (Berman 1998; Francis *et al.*, 1998), and safety and immunogenicity evaluation (Pitisuttithum *et al.*, 2000) of a bivalent recombinant gp120 HIV-1 vaccine (AIDSVAX®B/E; VaxGen, Inc.) made specifically for use in Thailand.

From March 1999 through June 2003, the world's first Phase III HIV vaccine efficacy trial outside the North America was conducted in Thailand by the Bangkok Vaccine Evaluation Group (BVEG), a team comprised of the BMA, Mahidol University, VaxGen, Inc., and the Collaboration. Recruitment and enrollment of 2546 HIV-negative IDU was completed in August 2000 (Vanichesni *et al.*, 2004). Volunteers received either AIDSVAX®B/E vaccine or placebo (1:1 ratio) at months 0, 1, and 6, with booster doses at months 12, 18, 24, and 30. Participants were followed for 36 months, immunization compliance exceeded 95%, and risk behavior counseling was shown to be effective throughout the conduct of the trial (van Griensven *et al.*, 2003a). Trial results were announced on November 12, 2003 (VaxGen, 2003); the vaccine failed to demonstrate efficacy for the prevention of HIV infection, and failed to demonstrate mitigation of clinical HIV disease progression prior to the initiation of highly active antiretroviral drug therapy (HAART), which was universally provided according to BMA treatment guidelines (Martin *et al.*, 2003). Although trial results were disappointing, the vaccine preparatory cohort and vaccine trial were successful in increasing Thailand's capacity to conduct future HIV vaccine trials, and proved that high-risk populations, such as IDU, can ethically participate in the evaluation of promising HIV vaccine candidates in large-scale trials.

Prevention of Mother-to-Child Transmission of HIV

Since 1992, the Collaboration has worked with the MoPH, Mahidol University, and other partners to conduct research directed at understanding and preventing mother-to-child HIV transmission (PMTCT). Early retrospective, descriptive work identified HIV infection to be an important factor for low birth weight deliveries (Srismith *et al.*, 1998), and that HIV prevalence at delivery increased rapidly from 1.3% in 1990 to 6.4% in 1994 (Bunnell *et al.*, 1999) in Chiang Rai province. Having more than one lifetime sex partner was found to be an important risk factor for HIV infection among pregnant women delivering at two large hospitals in Bangkok, and surprisingly, a quarter of all delivering women had current partners who were not HIV-infected (Siriwasin *et al.*, 1998). A prospective study of mother-to-child HIV transmission in these two hospitals during 1992–1994 found the risk of transmission to be 24.2% (Shaffer *et al.*, 1999b), with 75% of these infections arising intrapartum (Mock *et al.*, 1999), and with maternal viral load being the strongest predictor for transmission for both in utero and intrapartum transmission.

In 1994, the results of AIDS Clinical Trials Group (ACTG) protocol 076 were announced (Conner *et al.*, 1994). The study found that a complex regimen of zidovudine (076 regimen), given to HIV-infected women during pregnancy, labor and to the neonate for 6 weeks reduced mother-to child transmission by two-thirds in the absence of breastfeeding. However, most HIV-infected women live in Africa and Asia in settings where governments (including Thailand) could not afford the 076 regimen implementation costs (Stringer *et al.*, 1999). In order to find a safe, simple, and inexpensive regimen, the Collaboration, building on the infrastructure established during the 1992–1994 study, conducted a Phase III, randomized, placebo-controlled clinical trial of short-course zidovudine for PMTCT in Bangkok in 1996–1998 (CDC, 1998; Shaffer *et al.*, 1999a). HIV transmission was significantly lower (9%) among the 198 women who received zidovudine from 36 weeks' gestation until labor onset, then every 3 hours until delivery, than among the 199 women who did not (19%); adverse events were similar in the 2 groups (mild anemia at birth only), as was survival among HIV-infected children at 18 months follow-up (Chotpitayasunondh *et al.*, 2001). The trial results had a profound and immediate impact on Thailand and the world (Kanshana and Simonds, 2002). Several weeks after the results were announced, UNAIDS met and issued a recommendation to use the short course zidovudine regimen in countries that could not implement the 076 regimen. Additional findings from this trial included the detection of HIV in cervicovaginal lavage (CVL) specimens as an independent risk factor for mother–child transmission (Chuachoowong *et al.*, 2000), and the evaluation of the sensitivity and specificity of the Roche Amplicor RNA and DNA PCR tests for early diagnosis of HIV-1 infection (Young *et al.*; 2000); RNA PCR was more sensitive (47%) at birth than DNA PCR (38%), and both assays were 100% sensitive and specific by two months of age.

Since the late 1990s, nevirapine has received increasing attention in Thailand for PMTCT (either in combination with short-course zidovudine, or as an alternative to the 1- or 6-week infant component of modified national zidovudine regimen (Amornwichet *et al.*, 2002) due to its low cost, favorable pharmacokinetics, and simplicity and efficacy as monotherapy. Because there is limited data on the safety or efficacy of nevirapine in Thai women and children, the Collaboration conducted a Phase II, single-arm, open label clinical trial of providing nevirapine to 220 mothers and their children already receiving the short-course zidovudine regimen. Mothers received one 200 mg dose of nevirapine after presenting to the hospital in labor, and their infants received one 6mg (approximately 2 mg/kg) dose in the first three days of life. The perinatal transmission rate was 4.6%, and 93% of women had blood specimens that tested successfully for drug resistance; of these, 17% and 2% had nevirapine and zidovudine resistance mutations, respectively (Chaowanachan *et al.*, 2003). Data from this trial and others in Thailand prompted the MoPH to add nevirapine to the national short-course zidovudine regimen in late 2003.

Sexual Transmission of STIs, HIV, and the Study of Vaginal Microbicides

In 1991, the Collaboration established a field research station in Chiang Rai, Thailand's northernmost province where HIV infection rates have been among the highest in Asia (Kilmarx *et al.*, 2000b). Surveillance data from the first half of the decade found increasing prevalence of HIV infection among all risk groups, and in particular, female sex workers (Limpakarnjanarat *et al.*, 1991). STIs were common among female sex workers from Chiang Rai who were followed in a prospective cohort study. (Kilmarx *et al.*, 1998b; Limpakarnjanarat *et al.*, 1999), More than half were using medications they obtained from a source other than a STI clinic, such as a pharmacy, to treat symptomatic disease (Kilmarx *et al.*, 1997). From 1991–1994, HIV incidence among 285 female sex workers in this Chiang Rai cohort was 20.3 per 100 person-years among 126 brothel-based sex workers and 0.7 per 100 person-years among 159 sex workers who worked in other venues; risk factors for acquiring HIV infection were working in a brothel and having chlamydia cervicitis (Kilmarx *et al.*, 1998b). In addition, some female sex workers were using vaginal products with the perception that they might help to prevent STIs, rather than potentially facilitating acquisition of HIV/STI through damage to the vaginal and cervical mucosa (Kilmarx *et al.*, 1998a). Sex work was also found to be inconsistent, with a majority of sex workers having one or more quit-re-entry-quit cycles. These inconsistencies were determined by economic factors, relationship with a steady partner, attitudes towards sex work, and HIV/AIDS experience (Manopaiboon *et al.*, 2003). Disease progression and survival rates among 194 female sex workers in this cohort with HIV infection (96% subtype E) were shown to be similar to that found among populations elsewhere with HIV subtype B infection (Kilmarx *et al.*, 2000a), and the mortality risk among HIV-infected sex workers was more than 50-fold higher when compared to sex workers without HIV infection (Kilmarx *et al.*, 2000c). This cohort also provided the opportunity to identify genetic polymorphisms, such as HLA-A11, CCR5 59402GG promoter, and SDF-1 3′ UTR 801 A (Sriwanthana *et al.*, 2001), homozygosity of HHF*2 (the CCR2b-641 bearing haplogroup [Yang *et al.*, 2003]), and viral suppressive activity (Butera *et al.*, 2001) that might explain resistance to HIV infection among highly HIV-exposed, persistently seronegative female sex workers.

A 1991–1993 prospective cohort study of more than 1100 young, male military conscripts from northern Thailand identified sex with female sex workers as the dominant risk factor for HIV infection and identified other STIs as a major co-factor for transmission (Nopkesorn *et al.*, 1993; Nopkesorn *et al.*, 1998). A subsequent study also identified a relatively high per-sex-act HIV-1 transmission probability from female sex workers to young men, perhaps explaining in-part the rapid expansion of the HIV-1 epidemic in northern Thailand (Mastro *et al.*, 1994b) Although the "100% condom" campaign was effective in rapidly decreasing HIV prevalence among young male military conscripts (Rojanapithayakom and Hanenberg, 1996; Nelson *et al.*, 1996; Kilmarx *et al.*, 2000a; Mastro and Limpakarnjanarat, 1995; Weniger and Brown, 1996; Torgusa *et al.*, 2003), HIV prevalence remained high among our cohort of 508 women who entered sex work at different time intervals throughout the 1990s, suggesting ongoing infection risk in this population (Kilmarx *et al.*, 1999).

Vaginal microbicides are a promising new technology that if effective, could be used by women to protect themselves from infection with HIV and other STIs. Carraguard® (with 3% carrageenan), is the Population Council's lead candidate microbicide. Carrageenans are sulfated polymers with a large molecular weight derived from seaweed, and have been used extensively in the food, pharmaceutical, and cosmetics industries. Carraguard® has been shown to block infection from HIV and other STIs, and is thought to be noncontraceptive. A randomized, placebo-controlled, Phase II study of Carraguard® among 165 HIV-seronegative women was completed in Chiang Rai in December 2001, and a second Phase II clinical trial of this product among 55 HIV-seronegative couples was completed in Chiang Rai in June, 2002. Preliminary, blinded results from both studies revealed strong safety profiles and high rates of acceptability with product use (Manopaiboon *et al.*, 2002; Limpakarnjanarat *et al.*, 2002; Kilmarx *et al.*, 2002; Blanchard *et al.*, 2004; Kilmarx *et al.*, 2004). Some women who choose to use a microbicide may be HIV-infected, but may not be aware of their infection. Therefore, data from microbicide studies of HIV-infected women are important. Enrollment into a third Phase II trial of Carraguard® among 54 HIV-infected women in Chiang Rai was completed in March 2004 (McLean *et al.*, 2004b; McLean *et al.*, 2004a; Chaikummao *et al.*, 2004). Final, unblinded analyses for these three studies will be conducted following completion of companion studies in South Africa; results will be critical for moving forward the Population Council's planned Phase III efficacy trial of Carraguard® in South Africa. Heterosexual women attending postpartum and family planning clinics in Chiang Rai have low (3.1%) HIV prevalence (Xu *et al.*, 2002), and although they have expressed a willingness to participate in large-scale vaginal microbicide trials (Tharawan *et al.*, 2001), their annual incidence of HIV infection in not sufficient to conduct a Phase III trial (Xu *et al.*, 2000; Tharawan *et al.*, 2001; Xu *et al.*, 2002). The Phase II evaluation of promising new vaginal microbicide candidates, as well as other studies will continue in Chiang Rai with the strong support of the Provincial Public Health Office and Chiang Rai Regional Hospital.

Behavioral Science

In 1998, a behavioral science section was added to the Collaboration to increase behavioral research capacity, provide support for the development of procedures for protection of human subjects in research and to monitor risk behaviors in HIV clinical trials. In 1999, a rapid assessment of the "Prevalence of HIV, STD and sexual and drug use Risk behaviors among Adolescents and Young Adults" or PHRAYA Study was conducted in Chiang Rai (van Griensven *et al.*, 2001). In this study, an innovative audio-computer-assisted self-interviewing (ACASI) technique was used in conjunction with non-invasive HIV, STI and drug use testing methods (oral fluid and urine). The study enrolled 1725 students, and showed that northern Thai youth are at high risk for unsafe sex, early sexual initiation, unwanted pregnancy, STIs, sexual coercion, methamphetamine drug use and absence of motor cycle helmet use (Jenkins *et al.*, 2002; Allen *et al.*, 2003; Manopaiboon *et al.*, 2004b; Manopaiboon *et al.*, 2004a; Paz-Bailey *et al.*, 2003; van Greinsven *et al.*, 2003b; Sattah *et al.*, 2002; Pitaktong *et al.*, 2004). Although the study showed that ACASI provided high quality behavioral data, ACASI systems are relatively expensive and not easily transported.

In 2002, the Collaboration evaluated the reliability of use of hand-held mini-computers for behavioral risk surveillance among Chiang Rai adolescents (PalmPHRAYA study). In a randomized design, 1300 students were assigned to one of four data collection arms: face-to-face interview (FFI), self-administered questionnaire (SAQ), ACASI, and Palm-assisted self-interview (PASI). The study included drug-use urine testing to evaluate completeness of self-reports and reliability across arms. The PASI was found to be equivalent to ACASI, and both were superior FFI and SAQ in providing accurate and complete data to sensitive behavioral questions, and with fewer errors. Ongoing adolescent behavioral risk surveillance using PASI data collection methods is now under development with the MoPH. The low prevalence of methamphetamine use reactive urines in the PalmPHRAYA study, compared to the PHRAYA study (10.3% vs. 2.4%), prompted a qualitative assessment into trends in adolescent drug use, the results of which are currently being analyzed.

In April and May 2003, the behavioral section led the first cross-sectional assessment in men who have sex with men (MSM) in Thailand. In this venue-based assessment, 1121 MSM completed an interviewer-administered Palm based questionnaire and oral fluid specimens were collected for HIV testing. In this young (median age 26 years) and sexually active population (22% had recent sexual intercourse with a women), an HIV prevalence of 17.3% was found, which was associated with indicators of sexual activity and lower education. This data is essential to inform and develop preventive interventions and services for this group. In addition to research among adolescents and MSM, the behavioral science section was included in several studies in groups at elevated risk for HIV infection such as Myanmese migrants (Srithanaviboonchai *et al.*, 2002), fishermen (Entz *et al.*, 2001) and drug users with a history of incarceration (Buavirat *et al.*, 2003).

GLOBAL AIDS PROGRAM (GAP)

In 2001, GAP became a component of the Collaboration, with a mission of technical cooperation with the MoPH and BMA to strengthen programs for HIV/AIDS, TB, and STI prevention and care. Thailand is one of the 25 countries supported by CDC through this program. To develop GAP activities in Thailand, the Collaboration built on its existing strengths in epidemiology, laboratory science, and informatics; on existing relationships with the MoPH and BMA that were developed through many years of collaborative research; and on findings that emerged from research performed by the Collaboration and elsewhere that were important to introduce into programs.

Although Thailand already had great success in the 1990s with HIV prevention through the program for 100% condom use (Mastro and Limpakarnjanarat, 1995; Hanenberg *et al.*, 1994) and a model program for prevention of mother to child transmission, major challenges in prevention and care for HIV/AIDS, TB, and STIs were apparent in 2001 when GAP became part of the Collaboration. The new systems for monitoring coverage and impact of activities for PMTCT needed to be strengthened and institutionalized. HIV seroprevalence among IDU remained 40–50% in Bangkok (BMA) and elsewhere around the country (MoPH), and no program of community-based outreach for IDU was in place. In early 2000, data from behavioral surveillance performed by the MoPH indicated that rates of condom use, particularly among indirect sex workers (e.g., sex work occurring in relation to bars and massage parlors), were declining, coinciding with decreased support for prevention programs at the provincial level in some areas. Concerns regarding risk behavior in adolescents were growing based on behavioral surveillance data and studies such as the PHRAYA study that demonstrated high rates of unprotected sex, unwanted pregnancy, drug use and STIs in school-age adolescents (van Griensven *et al.*, 2001). Single and dual antiretroviral therapy regimens for treatment of HIV infection had become available in some provinces in the 1990s through programs of the MoPH, and a major program was undertaken to develop comprehensive HIV/AIDS care services. However, coverage and quality of these care and treatment services was limited, even as the government was developing plans to scale-up the availability of HAART through a combination drug produced by the Thai Government Pharmaceutical Organization (GPOvir), consisting of D4T, 3TC, and nevirapine. Thailand ranked 16th among the 22 TB high-burden countries identified by WHO, and coverage of programs for directly observed therapy, short-course (DOTS), and isoniazid prophylaxis for persons with HIV infection were low (World Health Organization , 2003). Although STIs had reportedly declined dramatically over the last decade, and rates of serologic syphilis were low, utilization of sensitive diagnostic testing for chlamydia infection, which is probably the most common bacterial STI in Thailand, were not generally available.

The GAP/Thailand 5-Year Country Plan, developed in collaboration with, and approved by the MoPH in 2002 calls for 1) supporting the work of the Departments of the MoPH centrally and 2) providing support for the development of province-level networks for support of activities in HIV/AIDS prevention, care, training and surveillance. The decision to develop mechanisms at the provincial level to strengthen technical work of HIV/AIDS, TB, and STI prevention and care by focusing initially on the development of activities in four to five provinces was based on the need to develop local models for addressing multiple complex issues in prevention and care. A major focus of the plan is on piloting new models, scaling up successful pilot projects nationally, and in some cases, filling gaps in existing programs. The major offices of the MoPH supported through GAP/Thailand are the Department of Disease Control (Bureau of AIDS, TB, and STI, and the Bureau of Epidemiology, which conducts national HIV/AIDS surveillance), and the Department of Health, (which is responsible for maternal and child health).

The first provinces selected for GAP/Thailand support in 2002 and 2003 were Bangkok, Chiang Rai, Ubon Ratchathani, and Phuket. The Collaboration's existing relationships with the BMA through the work on the BVEG AIDSVAX®B/E trial (Vanichesni *et al.*, 2004) led to the development of a new set of GAP-supported projects for strengthening HIV/AIDS programs in Thailand's largest city, with a major focus on interventions for IDU. Chiang Rai, one of the provinces most severely affected by HIV/AIDS in the 1990s, served as a key field site for collaborative research; longstanding relationships with the provincial health office and local hospitals made this a logical choice. Ubon Ratchathani was the first province to pilot the short course zidovudine intervention for PMTCT, with the support of the Collaboration for implementation and monitoring. Phuket was selected for support because of its increasing antenatal prevalence of HIV, high rates of TB, burgeoning populations of male and female sex workers, indigenous IDU and a large and transient Myanmese population with high rates of disease.

To support these activities, GAP/Thailand efforts are organized through seven technical areas: 1) training, communications and partnerships, 2) care and counseling, 3) prevention and care for families, 4) prevention and care for special populations, 5) surveillance, monitoring and evaluation, 6) laboratory services, and 7) informatics. These areas provide the structure for supporting a focused set of projects to strengthen MoPH activities, and are administered through GAP Coordinating Units established within the MoPH and BMA to administer cooperative agreement projects that address the following issues:

Preventing Mother-to-Child HIV Transmission

Activities to strengthen the national PMTCT program include support for the perinatal HIV implementation monitoring system, evaluation of a system for analyzing outcomes in infants, and two training programs to support the PMTCT program, in the context of evolving guidelines and the needs of health care workers and program managers.

Following the success of the short-course zidovudine study in 1998, the MoPH developed a plan to pilot the implementation of the short course regimen and provision of infant formula in a region covering seven northeastern provinces, where antenatal prevalence was about 1% (Kanshana *et al.*, 2000). The Collaboration was asked to work with the MoPH to evaluate this initial implementation, with the purpose of assessing the feasibility, effectiveness, and acceptability of a program consisting of routine antenatal counseling and voluntary HIV testing, zidovudine provided from 36 weeks' gestation and during labor, and free powder for preparation of infant formula for 12 months. This evaluation demonstrated that from July, 1998–June, 2000, 104,393 (86%) of 122,094 antenatal clinic clients had received HIV testing, 640 (69%) of HIV-infected pregnant women received antenatal zidovudine prophylaxis (CDC, 2001).

Analysis of HIV PCR testing performed on exposed infants after one month of age demonstrated that about 8% of infants whose mothers had received zidovudine were HIV infected, compared with 14% of infants whose mothers had not received zidovudine (CDC, 2001).

By 1999, HIV counseling and testing, zidovudine, and use of infant formula were used in many hospitals throughout Thailand for PMTCT, and in October 2000, a national system was established to monitor key PMTCT program indicators, with financial and technical support from the Collaboration. The system included logbooks maintained at the hospitals, monthly reports sent to provincial health offices where the data was computerized, regional aggregation of this data by 12 Health Promotion Centers, and final analysis and reporting by the MoPH in Nonthaburi. Standardized reports at each level were used to monitor coverage of each of the key components of the intervention. Data reported from October, 2000 through September 2001 demonstrated that of 93% of women receiving antenatal care were screened for HIV, 70% of HIV-positive women identified during screening received zidovudine before delivery, and 89% of HIV-exposed infants received prophylactic zidovudine and 83% were placed on infant formula (Amornwiclet *et al.*, 2002).

HIV/AIDS Care and Treatment

Support for the national program for improving access to care includes 1) development of systems for performance measurement of HIV care and treatment services, complemented by activities to improve the quality and coverage of these services, 2) expansion of CD4 testing, including provision of reagents and strengthening of laboratory quality assurance mechanisms, and 3) development of a model for ensuring referral of HIV-positive women identified during pregnancy, their infants, and partners into HIV care services. An initial GAP-supported assessment of HIV care and treatment services provided through public hospitals and community health centers in three northern provinces identified specific benchmarks for monitoring opportunistic infection prophylaxis, coverage, and antiretroviral therapy access (Lertpiriyasuwat *et al.*, submitted).

TB Surveillance and Strengthening of DOTS

Support is provided for strengthening TB surveillance and control activities and laboratory activities in Network provinces, and strengthening of systems for diagnostic testing, laboratory quality, and information systems at the National TB Reference Laboratory. Laboratory development includes an emphasis on increasing the availability of rapid TB culture and identification methods to facilitate surveillance and control activities. Increasing HIV testing of persons with TB is an important GAP/Thailand and MoPH objective.

STI Care

Support is provided for strengthening systems for STI care in Network provinces, and for increasing diagnostic and informatics capacity of the Division of STI. These activities include increasing the availability of diagnostic testing for *Chlamydia trachomatis* infection, which has been found in several studies to be the most common bacterial STI in Thailand, and increasing STI and cervical cytologic screening among HIV-positive women.

Interventions for IDU

A comprehensive set of assessments and interventions will be supported in Bangkok, including 1) estimation of the size of the IDU population, 2) a qualitative study of midazolam injection, 3) development of a program of community-level outreach for IDU, 4) an adult immunization program for prevention of hepatitis B and tetanus, and 5) strengthening of the system of HIV/AIDS care for Bangkok IDU, including support for a program to provided directly observed HAART to IDU with advanced HIV disease.

Interventions for Adolescents

Support is provided to strengthen interventions for adolescents, which have become a high priority for the MoPH, due in part to the findings of the Collaboration regarding increasing rates of unprotected sexual intercourse and high rates of STIs in adolescents (van Greinsven *et al.*, 2001). GAP/Thailand is providing support to the MoPH in designing and implementing a comprehensive clinical services model for youth in four provinces.

Surveillance, Monitoring, and Evaluation

Support is provided for reviewing existing AIDS surveillance activities, and developing new models for surveillance. This will include piloting implementing the use of the personal digital assistant or hand-held minicomputer for behavioral surveillance, evaluating the role of the IgG-capture, HIV-1 subtype B, E, and D enzyme immunoassay (or BED assay) (Parekh *et al.*, 2002) for incidence estimation as a component of national HIV serosurveillance, and development of population-based surveillance for TB. GAP/Thailand is also working with the MoPH to develop systems to monitor and evaluate GAP activities, and provide support to strengthen monitoring and evaluation capacity of the MoPH and National AIDS Committee.

Through a cooperative agreement between CDC and the American Red Cross, support was also provided to the Thai Red Cross AIDS Research Centre to expand their highly successful model for anonymous voluntary counseling and testing for HIV in Bangkok to three other provinces, and to include provision of CD4 testing to facilitate entry into the growing national systems for provision of opportunistic infection prophylaxis and antiretroviral therapy. Additionally, agreements were developed with the UNAIDS Regional Office in Bangkok to use GAP funds available through UNAIDS in Geneva to strengthen activities for public-private partnerships in the fight against AIDS in the Asia region, and to advocate for interventions for prevention and care of men who have sex with men in Cambodia, Thailand, and Vietnam.

CDC GAP ASIA REGIONAL ACTIVITIES

In 2002, the Collaboration received support from U.S. CDC to establish an organized program of regional activities. The first major event was a meeting held in Chiang Rai in December, 2002, attended by representatives from GAP country offices, senior ministry of health counterparts from China, Cambodia, India, Thailand and Vietnam, and representatives of UNAIDS, USAID, and Department for International Development (DFID) of the UK. At this meeting each country provided information on potential areas for regional collaboration, focusing on key topics in surveillance, monitoring and evaluation, laboratory services, informatics, prevention (including prevention of mother-to-child transmission) and care and treatment (CDC, 2003). The U.S. CDC designated GAP/Thailand as the GAP Asia Regional Office to continue to work with other countries of the region in developing this program, which will have an important role in facilitating country-to-country collaboration, and multi-country trainings, workshops, and projects (CDC, 2003).

Vietnam

CDC activities in Vietnam in support of HIV/AIDS prevention and care were initiated in 1999, two years prior to establishment of a GAP office in that country. Initial activities included a variety of multi-disciplinary HIV training courses and technical assistance to strengthen HIV surveillance and to conduct innovative assessments to better characterize the epidemic, especially among high-risk groups such as IDU and female sex workers. CDC supported Harvard Medical School to assist with training on HIV care and treatment and to establish VCHAP, the Vietnam-CDC-Harvard Medical School AIDS Partnership. The CDC/GAP office in Hanoi provides, through a cooperative agreement with the Ministry of Health, support to ten institutes of the Ministry and 40 provinces. The collaboration covers several areas in HIV prevention and care, with particular emphasis on voluntary counseling and testing; community outreach to high risk individuals through peer education programs; HIV treatment infrastructure including diagnosis, prophylaxis, and treatment of opportunistic infections; and support for HIV sentinel surveillance and STI surveillance.

Cambodia

A CDC/GAP assessment in Cambodia performed in 2001 recommended strengthening laboratory capacity for HIV and STI at the National Institute of Public Health and the National Center for HIV/AIDS, Dermatology, and STIs (NCHADS); supporting blood safety policy and program development, national capacity for monitoring and evaluation, a province-wide demonstration project that integrates prevention and care strategies, and training for capacity development (e.g., field epidemiology, laboratory, and program management). The CDC GAP office, established in 2002, worked directly with NCHADS to strengthen activities at the National Institute of Public Health, strengthen national STD clinical services, and develop an integrated model for interventions in Bantey Meanchay province, a province on the Thai border with high rates of HIV, TB, and STIs.

India

The GAP office in India was established in October 2001, with the primary goal of promoting integration and access to quality HIV/AIDS care and prevention in Tamil Nadu and elsewhere in India. Major activities have focused on building capacity and infrastructure for information systems and clinical and laboratory diagnosis, developing models for home-based community care, strengthening voluntary counseling and testing services, promoting a safe blood supply, and supporting training for HIV/AIDS care and prevention.

China

GAP activities in China were initiated in 2003, with establishment of a country office and a cooperative agreement with the Ministry of Health, focusing on strengthening interventions for injection drug users in heavily affected counties, with a primary emphasis on strengthening HIV serosurveillance, services for voluntary counseling and testing, and aspects of care and support. Strengthening of linkages between the China CDC and provincial and local systems for addressing the HIV/AIDS epidemic is an important focus of this effort.

INTERNATIONAL EMERGING INFECTIONS PROGRAM

CDC's first IEIP was launched in Thailand in October 2001. IEIPs were envisioned to be a center of excellence that would integrate disease surveillance, applied research, prevention and control activities (Dowell and Levitt, 2002). IEIP/Thailand maintains its relations with medical research institutes, local universities, the Thai FETP, U.S. military laboratories and WHO country and regional offices. IEIP/Thailand will strengthen national public health capacity and provide hands-on training in laboratory science, epidemiological science, and public health administration (Dowell *et al.*, 2004).

The long-term goal of the IEIP is to develop sustainable, in-country capacity for disease surveillance, outbreak investigation, and research on diseases of national, regional, or global importance by fostering the next generation of international public health leaders. In its initial years of operation, IEIP/Thailand initiated activities in each of the four priority areas described by CDC's global strategy: surveillance, research, training and capacity development, and outbreak support.

Surveillance

IEIP/Thailand initially focused its effort on establishing population-based surveillance as one of its core objectives. With additional support by CDC, the MoPH conducts high-quality surveillance and produces data to guide national and global infectious disease control priorities (Kanlayanaphotporn *et al.*, 2004, Olsen *et al.*, 2003a). The surveillance system also provides a broad platform to launch research projects and possibly evaluate new vaccines or other interventions in the future. Provinces are selected as sites for surveillance on the basis of several criteria, including representativeness of the Thai population, accessibility from Bangkok, feasibility of capturing the majority of hospitalizations through public health systems, availability of basic laboratory facilities, existence of epidemiologic capability, and interest and commitment from local public health authorities. Sakaeo province, with a population of 613,585, located 300 kilometers east of Bangkok on the Cambodian border was chosen by a MoPH and IEIP team in March 2002 as the first site. The province established a working group to conduct a review of existing systems and proposed data collection in consultation with a CDC expert, and developed a written action plan. Case reporting began in August 2002. Pneumonia was used as the first syndrome for this phase of surveillance since it is a leading cause of mortality worldwide and hospitalized patients may be infected with any of several pathogens. Some of these organisms are also leading opportunistic pathogens among HIV infected patients in Thailand. In July 2003, Nakorn Phanom province, with a polulation of 626,221, in the northeastern region, bordering Laos was selected to be the second surveillance site. In 2003, IEIP and collaborating MoPH and provincial health offices agreed to add jaundice as a second syndrome for surveillance. Over the next few years, Thailand may be able to share expertise in emerging infections with neighboring countries.

Research

IEIP sites are intended to provide platforms for conducting a broad range of research on infectious diseases of global importance. Priority for research in IEIP sites is placed on diseases that are identified by MoPH as important public health problems in the region. In 2001, the first research project was developed in response to a request from the Thai government to assist with an ongoing epidemic of leptospirosis (Tappero, 2002; Sejvar *et al.*, submitted). A subsequent project is evaluating field diagnostic tools for use at the hospital or national level and attempting to identify new pathogens that contribute to fever. During the first year, 749 febrile patients were enrolled at the four study hospitals and 98% returned after 4 to 6 weeks to provide a convalescent serum sample and complete the final questionnaire (Fisk *et al.*, 2003). Research plans for 2002–2003 included studies of encephalitis, respiratory pathogens, and hepatitis. Collaborative research projects ultimately improve surveillance, outbreak response, and control of priority communicable diseases. At the same time, they provide training in research strategies and principles that can later be applied to future emerging diseases and be transferred to other regions of the world.

Training and Capacity Development

Capacity development through training is a priority goal of IEIP. Training through IEIP includes opportunities for scientists from Thailand to obtain advanced training in CDC laboratories and for CDC scientists to obtain training and experience in an international setting. In its first year of operation, IEIP/Thailand developed capacity through training in laboratory science, epidemiology, case management and project management. In addition, in response to letter hoaxes with white powders purported to contain anthrax spores in late 2001, IEIP/Thailand conducted an anthrax training course with WHO's South-east Asia Regional Office and the Thai National Institute of Health for 64 participants from 16 countries (Simmerman *et al.*, 2002).

Outbreak Support

Bringing advanced laboratory diagnostic capability to a sophisticated field investigation is one way in which IEIP can further strengthen the already existing Thai capacity for outbreak investigation, especially of unknown etiology. In 2002, IEIP assisted MoPH in investigating outbreaks of gastroenteritis among foreign tourists at a resort hotel in southern Thailand and hand, foot, and mouth syndrome in Bangkok and six other provinces. The potential for IEIP to strengthen the outbreak response to emerging infections was realized during the recent outbreak of Severe Acute Respiratory Syndrome (SARS) in 2003. Epidemiologists from the Collaboration and the Thai MoPH worked together to set up mobile evaluation and training teams with checklists and information packets on infection control practices (Lee *et al.*, submitted). The first SARS patient in Thailand was confined to a negative pressure room with full personal protective equipment for all health care workers (Wongsawat *et al.*, 2004). Some 70 persons had contact with the patient but there were no secondary infections. Specimens from this patient were shipped to CDC and were the source for the first identification of a novel coronavirus as the cause for the worldwide outbreak (Ksiazek *et al.*, 2003). In part because of those efforts, Thailand was better able to control the spread of disease. IEIP/Thailand also served in a variety of roles for a regional SARS outbreak response, sending teams immediately in response to urgent requests from Taiwan, Laos, Hong Kong, Beijing and Singapore (Lee *et al.*, submitted; Twu *et al.*, 2003; Lim *et al.*, 2004). This regional perspective on the SARS outbreak response made possible the assembly of data from four countries on the transmission of SARS aboard aircraft (Olsen *et al.*, 2003b), and a report on differences in infection control practices in several countries (Lee, *et al.*, submitted).

CONCLUSION

For more than two decades, the Thai MoPH and U.S. CDC have worked closely together on public health and epidemiology training, capacity building, surveillance, prevention and clinical research, and public health program development. What started as general epidemiologic training in the 1980s, became focused on the exploding Thai HIV/AIDS epidemic in the 1990s, and has now broadened in the current decade to include diverse emerging infection threats in Thailand and Asia regional activities. The Thai MoPH–U.S. CDC Collaboration can serve as a model of international cooperation and capacity building with manifold benefits to public health in Thailand, Asia, and the world.

REFERENCES

Allen, D.R., Carey, J.W., Jenkins, R.A., Manopaiboon, C., Jenkins, R.A., Uthaivoravit, W., Kilmarx, P. (2003). Sexual health risks among young Thai women: implications for HIV/STD prevention and contraception. *AIDS & Behavior.* 7:9–21.

Amornwichet, P., Teeraratkul,A., Simonds, R.J., Naiwatanakul, T., Chantharojwong, N., Culnane, M., Tappero, J., Kanshana, S. (2002). Preventing mother-to-child HIV transmission-results from the first year of Thailand's national program. *JAMA.* 288:245–248.

Berman, P.W. (1998). Development of bivalent rgp120 vaccines to prevent HIV type 1 infection. *AIDS Res Hum Retroviruses* 14(Suppl 3):S277–S289.

Blanchard, K., Witwatwongwana, P., Supawitkul, S., Chaikummao, S., Friedland, B., Mock, P.A., Tappero, J.W., Kilmarx, P.H. (2004). Acceptability of Carraguard use among heterosexual couples in a six-month clinical trial Thailand. *Microbicides* London, UK, March 28–31, 2004.

Buavirat, A., Page-Shafer, K., van Griensven, G.J.P., Mandel, J.S., Evans, J., Chuaratanaphong, J., Chiamwongpat, S., Sacks, R., Moss, A. (2003). Risk of prevalent HIV infection associated with incarceration among injecting drug users in Bangkok, Thailand: case-control study. *BMJ.* 326:308–312.

Bunnell, R.E., Yanpaisarn,S., Kilmarx, P.H., Rhodes, P.H., Limpakarnjanarat, K., Srismith, R., Mastro, T.D. (1999). St. Louis ME. HIV-1 seroprevalence among childbearing women in northern Thailand: monitoring a rapidly evolving epidemic. *AIDS* 13:509–515.

Butera, S.T., Pisell,T.L., Limpakarnjanarat, K., Young, N.L., Hodge, T.W., Mastro, T.D., Folks, T.M. (2001). Production of a novel viral suppressive activity associated with resistance to infection among female sex workers exposed to human immunodeficiency virus-1. *AIDS Res Hum Retroviruses.* 17:735–744.

Centers for Disease Control and Prevention (CDC). (1998). Administration of zidovudine during late pregnancy and delivery to prevent perinatal HIV transmission—Thailand, 1996–1998. *MMWR.* 48:151–154.

Centers for Disease Control and Prevention (CDC). (2001). Evaluation of a regional pilot program to prevent mother-infant HIV transmission—Thailand, 1998–2000. *MMWR* 50:599–603.

Centers for Disease Control and Prevention (CDC). (2003). CDC Global AIDS Program Asia Regional Meeting. Thailand MoPH–U.S. CDC Collaboration, Nonthaburi, December 11–13.

Chaikummao, S. Uthaiworavit, W., Medtanavyn, T., Manopaiboon, C., Kilmarx, P.H., Braunstein, S., Srivirojana, N., Siraprapasiri, T., Tappero, J.W., McLean, C.A. (2004). Recruitment efforts for a clinical trial of microbicide safety and acceptability among HIV-infected women in northern Thailand. Microbicides 2004. London, UK, March 28–31.

Chaowanachan, T., Chotpitayasunondh, T., Vanprapar, N., Leelawiwat, W., Culnane, M., Teeraratkul, A., Jetsawang, B., Tasaneeyapan, T., Mock, P., Tappero, J., Simonds, R.J. (2003). Resistance mutations following a single-dose intrapartum administration of nevirapine to HIV-infected Thai women and their infants receiving short-course zidovudine. Session 107—Prevention of perinatal transmission; poster board #855. Tenth Conference on Retroviruses and Opportunistic Infections. Boston, MA, USA, February 10–14.

Chotpitayasunondh, T., Vanprapar, N., Simonds, R.J., Chokephaibulkit, K., Waranawat, N., Mock, P.A., Chuachoowong, R., Young, N.L., Mastro, T.D., Shaffer, N. (2001). Safety of Late in utero exposure to zidovudine in infants born to HIV-infected mothers, Bangkok. *Pediatrics* 107: http://www.pediatrics.org/chi/content/full/107/1/e5.

Chuachoowong, R., Shaffer, N., Siriwasin, W., Chaisilwattana, P., Young, N.L., Mock, P.A., Chearskul, S., Waranawat, N., Chaowanachan,T., Karon, J., Simonds, R.J., Mastro, T.D. (2000). Bangkok Collaborative Perinatal HIV Transmission Study Group. Short-course antenatal zidovudine reduces both cervicovaginal human immunodeficiency virus type 1 RNA levels and risk of perinatal transmission. *J Infect Dis.* 181:99–106.

Conner, E.M., Sperling, R.S., Gelber, R., Kiselev, P., Scott, G., O'Sullivan, M.J., VanDyke, R., Bey, M., Shearer, W., Jacobson, R.L., Jimenez, E., O'Neill, E., Bazin, B., Delfraissy, J-F., Culnane, M., Coombs, R., Elkins, M., Moye, J., Stratton, P., Balsley, J., for the Pediatric AIDS Clinical Trials Group Protocol 076 Study Group. (1994). Reduction of maternal–infant transmission of human immunodeficiency virus type 1 with zidovudine treatment. *N Engl J Med* 331:1173–1180.

Dowell, S.F., and Levitt, A.M. (2002). Protecting the Nation's Health in and Era of Globalization: CDC's Global Infectious Disease Strategy. Atlanta, GA: U.S. Department of Health and Human Services, 2002.

Dowell, S.F., Chunsuttiwat, S., Olsen, S.J., Sawanpanyalert, P., Simmerman, J.M., Fisk, T.L., Ungchusak K. (2004). The International Emerging Infections Program, Thailand—An Early Report. In: Emerging Infections 6. Scheld WM, Murray BE, Hughes JM, Editors. Washington D.C. ASM Press. 2004.

Entz, A., Prachuabmoh, V., van Griensven, F., Soskolne, V. (2001). STD history, self treatment and health care behaviors among fishermen in the Gulf of Thailand and the Andaman Sea. *Sex Transm Inf* 77:436–440.

Esparza, J., Osmanov, S., Kallings, L.O., Wigzell, H. (1991). Planning for HIV vaccine trails: The Wolrd Health Organization perspective. *AIDS* 5:S159–S163.

Fisk, T.L., Tangkanakul, W., Sawanpanyalert, P., Limpakarnjanarat, K., Ashford, D., Naigowit, P., Nisaluk, A., Mittenthal, S., Charn, K., Dasch, G., Dowell, S. (2003). Causes of febrile illness in rural Thailand. 43rd Interscience Conference on Antimicrobial Agents and Chemotherapy (ICAAC), Chicago, Illinois.

Francis, D.P., Gregory, T. McElrath, M.J., Belshe, R.B., Gorse, G.J., Migasena, S., Kitayaporn, D., Pitisuttitham, P., Matthews, T., Schwartz, D.H., Berman, P.W. (1998). Advancing AIDSVAX™ to phase 3. Safety, immunogenicity and plans for phase 3. *AIDS Res Hum Retroviruses* 14 (Suppl 3):S325–S331.

Hanenberg, R.S., Rojanapithayakorn, W., Kunasol, P., Sokal, D.C. (1994). Impact of Thailand's HIV-control programme as indicated by the decline of sexually transmitted diseases. *Lancet.* 344:243–245.

Heyward, W.L., Osmanov, S., Esparza, J. (1996). Establishment of WHO-sponsored field sites for HIV vaccine evaluation in developing countries. *Antibiot Chemother* 48:139–144.

Hu, D.J., Vanichseni, S., Mastro, T.D., Raktham, S., Young,N.L., Mock, P.A., Subbarao, S., Parekh, B.S., Srisuwanvilai, L., Sutthent, R., Wasi, C., Heneine, W., Choopanya, K. (2001). Viral load differences in early infection with two HIV-1 subtypes. *AIDS* 15:683–691.

Jenkins, R.A., Manopaiboon, C., Samuel, A.P., Jeeyapunt, S., Carey, J.W., Kilmarx, P.H., Utaivoravit, W., van Griensven, F. (2002). Condom use among vocational school students in Chiang Rai, Thailand. *AIDS Ed Prev* 14:228–245.

Kalish, M.L., Baldwin, A., Raktham, S., Wasi, C., Luo, C.C., Schochetman, G., Mastro, T.D., Young, N., Vanichseni, S., Rübsamen-Waigmann, H., von Briesen, H., Mullins, J.I., Delwart, E., Herring, B., Esparza, J., Heyward, W.L., Osmanov, S. (1995). The evolving molecular epidemiology of HIV-1 envelope subtypes in injecting drug users in Bangkok, Thailand: implications for HIV vaccine trials. *AIDS* 9:851–857.

Kanlayanaphotporn J., Brady, M.A., Chantate, P., Chantra, S., Siasiriwattana, S., Dowell, S.F., Olsen, S.J. (2004). Pneumonia Surveillance in Thailand: Current Practice and Future Needs. SE *Asian J Trop Med & Hyg*. In press.

Kanshana, S., and Simonds, R.J. (2002). National program for preventing mother-child HIV transmission in Thailand-successful implementation and lessons learned. *AIDS* 16:953–959.

Kanshana, S., Thewanda, D., Teeraratkul, A., Limpakarnjanarat, K., Amornwichet, P., Kullerk, N., Akksilp, S., Seresittipitak, V., Mastro, T.D., Simonds, R.J. (2000). Implementing short-course zidovudine to reduce mother–infant HIV transmission in a large regional pilot program in northeastern Thailand. *AIDS* 14:1617–1623.

Kilmarx, P.H., Limpakarnjanarat K. St. Louis, M.E., Supavitkul, S., Korattana, S., Mastro, T.D. (1997). Medication use by female sex workers for treatment and prevention of sexually transmitted diseases, Chiang Rai, Thailand. *Sex Trans Dis* 24: 593–598.

Kilmarx, P.H., Limpakarnjanarat, K., Supawitkul, S., Korattana, S., Young, N.L., Parekh, B.S., Respess, R.A., Mastro, T.D., St Louis, M.E. (1998a). Mucosal disruption due to a widely-distributed commercial vaginal product: Potential to facilitate HIV transmission. *AIDS* 12:767–773.

Kilmarx, P.H., Limpakarnjanarat, K., Mastro, T.D., Saisorn, S., Kaewkungwal, J., Korattana, S., Uthaivoravit, W., Young, N.L., Weniger, B.G., St. Louis, M.E. (1998b). HIV-1 seroconversion in a prospective study of female sex workers in northern Thailand: Continued high incidence among brothel-based women. *AIDS* 12:1889–1898.

Kilmarx, P.H., Palanuvej, T., Limpakarnjanarat, K., Chitvarakorn, A., St. Louis, M.E., Mastro, T.D. (1999). Seroprevalence of HIV among female sex workers in Bangkok: Evidence of ongoing infection risk after the "100% condom program" was implemented. *JAIDS* 21:313–316.

Kilmarx, P.H., Limpakarnjanarat, K., Kaewkungwal, J., Saisorn, S., Uthaivoravit, W., Young, N.L., Mastro, T.D. (2000a). Disease progression and survival with human immunodeficiency virus type 1 (HIV-1) subtype E infection among female sex workers in Thailand. *J Infect Dis* 181:1598–1606.

Kilmarx, P.H., Supawitkul, S., Wankrairoj, M., Uthaivoravit, W., Limpakarnjanarat, K., Saisorn, S., Mastro, T.D. (2000b). Explosive spread and effective control of human immunodeficiency virus in northernmost Thailand: The epidemic in Chiang Rai province, 1988–99. *AIDS* 14:2731–2740.

Kilmarx, P.H., Limpakarnajanarat, K., Saisorn, S., Mock, P.A., Mastro, T.D. (2000c). High mortality among women with human immunodeficiency virus type 1 (HIV-1) infection in Thailand. *Lancet.* 356:770–771.

Kilmarx, P.H., Supawitkul, S.,Yanpaisarn, S., Jones, H., Guest, P., Young, N.L., Srivirojana, N., van de Wijgert, J. (2002). A year-long, randomized, controlled clinical trial of a carrageenan gel as a vaginal microbicide: effect on reproductive tract infection rates. The Fourteenth International AIDS Conference. Barcelona, Spain, July 7–12.

Kilmarx, P.H., Wankrairoj, M., Achalapong, J., Blanchard, K., Chaikummao, S., Connolly, C., Friedland, B., Tappero, J.W. (2004). Safety of Carraguard use by heterosexual men in a six-month clinical trial in Thailand. *Microbicides* London, UK, March 28–31.

Kitayaporn, D., Vanichseni, S., Mastro, T.D., Raktham, S., Vaniyapongs, T., Des Jarlais, D.C., Wasi, C., Young, N.L., Sujarita, S., Heyward, W.L., Esparza, J. (1998). Infection with HIV-1 subtypes B and E in injecting drug users screened for enrollment into a prospective cohort in Bangkok, Thailand. *J Acquir Immune Defic Syndr Hum Retrovirol* 19:289–295.

Ksiazek, T.G., Erdman, D., Goldsmith, C.S., Zaki, S.R., Peret, T., Emery, S., Tong, S., Urbani, C., Comer, J.A., Lim, W., Rollin, P.E., Dowell, S.F., Ling, A.E., Humphrey, C.D., Shieh, W.J., Guarner, J., Paddock, C.D., Rota, P., Fields, B., DeRisi, J., Yang, J.Y., Cox, N., Hughes, J.M., LeDuc, J.W., Bellini, W.J., Anderson, L.J. (2003). SARS Working Group. A novel coronavirus associated with severe acute respiratory syndrome. *N Engl J Med* 348:1953–66.

Lee, N.E., Siriarayapon, P., Tappero, J.W., Chen, K-T., Shuey, D., Limpakarnjanarat, K., Chavavanich, A., Dowell, S.F. and the SARS Mobile Response Team Investigators. Infection control practices for Severe Acute Respiratory Syndrome (SARS) in Lao People's Democratic Republic, Taiwan and

Thailand—Experience from mobile SARS containment teams. (Submitted).

Lertpiriyasuwat, C., Thaprasertsuk, S., Leusaree, T., Sumanapan, S., Chariyalertsak, C., Panputtanakul, S., Simmons, N., Siraprasiri, T., Ellerbrock, T.V., Yachompoo, C., Yuktanon, P., Virapat, P., Supakalin, P., Srithanivaiboonchai, K., Mock, P., Supawitkul, S., Tappero, J.W., Levine, W.C. An assessment of HIV care and treatment in three provinces in Northern Thailand. (Submitted).

Lim, P.L., Kurup, A., Gopalakrishna, G., Chan, K.P., Wong, C.W., Ng, L.C., Se-Thoe, S.Y., Oon, L., Bai, X., Stanton, L.W., Ruan, Y., Miller, L.D., Vega, V.B., James, L., Ooi, P.L., Chew, S.K., Olsen, S.J., Ang, B., Leo, Y.S. (2004). Laboratory-Acquired Severe Acute Respiratory Syndrome (SARS)—Singapore 2003. *N Engl J Med.* In press.

Limpakarnjanarat, K., Wangrairoj, M., Sukaravetsiri, P., Thanprasertsuk, S. (1991). Epidemic of AIDS in Chiangrai-1990. *Thai AIDS Journal [Thai].* 3:61–71.

Limpakarnjanarat, K., Ungchusak, K., Mastro, T.D., Young, N.L., Likhityingvara, C., Sangwonloy, O., Weniger, B.G., Pau, C., Dondero, T.J. (1998). The epidemiologic evolution of HIV-1 subtypes B and E among heterosexuals and injecting drug users in Thailand, 1992–1997. *AIDS* 12:1108–1109.

Limpakarnjanarat, K., Mastro, T.D., Saisorn, S., Uthaivoravit, W., Kaewkungwal, J., Korattana, S., Young, N.L., Morse, S.A., Schmid, S., Weniger, B.G., Nieburg, P. (1999). HIV-1 and other sexually transmitted infections in a cohort of female sex workers in Chiang Rai, Thailand. *Sex Trans Infect* 75:30–35.

Limpakarnjanarat, K., Kilmarx, P.H., Supawitkul, S., Yanpaisarn, S., van de Wijgert, J., Blanchard, K., Mock, P.A., Mastro, T.D. (2002). A year-long, randomized, controlled clinical trial of a carrageenan gel as a vaginal microbicide: Incidence of irritation and genital lesions. The Fourteenth International AIDS Conference. Barcelona, Spain, July 7–12.

MacQueen, K.M., Vanichseni, S., Kitayaporn, D., Lin, L.S., Buavirat, A., Naiwatanakul, T., Raktham, S., Mock, P., Heyward, W.L., Des Jarlais, D.C., Choopanya, K., Mastro, T.D. (1999). Willingness of injecting drug users to participate in an HIV vaccine efficacy trial in Bangkok, Thailand. *J Acquir Immun Defic Syndr* 21:243–251.

Manopaiboon, C., Kilmarx, P.H., Watcharinyanond, K., Achalapong, J., Friedland, B., Chaikummao, S., Guest, P., Tappero, J.W. (2002). A year-long, randomized, controlled clinical trial of a carrageenan gel as a vaginal microbicide: Acceptability of gel and applicator use. Poster Presentation. The Fourteenth International AIDS Conference. Barcelona, Spain, July 7–12.

Manopaiboon, C., Bunnell, R.E., Kilmarx, P.H., Chaikummao, S., Limpakarnjanarat, K., Supawitkul, S., St. Louis, M.E., Mastro, T.D. (2003). Leaving sex work: barriers, facilitating factors and consequences for female sex workers in northern Thailand. *AIDS Care* 15:39–52.

Manopaiboon, C., Kilmarx, P.H., Limpakarnjanarat, K., Jenkins, R.A., Chaikummao, S., Somsak, S., van Griensven, F. (2004a). Sexual Coercion Among Adolescents in Northern Thailand: Prevalence and Associated Factors. *South East Asian J Trop Med & Pub Health* (In Press).

Manopaiboon, C., Kilmarx, P.H., van Griensven, F., Chaikummao, S., Jeeyapant, S., Limpakarnjanarat, K., Uthaiworavit, W. (2004b). High rates of pregnancy among vocational school students: results of audio-assisted computer self-interview survey in Chiang Rai, Thailand. *J Adolescence* (In Press).

Martin, M., Mansakul, W., Tappero, J., Sangkum, U., Vanichseni, S., Prasitiphol, B., Pitisuttithum, P., Orelind, K., van Griensven, F., Choopanya, K. (2003). Care and treatment of HIV-infected persons during an HIV vaccine efficacy trial, Bangkok, Thailand. Session 62—Clinical trials: risk factors; poster abstract no. 502. AIDS Vaccine 2003 Conference, New York, U.S.A., September 18–21.

Mastro, T.D., and Limpakarnjanarat, K. (1995). Condom use in Thailand: How much is it slowing the HIV/AIDS epidemic? *AIDS.* 9:523–525.

Mastro, T.D., Kitayaporn, D., Weniger, B.G., Vanichseni, S., Laosunthorn, V., Uneklabh T., Uneklabh, C., Choopanya, K., Limpakarnjanarat, K. (1994a). Estimating the number of HIV-infected injection drug users in Bangkok: A capture-recapture method. *Am J Public Health* 84:1094–1099.

Mastro, T.D., Satten, G.A., Nopkesorn, T., Sangkharomya, S., Longini, I.M. Jr. (1994b). Probability of female-to-male transmission of HIV-1 in Thailand. *Lancet* 343:204–207.

McLean C., Kantipong, P., Chaowanachan, T., van de Wijgert, J., Medtanavyn, T., Braunstein, S., Whitehead, S.J., Siraprapasiri, T., Tappero, J.W. (2004a). Clinical evaluation of women screened for participation in a Phase I/II clinical trial of candidate microbicide safety and acceptability among HIV-infected women in northern Thailand. Microbicides 2004. London, UK, March 28–31.

McLean C., Kilmarx, P.H., van de Wijgert J., Chaikummao, S., Sternberg, M., Achalapong, J., Bollen, L.J.M., Markowitz, L.E., Tappero, J.W. (2004b). Clinical trial of microbicide safety and acceptability among HIV-infected women in northern Thailand—A cross-over design. *Microbicides 2004.* London, UK, March 28–31.

Mock, P.A., Shaffer, N., Bhadrakom, C., Siriwasin, W., Chotitayasunondh, T., Chearskul, S., Young, N.L., Roongpisuthipong, A., Chinayon, P., Kalish, M.L., Parekh, B., Mastro, T.D., Bangkok Collaborative Perinatal HIV Transmission Study Group.

(1999). Maternal viral load and timing of mother-to-child HIV transmission, Bangkok, Thailand. *AIDS* 13:407–414.

Nelson, K.E., Celetano, D.D., Eiumtrakul, S., Hoover, D., Beyrer, C., Suprasert, S., Kuntolbutra, S., Khambooruang, C. (1996). Changes in sexual behavior and a decline in HIV infection among young men in Thailand. *N Engl J Med* 35:297–303.

Nopkesorn, T., Mastro, T.D., Sangkharomya, S., Sweat, M., Singharaj, P., Limpakarnjanarat, K., Gayle, H., Weniger, B.G. (1993). HIV-1 infection in young men in northern Thailand. *AIDS* 7:1233–1239.

Nopkesorn, T., Mock, P.A., Mastro, T.D., Sangkharomya, S., Sweat, M., Limpakarnjanarat, K., Laosakkitiboran, J., Young, N.L., Morse, S.A., Schmid, D.S., Weniger, B.G. (1998). HIV-1 subtype E incidence and sexually transmitted diseases in a cohort of military conscripts in northern Thailand. *AIDS Hum Retroviriology* 18:372–379.

Olsen, S.J., Premsri, N., Kanlayanaphotporn, J., Burapat, C., Wannachaiwong, Y., Siasiriwattana, S., Ungchusak, K., Sawanpanyalert, P., Chunsuttiwat, S., Dowell, S.F. (2003a). Active, population-based surveillance for chest x-ray confirmed pneumonia in Thailand. 41st Meeting of the Infectious Diseases Society of America, San Diego, CA, 2003.

Olsen, S.J., Chang, H.L., Cheung, T.Y., Tang, A.F., Fisk, T.L., Ooi, S.P., Kuo, H.W., Jiang, D.D., Chen, K.T., Lando, J., Hsu, K.H., Chen, T.J., Dowell, S.F. (2003b). Transmission of the Severe Acute Respiratory Syndrome on Aircraft. *N Engl J Med.* 349:2414–2420.

Ou, C-Y., Takebe, Y., Weniger, B.G., Luo, C-C., Kalish, M., Auwanit, W., Yamazaki, S., Gayle, H.D., Young, N.L., Schochetman, G., Laboratory Investigation Group. (1993). Independent introduction of two major HIV-1 genotypes into distinct high risk populations in Thailand. *Lancet* 341:1171–1174.

Parekh, B.S., Kennedy, M.S., Dobbs, T., Pau, C-P., Byers, R., Green, T., Hu, D.J., Vanichseni, S., Young, N.L., Choopanya, K., Mastro, T.D., McDougal, J.S. (2002). Quantitative detection of increasing HIV-1-antibodies following seroconversion: a simple assay for detecting recent HIV infection and estimating incidence. AIDS Research and Human Retroviruses. 18:295–307.

Paz-Bailey, G., Kilmarx, P.H., Supawitkul, S., Chaowanachan, T., Jeeyapant, S., Sternberg, M., Markowitz, L., Mastro, T.D., van Griensven, F. (2003). Risk factors for sexually transmitted diseases in northern Thai adolescents: an audio-computer–assisted self-interview with noninvasive specimen collection. *Sex Trans Dis* 30:320–326.

Phan, K-O., Callahan, M.E., Vanichseni, S., Hu, D.J., Raktham, S., Young, N.L., Choopanya, K., Mastro, T.D, Subbarao, S. (2000). A comparison of full-length gp120 from incident HIV-1 subtype E and B infections in Bangkok injecting drug users to prototype E and B strains that are components of a candidate vaccine. *AIDS Res Hum Retroviruses* 16:1445–1450.

Phoolcharoen, W., Ungchusak, K., Sittitrai, W., Brown, T. (1998). Thailand: lessons from a strong national response to HIV/AIDS. *AIDS* 12:S123–S135.

Pitisuttithum, P., Chernow, M., Berman, P., Francis, D., Phonrat, B., Suntharasamai, P., Raktham, S., Srisuwanvilai, L., Kitayaporn, D., Kaewkangwal, J., Migasena, S. (2000). Initial report of a Phase I/II trial of AIDSVAX™ B/E rgp120 HIV vaccine. Bangkok, Thailand. Poster Presentation [WePpA1362]. The Thirteenth International AIDS Conference. Durban, South Africa, July 9–14.

Pitaktong, U., Manopaiboon, C., Kilmarx, P., Jeeyapant, S., Jenkins, R., Tappero, J., Uthaivoravit, W., van Griensven, F. (2004). Motorcycle helmet use and related risk behaviors among adolescents and young adults in northern Thailand. *South East Asian J Trop Med & Pub Health.* (in press).

Ramos, A., Hu, D.J., Nguyen, L., Phan, K-O., Vanichseni, S., Promadej, N., Choopanya, K., Callahan, M., Young, N.L., McNicholl, J., Mastro, T.D., Folks, T.M., Subbarao, S. (2002). Intersubtype human immunodeficiency virus type 1 superinfection following seroconversion to primary infection in two injection drug users. *J Virol* 76:7444–7452.

Rojanapithayakorn, W., and Hanenberg, R. (1996). The 100% condom program in Thailand. AIDS 10:1–7.

Sattah, M.V., Supawitkul, S., Dondero, T.J., Kilmarx, P.H., Young, N.L., Mastro, T.D., Chaikummao, S., Manopaiboon, C., van Griensven, F. (2002). Prevalence of and risk factors for methamphetamine use in northern Thai youth: Results of an audio-computer-assisted self-interviewing survey with urine testing. *Addiction* 97:801–808.

Sejvar, J., Tangkanakul, W., Ratanasang, P., Dowell, S., Sangjun, N., Bragg, S., Ashford D., Tappero, J.W. An outbreak of leptospirosis, Thailand—the importance of the laboratory. (Submitted).

Shaffer, N., Chuachoowong, R., Mock, P., Bhadrakom, C., Siriwasin, W., Young, N.L., Chotpitayasunondh, T., Chearskul, S., Roongpisuthipong, A., Chinayon, P., Karon, J., Mastro, T.D., Simonds, R.J., Bangkok Collaborative Perinatal HIV Transmission Study Group. (1999a). Short-course zidovudine for perinatal HIV-1 transmission in Bangkok, Thailand: a randomised controlled trial. *Lancet* 353: 773–780.

Shaffer, N., Roongpisuthipong, A., Siriwasin, W., Chotpitayasunondh, T., Chearskul, S., Young, N.L., Parekh, B., Mock, P.A., Bhadrakom, C., Chinayon, P., Kalish, M.L., Phillips, S.K., Granade, T.C., Subbarao, S., Weniger, B.G., Mastro, T.D., Bangkok

Collaborative Perinatal HIV Transmission Study Group. (1999b). Maternal viral load and perinatal HIV-1 subtype E transmission, Thailand. *J Infect Dis* 179:590–599.

Simmerman, J.M., Kumari, S., Bhatia, R., Dejsirilert, S., Sangsuk, L., Sawanpanyalert, P., Fisk, T., Tima, N., Dowell, S.F. (2002). Strengthening Public Health Response to Anthrax in Southern Asia. International Conference on Infectious Diseases, Kuala Lumpur, Malaysia.

Siriwasin, W., Shaffer, N., Roongpisuthipong, A., Bhiraleus, P., Wasi, C., Singhanati, S., Chotpitayasunondh, T., Chearskul, S., Pokapanichwong, W., Mock, P., Weniger, B.G., Mastro, T.D. Bangkok Collaborative Perinatal HIV Transmission Study Group. (1998). HIV prevalence, risk factors and partner serodiscordance among pregnant women, Bangkok, Thailand. *JAMA*. 280:49–54.

Srismith, R., Yanpaisarn, S., Wangwinyoo, J., Korattana, S., Kilmarx, P.H., Limpakarnjanarat, K. (1998). Trend and risk factors of low birth weight in Chiang Rai Regional Hospital, 1990–June 1997. *Health Sciences [Thai]* 7:32–39.

Srithanaviboonchai, K., Choi, K., van Griensven, F., Hudes, E.S., Visaruratana, S., Mandel, J.S. (2002). HIV-1 in ethnic Shan migrant workers in northern Thailand. *AIDS*. 16:929–931.

Sriwanthana, B., Hodge, T.W., Mastro, T.D., Dezutti, C.S., Bond, K.B., Stephens, H., Kostrikis, L.G., Limpakarnjanarat, K., Young, N.L., Qari, R.B., Lal, S.H., Chandanayingyong, D., McNicholl, J.M. (2001). HIV-specific cytotoxic T lymphocytes, HLA-A11 and chemokine related factors may act synergistically to determine HIV resistance in CCR5 Δ32 negative female sex workers in Chiang Rai, northern Thailand. *AIDS Res Hum Retroviruses* 17:719–734.

Stringer, J.S.A., Stringer, E.M., Phanuphak, P., Jetwana, P., Reinprayoon, D., Funkhouser, E.M., Vermund, S.H. (1999). Prevention of mother-to-child transmission of HIV in Thailand: Physicians' attitudes on zidovudine use, pregnancy transmission, and willingness to provide care. *JAIDS*. 21:217–222.

Subbarao, S., Limpakarnjanarat, K., Mastro, T.D., Bhumisawasdi, J., Warachit, P., Jayavasu, C., Young, N.L., Luo, C-C., Shaffer, N., Kalish, M.L., Schochetman, G. (1998). HIV-1 in Thailand, 1994–1995: Persistence of two subtypes with low genetic diversity. *AIDS Res Hum Retroviruses*. 14:319–327.

Subbarao, S., Vanichseni, S., Hu, D.J., Kitayaporn, D., Choopanya, K., Raktham, S., Young, N.L., Wasi, C., Sutthent, R., Luo, C-C., Ramos, A., Mastro, T.D. (2000). Genetic characterization of HIV-1 subtype E and B strains from a prospective cohort of injecting drug users in Bangkok, Thailand. *AIDS Res Hum Retroviruses* 16:699–707.

Tappero, J.W. (2002). Emerging infectious diseases in Asia: leptospirosis. Symposium 12: TU-S12-3. First Asian Congress of Pediatric Infectious Diseases. Pattaya, Thailand, November 10–13.

Thai Ministry of Public Health (MoPH). (2002, June). HIV serosurveillance in Thailand: result of the 20th round. *Mthly Epidemiol Surveil Rep*.

Tharawan, K., Manopaiboon, C., Ellertson, C., Limpakarnjanarat, K., Korattana, S., Kilmarx, P.H., Blanchard, K., Coggins, C., Mastro, T.D., Elias, C. (2001). Women's willingness to participate in microbicide trials, northern Thailand. *JAIDS*. 28:180–186.

The Thai Working Group on HIV/AIDS Projection. (2001). Projections for HIV/AIDS in Thailand: 2000–2020. Division of AIDS, Department of Communicable Disease Control, Ministry of Public Health, Nonthaburi.

Torugsa, K., Anderson, S., Thongsen, N., Sirisopana, N., Jugsudee, A., Junlananto, P., Nitayaphan, S., Sangkharomya, S., Brown, A.E. (2003). HIV epidemic among young Thai men, 1991–2000. *Emerg Infect Dis*. 9:881–883.

Twu, S.J., Chen, T.J., Chen, C.J., Olsen, S.J., Lee, L.T., Fisk, T., Hsu,K.H., Chang, S.C., Chen, K.T., Chiang, I.H., Wu, Y.C., Wu, J.S., Dowell, S.F. (2003). Control Measures for Severe Acute Respiratory Syndrome (SARS) in Taiwan. *Emerg Infect Dis*. 9:718–720.

van Griensven, F., Supawitkul, S., Kilmarx, P.H., Limpakarnjanarat, K., Young, N.L., Manopaiboon,C., Mock, P.A., Korattana, S., Mastro, T.D. (2001). Rapid assessment of sexual behavior, drug use, human immunodeficiency virus, and sexually transmitted diseases in northern Thai youth using audio-computer-assisted self-interviewing and noninvasive specimen collection. *Pediatrics*. Jul;108(1):E13.

van Griensven, F., Keawkungwal, J., Tappero, J.W., Sangkum, U., Pitisuttithum, P., Vanichseni, S., Suntharasamai, P., Orelind, K., Gee, C., and Choopanya, K. for the Bangkok Vaccine Evaluation Group. (2003a). Lack of increased HIV risk behavior among injecting drug users participating in the AIDSVAX®B/E HIV vaccine trial in Bangkok, Thailand. *AIDS* 2003; 18:295–301.

van Griensven, F., Kilmarx, P.H., Jeeyapant, S., Manopaiboon, C., Korattana, S., Jenkins R.A., Uthaivoravit, W., Limpakarnjanarat, K., Mastro, T.D. (2003b). The prevalence of homosexual and bisexual orientation and related health risks among adolescents in northern Thailand. *Arch Sex Behavior*. 2003; 18:295–301.

Vanichseni, S., Kitayaporn, D., Mastro, T.D., Mock, P.A., Raktham, S., Des Jarlais, D.C., Sujarita, S., et al. (2001). Continued high HIV-1 incidence in a vaccine trial preparatory cohort of injection drug users in Bangkok, Thailand. *AIDS.* 15:397–405.

Vanichseni, S., Tappero, J.W., Pitisuttithum, P., Kitayaporn, D., Mastro, T.D., Vimutisunthorn, E., van Griensven, F., Heyward, W.L., Francis, D.P. and Choopanya K for the Bangkok Vaccine Evaluation Group. (2004). Recruitment, screening and characteristics of injection drug users participating in the AIDSVAX®B/E HIV vaccine trial, Bangkok, Thailand. *AIDS.* 2004; 18:311–316.

VaxGen. (2003). VaxGen announces results of its Phase III HIV vaccine trial in Thailand: vaccine fails to meet endpoints. http://www.vaxgen.com/pressroom/index.html (accessed Nov. 12, 2003).

Wasi, C., Herring, B., Raktham, S., Vanichseni, S., Mastro, T.D., Young, N., Rübsamen-Waigmann, H., von Briesen, H., Kalish, M.L., Luo, C-C., Pau, C-P., Baldwin, A., Mullins, J.I., Delwart, E., Esparza, J., Heyward, W.L., Osmanov, S. (1995). Determination of HIV-1 subtypes in injecting drug users in Bangkok, Thailand, using peptide binding enzyme immunoassay and the heteroduplex mobility assay: Evidence of increasing infection with HIV-1 subtype E. *AIDS* 9: 843–849.

Weniger, B.G., Limpakarnjanarat, K., Ungchusak, K., Thanprasertsuk, S., Choopanya, K., Vanichseni, S., Uneklabh, T., Thongcharoen, P., Wasi, C. (1991). The epidemiology of HIV infection and AIDS in Thailand. *AIDS.* 5(Suppl 2):S71–S85.

Weniger, B.G., and Brown, T. (1996). The March of AIDS through Asia. *N Engl J Med* 335:343–345.

Wongsawat, J., Chaovavanich, A., Uvanich, W., Melgaard, B., Limpakarnjanarat, K., Martin, M.T., Dowell, S.F. (2004). Early Containment of SARS; Experience from Bamrasnaradura Institute, Thailand. International Conference on Emerging Infectious Diseases, Atlanta, GA.

World Bank Thailand Office, Bangkok. (2000). *The World Bank Social Monitor.* Thailand's Response to AIDS: Building on success, confronting the future.

World Health Organization. (2003). *Global Tuberculosis Control: Surveillance, Planning, Financing. WHO Report 2003.* Geneva, Switzerland, WHO/CDS/TB/2003.316.

Xu, F., Kilmarx, P.H., Supawitkul, S., Yanpaisarn, S., Limpakarnjanarat, K., Manopaiboon, C., Korattana, S., Mastro, T.D., St. Louis, M.E. (2000). HIV-1 seroprevalence, risk factors, and preventive behaviors among women in northern Thailand. *JAIDS.* 25:353–359.

Xu, F., Kilmarx, P.H., Supawitkul, S., Manopaiboon, C., Yanpaisarn, S., Limpakarnjanarat, K., Korattana, S., Mock, P.A., Young, N.L., Mastro, T.D. (2002). Incidence of HIV-1 infection and effects of clinic-based counseling on HIV preventive behaviors among married women in northern Thailand. *JAIDS.* 29:284–288.

Yang, C., Li, M., Limpakarnjanarat, K., Young, N.L., Hodge, T., Butera, S.T., McNicholl, J.M., Mastro, T.D., Lal, R.B. (2003). Polymorphisms in the CCR5 coding and noncoding regions among HIV-1-exposed, persistently seronegative female sex workers from Thailand. *AIDS Res Hum Retroviruses.* 19:661–665.

Young, N.L., Shaffer, N., Chaowanachan, T., Chotpitayasunondh, T., Vanprapar, N., Mock, P.A., Waranawat, N., Chokephaibulkit, K., Chuachoowong, R., Wasinrapee, P., Mastro, T.D., Simonds, R.J. (2000). Early diagnosis of HIV-1 infected infants in Thailand using RNA and DNA PCR assays sensitive to non-B subtypes. *J Acquir Immune Defic Syndr.* 24:401–407.

38

Japan's Collaboration with Thailand in the Development of an HIV/AIDS Vaccine

Kazuhiro Matsuo[1], Pilaipan Puthavathana[2], Duanthanorm Promkhatkaew[3], Kruavon Balachandra[3], Kiat Ruxrungtham[4], Takaichi Hamano[1], Ruengpung Sutthent[2], Nopporn Sittisombut[5], Raywadee Butraporn[3], Bussarawan Sriwanthana[3], Jotika Boonlong[3], Yasuyuki Izumi[1], Shudo Yamazaki[1], Naoki Yamamoto[1], Paijit Warachit[6], and Mitsuo Honda[1]

[1]*AIDS Research Center, National Institute of Infectious Diseases, Tokyo, Japan*
[2]*Siriraj Hospital, Mahidol University, Bangkok, Thailand*
[3]*Department of Medical Sciences, Ministry of Public Health, Nonthaburi, Thailand*
[4]*Chulalongkorn University, Bangkok, Thailand*
[5]*Chiang Mai University, Chiang Mai, Thailand*
[6]*Ministry of Public Health, Nonthaburi, Thailand*

INTRODUCTION

On March 26, 1998, the Japan Science and Technology Corporation, Japan's Ministry of Education, Science and Culture, Ministry of Health, Labor and Welfare, and Thailand's Department of Medical Sciences and Ministry of Public Health jointly launched a bilateral collaborative HIV vaccine project with equal partnership. This international collaboration primarily focused on in-country capacity building for HIV vaccine research and development, and preclinical development of the Thailand-Japan AIDS vaccine candidates that targeted the prevalent HIV-1 subtype in Thailand—HIV CRF01_AE—with potential for work with other types of vaccines as well in Thailand.

The Thailand-Japan Cooperative AIDS Vaccine Research Project (T-J CAVRP) initially targeted development of a recombinant Bacillus Calmette-Guérin (rBCG)-based HIV CRF01_AE *env* vaccine (Chujoh *et al.*, 2002). However, a more realistic goal of a preventive HIV vaccine may be to limit HIV infection by producing a cellular immune response to control viral load and prevent disease progression (Nabel, 2001; Schultz and Bradac, 2001). Therefore, the vaccine strategy was changed to apply the experimental results of a prime-boost regimen consisting of rBCG-SIV priming followed by recombinant vaccinia virus DIs (rDIs)-SIV boost. The vaccine candidates in this prime-boost regimen were developed primarily by another project of the Organization for Pharmaceutical Safety and Research (OPSR) from 1996 to 2001 and the Japan Health Sciences Foundation (JHSF) since 1993, and introduced into an HIV CRF01_AE vaccine in 2000.

This chapter provides a brief summary for each of the four main groups of research activities in the T-J CAVRP. They include: (i) molecular epidemiology studies of HIV CRF01_AE infection in Thailand, (ii) Japanese CRF01_AE vaccine constructions designed for Thailand, (iii) HIV/AIDS pathogenesis studies in Thailand, and (iv) safety and efficacy evaluation of the Thailand-Japan candidate vaccines in macaque models.

STRUCTURE OF THE THAILAND-JAPAN COOPERATIVE AIDS VACCINE RESEARCH PROJECT

The structure of the T-J CAVRP is illustrated in Figure 1. The National Institute of Infectious Diseases (NIID) in Tokyo, Japan served as the organizing institution for this project. The Japan Science and Technology Corporation and different ministries of the Japanese government provided the primary funding. Various research groups within NIID that were supported by OPSR and JHSF applied the results of their basic research on SIV, HIV, and vaccine development for the T-J CAVRP and provided the major technical resources and expertise. The T-J CAVRP was also financially supported by the Japanese Foundation for AIDS Prevention (JFAP), and the Sasakawa Memorial Health Foundation, Japan.

MOLECULAR EPIDEMIOLOGY STUDIES OF HIV-1 INFECTION IN THAILAND

In order to develop HIV vaccine candidates that were specifically designed for Thailand, a series of molecular epidemiology studies were conducted to further characterize the HIV infections in different populations in Thailand. Clinical specimens were

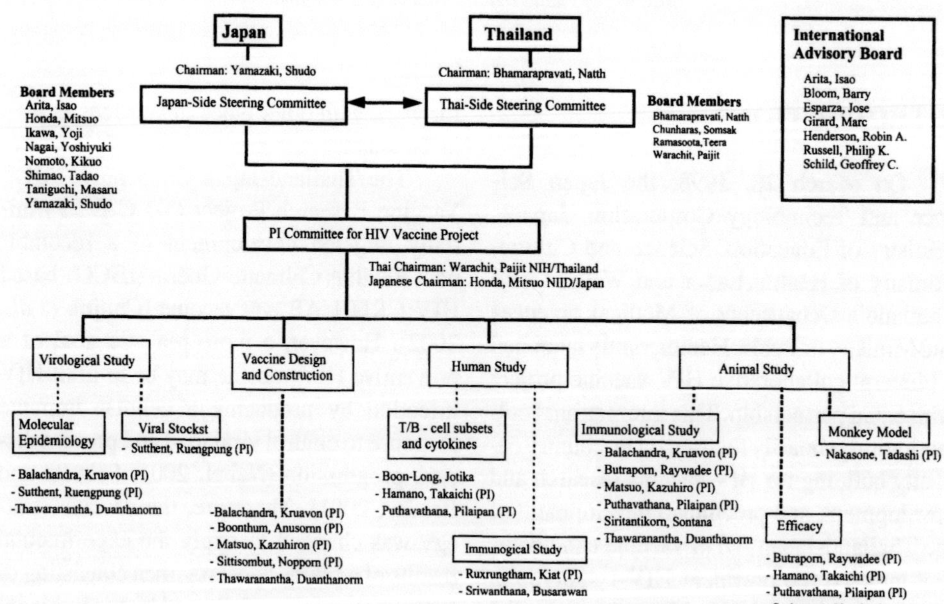

FIGURE 1. Structure of the Thailand–Japan Collaborative AIDS Vaccine Research Project.

collected and virus was isolated from HIV-1-infected individuals throughout Thailand by various local hospitals and institutions, including the Siriraj Hospital, Bamurasnaradura Hospital, Rajavithi Hospital, the Queen Sirikit National Institute of Child Health, and others. Sequence analysis of HIV-1 genes *env*, *env*-V3 (the variable loop 3 of the *env* gene), *pol, gag, tat,* and *nef* were performed. These studies demonstrated that HIV CRF01_AE is spreading all over Thailand. Most of these viruses had the amino acid sequence GPGQ at the tip of V3 of their *env* genes (Naganawa *et al.*, 1997; Sutthent *et al.*, 2001; Balachandra *et al.*, 2002). It was also shown that the HIV CRF01_AE isolates from genital fluid samples appeared to have less genetic divergence than those from the blood samples of the same individuals (Sutthent *et al.*, 2001). Moreover, the sero-reactivity of an HIV-infected individual appeared to decrease when the GPGQ sequence at the tip of V3 was substituted, and its reactivity in AIDS patients was inversely correlated with their tip sequences. The sequence substitutions at the V3 also seemed to correlate with the appearance of HIV-1 mutants that become unrecognizable by the neutralizing antibody in the hosts (Balachandra *et al.*, 2002). HIV CRF01_AE in cerebrospinal fluid was defined to be non-syncytium-inducing even when the patients progressed to the disease state, suggesting that central nervous tissue cells may be one of the reservoirs of CCR5-tropic virus in individuals with advanced disease (Albright *et al.*, 1999). The Gag sequence of HIV CRF01_AE also had a characteristic deletion of six amino acids in the p15 peptide, which was approximately 90% homologous to that of HIV-1 subtype B primary isolates. Another recent study of HIV-1 CRF01_AE showed that the consensus sequence of the *gag* and *env*-V3 region was very close to the consensus sequence of sero-converters in the early epidemic period in Thailand. These data suggest that CRF01_AE might have evolved randomly, and the consensus sequence strategy should be applicable to selecting appropriate vaccine antigens (Hamano *et al.*, 2004).

Various HIV-1 subtypes spread predominantly in different human populations in the world. Our studies, together with studies from many other investigators, showed that the predominant HIV-1 subtype in Thailand, CRF01_AE, has significant genetic differences from the predominant HIV-1 subtype B in Japan (Weniger *et al.*, 1994; Kitsutani *et al.*, 1998; Kusagawa *et al.*, 2002). In order to make the candidate Thailand-Japan HIV-1 vaccines beneficial for the people in Thailand where future vaccine efficacy trials will be conducted, we devoted our efforts to match the origins of HIV-1 antigens in our vaccine designs with the HIV CRF01_AE that is prevalent in Thailand. In our opinion, in the absence of convincing evidence showing that the subtype of HIV-1 antigens in a vaccine design has nothing to do with potential vaccine efficacy, developing the Thailand-Japan HIV-1 vaccines that include CRF01_AE was the only ethically correct way to proceed.

HUMAN GENETICS, CELLULAR IMMUNE RESPONSES, AND HIV VACCINE DESIGN

Numerous factors and cofactors are believed to affect the infectivity of HIV and the disease progression of AIDS, some of which warrant special consideration in the HIV/AIDS vaccine design for Thailand. The design was focused on specifically mapping the HIV viral epitopes that are responsible for eliciting HLA restricted anti-HIV cytotoxic T lymphocytes (CTL) responses in HIV-infected people in Thailand. Using the classical chromium release CTL assay, intracellular cytokine staining, and ELISPOT assays, new CTL epitopes were identified in HIV-infected people in Thailand that differed from the dominant CTL epitopes in HIV-infected people in the United States (Ruxrungtham and Phanuphak, 2001; Ariyoshi *et al.*, 2002; Ananworanich *et al.*, 2003). Significant cross-clade CTL responses were also found in Thai HIV-infected people, characterized by reactions to peptide epitopes derived from different subtypes, including Gag, Env, Pol and Tat antigens (Ruxrungtham *et al.*, 2003). HLA typing in Thai people revealed that the frequencies of HLA-A2, -A11, -B46, -B57 and DQB1*0303 were significantly increased as compared to controls from other populations ($p < 0.05$) (Ward *et al.*, 1995; Vejbaesya *et al.*, 1998; Fukada *et al.*, 2002; Pimtanothai *et al.*, 2003).

These studies provided additional support to the designing principle of the T-J CAVRP that the proposed HIV vaccine candidates for Thailand should be based on CRF01_AE rather than the HIV-1 subtype B that is prevalent in the United States and Japan. By characterizing the immune responses of Thai infected people to CRF01_AE, we also obtained useful information about potential CTL responses in Thailand where the proposed HIV vaccine would be evaluated. Moreover, by collaboratively conducting these state-of-art immunology and molecular virology studies in Thailand with necessary laboratory and clinical capacity and infrastructure building, new vaccine research capability was introduced into Thailand to benefit future vaccine studies in the country.

HIV VACCINE DEVELOPMENT STRATEGY SPECIFICALLY DESIGNED FOR THAILAND

Increasing evidence suggests that cell-mediated immune responses play critical roles in controlling HIV-1 replication and disease progression. It is widely believed that an effective HIV vaccine should elicit both humoral and cell-mediated immunity in order to provide protection against HIV. Our approach to develop an HIV vaccine for Thailand is mainly focused on the induction of protective cellular immune responses to HIV. In the past five years, T-J CAVRP focused primarily on two types of recombinant vectors: *Mycobacterium bovis* BCG, which has been used in Thailand and Japan for many years as the vaccine against tuberculosis (TB), and vaccinia virus DIs (Tagaya *et al.*, 1961; Kitamura *et al.*, 1967), which had been tested in Japan as the vaccine against smallpox. These two vaccines not only have had excellent safety records for human use, they also have a number of features that are highly desirable for practical use in Thailand. BCG is known to induce long-lasting T helper type 1 responses, which are preferable for induction and maintenance of antigen-specific CTL responses. In addition, BCG can be produced at low cost and can be given by oral, nasal, and rectal administration for targeting mucosal delivery of recombinant antigens to induce effective mucosal immunity (Lagranderie *et al.*, 1997).

Based on the reports that previously used vaccinia strains posed potential safety hazards associated with replication of the viruses in immune-compromised individuals, we sought to select and evaluate highly attenuated vaccinia virus (DIs) as another vaccine vector for T-J CAVRP. One desirable feature of this particular virus vector is its lack of replication capacity in mammalian cells.

The strategy of using recombinant BCG-Tokyo 172 and attenuated vaccinia virus DIs as the vectors for the proposed Thailand-Japan HIV vaccine also resulted from considerations beyond the proposed clinical testing. If these vaccine candidates turn out to be effective in future large-scale vaccine efficacy trials in Thailand, they should be made available immediately for the Thai government to use. Based on this principle, the transfers of these two recombinant vaccine technologies from Japan to Thailand, including molecular construction, pilot production, and quality control and assurances, has been a major goal of the T-J CAVRP. Moreover, the organizing committee of the T-J CAVRP has also initiated discussions about the intellectual property issues that will affect the use of these vaccines in Thailand. The intellectual property covering any new vaccine of the prime-boost regimen targeting HIV CRF01_AE Gag, achieved by the Thailand-Japan Collaborative

Project, will be equally shared by both countries.

The experimental part of T-J CAVRP has produced encouraging results. First, it was established that whole HIV-1 *gag* genes from subtype B, CRF01_AE, and SIV could be productively expressed by the recombinant BCG-vector. After optimizing the codon usage for viral antigen expression in mycobacteria, we demonstrated that the expression of the HIV-1 p24 antigen by the recombinant BCG increased more than 20-fold (Kanekiyo *et al.*, 2003). We obtained similar results using recombinant non-replicative vaccinia vector DIs, which productively expressed the Gag proteins from HIV subtype B, CRF01_AE, and SIV (Ishii *et al.*, 2002; Izumi *et al.*, 2003). In small animal experiments, these potential HIV vaccine candidates were shown to effectively induce strong anti-HIV specific CTL responses in mice (Ishii *et al.*, 2002).

The same prime-boost regimen, in which the recombinant BCG bacteria were used first and followed by a boost immunization with the recombinant vaccinia DIs that expressed the same HIV antigens, also showed a strong ability to induce CTL in immunized macaque monkeys (Matsuo *et al.*, 2002). This result was critically important to advance the T-J CAVRP into the preclinical testing stage of the HIV vaccine candidates.

PRECLINICAL EVALUATION OF THE THAILAND-JAPAN AIDS VACCINE CANDIDATES

As part of the research capacity building efforts of the T-J CAVRP, facilities and expertise were collaboratively established in the Sasakawa Memorial Animal Facility Building, Nonthaburi, Thailand, where the HIV vaccines would be evaluated in a hu-PBL-NOD-SCID mouse model. Such a complicated but useful animal model enabled us to demonstrate the capability of our prime-boost regimen to induce the desirable neutralizing antibodies that would be required in order to protect human vaccinees from HIV/AIDS. In one particular experiment, the IgG fraction collected from HIV-1-positive individuals, which has neutralizing activity *in vitro* checked by the MAG1C5 cell line, inhibited virus growth in hu-PBL-NOD-SCID mice more than 100 times compared to negative controls (Ogura *et al.*, 1996; Okamoto *et al.*, 1997; Okamoto *et al.*, 1998).

Next, we established the macaque monkey HIV/AIDS models using chimeric human-simian immunodeficiency virus (SHIV) that was specifically developed for this project. A panel of challenging SHIV stocks was prepared for the proposed vaccine efficacy studies, including the nonpathogenic SHIV-MN, SHIV-HXB, the pathogenic SHIV-C2/1, and its molecular clone, SHIV-C2/1 KS661 (Shinohara *et al.*, 1999; Sakai *et al.*, 2001). In order to demonstrate the potential vaccine efficacy for candidates with the SHIV model, we constructed new recombinant BCG and non-replicative vaccinia DIs that productively express the SIV *gag* protein to match the SIV *gag* gene in the challenging SHIV viruses. Results showed that the recombinant BCG-vectored and recombinant non-replicative vaccinia virus DIs-vectored SIV Gag vaccines induced strong CTL responses in immunized monkeys, respectively. However, the best immune responses in monkeys were obtained when the two vaccines were used in combination as a prime-boost regimen. When the immunized monkeys were challenged with the pathogenic SHIV-C2/1, the vaccination provided full protection for the monkey hosts from developing simian AIDS (Matsuo *et al.*, 2002). The CD4 T-cell decline in the vaccinated monkeys after the lethal challenge of SHIV, which is the hallmark of simian AIDS as well as AIDS in humans, was prevented. The plasma virus load in the vaccinated monkeys after the SHIV challenge also showed approximately 100- to 1000-fold reductions in comparison with unvaccinated monkeys (Matsuo *et al.*, 2002). Moreover, it was demonstrated that oral administration of the recombinant

BCG-based vaccines with two doses of 80 mg in guinea pigs was sufficient to induce the desired virus-specific cell-mediated immune responses, thus presenting the possibility of using the vaccine candidates orally in humans (Kawahara *et al.*, 2002).

These studies also demonstrated that the proposed prime-boost regimen was safe to use in the non-human primate hosts: no detectable adverse effects resulted from vaccination in any of the immunized monkeys. One of the concerns regarding the use of recombinant BCG in Thailand was possible side effects or reduced efficiency in people who were previously immunized with BCG. A series of animal experiments were conducted to address these issues. We showed that prior immunization with BCG did not affect the induction of HIV p24 antigen-specific cellular immunity in monkeys that were immunized with the recombinant BCG/DIs-based HIV vaccines. However, previous exposure to BCG vaccination in monkeys did seem to reduce Gag-specific cellular immune responses in the immunized monkeys by about 50%.

We believe that the recombinant BCG-based HIV vaccines would be safe to use in Thailand. To date, more than two billion people worldwide have been vaccinated with BCG against TB with a proven safety record. With regard to the use of the recombinant vaccinia virus-based HIV vaccines, we believe that the non-replicative DIs strain presents a safer alternative to the MVA (modified vaccinia Ankara) that is being widely used in HIV-1 vaccine development elsewhere. Like the MVA-based HIV-1 vaccines, the recombinant non-replicative vaccinia virus DIs is capable of efficiently expressing the HIV-1 antigens in mammalian host cells. However, the DIs-based viruses lack the replicative ability in these cells, thus producing no infectious viruses. In contrast, MVA is able to replicate in mammalian cells like BHK and CV-1 following infection (Carroll and Moss, 1997). Although the deleted region in DIs is larger than that of MVA, the structural basis for this distinction between the DIs virus and MVA is not yet known. It was shown that the DIs virus as a smallpox vaccine failed to induce a skin reaction in inoculated infants and permitted revaccination by another smallpox vaccine strain without complications, demonstrating a safety advantage over the use of MVA as a recombinant vaccinia vector (Fujii and Minamitani, 1968).

In order to assure the safety of the T-J CAVRP candidate vaccines, the pilot products of these vaccines are evaluated in baby monkeys, as well as in adult monkeys. Studies showed that as much as 800 mg of the recombinant BCG-based HIV vaccines by oral administration, or repeated subcutaneous injections of 50 mg of the vaccine, did not cause any detectable adverse effects when compared directly with the standard BCG vaccine (Sukpanichnant *et al.*, Department of Pathology, Faculty of Medicine, Siriraj Hospital, Mahidol University, December 2003, unpublished data). Similar safety experiments are underway to evaluate the recombinant non-replicative vaccinia DIs-based HIV vaccines.

FUTURE PLANS

The above-mentioned first generation candidate vaccine incorporates the *gag* gene only, and does not induce sterile immunity because the immunized monkeys do not suppress primary viremia completely after the SHIV challenge. The *gag* gene product cannot induce neutralizing antibodies that block virus entry. Therefore, introduction of the *env* gene to current constructs may be important to enable the vaccines to prevent both HIV-1 infection and disease progression. Furthermore, the construct of a single *gag* gene would have a restricted range of CTL responder population in which the HLA type is involved. To address these issues, future research may be conducted to improve the capacity and expression level of incorporated HIV-1 *env* genes in rBCG and rDIs.

To improve immunogenicity of the vaccine constructs, antigen expression in BCG or in DIs should be optimized. Regarding rBCG, we have already found that the codon-optimized *gag* p24 gene is expressed at a drastically higher level than the native *gag*; this strategy can be applied to other rBCG constructs to make them more immunogenic (Kanekiyo *et al.*, unpublished data). Such investigations are continuing now through collaboration between Japan and Thailand. These approaches are of particular importance to obtain an HIV vaccine that is highly effective.

Acknowledgements. We would like to thank Drs. Bonnie Mathieson, Jorge Flores and Rebecca Sheets, Division of AIDS, National Institute of Allergy and Infectious Diseases (NIAID), National Institutes of Health (NIH), Bethesda, MD, USA; Dr. Bernard Moss, Laboratory of Viral Diseases, NIAID, for their helpful discussions; and Drs. Hidemi Takahashi, and Yohko Nakagawa, Department of Microbiology and Immunology, Nippon Medical School, Tokyo, for their helpful discussions. Japan Science and Technology Corporation, thc Organization of Pharmaceutical Safety and Research, the "Panel on AIDS" of the US-Japan Cooperative Medical Science Program, Japan Health Sciences Foundation, and the Japanese Ministry of Health, Labor and Welfare also supported this work. This study was also supported by the AIDS vaccine project in conjunction with Japan Science and Technology Corporation.

REFERENCES

Albright, A.V., Shieh, J.T., Itoh, T., Lee, B., Pleasure, D., O'Connor, M.J., Doms, R.W., and Gonzalez-Scarano, F. (1999). Microglia express CCR5, CXCR4, and CCR3, but of these, CCR5 is the principal coreceptor for human immunodeficiency virus type 1 dementia isolates. *J Virol* 73:205–213.

Ananworanich, J., Nuesch, R., Teeratakulpisarn, S., Srasuebkul, P., Chuenyam, T., Siangphoe, U., Ungsedhaphand, C., Phanuphak, P., and Ruxrungtham, K. (2003). In vivo cell-mediated immunity in subjects with undetectable viral load on protease inhibitor-based versus non-protease inhibitor-based highly active antiretroviral therapy. *J Acquir Immun Defic Syndr* 32:570–572.

Ariyoshi, K., Promadej, N., Ruxrungtham, K., and Sutthent, R. (2002). Toward improved evaluation of cytotoxic T-lymphocyte (CTL)-inducing HIV vaccines in Thailand. *AIDS Res. Hum. Retroviruses* 18:737–739.

Balachandra, K., Matsuo, K., Sutthent, R., Hoisanka, N., Boonsarthorn, N., Sawanpanyalert, P., Warachit, P., Yamazaki, S., and Honda, M. (2002). Characteristic of HIV-1 in V3 loop region based on seroreactivity and amino acid sequences in Thailand. *Asian Pac J Allergy Immunol* 20: 93–98.

Carroll, M.W. and Moss, B. (1997). Host range and cytopathogenicity of the highly attenuated MVA strain of vaccinia virus: propagation and generation of recombinant viruses in a nonhuman mammalian cell line. *Virology* 238:198–211.

Chujoh, Y., Matsuo, K., Yoshizaki, H., Nakasatomi, T., Someya, K., Okamoto, Y., Naganawa, S., Haga, S., Yoshikura, H., Yamazaki, A., Yamazaki, S., and Honda, M. (2002). Cross-clade neutralizing antibody production against human immunodeficiency virus type 1 clade E and B′ strains by recombinant *Mycobacterium bovis* BCG-based candidate vaccine. *Vaccine* 20: 797–804.

Fujii, R., and Minamitani, M. (1968). Virus infections with exanthema. *Saishin Igaku* 23:1146–1155. In Japanese.

Fukada, K., Tomiyama, H., Wasi, C., Matsuda, T., Kusagawa, S., Sato, H., Oka, S., Takebe, Y., and Takiguchi, M. (2002). Cytotoxic T-cell recognition of HIV-1 cross-clade and clade-specific epitopes in HIV-1-infected Thai and Japanese patients. *AIDS* 16:701–711.

Hamano, T., Sawanpanyalert, P., Yanai, H., Piyaworawong, S., Hara, T., Sapsutthipas, S., Phromjai, J., Yamazaki, S., Yamamoto, N., Warachit, P., Honda, M., and Matsuo, K. (2004). Determination of HIV-1 CRF01_AE gag p17 and env-V3 consensus sequences for HIV/AIDS vaccine design. *AIDS Res Hum Retroviruses* (in press)

Ishii, K., Ueda, Y., Matsuo, K., Matsuura, Y., Kitamura, T., Kato, K., Izumi, Y., Someya, K., Ohsu, T., Honda, M., and Miyamura, T. (2002). Structural analysis and application of vaccinia virus DIs strain as a completely replication-deficient viral vector for HIV vaccine. *Virology* 302:433–444.

Izumi, Y., Ami, Y., Matsuo, K., Someya, K., Sata, T., Yamamoto, N., and Honda, M. (2003). Intravenous inoculation of replication-deficient recombinant vaccinia virus DIs expressing simian immunodeficiency virus gag controls highly pathogenic simian-human immunodeficiency virus in monkeys. *J Virol* 77:13248–13256.

Kanekiyo, M., Matsuo, K., Hamatake, M., Yamamoto, N., Honda, M. (2003). Optimization of codon usage confers vigorous expression in recombinant *Mycobacterium bovis* BCG vaccine. Proceedings of the International Symposium on Research and Development of Recombinant BCG and Vaccinia Virus-based HIV Vaccine. Tokyo, Japan; 21–24.

Kawahara, M., Hashimoto, A., Toida, I., and Honda, M. (2002). Oral recombinant *Mycobacterium bovis* bacillus Calmette-Guerin expressing HIV-1 antigens as a freeze-dried vaccine induces long-term, HIV-specific mucosal and systemic immunity. *Clin Immunol* 105:326–331.

Kitamura, T., Kitamura, Y., and Tagaya, I. (1967). Immunogenicity of an attenuated strain of vaccinia virus on rabbits and monkeys. *Nature* 215:1187–1188.

Kitsutani, P. T., Naganawa, S., Shiino, T., Matsuda, M., Honda, M., Yamada, K., Taki, M., and Sugiura, W. (1998). HIV type 1 subtypes of nonhemophiliac patients in Japan. *AIDS Res Hum Retroviruses* 14:1099–1103.

Kusagawa, S., Sato, H., Tomita, Y., Tatsumi, M., Kato, K., Motomura, K., Yang, R., and Takebe, Y. (2002). Isolation and characterization of replication-competent molecular DNA clones of HIV type 1 CRF01_AE with different coreceptor usages. *AIDS Res Hum Retroviruses* 18:115–122.

Lagranderie, M., Balazuc, A.M., Gicquel, B., and Gheorghiu, M. (1997). Oral immunization with recombinant *Mycobacterium bovis* BCG simian immunodeficiency virus nef induces local and systemic cytotoxic T-lymphocyte responses in mice. *J Virol* 71: 2303–2309.

Matsuo, K., Nakasone, T., Izumi, Y., Ami, Y., Ohsu, T., Hamano, T., Yamamoto, N., Yamazaki, S., and Honda, M. (2002). SIV Gag-expressing recombinant BCG-prime and recombinant vaccinia virus DIs strain-boost regimen evokes protective immune response in monkey. XIV International AIDS Conference; July 2002. Barcelona, Spain. TuOrA1222.

Nabel, G.J. (2001). Challenges and opportunities for development of an AIDS vaccine. *Nature* 410:1002–1007.

Naganawa, S., Na Ayuttaya, P.I., Duangchanda, S., Auwanit, W., Warachit, P., Miyamura, K., Yamazaki, S., and Honda, M. (1997). A characteristic change of consensus core motif in the V3 region of HIV type 1 clade B, but not in clade E, in Thailand. *AIDS Res Hum Retroviruses* 13:271–273.

Ogura, A., Noguchi, Y., Yamamoto, Y., Shibata, S., Asano, T., Okamoto, Y., and Honda, M. (1996). Localization of HIV-1 in human thymic implant in SCID-hu mice after intravenous inoculation. *Int J Exp Pathol* 77:201–206.

Okamoto, Y., Ogura, A., Shibata, S., Amagai, T., Katsura, Y., Asano, T., and Honda, M. (1997). Simple i.v. inoculation of HIV-1 to Thy/Liv SCID-hu mice induce reproducible HIV infection with narrowing of medulla in human thymic implant. *J Vet Med Sci.* 59:259–263.

Okamoto, Y., Eda, Y., Ogura, A., Shibata, S., Amagai, T., Katsura, Y., Asano, T., Kimachi, K., Makizumi, K., and Honda, M. (1998). In SCID-hu mice, passive transfer of a humanized antibody prevents infection and atrophic change of medulla in human thymic implant due to intravenous inoculation of primary HIV-1 isolate. *J Immunol* 160:69–76.

Pimtanothai, N., Kangwanshiratada, O., and Charoenwongse, P. (2003). Serological analysis of human leukocyte antigens-A and -B antigens in Thai patients with nasopharyngeal carcinoma. *J Med Assoc Thai* 86 Suppl 2:S237–S241.

Ruxrungtham, K., and Phanuphak, P. (2001). Update on HIV/AIDS in Thailand. *J Med Assoc Thai* 84 Suppl 1:S1–S17.

Ruxrungtham, K., Buranapraditkul, S., Kosonsiriluk, S., Kerdsanti, S., Hansasutha, P., Sirivichaykul, S., Rowland-Jones, S., and Phanuphak, P. (2003). HIV-1 specific cytotoxic T-lymphocytes (CTLs) study. Proceedings of the International Symposium on Research and Development of Recombinant BCG and Vaccinia Virus-based HIV Vaccine. Tokyo, Japan; 43–52.

Sakai, K., Shinohara, K., Takahashi, E., Izumi, Y., Ami, Y., Sasaki, Y., Nakasone, T., and Honda, M. (2001). Molecular cloning of a pathogenic simian-human immunodeficiency virus for HIV/AIDS monkey model. Sixth International Congress on AIDS in Asia and the Pacific; 2001 Oct 5–10. Melbourne, Australia. Abstract p. 84. *Proc Int Cong AIDS Asia Pacific* 6:84.

Schultz, A.M., and Bradac, J.A. (2001). The HIV vaccine pipeline, from preclinical to phase III. *AIDS* 15: 8147–8158.

Shinohara, K., Sakai, K., Ando, S., Ami, Y., Yoshino, N., Takahashi, E., Someya, K., Suzaki, Y., Nakasone, T., Sasaki, Y., Kaizu, M., Lu, Y., and Honda, M. (1999). A highly pathogenic simian/human immunodeficiency virus with genetic changes in cynomolgus monkey. *J Gen Virol* 80:1231–1240.

Sutthent, R., Sumrangsurp, K., Wirachsilp, P., Chaisilwattana, P., Roongpisuthipong, A., Chaiyakul, P., Nooma, P, Honda, M., and Warachit, P. (2001). Diversity of HIV-1 subtype E in semen and cervicovaginal secretion. *J Hum Virol* 4:260–268.

Tagaya, I., Kitamura, T., and Sano, Y. (1961). A new mutant of dermovaccinia virus. *Nature* 192: 381–382.

Vejbaesya, S., Eiermann, T.H., Suthipinititharm, P., Bancha, C., Stephens, H.A., Luangtrakool, K., and Chandanayingyong, D. (1998). Serological and molecular analysis of HLA class I and II alleles in Thai patients with psoriasis vulgaris. *Tissue Antigens* 52:389–392.

Ward, F.E., Tuan, S., and Haynes, B.F. (1995). Analysis of HLA Frequencies in Population Cohorts for Design of HLA-Based HIV Vaccines. In: Korber, B., Brander, C., Walker, B.D., Koup, R., Moore, J.P., Haynes, B.F., and Myers, G. (eds.), *HIV Molecular Immunology Database 1995*, Theoretical Biology and Biophysics Group, Los Alamos National Laboratory, Los Alamos, NM. pp. IV-10–16.

Weniger, B.G., Takebe, Y., Ou, C.Y., and Yamazaki, S. (1994). The molecular epidemiology of HIV in Asia. *AIDS* 8 Suppl 2:S13–S28.

39

Developing Countries

A Force in the Global Fight against HIV/AIDS

Xiaojun Lin[1], Bryan Roberts[2], and Yichen Lu[3,4]

[1]*Eastern Home Pharmaceuticals, Chengdu, China*
[2]*Parallel Solutions, Inc., Cambridge, Massachusetts, USA*
[3]*The Harvard AIDS Institute, Boston, Massachusetts, USA*
[4]*Nankai University Vaccine Laboratory, Tianjin, China*

INTRODUCTION

Infectious diseases at the start of the 21st century are responsible for 13 million deaths annually, of which two thirds are children, mainly in the developing world. In 2002, AIDS, malaria, and tuberculosis were responsible for six million deaths, and the immune deficiency caused by HIV is accelerating the spread and pathogenicity of both malaria and tuberculosis (TB). The global estimates of HIV infections exceed 42 million people, and this pandemic is most advanced in sub-Saharan Africa. The average rate of HIV infection in southern African countries has reached at least 10% of the general population. In Botswana, the average life span has been reduced from 77 to 29 years because of HIV/AIDS (Stanecki and Walker, 2002). A UNAIDS report estimated that the chance a 15-year-old boy in Botswana would die of AIDS before he reached adulthood (30 years) was about 90% (Piot and Bartos, 2002). The African epidemic demonstrates the social and economic consequences incurred by the directional transmission of this lethal infection by sex and blood contact targeting the major workforce and child-rearing age segment of society. The social impact of the efficient extinction of the sexually active segment of society is the generation of 11 million orphans by 2002 and an expectation that this number will exceed 20 million by 2010. Moreover, the directed infection of the major workforce has profound economic consequences, together with the associated spiraling burden of their health care. Vaccine development for AIDS is a low priority for the major vaccine manufacturers in developed countries and currently early stage clinical evaluation of vaccine candidates is spearheaded by publicly funded non profit groups. This picture of HIV/AIDS in Africa will be repeated in other developing countries unless a coordinated, proactive international effort is organized.

In 1996, Weniger and Brown proposed that evidence suggested that Asia would become the new battle ground in the war between humanity and AIDS (Weniger and Brown, 1996). This prediction was accurate and currently Asia faces a crisis similar to that confronted by Sub Saharan Africa in the early 1990's. In 1997, China reported less than one thousand cases of HIV. In response the "Chinese National Medium- and Long-Term Strategic Plan for HIV/AIDS prevention and control (1998–2010)", was to limit the HIV/AIDS cases to 1 million by the year of 2010. However, by the end of 2003, the Chinese Ministry of Health (MOH) estimated that HIV-1 might have already infected 840,000 people in China (UNAIDS 2003). China, India and Indonesia comprise more than half the world's population and have considerable financial resources, expertise in high technology, preventative medicine and public health. To control this economic and socially devastating disease, it remains to be seen whether they will entrust the development of an effective vaccine to poorly motivated manufactures in the developed world or will they devote national resources and expertise to develop an HIV vaccine on their own timetable. It is difficult to imagine that countries that have thriving high technology industries, nuclear and space programs and undertake major hydroelectric programs cannot coordinate with international collaborators the development of an effective HIV vaccine.

This chapter investigates the requirements for developing countries to take a leadership role in solving major infectious disease problems, such as those posed by AIDS. This will be attempted by evaluating:

1. the capacity to develop and manufacture safe and effective vaccines;
2. the infrastructure required to evaluate and distribute vaccines; and
3. the long-term commitment of government and public health officials to the production of high quality vaccines.

This evaluation will focus on China since it is a developing country with an emerging AIDS epidemic and has the capacity to attempt the development of an AIDS vaccine.

The Capacity to Develop and Manufacture Safe and Effective Vaccines

Vaccine production was initiated in China in 1919 and significantly expanded in the 1950's by the establishment of six major vaccine development and production facilities throughout the country, which were directly affiliated with the MOH in Beijing. These new institutes developed and produced a number of vaccines, including the large-scale production of Tiantan strain of vaccinia virus as the vaccine against smallpox, large-scale production of BCG as the vaccine against TB, live attenuated *Brucella* vaccine, live attenuated anthrax vaccine, and live attenuated yellow fever vaccine. In 1950, the Chinese Government published "the temporary measures for vaccination." The most notable success of these measures was the smallpox vaccination program. Within a decade, public health workers in the newly established epidemics preventive stations throughout the country were able to implement an effective nationwide vaccination drive using the Tiantan vaccinia virus as the vaccine. Together with the establishment of the nationwide smallpox case reporting and control network during the same ten year period, the last case of smallpox infection in China was reported in 1959 and was claimed to be eradicated in the country after an examination by the World Health Organization (WHO) (Wang *et al.*, 2000).

Another achievement of the Chinese vaccine production and national immunization programs in the 1950s was the use of BCG as the vaccine against TB in China. In 1950, the Ministry of Health decided to provide the BCG vaccine in Chinese cities free of charge, which in fact became the prologue of the national immunization program that was expanded in the following five decades. Although many vaccine experts and public health officials consider that the real

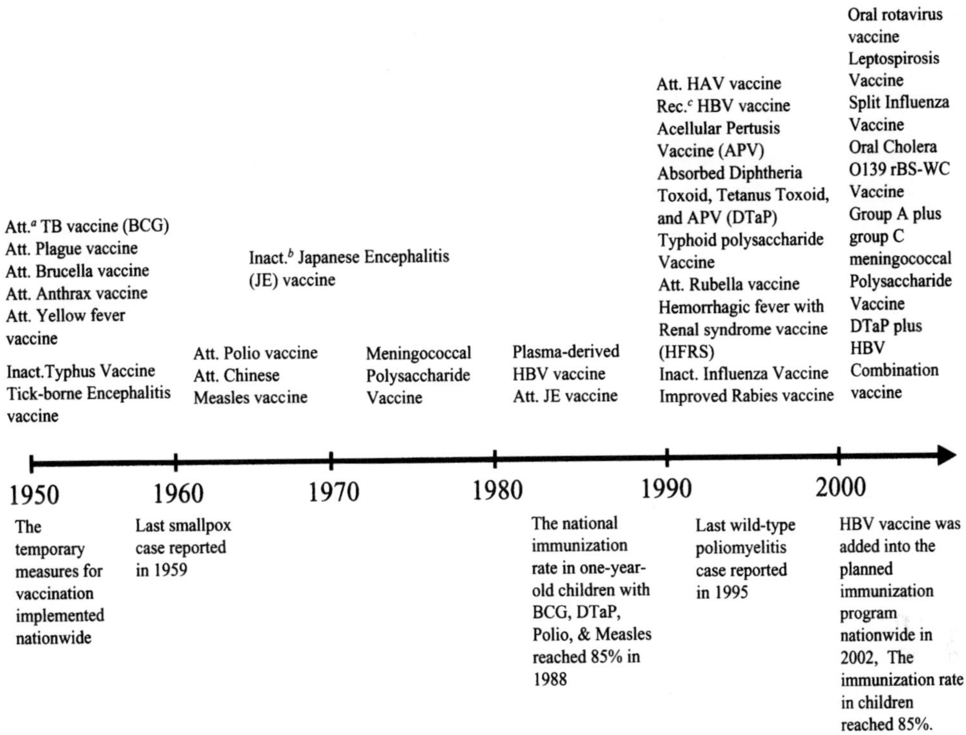

FIGURE 1. Vaccine production in developing countries: a case study (adapted from Lu *et al.*, 1995).
[a]live attenuated [b]inactivated [c]recombinant protein-based

effectiveness of BCG vaccination against TB is still scientifically questionable, the effort of the government trying to protect its people through a 50 year long national program should be commended.

In the 1960s, as shown in Figure 1, two notable new vaccine products were the vaccines against poliomyelitis and measles. The Beijing Institute for Biological Products introduced into China from the US the oral trivalent poliomyelitis vaccine (the Sabin strain). Within a short period of time, the Beijing Institute for Biological Products and the Kunming Biological Research Institute were able to achieve 1 hundred million doses per year, respectively. Like the successful eradication of smallpox in China through the nationwide vaccination program in the previous decade, the last case of poliomyelitis in China that was caused by wild strain virus infection was reported in 1995, and it has not been found since then (Wang *et al.*, 2000).

In 1965, the live attenuated measles vaccine of Chinese origin was developed (Lu *et al.*, 1995). The new live attenuated Chinese measles vaccine was soon proved to be safe and effective and used widely in the nationwide vaccination program. By 1987, the vaccination rate of this vaccine for children under age one reached about 77% nationwide, and the incidence rate for measles in the general population decreased 92% in comparison with that in 1980. By 2001, the Chinese vaccine industry was able to meet the need of vaccinating nearly 98% of all Chinese children under age five (MOH, 2002).

Since the early 1950s, China has managed to produce and supply a massive amount of childhood vaccines in a nationwide immunization program through its domestic vaccine manufacturers that are owned and operated by the government. As the Chinese vaccine industry has undertaken a self-sufficient proactive vaccination program that covers a vastly populous nation of 1.3 billion people, it is conceivable that the industry may also enable China to play a significant role in the fight against AIDS. As shown in Figure 1, the Chinese vaccine industry entered into a rapid-growth period in the 1980s as a result of the country's economic reform. The production of the combination vaccine for prevention of diphtheria, tetanus, and pertussis (DTP) finally reached a massive scale that enabled the government to launch an initiative to immunize all newborns with four vaccines, including BCG, polio, measles, and DTP. The initiative later became known as the National Planned Vaccines in China. The immunization coverage rate of the planned vaccines in Chinese children under age one was 85% in 1988 for the first time. Two years later, the rate reached 90%. In 2001, the rate of the planned vaccination in children under age one was 97% nationwide (MOH, 2002). The annual production output by the Chinese vaccine industry is at average 110 million doses for each one of these four vaccines, respectively.

The Infrastructure Required to Evaluate and Distribute Vaccines

By 1997, there were 280,558 public health professionals working in 3619 Centers for Disease Control nationwide, plus 1893 special disease prevention and treatment centers in China (Wang *et al.*, 2000). These centers and their public health workers are mainly responsible for disease control and monitoring, sanitary inspection, health education and promotion, scientific research and personnel training, and annual immunization drives that inoculate millions of infants and children nationwide. It is worth noting that unlike many countries in the world, the vaccination program in China, including the vaccine production and planning, product distribution and pricing, and vaccine inoculation, has always been the responsibility of the government. Every year, the vaccine inoculation is conducted at the state-assigned hospitals and epidemic prevention centers, and various vaccines are purchased by local governmental health bureaus and distributed by their public health workers.

This huge and complex public health network in China has played an essential role in various national and local planned vaccination programs. After receiving vaccines from the state-owned vaccine manufacturers in their region (each of the six state-owned Institutes for Biological Products is assigned a number of neighboring provinces), the provincial CDC (Center for Disease Control, formerly known as the Disease Prevention Station) is responsible for proper storage of the vaccines and their distribution to the county and village level CDC. Each CDC, regardless of its level, must have designated public health workers responsible for individual tasks such as record-keeping, proper cold-chain storage and transportation, and safekeeping of the biological potencies of each vaccine according to the manufacturer's specific requirement.

The threat of Japanese Encephalitis (JE) virus infections in China lead to the development and field evaluation of an effective vaccine, SA14-14-2, which was used to stem the national epidemics of JE infections (Tsai *et al.*, 1999, Zhou *et al.*, 2001). The successful development of JE vaccine in China demonstrated a number of interesting features of the Chinese public health system and its vaccine industry. Firstly, it showed that when the country was threatened with a serious epidemic, it was capable of effectively mobilizing sufficient national resources to successfully combat the disease. Secondly, it showed that China has the scientific capability, the material resource, and the public health infrastructure to conduct large-scale vaccine efficacy trials with hundreds of thousands of participants.

Like in many other developing countries, the Chinese pubic health system lacks the ability and resources for the early detection and prevention of the epidemics that spread by chronic or "silent" infections. A devastating example is the wide spread of Hepatitis B infection in the country in the past three to four decades. According to government statistics, as many as 58.1% of Chinese are infected with the Hepatitis B virus and 10.8% of Chinese are "carriers", who are at high risk of developing viral hepatitis disease in their lifetime (Lu *et al.*, 1995). An effective HBV vaccine (plasma-derived) was licensed in the US in 1982, and followed by the recombinant protein-based HBV vaccine (Mahoney and Kane, 1999). In 2002, the same recombinant protein-based HBV was listed as one of the planned vaccines for children nationwide in China, and the long-anticipated object of immunizing 90% of neonates in cities and towns was finally reached. In metropolitan areas such as Beijing and Shanghai, the HBV rate of infection in children under 5 years old for the first time has dipped below 1%. The development of the recombinant HBV vaccine in China was a slow process, yet it demonstrated the ability to transfer new technologies into the national vaccination program. It is anticipated that this and similar experiences will facilitate the transfer of new technologies that will be associated with the development of HIV vaccines.

The Long-Term Commitment of Government and Public Health Officials to the Production of High Quality Vaccines

Another example of infrastructure building in the Chinese public health system is the establishment of a functional system that regulates vaccines and other biological products. In the early 1960s, the government established the National Institute for the Control of Pharmaceutical and Biological Products (NICPBP) in Beijing in order to control the quality of pharmaceutical and biological products nationwide. In 1989, the Chinese Committee for the Standardization of Biological Products (CCSBP) was established, which has five branches with respective responsibility for virus products, bacterial products, blood products, bioengineering products, and diagnostic reagents. The main function of this new government agency was to establish a new set of regulatory standards known as *The Standards for Chinese Biological Products*, for all of biological products that were made or used in China. With regard to the vaccine industry, these standards are applied to the development of new products and the improvement of manufacturing technologies and quality control procedures. CCSBP amends *The Standards for Chinese Biological Products* every five years. For example, the latest edition of *The Standards for Chinese Biological Products* was published on October 1, 2000 and is still in effect.

In 1998, the State Drug Administration (SDA) was established, which published *The Regulations for Examination and Approval of New Biological Products* in order to differentiate biological products from chemical drugs and traditional Chinese medicines. In these regulations, biological products are defined as the products made from microorganisms (yeast, bacteria, viruses, etc.), cells, and various animal and human tissues and fluids. These include all vaccine products, blood-derived products, medicines, and diagnostic reagents. For example, the number of biological products listed in the year 2000 edition of *The Standards for Chinese Biological Products* was 137, which was divided into 36 preventive products, 39 therapeutic products, and 62 diagnostic products. However, this publication also listed ten preventive or therapeutic products that still need to be inspected due to unsatisfactory quality control standards and determination methods. If further improvement of these products by the manufacturers does not meet the deadline set up by the SDA, they will be deleted from the list in the next edition.

In July 1993, MOH issued The Management Rules of Biological Products, which stated that all of biological products were subject to governmental regulation and management, and principally listed the requirements for the ordering, supplying, cold-chain storage and abnormal reaction accident handling of biological products, especially preventive vaccines. In the following year, the ministry further issued The Manufacture and Supply Management Rules of Preventive Biological Products, stating that preventive biological products are under the management system of the government-owned vaccine manufacturers and their supply chains. But, fitting the fifty-year-old Chinese public health system into the new market economy in China has been a real challenge to the Chinese political leadership. For example, the Chinese central government in 1989 created the China National Biological Products Company as an attempt to reorganize the national vaccine industry as a market-oriented business company instead of being just a government agency. Then in August 2003, this company was reorganized again as the China National Biotech Corporation (CNBC), a state-owned enterprise governed by the State-owned Assets Supervision and Administration Commission of the State Council (SASAC). This new corporation consists of the China National Scientific Instruments and Materials Import/Export Corporation (China Scientific), Beijing Tiantan Biological Products Company Ltd., and the six institutes of biological products. As aforementioned, these six institutes in Beijing, Changchun, Chengdu, Lanzhou, Shanghai and Wuhan were the backbone of the Chinese vaccine industry in the past fifty years. And they played major roles in the development and production of various vaccines that have protected hundreds millions of Chinese from several dreadful infectious diseases. As the largest corporation in the Chinese vaccine industry, CNBC aims at integrating vaccine development and production with marketing strategy. As a government-owned enterprise, CNBC also has the responsibility of producing and supplying various biological products, including vaccines, to meet the public health demands of the most populous nation in the world.

CNBC has more than 80 production lines that are in compliance with the national GMP (Good Manufacture Practice) and collectively produces more than 50 different vaccines with an annual output over three hundred million doses. The current vaccine product lines in CNBC are divided into three groups. The first group of vaccines are those that are listed in the national planned vaccination program, including BCG, polio vaccine, DTP, measles vaccine, and Hepatitis B Vaccine. These vaccines are mainly for newborns and children under school age and manufactured for the government with the pricing policy that is determined by the government. The second group of vaccines includes those that are listed or to-be-listed in the planned vaccination programs for children by each individual province in the country. These vaccines include the group A meningococcal polysaccharide vaccine, JE vaccine, and others. Unlike the vaccines in the national planned vaccine group, this group of vaccines has a more flexible price range, thus having possible profit margins. The vaccines in this group that are produced by CNBC has about 90% share of the Chinese domestic market. The third group is the so-called "market vaccines (shi-chang-miao)" such as Varicella, Rabies, Hepatitis A, Influenza, Pneumonia, epidemic hemorrhagic fever, and Typhoid. The vaccines in this group are profitable for the vaccine manufacturers. The price difference between a vaccine in the planned vaccination program and the others can be as much as 100 fold.

However, it became inevitable that the profound social and economic reforms in China since the early 1980s would change the monopoly status of the state-owned vaccine industry. By the year 2000, there were more than 200 private biotechnology companies that produced various biological products, including vaccines. Among these new companies, there were about 30 producing various vaccines as their main products. Because of their for-profit nature, these companies only focused on the profitable vaccines such as Rabies, Hepatitis A, Influenza and epidemic hemorrhagic fever. It is anticipated that the positive aspects of both the established CNBC and the new wave of for profit biotechnology companies can be exploited in a concerted effort to produce an HIV vaccine. Moreover, during the evolution of the market driven economy, it would be desirable for the government to maintain its national planned vaccination program and expand it to include new vaccines for future generations of Chinese children.

Another essential component is that governments and public health officials adopt an open and honest approach to outbreaks of infectious diseases. In the past it was traditional for governments to try to conceal information on epidemics or deny the emergence of new diseases for reasons of pride or economy. Recent experience in both developed and developing countries has demonstrated the risks of such behavior, in particular with diseases like AIDS, that lead to the loss of the opportunity to control the disease before it becomes established and widespread in the society.

CONCLUSION

The challenge for China is how to immediately and proactively initiate a nationwide HIV vaccine research and development program, which will allow the Chinese vaccine industry to be on the front line of the international collaboration on the most advanced HIV vaccine development programs. In so doing, China may not only avoid becoming one of the biggest victims of this dreadful pandemic, but also play an important role in the global fight against AIDS. Following are some reasons why we believe that achieving such a goal is possible.

First of all, China has one of the biggest vaccine industries in the world in terms of the production capacity and capability of producing various classes of modern vaccines as illustrated in this chapter. Suppose that a future HIV/AIDS vaccine comes from those vaccine candidates currently in development around the world—the Chinese vaccine industry will have the capacity to produce several hundred million doses in compliance with GMP. These potential products include the DNA-based, recombinant vaccinia or other live viral vector-based, live bacterial vector-based, and recombinant protein-based, all of which can be made in China in a price range affordable for use in developing countries. Considering the future need for the international community to make hundreds of millions of high quality, affordable AIDS vaccines annually available to the vast majority of people at risk of being infected worldwide, producing enormous amounts of vaccine in China with low cost and acceptable quality standards is perhaps the ideal solution.

Proactively engaging in international HIV vaccine development will also help China to sustain its state-owned vaccine industry at the current level and provide a new public health model in the world market economy. The Chinese vaccine industry is currently at a crossroads. All of the state-owned vaccine manufacturers have been trying to readjust themselves in the new environment of a market economy and to become financially self-sufficient. The challenges for them are formidable. On one hand, they must fulfill their responsibility of producing hundreds of millions of vaccines for the national planned vaccination programs that have little or negative profit margins. On the other hand, they cannot continue to rely on government subsidies for the development cost of more profitable new vaccines or biological products. With an increasing loss of their most experienced and talented workforce to the private sector and foreign competitors, and a lack of the brightest young graduates to join the state enterprises like they used to, these state-owned manufacturers are gradually losing their competitive edge and their monopoly status. Some even worry about becoming financial burdens for the government if the current downward trend continues. One can imagine that through HIV vaccine development, the Chinese vaccine industry will become a significant part of the international vaccine industry and participate in international competitive bidding to provide high-quality and low-price vaccines for millions of people in developing countries.

Secondly, China has one of the biggest functional public health networks in the world. Such a network is capable of conducting multiple large-scale vaccine efficacy trials, as illustrated in the development of JE vaccine in the past. Unlike other developing countries where the candidate HIV vaccines are to be tested, China has the infrastructure and workforce that can be mobilized rapidly for HIV vaccine development. With the increasing risk of HIV infection in many regions of China, it is conceivable that once China develops its own candidate vaccines for HIV, Chinese vaccine researchers will be able to test them effectively and expeditiously, thus facilitating the current international HIV vaccine development process. By adapting the international standard of GLP (Good Laboratory Practice) and GCP (Good Clinical Practice) for HIV vaccine testing, the current public health network will be able to improve itself for other vaccine tests that are urgently needed for China and the world. Moreover, with increasing cultural and economic globalization, the threats of global spread of newly emerging and re-emerging infectious diseases will undoubtedly increase in the 21st century. The world needs new vaccines, and research and development of new vaccines will become more and more important. Unlike drug development for medical treatment, vaccine development is unique in that it not only requires innovative basic and applied research, industrial capability to produce, and clinical infrastructure to test, it also needs populations in relative high risk of getting various infectious diseases. This is why many new preventive vaccines have to be tested in developing countries where the rate of infection for a particular disease is sufficiently high for demonstration of proposed vaccine efficacy.

Thirdly, there are thousands of qualified vaccine researchers in China who have advanced knowledge of molecular biology, virology, cell biology, immunology, and the state-of-art industrial biotechnology. In 1999, the newly established National Center for AIDS (NCAIDS) invited members of many of the key HIV vaccine research institutions and funding agencies in the world to attend the first international AIDS vaccine workshop in Beijing. The workshop focused on reviewing the development status of various candidate HIV vaccines in the advance stages of testing around the world, thus trying to formulate a national HIV vaccine development strategy that would be suitable for China. In the following year, an official delegation from the US National Institutes of Health (NIH) visited China to assess the possibilities of establishing a formal collaboration on the development of HIV vaccine in China. Afterwards, a team of American AIDS investigators was assembled by the NIH to collaborate with NCAIDS on preparation of a Comprehensive International Program for Research on AIDS (CIPRA), including plans that will launch an active international HIV vaccine collaboration in China. In the summer of 2001, a CIPRA working group was assembled with both Chinese and American principal investigators under the auspices of the MOH, and subsequently submitted a formal grant application to NIH. In May 2002, the governments of the US and China signed a memorandum of understanding on the governmental collaboration of HIV/AIDS in China and announced that NCAIDS was awarded $14.8 million as the first international recipient of the NIH's newly established CIPRA program. The significance of the Chinese CIPRA program is almost self-evident. It was built on the foundation of more than a decade of remarkable scientific research on HIV/AIDS in the US that included the most advanced knowledge in five key areas: epidemiology, behavior research, immunology and clinical laboratory assays, treatment, and vaccine development. Such a collaboration ensured that China, although a newcomer in the fight against AIDS, would begin its national AIDS program not from scratch, but in the frontier of the field with the most advanced knowledge and the best expertise available in the world. This notion is further supported by the fact that the Chinese CIPRA was co-written by American investigators and awarded through the NIH's critical peer review system.

In order to help China proactively participate in the international collaboration of HIV vaccine research and development, many participants of the 1999 Beijing vaccine workshop suggested to jump-start the Chinese HIV vaccine effort by working closely together with various international collaborators. This strategy allowed Chinese vaccine investigators to take advantage of the success and lessons in vaccine basic research in the US and build their new programs with the most advanced knowledge and technology available. Since 1999, such a strategy has proved to be successful with the support of the international scientific community and the US government. The current HIV vaccine prototypes for China utilize the most advanced technologies and discoveries available in the world by collaborating with the best research institutions and individual investigators in the world. They indeed include all of the most hopeful approaches in the current field of HIV vaccine development.

The fourth reason why China can rapidly develop HIV vaccines is that unlike a typical developing country, China has sufficient national resources and wealth to finance such an initiative. Development of a new vaccine usually costs millions of dollars and takes many years by a vaccine company in the west. However, unlike the vaccine industry in the developed world where the expertise and resources for vaccine development are in the private sector, the Chinese vaccine industry is still owned by the government. It is possible, therefore, for the Chinese government to take the advantage of this structural difference and quickly put together a national HIV vaccine initiative. In fact, when governments in the world face continuing public health crises such as HIV/AIDS, malaria, tuberculosis, pandemic influenza, SARS, and the threat of bio-terrorism, many wonder if the task of developing new vaccines should be the responsibility of governments rather than the for-profit vaccine industry.

Finally, China has a functional and powerful central government that is capable of launching an effective national program to stop the spread of infectious diseases, if it really feels the threat. The SARS epidemic in China during the spring of 2003 was a perfect example. Unfortunately, China lacks the ability to detect the spread of chronic infections that hide their devastating effects for years. The spread of HBV in China was a painful example. As aforementioned, HIV/AIDS is much worse than HBV in terms of its lethality. If 2% of the Chinese population contract HIV, their treatment will overburden the Chinese health care system and destroy the fruits of the economic reforms of the past decades. The government of China can make a huge difference in the global fight against HIV/AIDS, as well as all other infectious diseases.

In conclusion, with the full commitment of the government, China is not only capable of developing HIV vaccines, but also has an opportunity to lead in the production of this essential vaccine.

Acknowledgements. We thank our student assistants Li Shu and Leng Jin at Nankai University for their contribution to this work.

REFERENCES

Lu, J., Zhang, and Y., Zhao, K. (1995). In: Biomedical Products, People's Medical Publishing House.

Mahoney, F., and Kane, K. (1999). Hepatitis B vaccine, In: Plotkin, S., and Orenstein, W. (eds.), *Vaccines*, 3rd ed. W.B. Saunders & Co., Philidelphia, pp. 158–182.

Ministry of Health, China (MOH). (2002). Statistic Information Center of the Ministry of Health (May, 2002), Beijing.

Stanecki, K.A., and Walker, N. (2002). Current estimate and projections for the epidemic. In: Essex, M., Mboup, S., Kanki, P., Marlink, R., Tlou, S. (eds.),

AIDS in Africa, Kluwer Academic/Plenum Publishers, NewYork, pp. 281–296.

Tsai, T., Chang, G., and Yu, Y. (1999). Japanese Encephalitis Vaccines. In: Plotkin, S., and W. Orenstein (eds.), *Vaccines,* 3rd ed. W.B. Saunders & Co., Philidelphia, pp. 672–710.

UNAIDS (2003). www.unaids.org/en/geographical+area/by+country/china.asp (assessed January 2004)

Wang, S., Zheng, G., Xu, C., and Zhang, J. (2000). Achievement of the Chinese Public Health Prevention and immunization benefits people. *Chinese Journal of Epidemiology* 21(2): 147–149.

Weniger, B., and Brown, T. (1996). The march of AIDS through Asia. *N Eng J Med* 335:343–345.

Piot, P., and Bartos, M. (2002). The epidemiology of HIV and AIDS in Africa. In: Essex, M., Mboup, S., Kanki, P., Marlink, R., Tlou, S. (eds.), *AIDS in Africa,* Kluwer Academic/Plenum Publishers, NewYork, pp. 200–217.

Zhou, B., Zhang, M., Chen, P., Jiang, X., Zhang, L. (2001). An 11-year study on the epidemiological efficacy of Japanese encephalitis live vaccine (SA14-14-2). *Chinese Journal of Biologicals* 14(3):183–186.

Index